ESTHETIC DENTISTRY

A Clinical Approach to Techniques and Materials

Third Edition

Kenneth W. Aschheim, DDS
Associate Clinical Professor
New York University
College of Dentistry
Associate Clinical Professor
Mount Sinai Medical Center
New York, New York

ELSEVIER
MOSBY

3251 Riverport Lane
St. Louis, Missouri 63043

ESTHETIC DENTISTRY: A CLINICAL APPROACH TO TECHNIQUES
AND MATERIALS, THIRD EDITION

ISBN: 978-0-323-09176-3

Notices

Knowledge and best practice in this field are constantly changing. As new research and experience broaden our understanding, changes in research methods, professional practices, or medical treatment may become necessary.

Practitioners and researchers must always rely on their own experience and knowledge in evaluating and using any information, methods, compounds, or experiments described herein. In using such information or methods they should be mindful of their own safety and the safety of others, including parties for whom they have a professional responsibility.

With respect to any drug or pharmaceutical products identified, readers are advised to check the most current information provided (i) on procedures featured or (ii) by the manufacturer of each product to be administered, to verify the recommended dose or formula, the method and duration of administration, and contraindications. It is the responsibility of practitioners, relying on their own experience and knowledge of their patients, to make diagnoses, to determine dosages and the best treatment for each individual patient, and to take all appropriate safety precautions.

To the fullest extent of the law, neither the Publisher nor the authors, contributors, or editors, assume any liability for any injury and/or damage to persons or property as a matter of products liability, negligence or otherwise, or from any use or operation of any methods, products, instructions, or ideas contained in the material herein.

International Standard Book Number: 978-0-323-09176-3

Executive Content Strategist, Professional/Reference: Kathy Falk
Senior Content Development Specialist: Courtney Sprehe
Publishing Services Manager: Julie Eddy
Senior Project Manager: Marquita Parker
Designer: Ashley Miner

Printed in the United States

Last digit is the print number: 9 8 7 6 5 4 3 2 1

Working together
to grow libraries in
developing countries

www.elsevier.com • www.bookaid.org

In memory of my parents, David and Edith — together they pointed me in the right direction. And to my wife, Susan, her parents, Herb and Edith, and my children, Sara and Joshua, who have joined me along that path and without whom I could not continue to find the way.

Contributors

* Deceased

Fred B. Abbott, DDS, MDS, FACD*

Life Member, American College of Prosthodontics
Former Associate Professor
Northwestern University
School of Dentistry
Chicago, Illinois
Practice Limited to Prosthodontics
Salisbury, Maryland

Nellie Abbott, PhD, RN

Former Associate Administrator
Nursing Hospital of University of Pennsylvania
Former Associate Dean
Nursing Practice
University of Pennsylvania
School of Nursing
Philadelphia, Pennsylvania

Yakir A. Arteaga, DDS

Clinical Instructor
Department of Cariology and Comprehensive Care
College of Dentistry
New York University
Mount Sinai Medical Center
Private Practice
New York, New York

Milton B. Asbell, DDS, MSc, MA*

Former Clinical Associate Professor
Department of Community Dentistry
Temple University School of Dentistry
Staff, Department of Dental Medicine
Einstein Medical Center
Philadelphia, Pennsylvania

Kenneth W. Aschheim, DDS, FAAFS, FACD, FICD

Associate Clinical Professor
New York University
College of Dentistry
Associate Clinical Professor
Mount Sinai Medical Center
New York, New York

Ali B. Attaie, DDS, FAAPD

Assistant Clinical Professor of Pediatrics & Dentistry
Director, Division of Pediatric Dental Medicine
Icahn School of Medicine at Mount Sinai
New York, New York

William Baum, CDT, MDT

Instructor
Department of Prosthodontics
College of Dentistry
New York University
New York, New York
President, Dental Laboratory Association of New York

Jerry B. Black, DMD, MS, FACD

Private Practice
Birmingham, Alabama

Stanley Bodner, PhD

Practicing Psychologist
Senior Adjunct Faculty
Department of Social Science
Adelphi University-University College
Garden City, New York

Daniel Buchbinder, DMD, MD

Professor and Chief, Maxillofacial Surgery
Department of Otolaryngology, Head and Neck Surgery
Mount Sinai Health System
New York, New York

Vincent Celenza, DMD

Private Practice
New York, New York

Paul R. Chalifoux, DDS

Private Practice
Wellesley, Massachusetts

Chelsea Dale, BA

Colgate University
Hamilton, New York

Paul Federico, CDT, MDT

Adjunct Assistant Clinical Professor
Department of Prosthodontics
College of Dentistry
New York University
New York, New York
President, Association of Master Dental Technicians

Masly Harsono, DMD

Assistant Professor
Department of Research Administration
School of Dental Medicine
Tufts University
Boston, Massachusetts

Joseph Hung, DMD

Private Practice
New York, New York

Mark E. Jensen, DDS, PhD

Private Practice
Diamondhead, Mississippi

Gerard Kugel, DMD, MS, PhD

Professor of Prosthodontics and Operative Dentistry
Associate Dean for Research
School of Dental Medicine
Tufts University
Boston, Massachusetts

Kenneth S. Kurtz DDS, FACP

Clinical Associate Professor
Department of Prosthodontics
College of Dentistry
New York University
New York, New York
Private Practice Limited to Prosthodontics
New Hyde Park, New York

Dawn LaFrance, PsyD

Associate Director
Counseling and Psychological Services
Colgate University
Hamilton, New York

Frank Lauciello, DDS

Associate Clinical Professor
The State University of New York
University at Buffalo
Buffalo, New York
Director of Removable Prosthodontics
Ivoclar Vivadent
Amherst, New York

John P. Little, DMD, JD, MPA

Private Practice
Sea Girt, New York

Howard N. Livers, DDS

Private Practice
New York, New York

Kenneth S. Magid, DDS

Clinical Associate Professor
Director of Pre-Doctoral Laser Dentistry
Assistant Director Honors Esthetics
Department of Cariology and Comprehensive Care
College of Dentistry
New York University
New York, New York

Stanley Markovits, BS, DDS, MAGD

Clinical Professor
Department of Cariology and Comprehensive Care
College of Dentistry
New York University
New York, New York

Edward C. McNulty, DMD, MDS, FACD, FICD*

Former Clinical Associate Professor
Former Chairman, Orthodontic Department
New York University College of Dentistry
New York, New York
Former Co-Chief, Orthodontic Division
Department of Surgery (Dental)
Lenox Hill Hospital
New York, New York
Former Senior Attending Staff
Dental Clinic
Greenwich Hospital
Greenwich, Connecticut

Richard D. Miller, DDS

Former Clinical Associate Professor
Department of Prosthodontics
College of Dentistry
New York University
New York, New York

Ross Nash, DDS

Co-founder and President, Nash Institute
Charlotte, North Carolina

Nabil Ouatik, DMD, MSc, FRCD(C)

Faculty Lecturer
Faculty of Dentistry
McGill University
Montréal, QC, Canada
Head, Pediatric Dentistry
Janeway Child Health and Rehabilitation Centre
St. John's, NL, Canada

Mitchell S. Pines, DDS*

Former Clinical Professor, Department of Biomaterials and Biomimetics
Former Co-Director, Graduate Studies
Department of Biomaterials and Biomimetics
College of Dentistry
New York University
New York, New York

Burton R. Pollack, DDS, JD, MPH

Professor and Dean Emeritus
School of Dental Medicine
Stony Brook University
Stony Brook, New York

Gregory E. Rauscher, MD

Professor of Plastic Surgery
New Jersey Medical School
Rutgers University
Hackensack, New Jersey

Patrick E. Reid, CDT, MDT

Adjunct Associate Professor
Department of Prosthodontics
College of Dentistry
New York University
New York, New York

Edwin S. Rosenberg, BDS, HDipDent, DMD

Professor
Department of Prosthodontics, Periodontics, and Implant Dentistry
College of Dentistry
New York University
New York, New York
Visiting Professor
Hadassh School of Dental Medicine
The Hebrew Univesity of Jerusalem
Jerusalem, Israel

Yale E. Schnader DDS

Associate Clinical Professor
Department of Prosthodontics
College of Dentistry
New York University
New York, New York

Zev Schulhof, DMD, MD

Diplomate, American Board of Oral and Maxillofacial Surgery
President, American Academy of Facial Cosmetics
Clinical Instructor
Mount Sinai Hospital
New York, New York
Private Practice, Teaneck, New Jersey

Gail E. Schupak, DMD

Clinical Assistant Professor of Orthodontics
College of Dentistry
New York University
Private Practice, Orthodontics
New York, New York

Bruce A. Singer, BS, DDS*

Former Clinical Assistant Professor
Department of General Restorative Dentistry
University of Pennsylvania
School of Dental Medicine
Philadelphia, Pennsylvania
Albert Einstein Medical Center, North Division
Jenkintown, Pennsylvania

Robert A. Strauss, DDS, MD

Professor and Director
Residency Training Program
Department of Oral and Maxillofacial Surgery
Virginia Commonwealth University Medical Center
Richmond, Virginia

James Torosian, DMD

Clinical Associate Professor
Department of Periodontology
Kornberg School of Dentistry
Temple University
Philadelphia, Pennsylvania

Richard D. Trushkowsky, FAGD, FADM, FICD, FACD, DDS

Clinical Associate Professor and Associate Director
Advanced Program for International Dentists in Aesthetic
Dentistry
College of Dentistry
New York University
New York, New York
Private Practice
Staten Island, New York

DeWitt C. Wilkerson, III, DMD

Adjunct Professor of Graduate Studies
College of Dentistry
University of Florida
Gainesville, Florida
Senior Lecturer and Director of Dental Medicine
Dawson Academy for Advanced Dental Study
St Petersburg, Florida

Franklin D. Wright, DMD, FAAFS, D-ABFO

Forensic Odontology Consultant
Private Practice
Cincinnati, Ohio

Jung Yi, EdMA, PsyD

Licensed Psychologist
University of California
Neuropsychological Testing
Spectrum Practice of Berkeley
Educational Consultant
Daisiful Consulting, LLC
Berkley, California

Ira D. Zinner, DDS, MSD

Clinical Professor
Department of Prosthodontics
College of Dentistry
New York University
New York, New York

Edward Zuckerberg, DDS, FAGD

CEO, Painless Social Media, LLC
Private Practice
Palo Alto, California

Foreword

The Great Recession caused those in every aspect of the dental profession to re-examine their priorities, overall goals, techniques and materials, purchases of devices and equipment, and patient public relations. Fixed prosthodontic procedures were reduced significantly; many elective procedures in all areas of dentistry were delayed or reduced and many dentists had far less clinical activity.

However, what area of dentistry was still in high demand during this economic down? Esthetic dentistry concepts and procedures were still near the top of all oral procedures in demand by patients. Were the esthetic procedures the same as before the recession? No, they were somewhat different. They were more conservative. The procedures were segmented and spread over time instead of accomplished all at once. Often, the materials used for the procedures were different, such as the placement of direct resin veneers instead of indirect ceramic veneers.

A very clear conclusion can be made relative to the changes in esthetic dentistry during those few years of economic frustration.

Esthetic dentistry is a major and permanent patient desire. Patients want to look better, feel better about themselves, have higher self-esteem, and be able to smile without hesitation.

Esthetic dentistry has become high on the wish lists of most people and they will seek and find those practitioners who will provide the esthetic procedures they desire.

The third edition of *Esthetic Dentistry* provides to dentists the entire gamut of eclectic esthetic procedures to satisfy those patients with and without economic challenges. The concepts and techniques are timely, authoritative, easy to understand, and implement.

Gordon J. Christensen, DDS, MSD, PhD
Diplomate American Board of Prosthodontics

Preface

Dental materials and techniques have significantly changed since the first edition of *Esthetic Dentistry: A Clinical Approach to Techniques and Materials* was published over 20 years ago. However, the need for precise step-by-step presentations including nuanced clinical tips—two of the hallmarks of this textbook - has not. Dental restorations exhibiting exquisite esthetics and physiologic function are now not only well within the province of today's dentist, but are considered the "standard of care." In keeping with the successful formula of the previous two editions we have created a definitive, all encompassing, single source of information presented in a clinically relevant, user-friendly format.

Resolution of a cosmetic dental problem requires the practitioner to determine a diagnosis, formulate a treatment plan, and select the appropriate instruments and materials. Treatment must then be performed in an orderly fashion with an understanding of proper clinical technique and specific material manipulations. The competent clinician will approach any cosmetic dilemma in this manner. We therefore organized this text to duplicate this sequence of thought processes and clinical operations.

A Troubleshooting Guide (Part 1) quickly directs the practitioner to appropriate information in this textbook. It permits diagnosis and treatment planning at a glance and provides cross-references to more detailed discussions of material selection and clinical technique.

Part 2, Principles of Esthetics, lays the foundation of basic esthetic principles. A detailed discussion of the fundamentals of esthetics and the relevancy to dentistry is presented. The principles are referred to throughout the textbook to link clinical relevancy to basic theory. A section on facial and tooth biometrics has been added.

Part 3, Esthetic Materials and Techniques, aids in selecting the correct materials for a specific clinical situation. The concise discussion of basic material science enables the clinician to fully understand the ramifications of using the various materials currently available. Furthermore, this serves as a basis of comparison enabling an effective evaluation of new materials as they are introduced. Detailed step-by-step clinical techniques delineate appropriate armamentarium and include specific procedural nuances and numerous highlighted Clinical Tips. This facilitates a sound clinical approach. Also included is a comprehensive discussion of special considerations, indications, and contraindications for each technique and material presented, as well as numerous case presentations. A new chapter on Luting Agents has also been added.

Part 4, Esthetics and Other Clinical Applications, is a specialty-oriented section that presents an overview of other clinical applications by eminent practitioners. Included are such dental specialties as orthodontics, periodontics, and oral and maxillofacial surgery. This edition includes entirely new chapters covering implant surgery, implant prosthetics, and CAD/CAM technology, as well as extensive updates of other clinically relevant topics such as laser surgery and dental photography. As with the previous editions, the clinical relevance to the esthetic dentist is stressed by using case studies, office forms, and clinical techniques. Advanced techniques and criteria are presented to aid the dentist in determining when to refer a patient for specialty care.

Part 5, Esthetic Practice Management, details important patient psychology, marketing, and jurisprudence information. Today's clinician will find this section helpful in meeting the challenges facing dentistry and in managing a successful dental practice. A new section on social media has been included to cover this emerging field.

A new Part 6, Esthetics and Social Issues, covers some of the challenges that appear when treating unique dental and social issues such as eating disorders and domestic violence. The goal of these chapters is to not only heighten the awareness of these problems, but also to gain an understanding of their recognition and management.

As our profession proceeds through the twenty-first century, esthetic dentistry offers a new era of doctor and patient satisfaction and excitement. We hope we have shared our own enthusiasm in the pages of this text.

Kenneth W. Aschheim, DDS

Acknowledgments

A textbook of this magnitude requires the combined efforts of many talented individuals. As with the previous editions, I am cognizant that this work was built on the "shoulders of giants" in the field of esthetic dentistry and dental materials. Their collective expertise and the diligence and knowledge of the contributors made this book possible. These learned colleagues surpassed all expectations resulting in a "state-of the-art" textbook. I feel privileged to have had the opportunity to work closely with such a talented group of individuals.

I also want to thank my co-editor of the first two editions, Dr. Barry Dale. Without his support, guidance, and editorial skills neither would have ever seen the light of day. The knowledge he bestowed on me during our previous collaboration has guided me through this edition. I also want to extend a special thank you to Dr. Gordon J. Christensen, who, for the third time, has honored the book by authoring the foreword.

Despite advances in technology, the need for the assistance of a seasoned editorial staff has never been greater. Elsevier has again provided me with such guidance, in particular Courtney Sprehe, my Senior Content Development Specialist, Linda Wood, my freelance Content Development Specialist, and Marquita Parker, Senior Project Manager. I also wish to thank Kathy Falk, my executive content strategist, and John Dolan for agreeing to undertake this third edition. Elsevier's continued support of the project, the staff's high degree of professionalism, and the positive attitude they conveyed made this arduous task easier. I would also like to thank Elsevier's design and production departments, who transformed a manuscript and some photographs into a true work of art.

A note of appreciation must also be extended to the textbook's medical illustrators, Jodie Bernard of Lightbox Visual Communications, Inc. and Ken Vanderstoep, who were tasked with creating the 3-D illustrations. Jodie's positive attitude, combined with her excellent technical editing skills and Ken's creative talents, were vital in creating the new illustrations that are a hallmark of this edition.

I also wish to thank all the laboratory technicians and manufacturers' representatives who supplied the textbook with much of the necessary technical information. I must extend a special thank you to Rafael Babekov of Golden Cusp Studios, George Song of MK Restoration, and all the contributors' lab technicians who were reservoirs of information for some of the laboratory aspects of dental esthetics. Additional thanks to Fred Gebert of Benco Inc., Steve Sloan of Brasseler USA Inc., Kenneth J. Cathers and Gary Osborn of Ivoclar / Vivadent Inc., and Jim McGuire of Vident Inc., for providing me with information and equipment for some of the products in this textbook.

A special note of gratitude must be extended to Michelle Otero, Marcel McGuire, Agata Ehrlinger, and Marianela Castillo as well as my former and present dental assistants and office managers who helped "mind the store" while the textbook was being produced and who aided me in compiling many of the clinical cases. I also owe particular gratitude to my former partner Dr. Jack Hirsch, who previously supported my "bookwork," as well as my current partner, Dr. Yakir Arteaga, who not only provided me with support, but also much appreciated insight and guidance, as well authorship of a chapter.

I would also like to thank the individuals in the Department of Dentistry of The Mount Sinai Medical Center, especially the former chairman, Dr. Daniel Buchbinder, the current chairman, Dr. John Pfail, the attending staff, and the many residents for laying the foundation, providing the resources, and posing the intellectual challenges that motivated me to produce this text.

I also owe much to my colleagues at the New York University College of Dentistry International Esthetics Program for their continued support and guidance. A special note of gratitude goes to Dr. Steven David, Dr. Richard Trushkowsky, Dr. Anabella Oquendo, Dr. Louis Brea, and Larry Passaro and all the student colleagues that I have had the privilege to teach. My informal dental discussions with them provided me with many pearls of wisdom that were included in the book.

Finally, I wish to thank my wife, Susan, and my children, Sara and Joshua. When I began the first edition, my children were infants. During production of the second edition they were in middle school, and as I complete this edition they have graduated from college and embarked on careers of their own. They have all always provided me with unwavering love, encouragement, guidance, and moral support that ensured that this book would be successful.

I hope it has succeeded in clearly and comprehensively discussing the state of esthetic dentistry today and perhaps it will lay a basic framework for the esthetic dentist of tomorrow.

Kenneth W. Aschheim, DDS

Contents

Part 1

Troubleshooting
Troubleshooting Guide

TABLE OF CONTENTS FOR TROUBLESHOOTING GUIDE

Problem	Solution	Chapter Number and Title
	Tooth-Related Problems	
Size and Shape Problems		
Abrasion	Direct composite resin restoration	Ch 3 Dentin Bonding Agents Ch 4 Color Modifiers and Opaquers Ch 5 Composite Resin: Fundamentals and Direct Technique Restorations
	Indirect composite resin restoration	Ch 3 Dentin Bonding Agents Ch 4 Color Modifiers and Opaquers Ch 6 Composite Resin: Indirect Technique Restorations
	Ceramometal restoration	Ch 9 Ceramometal Full Coverage Restorations Ch 12 Esthetic Dentistry and Luting Agents Ch App A Custom Staining
	All-porcelain restoration	Ch 3 Dentin Bonding Agents Ch 4 Color Modifiers and Opaquers Ch 8 Porcelain-Full Coverage and Partial Coverage Restorations Ch 12 Esthetic Dentistry and Luting Agents Ch 23 Esthetics and Computer-Aided Design and Computer-Aided Manufacturing (CAD/CAM) Systems Ch App A Custom Staining
	Porcelain laminate veneer	Ch 3 Dentin Bonding Agents Ch 4 Color Modifiers and Opaquers Ch 7 Porcelain Laminate Veneers Restorations Ch 12 Esthetic Dentistry and Luting Agents Ch 23 Esthetics and Computer-Aided Design and Computer-Aided Manufacturing (CAD/CAM) Systems Ch App A Custom Staining
Aged teeth—worn	Direct composite resin restorations	Ch 3 Dentin Bonding Agents Ch 4 Color Modifiers and Opaquers Ch 5 Composite Resin: Fundamentals and Direct Technique Restorations
	Indirect composite resin restorations	Ch 3 Dentin Bonding Agents Ch 4 Color Modifiers and Opaquers Ch 6 Composite Resin: Indirect Technique Restorations
	Ceramometal restoration	Ch 9 Ceramometal Full Coverage Restorations Ch 12 Esthetic Dentistry and Luting Agents Ch App A Custom Staining
	All-porcelain restoration	Ch 3 Dentin Bonding Agents Ch 4 Color Modifiers and Opaquers Ch 8 Porcelain-Full Coverage and Partial Coverage Restorations Ch 12 Esthetic Dentistry and Luting Agents Ch 23 Esthetics and Computer-Aided Design and Computer-Aided Manufacturing (CAD/CAM) Systems Ch App A Custom Staining
	Porcelain laminate veneers	Ch 3 Dentin Bonding Agents Ch 4 Color Modifiers and Opaquers Ch 7 Porcelain Laminate Veneers Restorations Ch 12 Esthetic Dentistry and Luting Agents Ch 23 Esthetics and Computer-Aided Design and Computer-Aided Manufacturing (CAD/CAM) Systems Ch App A Custom Staining

Continued

Problem	Solution	Chapter Number and Title
		Tooth-Related Problems
Anterior tooth—chipped or fractured	Cosmetic recontouring	Ch 2 Fundamentals of Esthetics and Smile Analysis
	Direct composite resin restoration	Ch 3 Dentin Bonding Agents Ch 4 Color Modifiers and Opaquers Ch 5 Composite Resin: Fundamentals and Direct Technique Restorations
	Indirect composite resin restoration	Ch 3 Dentin Bonding Agents Ch 4 Color Modifiers and Opaquers Ch 6 Composite Resin: Indirect Technique Restorations
	All-porcelain restoration	Ch 3 Dentin Bonding Agents Ch 4 Color Modifiers and Opaquers Ch 8 Porcelain-Full Coverage and Partial Coverage Restorations Ch 12 Esthetic Dentistry and Luting Agents Ch 23 Esthetics and Computer-Aided Design and Computer-Aided Manufacturing (CAD/CAM) Systems Ch App A Custom Staining
	Ceramometal restoration	Ch 9 Ceramometal Full Coverage Restorations Ch 12 Esthetic Dentistry and Luting Agents Ch App A Custom Staining
	Porcelain laminate veneer	Ch 3 Dentin Bonding Agents Ch 4 Color Modifiers and Opaquers Ch 7 Porcelain Laminate Veneers Restorations Ch 12 Esthetic Dentistry and Luting Agents Ch 23 Esthetics and Computer-Aided Design and Computer-Aided Manufacturing (CAD/CAM) Systems Ch App A Custom Staining
	Domestic violence	Ch 30 Esthetic Dentistry and Domestic Violence
Attrition	Direct composite resin restoration (in selected cases)	Ch 3 Dentin Bonding Agents Ch 4 Color Modifiers and Opaquers Ch 5 Composite Resin: Fundamentals and Direct Technique Restorations
	Indirect composite resin restoration (in selected cases)	Ch 3 Dentin Bonding Agents Ch 4 Color Modifiers and Opaquers Ch 6 Composite Resin: Indirect Technique Restorations
	Ceramometal restoration	Ch 9 Ceramometal Full Coverage Restorations Ch 12 Esthetic Dentistry and Luting Agents Ch App A Custom Staining
	All-porcelain restoration (in selected cases)	Ch 3 Dentin Bonding Agents Ch 4 Color Modifiers and Opaquers Ch 7 Porcelain Laminate Veneers Restorations Ch 12 Esthetic Dentistry and Luting Agents Ch 23 Esthetics and Computer-Aided Design and Computer-Aided Manufacturing (CAD/CAM) Systems Ch App A Custom Staining
	Porcelain laminate veneer (in selected cases)	Ch 3 Dentin Bonding Agents Ch 4 Color Modifiers and Opaquers Ch 7 Porcelain Laminate Veneers Restorations Ch 12 Esthetic Dentistry and Luting Agents Ch 23 Esthetics and Computer-Aided Design and Computer-Aided Manufacturing (CAD/CAM) Systems Ch App A Custom Staining

Problem	Solution	Chapter Number and Title
		Tooth-Related Problems
Chipped tooth	Cosmetic recontouring	Ch 2 Fundamentals of Esthetics and Smile Analysis
	Direct composite resin restoration	Ch 3 Dentin Bonding Agents Ch 4 Color Modifiers and Opaquers Ch 5 Composite Resin: Fundamentals and Direct Technique Restorations
	Indirect composite resin restoration	Ch 3 Dentin Bonding Agents Ch 4 Color Modifiers and Opaquers Ch 6 Composite Resin: Indirect Technique Restorations
	Ceramometal restoration	Ch 9 Ceramometal Full Coverage Restorations Ch 12 Esthetic Dentistry and Luting Agents Ch App A Custom Staining
	Porcelain laminate veneer	Ch 3 Dentin Bonding Agents Ch 4 Color Modifiers and Opaquers Ch 7 Porcelain Laminate Veneers Restorations Ch 12 Esthetic Dentistry and Luting Agents Ch 23 Esthetics and Computer-Aided Design and Computer-Aided Manufacturing (CAD/CAM) Systems Ch App A Custom Staining
	Domestic violence	Ch 30 Esthetic Dentistry and Domestic Violence
Erosion	Direct composite resin restoration	Ch 3 Dentin Bonding Agents Ch 4 Color Modifiers and Opaquers Ch 5 Composite Resin: Fundamentals and Direct Technique Restorations
	Indirect composite resin restoration	Ch 3 Dentin Bonding Agents Ch 4 Color Modifiers and Opaquers Ch 6 Composite Resin: Indirect Technique Restorations
	Ceramometal restoration	Ch 9 Ceramometal Full Coverage Restorations Ch 12 Esthetic Dentistry and Luting Agents Ch App A Custom Staining
	All-porcelain restoration	Ch 3 Dentin Bonding Agents Ch 4 Color Modifiers and Opaquers Ch 8 Porcelain-Full Coverage and Partial Coverage Restorations Ch 12 Esthetic Dentistry and Luting Agents Ch 23 Esthetics and Computer-Aided Design and Computer-Aided Manufacturing (CAD/CAM) Systems Ch App A Custom Staining
	Porcelain laminate veneer	Ch 3 Dentin Bonding Agents Ch 4 Color Modifiers and Opaquers Ch 8 Porcelain-Full Coverage and Partial Coverage Restorations Ch 12 Esthetic Dentistry and Luting Agents Ch 23 Esthetics and Computer-Aided Design and Computer-Aided Manufacturing (CAD/CAM) Systems Ch App A Custom Staining
	Eating disorders	Ch 29 Esthetic Dentistry and Eating Disorders
Extruded tooth	Cosmetic recontouring	Ch 2 Fundamentals of Esthetics and Smile Analysis
	Ceramometal restoration (possibly combined with endodontic and periodontal therapy)	Ch 9 Ceramometal Full Coverage Restorations Ch 12 Esthetic Dentistry and Luting Agents Ch App A Custom Staining
	Indirect composite resin restoration	Ch 3 Dentin Bonding Agents Ch 4 Color Modifiers and Opaquers Ch 6 Composite Resin: Indirect Technique Restorations

Continued

Problem	Solution	Chapter Number and Title
Tooth-Related Problems		
Extruded tooth–cont'd	All-porcelain restoration (possibly combined with endodontic and periodontal therapy)	Ch 3 Dentin Bonding Agents Ch 4 Color Modifiers and Opaquers Ch 8 Porcelain–Full Coverage and Partial Coverage Restorations Ch 12 Esthetic Dentistry and Luting Agents Ch 23 Esthetics and Computer-Aided Design and Computer-Aided Manufacturing (CAD/CAM) Systems Ch App A Custom Staining
	Porcelain laminate veneer (sufficient tooth structure must be present)	Ch 3 Dentin Bonding Agents Ch 4 Color Modifiers and Opaquers Ch 7 Porcelain Laminate Veneers Restorations Ch 12 Esthetic Dentistry and Luting Agents Ch 23 Esthetics and Computer-Aided Design and Computer-Aided Manufacturing (CAD/CAM) Systems Ch App A Custom Staining
	Gingival recontouring—surgical (if necessary)	Ch 14 Esthetics and Periodontics
	Gingival recontouring—laser surgery (if necessary)	Ch 21 Esthetics and Laser Surgery
	Gingival grafting (if accompanied by recession)	Ch 14 Esthetics and Periodontics
	Artificial gingiva (if accompanied by recession) (pink porcelain)	Ch 3 Dentin Bonding Agents Ch 4 Color Modifiers and Opaquers Ch 6 Composite Resin: Indirect Technique Restorations Ch 7 Porcelain Laminate Veneers Restorations Ch 8 Porcelain–Full Coverage and Partial Coverage Restorations Ch 9 Ceramometal Full Coverage Restorations Ch 12 Esthetic Dentistry and Luting Agents Ch 23 Esthetics and Computer-Aided Design and Computer-Aided Manufacturing (CAD/CAM) Systems Ch App A Custom Staining
	Orthodontic therapy	Ch 15 Esthetics and Orthodontics
	Orthognathic surgery	Ch 18 Esthetics and Oral and Maxillofacial Surgery
	Cosmetic recontouring	Ch 2 Fundamentals of Esthetics and Smile Analysis
Feminine teeth—excessive	Cosmetic recontouring	Ch 2 Fundamentals of Esthetics and Smile Analysis
Fractured tooth	Direct composite resin restoration	Ch 3 Dentin Bonding Agents Ch 4 Color Modifiers and Opaquers Ch 5 Composite Resin: Fundamentals and Direct Technique Restorations
	Indirect composite resin restoration	Ch 3 Dentin Bonding Agents Ch 4 Color Modifiers and Opaquers Ch 6 Composite Resin: Indirect Technique Restorations
	Ceramometal restoration	Ch 9 Ceramometal Full Coverage Restorations Ch 12 Esthetic Dentistry and Luting Agents Ch App A Custom Staining
	All-porcelain restoration	Ch 3 Dentin Bonding Agents Ch 4 Color Modifiers and Opaquers Ch 8 Porcelain–Full Coverage and Partial Coverage Restorations Ch 12 Esthetic Dentistry and Luting Agents Ch 23 Esthetics and Computer-Aided Design and Computer-Aided Manufacturing (CAD/CAM) Systems Ch App A Custom Staining
	Porcelain laminate veneer	Ch 3 Dentin Bonding Agents Ch 4 Color Modifiers and Opaquers Ch 8 Porcelain–Full Coverage and Partial Coverage Restorations Ch 12 Esthetic Dentistry and Luting Agents Ch 23 Esthetics and Computer-Aided Design and Computer-Aided Manufacturing (CAD/CAM) Systems Ch App A Custom Staining

Problem	Solution	Chapter Number and Title
Tooth-Related Problems		
Fractured tooth-cont'd	Cosmetic recontouring	Ch 2 Fundamentals of Esthetics and Smile Analysis
	Domestic violence	Ch 30 Esthetic Dentistry and Domestic Violence
Large tooth	Direct composite resin restoration	Ch 3 Dentin Bonding Agents Ch 4 Color Modifiers and Opaquers Ch 5 Composite Resin: Fundamentals and Direct Technique Restorations
	Indirect composite resin restoration	Ch 3 Dentin Bonding Agents Ch 4 Color Modifiers and Opaquers Ch 6 Composite Resin: Indirect Technique Restorations
	Ceramometal restoration	Ch 9 Ceramometal Full Coverage Restorations Ch 12 Esthetic Dentistry and Luting Agents Ch App A Custom Staining
	All-porcelain restoration	Ch 3 Dentin Bonding Agents Ch 4 Color Modifiers and Opaquers Ch 8 Porcelain-Full Coverage and Partial Coverage Restorations Ch 12 Esthetic Dentistry and Luting Agents Ch 23 Esthetics and Computer-Aided Design and Computer-Aided Manufacturing (CAD/CAM) Systems Ch App A Custom Staining
	Direct composite resin restoration	Ch 3 Dentin Bonding Agents Ch 4 Color Modifiers and Opaquers Ch 12 Esthetic Dentistry and Luting Agents
	Porcelain laminate veneer	Ch 3 Dentin Bonding Agents Ch 4 Color Modifiers and Opaquers Ch 8 Porcelain-Full Coverage and Partial Coverage Restorations Ch 12 Esthetic Dentistry and Luting Agents Ch 23 Esthetics and Computer-Aided Design and Computer-Aided Manufacturing (CAD/CAM) Systems Ch App A Custom Staining
Long tooth	Cosmetic recontouring	Ch 2 Fundamentals of Esthetics and Smile Analysis
	Direct composite resin restoration	Ch 3 Dentin Bonding Agents Ch 4 Color Modifiers and Opaquers Ch 5 Composite Resin: Fundamentals and Direct Technique Restorations
	Indirect composite resin restoration (possibly combined with endodontic and periodontal therapy)	Ch 3 Dentin Bonding Agents Ch 4 Color Modifiers and Opaquers Ch 6 Composite Resin: Indirect Technique Restorations
	Ceramometal restoration (possibly combined with endodontic and periodontal therapy)	Ch 9 Ceramometal: Full Coverage Restorations Ch 12 Esthetic Dentistry and Luting Agents Ch App A Custom Staining
	All-porcelain restoration (possibly combined with endodontic and periodontal therapy)	Ch 3 Dentin Bonding Agents Ch 4 Color Modifiers and Opaquers Ch 8 Porcelain-Full Coverage and Partial Coverage Restorations Ch 12 Esthetic Dentistry and Luting Agents Ch 23 Esthetics and Computer-Aided Design and Computer-Aided Manufacturing (CAD/CAM) Systems Ch App A Custom Staining
	Porcelain laminate veneer (possibly combined with endodontic and periodontal therapy) (sufficient tooth structure must be present)	Ch 3 Dentin Bonding Agents Ch 4 Color Modifiers and Opaquers Ch 7 Porcelain Laminate Veneers Restorations Ch 12 Esthetic Dentistry and Luting Agents Ch 23 Esthetics and Computer-Aided Design and Computer-Aided Manufacturing (CAD/CAM) Systems Ch App A Custom Staining

Continued

Problem	Solution	Chapter Number and Title
Tooth-Related Problems		
Long tooth-cont'd	Artificial gingiva (pink porcelain)	Ch 3 Dentin Bonding Agents Ch 4 Color Modifiers and Opaquers Ch 6 Composite Resin: Indirect Technique Restorations Ch 7 Porcelain Laminate Veneers Restorations Ch 8 Porcelain-Full Coverage and Partial Coverage Restorations Ch 9 Ceramometal Full Coverage Restorations Ch 12 Esthetic Dentistry and Luting Agents Ch 23 Esthetics and Computer-Aided Design and Computer-Aided Manufacturing (CAD/CAM) Systems Ch App A Custom Staining
	Orthodontic therapy	Ch 15 Esthetics and Orthodontics
	Orthognathic surgery	Ch 18 Esthetics and Oral and Maxillofacial Surgery
Malformed teeth—mild	Cosmetic recontouring	Ch 2 Fundamentals of Esthetics and Smile Analysis
	Direct composite resin restorations	Ch 3 Dentin Bonding Agents Ch 4 Color Modifiers and Opaquers Ch 5 Composite Resin: Fundamentals and Direct Technique Restorations
	Indirect composite resin restorations	Ch 3 Dentin Bonding Agents Ch 4 Color Modifiers and Opaquers Ch 6 Composite Resin: Indirect Technique Restorations
	Ceramometal restoration	Ch 9 Ceramometal Full Coverage Restorations Ch 12 Esthetic Dentistry and Luting Agents Ch App A Custom Staining
	All-porcelain restoration	Ch 3 Dentin Bonding Agents Ch 4 Color Modifiers and Opaquers Ch 8 Porcelain-Full Coverage and Partial Coverage Restorations Ch 12 Esthetic Dentistry and Luting Agents Ch 23 Esthetics and Computer-Aided Design and Computer-Aided Manufacturing (CAD/CAM) Systems Ch App A Custom Staining
	Porcelain laminate veneers	Ch 3 Dentin Bonding Agents Ch 4 Color Modifiers and Opaquers Ch 7 Porcelain Laminate Veneers Restorations Ch 12 Esthetic Dentistry and Luting Agents Ch 23 Esthetics and Computer-Aided Design and Computer-Aided Manufacturing (CAD/CAM) Systems Ch App A Custom Staining
Malformed teeth—severe	Direct composite resin restorations	Ch 3 Dentin Bonding Agents Ch 4 Color Modifiers and Opaquers Ch 5 Composite Resin: Fundamentals and Direct Technique Restorations
	Indirect composite resin restorations	Ch 3 Dentin Bonding Agents Ch 4 Color Modifiers and Opaquers Ch 6 Composite Resin: Indirect Technique Restorations
	Ceramometal restoration	Ch 9 Ceramometal Full Coverage Restorations Ch 12 Esthetic Dentistry and Luting Agents Ch App A Custom Staining
	All-porcelain restorations	Ch 3 Dentin Bonding Agents Ch 4 Color Modifiers and Opaquers Ch 8 Porcelain-Full Coverage and Partial Coverage Restorations Ch 12 Esthetic Dentistry and Luting Agents Ch 23 Esthetics and Computer-Aided Design and Computer-Aided Manufacturing (CAD/CAM) Systems Ch App A Custom Staining

Problem	Solution	Chapter Number and Title
		Tooth-Related Problems
Malformed teeth— severe-cont'd	Porcelain laminate veneers	Ch 3 Dentin Bonding Agents Ch 4 Color Modifiers and Opaquers Ch 7 Porcelain Laminate Veneers Restorations Ch 12 Esthetic Dentistry and Luting Agents Ch 23 Esthetics and Computer-Aided Design and Computer-Aided Manufacturing (CAD/CAM) Systems Ch App A Custom Staining
Masculine teeth— excessive	Cosmetic recontouring	Ch 2 Fundamentals of Esthetics and Smile Analysis
Narrow tooth	Cosmetic recontouring	Ch 2 Fundamentals of Esthetics and Smile Analysis
	Direct composite resin restoration	Ch 3 Dentin Bonding Agents Ch 4 Color Modifiers and Opaquers Ch 5 Composite Resin: Fundamentals and Direct Technique Restorations
	Indirect composite resin restoration	Ch 3 Dentin Bonding Agents Ch 4 Color Modifiers and Opaquers Ch 6 Composite Resin: Indirect Technique Restorations
	Ceramometal restoration	Ch 9 Ceramometal Full Coverage Restorations Ch 12 Esthetic Dentistry and Luting Agents Ch App A Custom Staining
	All-porcelain restoration	Ch 3 Dentin Bonding Agents Ch 4 Color Modifiers and Opaquers Ch 8 Porcelain-Full Coverage and Partial Coverage Restorations Ch 12 Esthetic Dentistry and Luting Agents Ch 23 Esthetics and Computer-Aided Design and Computer-Aided Manufacturing (CAD/CAM) Systems Ch App A Custom Staining
	Porcelain laminate veneer	Ch 3 Dentin Bonding Agents Ch 4 Color Modifiers and Opaquers Ch 8 Porcelain-Full Coverage and Partial Coverage Restorations Ch 12 Esthetic Dentistry and Luting Agents Ch 23 Esthetics and Computer-Aided Design and Computer-Aided Manufacturing (CAD/CAM) Systems Ch App A Custom Staining
Peg lateral incisor	Direct composite resin restoration	Ch 3 Dentin Bonding Agents Ch 4 Color Modifiers and Opaquers Ch 5 Composite Resin: Fundamentals and Direct Technique Restorations
	Indirect composite resin restoration	Ch 3 Dentin Bonding Agents Ch 4 Color Modifiers and Opaquers Ch 6 Composite Resin: Indirect Technique Restorations
	Ceramometal restoration	Ch 9 Ceramometal Full Coverage Restorations Ch 12 Esthetic Dentistry and Luting Agents Ch App A Custom Staining
	All-porcelain restoration	Ch 3 Dentin Bonding Agents Ch 4 Color Modifiers and Opaquers Ch 8 Porcelain-Full Coverage and Partial Coverage Restorations Ch 12 Esthetic Dentistry and Luting Agents Ch 23 Esthetics and Computer-Aided Design and Computer-Aided Manufacturing (CAD/CAM) Systems Ch App A Custom Staining
	Porcelain laminate veneer	Ch 3 Dentin Bonding Agents Ch 4 Color Modifiers and Opaquers Ch 7 Porcelain Laminate Veneers Restorations Ch 12 Esthetic Dentistry and Luting Agents Ch 23 Esthetics and Computer-Aided Design and Computer-Aided Manufacturing (CAD/CAM) Systems Ch App A Custom Staining

Continued

Problem	Solution	Chapter Number and Title
Tooth-Related Problems		
Short tooth	Cosmetic recontouring	Ch 2 Fundamentals of Esthetics and Smile Analysis
	Direct composite resin restoration	Ch 3 Dentin Bonding Agents Ch 4 Color Modifiers and Opaquers Ch 5 Composite Resin: Fundamentals and Direct Technique Restorations
	Indirect composite resin restoration	Ch 3 Dentin Bonding Agents Ch 4 Color Modifiers and Opaquers Ch 6 Composite Resin: Indirect Technique Restorations
	Ceramometal restoration	Ch 9 Ceramometal Full Coverage Restorations Ch 12 Esthetic Dentistry and Luting Agents Ch App A Custom Staining
	All-porcelain restoration	Ch 3 Dentin Bonding Agents Ch 4 Color Modifiers and Opaquers Ch 8 Porcelain-Full Coverage and Partial Coverage Restorations Ch 12 Esthetic Dentistry and Luting Agents Ch 23 Esthetics and Computer-Aided Design and Computer-Aided Manufacturing (CAD/CAM) Systems Ch App A Custom Staining
	Porcelain laminate veneer	Ch 3 Dentin Bonding Agents Ch 4 Color Modifiers and Opaquers Ch 7 Porcelain Laminate Veneers Restorations Ch 12 Esthetic Dentistry and Luting Agents Ch 23 Esthetics and Computer-Aided Design and Computer-Aided Manufacturing (CAD/CAM) Systems Ch App A Custom Staining
	Gingival recontouring—surgical	Ch 14 Esthetics and Periodontics
	Gingival recontouring—laser surgery	Ch 21 Esthetics and Laser Surgery
Small tooth	Direct composite resin restoration	Ch 3 Dentin Bonding Agents Ch 4 Color Modifiers and Opaquers Ch 12 Esthetic Dentistry and Luting Agents
	Indirect composite resin restoration	Ch 3 Dentin Bonding Agents Ch 4 Color Modifiers and Opaquers Ch 6 Composite Resin: Indirect Technique Restorations
	Ceramometal restoration	Ch 9 Ceramometal Full Coverage Restorations Ch 12 Esthetic Dentistry and Luting Agents Ch App A Custom Staining
	All-porcelain restoration	Ch 3 Dentin Bonding Agents Ch 4 Color Modifiers and Opaquers Ch 8 Porcelain-Full Coverage and Partial Coverage Restorations Ch 12 Esthetic Dentistry and Luting Agents Ch 23 Esthetics and Computer-Aided Design and Computer-Aided Manufacturing (CAD/CAM) Systems Ch App A Custom Staining
	Porcelain laminate veneer	Ch 3 Dentin Bonding Agents Ch 4 Color Modifiers and Opaquers Ch 8 Porcelain-Full Coverage and Partial Coverage Restorations Ch 12 Esthetic Dentistry and Luting Agents Ch 23 Esthetics and Computer-Aided Design and Computer-Aided Manufacturing (CAD/CAM) Systems Ch App A Custom Staining
	Gingival recontouring—surgical	Ch 14 Esthetics and Periodontics
	Gingival recontouring—surgical	Ch 21 Esthetics and Laser Surgery

Problem	Solution	Chapter Number and Title
Tooth-Related Problems		
Wide tooth	Cosmetic recontouring	Ch 2 Fundamentals of Esthetics and Smile Analysis
	Direct composite resin restoration	Ch 3 Dentin Bonding Agents Ch 4 Color Modifiers and Opaquers Ch 5 Composite Resin: Fundamentals and Direct Technique Restorations
	Indirect composite resin restoration	Ch 3 Dentin Bonding Agents Ch 4 Color Modifiers and Opaquers Ch 6 Composite Resin: Indirect Technique Restorations
	Ceramometal restoration	Ch 9 Ceramometal Full Coverage Restorations Ch 12 Esthetic Dentistry and Luting Agents Ch App A Custom Staining
	All-porcelain restoration	Ch 3 Dentin Bonding Agents Ch 4 Color Modifiers and Opaquers Ch 8 Porcelain-Full Coverage and Partial Coverage Restorations Ch 12 Esthetic Dentistry and Luting Agents Ch 23 Esthetics and Computer-Aided Design and Computer-Aided Manufacturing (CAD/CAM) Systems Ch App A Custom Staining
	Porcelain laminate veneer	Ch 3 Dentin Bonding Agents Ch 4 Color Modifiers and Opaquers Ch 8 Porcelain-Full Coverage and Partial Coverage Restorations Ch 12 Esthetic Dentistry and Luting Agents Ch 23 Esthetics and Computer-Aided Design and Computer-Aided Manufacturing (CAD/CAM) Systems Ch App A Custom Staining
Position Problems		
Anterior flared teeth—major	Orthodontic therapy	Ch 15 Esthetics and Orthodontics
Anterior flared teeth—minor	Direct composite resin restoration	Ch 3 Dentin Bonding Agents Ch 4 Color Modifiers and Opaquers Ch 5 Composite Resin: Fundamentals and Direct Technique Restorations
	Indirect composite resin restoration	Ch 3 Dentin Bonding Agents Ch 4 Color Modifiers and Opaquers Ch 6 Composite Resin: Indirect Technique Restorations
	Ceramometal restoration	Ch 9 Ceramometal Full Coverage Restorations Ch 12 Esthetic Dentistry and Luting Agents Ch App A Custom Staining
	All-porcelain restorations	Ch 3 Dentin Bonding Agents Ch 4 Color Modifiers and Opaquers Ch 8 Porcelain-Full Coverage and Partial Coverage Restorations Ch 12 Esthetic Dentistry and Luting Agents Ch 23 Esthetics and Computer-Aided Design and Computer-Aided Manufacturing (CAD/CAM) Systems Ch App A Custom Staining
	Porcelain laminate veneers	Ch 3 Dentin Bonding Agents Ch 4 Color Modifiers and Opaquers Ch 7 Porcelain Laminate Veneers Restorations Ch 12 Esthetic Dentistry and Luting Agents Ch 23 Esthetics and Computer-Aided Design and Computer-Aided Manufacturing (CAD/CAM) Systems Ch App A Custom Staining
	Orthodontic therapy	Ch 15 Esthetics and Orthodontics

Continued

Problem	Solution	Chapter Number and Title
Tooth-Related Problems		
Crowding	Cosmetic recontouring	Ch 2 Fundamentals of Esthetics and Smile Analysis
	Direct composite resin restorations	Ch 3 Dentin Bonding Agents Ch 4 Color Modifiers and Opaquers Ch 5 Composite Resin: Fundamentals and Direct Technique Restorations
	Indirect composite resin restorations	Ch 3 Dentin Bonding Agents Ch 4 Color Modifiers and Opaquers Ch 6 Composite Resin: Indirect Technique Restorations
	Ceramometal restoration	Ch 9 Ceramometal Full Coverage Restorations Ch 12 Esthetic Dentistry and Luting Agents Ch App A Custom Staining
	All-porcelain restoration	Ch 3 Dentin Bonding Agents Ch 4 Color Modifiers and Opaquers Ch 8 Porcelain-Full Coverage and Partial Coverage Restorations Ch 12 Esthetic Dentistry and Luting Agents Ch 23 Esthetics and Computer-Aided Design and Computer-Aided Manufacturing (CAD/CAM) Systems
	Porcelain laminate veneers	Ch 3 Dentin Bonding Agents Ch 4 Color Modifiers and Opaquers Ch 7 Porcelain Laminate Veneers Restorations Ch 12 Esthetic Dentistry and Luting Agents Ch 23 Esthetics and Computer-Aided Design and Computer-Aided Manufacturing (CAD/CAM) Systems Ch App A Custom Staining
	Orthodontic therapy	Ch 15 Esthetics and Orthodontics
Diastemata	Direct composite resin restorations	Ch 3 Dentin Bonding Agents Ch 4 Color Modifiers and Opaquers Ch 5 Composite Resin: Fundamentals and Direct Technique Restorations
	Indirect composite resin restoration	Ch 3 Dentin Bonding Agents Ch 4 Color Modifiers and Opaquers Ch 6 Composite Resin: Indirect Technique Restorations
	Ceramometal restoration	Ch 9 Ceramometal Full Coverage Restorations Ch 12 Esthetic Dentistry and Luting Agents Ch App A Custom Staining
	All-porcelain restoration	Ch 3 Dentin Bonding Agents Ch 4 Color Modifiers and Opaquers Ch 8 Porcelain-Full Coverage and Partial Coverage Restorations Ch 12 Esthetic Dentistry and Luting Agents Ch 23 Esthetics and Computer-Aided Design and Computer-Aided Manufacturing (CAD/CAM) Systems Ch App A Custom Staining
	All-porcelain restorations	Ch 3 Dentin Bonding Agents Ch 4 Color Modifiers and Opaquers Ch 8 Porcelain-Full Coverage and Partial Coverage Restorations Ch 12 Esthetic Dentistry and Luting Agents Ch 23 Esthetics and Computer-Aided Design and Computer-Aided Manufacturing (CAD/CAM) Systems Ch App A Custom Staining
	Porcelain laminate veneers	Ch 3 Dentin Bonding Agents Ch 4 Color Modifiers and Opaquers Ch 7 Porcelain Laminate Veneers Restorations Ch 12 Esthetic Dentistry and Luting Agents Ch 23 Esthetics and Computer-Aided Design and Computer-Aided Manufacturing (CAD/CAM) Systems Ch App A Custom Staining
	Orthodontic therapy	Ch 15 Esthetics and Orthodontics

Problem	Solution	Chapter Number and Title
Tooth-Related Problems		
Excessive spacing	Direct composite resin restorations	Ch 3 Dentin Bonding Agents Ch 4 Color Modifiers and Opaquers Ch 5 Composite Resin: Fundamentals and Direct Technique Restorations
	Indirect composite resin restorations	Ch 3 Dentin Bonding Agents Ch 4 Color Modifiers and Opaquers Ch 6 Composite Resin: Indirect Technique Restorations
	Ceramometal restoration	Ch 9 Ceramometal Full Coverage Restorations Ch 12 Esthetic Dentistry and Luting Agents Ch App A Custom Staining
	All-porcelain restorations	Ch 3 Dentin Bonding Agents Ch 4 Color Modifiers and Opaquers Ch 8 Porcelain-Full Coverage and Partial Coverage Restorations Ch 12 Esthetic Dentistry and Luting Agents Ch 23 Esthetics and Computer-Aided Design and Computer-Aided Manufacturing (CAD/CAM) Systems Ch App A Custom Staining
	Porcelain laminate veneers	Ch 3 Dentin Bonding Agents Ch 4 Color Modifiers and Opaquers Ch 7 Porcelain Laminate Veneers Restorations Ch 12 Esthetic Dentistry and Luting Agents Ch 23 Esthetics and Computer-Aided Design and Computer-Aided Manufacturing (CAD/CAM) Systems Ch App A Custom Staining
	Orthodontic therapy	Ch 15 Esthetics and Orthodontics
Extruded tooth	Cosmetic recontouring	Ch 2 Fundamentals of Esthetics and Smile Analysis
	Indirect composite resin restoration (possibly combined with endodontic and periodontal therapy)	Ch 3 Dentin Bonding Agents Ch 4 Color Modifiers and Opaquers Ch 6 Composite Resin: Indirect Technique Restorations
	Ceramometal restoration (possibly combined with endodontic and periodontal therapy)	Ch 9 Ceramometal Full Coverage Restorations Ch 12 Esthetic Dentistry and Luting Agents Ch App A Custom Staining
	All-porcelain restoration (possibly combined with endodontic and periodontal therapy)	Ch 3 Dentin Bonding Agents Ch 4 Color Modifiers and Opaquers Ch 8 Porcelain-Full Coverage and Partial Coverage Restorations Ch 12 Esthetic Dentistry and Luting Agents Ch 23 Esthetics and Computer-Aided Design and Computer-Aided Manufacturing (CAD/CAM) Systems Ch App A Custom Staining
	Porcelain laminate veneer (possibly combined with endodontic and periodontal therapy) (sufficient tooth structure must be present)	Ch 3 Dentin Bonding Agents Ch 4 Color Modifiers and Opaquers Ch 7 Porcelain Laminate Veneers Restorations Ch 12 Esthetic Dentistry and Luting Agents Ch 23 Esthetics and Computer-Aided Design and Computer-Aided Manufacturing (CAD/CAM) Systems Ch App A Custom Staining
	Gingival recontouring (if necessary)	Ch 14 Esthetics and Periodontics
	Cosmetic recontouring	Ch 21 Esthetics and Laser Surgery
	Gingival grafting (if accompanied by recession)	Ch 14 Esthetics and Periodontics

Continued

Problem	Solution	Chapter Number and Title
		Tooth-Related Problems
Extruded tooth-cont'd	Artificial gingiva (if accompanied by recession) (pink porcelain)	Ch 3 Dentin Bonding Agents Ch 4 Color Modifiers and Opaquers Ch 7 Porcelain Laminate Veneers Restorations Ch 12 Esthetic Dentistry and Luting Agents Ch 23 Esthetics and Computer-Aided Design and Computer-Aided Manufacturing (CAD/CAM) Systems Ch App A Custom Staining
	Orthodontic therapy	Ch 15 Esthetics and Orthodontics
	Orthognathic surgery	Ch 18 Esthetics and Oral and Maxillofacial Surgery
Generalized spacing	Direct composite resin restorations	Ch 3 Dentin Bonding Agents Ch 4 Color Modifiers and Opaquers Ch 5 Composite Resin: Fundamentals and Direct Technique Restorations
	Indirect composite resin restorations	Ch 3 Dentin Bonding Agents Ch 4 Color Modifiers and Opaquers Ch 6 Composite Resin: Indirect Technique Restorations
	Ceramometal restoration	Ch 9 Ceramometal—Full Coverage Restorations Ch 12 Esthetic Dentistry and Luting Agents Ch App A Custom Staining
	All-porcelain restorations	Ch 3 Dentin Bonding Agents Ch 4 Color Modifiers and Opaquers Ch 8 Porcelain-Full Coverage and Partial Coverage Restorations Ch 12 Esthetic Dentistry and Luting Agents Ch 23 Esthetics and Computer-Aided Design and Computer-Aided Manufacturing (CAD/CAM) Systems Ch App A Custom Staining
	Porcelain laminate veneers	Ch 3 Dentin Bonding Agents Ch 4 Color Modifiers and Opaquers Ch 7 Porcelain Laminate Veneers Restorations Ch 12 Esthetic Dentistry and Luting Agents Ch 23 Esthetics and Computer-Aided Design and Computer-Aided Manufacturing (CAD/CAM) Systems Ch App A Custom Staining
	Orthodontic therapy	Ch 15 Esthetics and Orthodontics
High smile line	Cosmetic recontouring	Ch 2 Fundamentals of Esthetics and Smile Analysis
	Gingival recontouring (if necessary)	Ch 14 Esthetics and Periodontics
	Gingival recontouring—laser surgery (if necessary)	Ch 21 Esthetics and Laser Surgery
	Gingival grafting (if accompanied by recession)	Ch 15 Esthetics and Orthodontics
	Orthognathic surgery	Ch 18 Esthetics and Esthetics and Oral and Maxillofacial Surgery
	Artificial gingiva (if accompanied by recession) (pink porcelain)	Ch 3 Dentin Bonding Agents Ch 4 Color Modifiers and Opaquers Ch 6 Composite Resin: Indirect Technique Restorations Ch 7 Porcelain Laminate Veneers Restorations Ch 8 Porcelain-Full Coverage and Partial Coverage Restorations Ch 9 Ceramometal Full Coverage Restorations Ch 12 Esthetic Dentistry and Luting Agents Ch 23 Esthetics and Computer-Aided Design and Computer-Aided Manufacturing (CAD/CAM) Systems Ch App A Custom Staining

Problem	Solution	Chapter Number and Title
Tooth-Related Problems		
Long tooth	Cosmetic recontouring	Ch 2 Fundamentals of Esthetics and Smile Analysis
	Direct composite resin restoration (if necessary following tooth reduction)	Ch 3 Dentin Bonding Agents Ch 4 Color Modifiers and Opaquers Ch 5 Composite Resin: Fundamentals and Direct Technique Restorations
	Indirect composite resin restoration (if necessary following tooth reduction)	Ch 3 Dentin Bonding Agents Ch 4 Color Modifiers and Opaquers Ch 6 Composite Resin: Indirect Technique Restorations
	Ceramometal restoration (if necessary following tooth reduction)	Ch 9 Ceramometal Full Coverage Restorations Ch 12 Esthetic Dentistry and Luting Agents Ch App A Custom Staining
	All-porcelain restorations (if necessary following tooth reduction)	Ch 3 Dentin Bonding Agents Ch 4 Color Modifiers and Opaquers Ch 8 Porcelain-Full Coverage and Partial Coverage Restorations Ch 12 Esthetic Dentistry and Luting Agents Ch 23 Esthetics and Computer-Aided Design and Computer-Aided Manufacturing (CAD/CAM) Systems Ch App A Custom Staining
	Porcelain laminate veneer (if necessary following tooth reduction)	Ch 3 Dentin Bonding Agents Ch 4 Color Modifiers and Opaquers Ch 7 Porcelain Laminate Veneers Restorations Ch 12 Esthetic Dentistry and Luting Agents Ch 23 Esthetics and Computer-Aided Design and Computer-Aided Manufacturing (CAD/CAM) Systems Ch App A Custom Staining
	Gingival augmentation (with restoration if necessary)	Ch 14 Esthetics and Periodontics Ch 18 Esthetics and Oral and Maxillofacial Surgery
	Orthodontic therapy	Ch 15 Esthetics and Orthodontics
	Orthognathic surgery (repositioning only)	Ch 18 Esthetics and Oral and Maxillofacial Surgery
Midline disharmony	Cosmetic recontouring	Ch 2 Fundamentals of Esthetics and Smile Analysis
	Direct composite resin veneers	Ch 3 Dentin Bonding Agents Ch 4 Color Modifiers and Opaquers Ch 5 Composite Resin: Fundamentals and Direct Technique Restorations
	Indirect composite resin veneers	Ch 3 Dentin Bonding Agents Ch 4 Color Modifiers and Opaquers Ch 6 Composite Resin: Indirect Technique Restorations
	Ceramometal restoration	Ch 9 Ceramometal Full Coverage Restorations Ch 12 Esthetic Dentistry and Luting Agents Ch App A Custom Staining
	All-porcelain restoration	Ch 3 Dentin Bonding Agents Ch 4 Color Modifiers and Opaquers Ch 8 Porcelain-Full Coverage and Partial Coverage Restorations Ch 12 Esthetic Dentistry and Luting Agents Ch 23 Esthetics and Computer-Aided Design and Computer-Aided Manufacturing (CAD/CAM) Systems Ch App A Custom Staining
	Porcelain laminate veneer	Ch 3 Dentin Bonding Agents Ch 4 Color Modifiers and Opaquers Ch 7 Porcelain Laminate Veneers Restorations Ch 12 Esthetic Dentistry and Luting Agents Ch 23 Esthetics and Computer-Aided Design and Computer-Aided Manufacturing (CAD/CAM) Systems Ch App A Custom Staining
	Orthodontic therapy	Ch 15 Esthetics and Orthodontics

Continued

Problem	Solution	Chapter Number and Title
Tooth-Related Problems		
Migrated teeth	Orthodontic therapy	Ch 15 Esthetics and Orthodontics
Multiple diastemata	Direct composite resin restorations	Ch 3 Dentin Bonding Agents Ch 4 Color Modifiers and Opaquers Ch 5 Composite Resin: Fundamentals and Direct Technique Restorations
	Indirect composite resin restorations	Ch 3 Dentin Bonding Agents Ch 4 Color Modifiers and Opaquers Ch 6 Composite Resin: Indirect Technique Restorations
	Ceramometal restoration	Ch 9 Ceramometal Full Coverage Restorations Ch 12 Esthetic Dentistry and Luting Agents Ch App A Custom Staining
	All-porcelain restorations	Ch 3 Dentin Bonding Agents Ch 4 Color Modifiers and Opaquers Ch 8 Porcelain-Full Coverage and Partial Coverage Restorations Ch 12 Esthetic Dentistry and Luting Agents Ch 23 Esthetics and Computer-Aided Design and Computer-Aided Manufacturing (CAD/CAM) Systems Ch App A Custom Staining
	Porcelain laminate veneers	Ch 3 Dentin Bonding Agents Ch 4 Color Modifiers and Opaquers Ch 7 Porcelain Laminate Veneers Restorations Ch 12 Esthetic Dentistry and Luting Agents Ch 23 Esthetics and Computer-Aided Design and Computer-Aided Manufacturing (CAD/CAM) Systems Ch App A Custom Staining
	Orthodontic therapy	Ch 15 Esthetics and Orthodontics
Open bite—mild	Direct composite resin restorations	Ch 3 Dentin Bonding Agents Ch 4 Color Modifiers and Opaquers Ch 12 Esthetic Dentistry and Luting Agents
	Indirect composite resin restorations	Ch 3 Dentin Bonding Agents Ch 4 Color Modifiers and Opaquers Ch 6 Composite Resin: Indirect Technique Restorations
	Ceramometal restoration	Ch 9 Ceramometal Full Coverage Restorations Ch 12 Esthetic Dentistry and Luting Agents Ch App A Custom Staining
	Porcelain laminate veneers	Ch 3 Dentin Bonding Agents Ch 4 Color Modifiers and Opaquers Ch 7 Porcelain Laminate Veneers Restorations Ch 12 Esthetic Dentistry and Luting Agents Ch 23 Esthetics and Computer-Aided Design and Computer-Aided Manufacturing (CAD/CAM) Systems Ch App A Custom Staining
	Orthodontic therapy	Ch 15 Esthetics and Orthodontics
Open bite—severe	Orthodontic therapy	Ch 15 Esthetics and Orthodontics
	Orthognathic surgery	Ch 18 Esthetics and Oral and Maxillofacial Surgery
Overbite/overjet	Orthodontic therapy	Ch 15 Esthetics and Orthodontics
	Orthognathic surgery	Ch 18 Esthetics and Oral and Maxillofacial Surgery
Spacing	Direct composite resin restorations	Ch 3 Dentin Bonding Agents Ch 4 Color Modifiers and Opaquers Ch 5 Composite Resin: Fundamentals and Direct Technique Restorations

Problem	Solution	Chapter Number and Title
Tooth-Related Problems		
Spacing-cont'd	Indirect composite resin restorations	Ch 3 Dentin Bonding Agents Ch 4 Color Modifiers and Opaquers Ch 6 Composite Resin: Indirect Technique Restorations
	Ceramometal restoration	Ch 9 Ceramometal Full Coverage Restorations Ch 12 Esthetic Dentistry and Luting Agents Ch App A Custom Staining
	All-porcelain restorations	Ch 3 Dentin Bonding Agents Ch 4 Color Modifiers and Opaquers Ch 8 Porcelain-Full Coverage and Partial Coverage Restorations Ch 12 Esthetic Dentistry and Luting Agents Ch 23 Esthetics and Computer-Aided Design and Computer-Aided Manufacturing (CAD/CAM) Systems Ch App A Custom Staining
	Porcelain laminate veneer	Ch 4 Color Modifiers and Opaquers Ch 7 Porcelain Laminate Veneers Restorations Ch 12 Esthetic Dentistry and Luting Agents Ch 23 Esthetics and Computer-Aided Design and Computer-Aided Manufacturing (CAD/CAM) Systems Ch App A Custom Staining
	Orthodontic therapy	Ch 15 Esthetics and Orthodontics
Traumatic injury— luxation	Temporary splinting	Ch 19 Esthetics and Pediatric Dentistry
	Domestic violence	Ch 30 Esthetic Dentistry and Domestic Violence
Color Problems		
Aged (dark) teeth	Direct composite resin veneers	Ch 3 Dentin Bonding Agents Ch 4 Color Modifiers and Opaquers Ch 5 Composite Resin: Fundamentals and Direct Technique Restorations
	Indirect composite resin veneers	Ch 3 Dentin Bonding Agents Ch 4 Color Modifiers and Opaquers Ch 6 Composite Resin: Indirect Technique Restorations
	Ceramometal restorations	Ch 9 Ceramometal Full Coverage Restorations Ch 12 Esthetic Dentistry and Luting Agents Ch App A Custom Staining
	All-porcelain restorations	Ch 3 Dentin Bonding Agents Ch 4 Color Modifiers and Opaquers Ch 8 Porcelain-Full Coverage and Partial Coverage Restorations Ch 12 Esthetic Dentistry and Luting Agents Ch 23 Esthetics and Computer-Aided Design and Computer-Aided Manufacturing (CAD/CAM) Systems Ch App A Custom Staining
	Porcelain laminate veneers	Ch 3 Dentin Bonding Agents Ch 4 Color Modifiers and Opaquers Ch 7 Porcelain Laminate Veneers Restorations Ch 12 Esthetic Dentistry and Luting Agents Ch 23 Esthetics and Computer-Aided Design and Computer-Aided Manufacturing (CAD/CAM) Systems Ch App A Custom Staining
	Bleaching	Ch 13 Bleaching and Related Agents

Continued

Problem	Solution	Chapter Number and Title
	Color Problems	
Coloration	Direct composite resin veneers	Ch 3 Dentin Bonding Agents Ch 4 Color Modifiers and Opaquers Ch 5 Composite Resin: Fundamentals and Direct Technique Restorations
	Indirect composite resin veneers	Ch 3 Dentin Bonding Agents Ch 4 Color Modifiers and Opaquers Ch 6 Composite Resin: Indirect Technique Restorations
	Ceramometal restoration	Ch 9 Ceramometal Full Coverage Restorations Ch 12 Esthetic Dentistry and Luting Agents Ch App A Custom Staining
	All-porcelain restorations	Ch 3 Dentin Bonding Agents Ch 4 Color Modifiers and Opaquers Ch 8 Porcelain-Full Coverage and Partial Coverage Restorations Ch 12 Esthetic Dentistry and Luting Agents Ch 23 Esthetics and Computer-Aided Design and Computer-Aided Manufacturing (CAD/CAM) Systems Ch App A Custom Staining
	Porcelain laminate veneers	Ch 3 Dentin Bonding Agents Ch 4 Color Modifiers and Opaquers Ch 7 Porcelain Laminate Veneers Restorations Ch 12 Esthetic Dentistry and Luting Agents Ch 23 Esthetics and Computer-Aided Design and Computer-Aided Manufacturing (CAD/CAM) Systems Ch App A Custom Staining
	Bleaching	Ch 13 Bleaching and Related Agents
	Prophylaxis (extrinsic stains)	Ch 13 Bleaching and Related Agents
Congenital discoloration	Direct composite resin veneers	Ch 3 Dentin Bonding Agents Ch 4 Color Modifiers and Opaquers Ch 5 Composite Resin: Fundamentals and Direct Technique Restorations
	Indirect composite resin veneers	Ch 3 Dentin Bonding Agents Ch 4 Color Modifiers and Opaquers Ch 6 Composite Resin: Indirect Technique Restorations
	Ceramometal restoration	Ch 9 Ceramometal Full Coverage Restorations Ch 12 Esthetic Dentistry and Luting Agents Ch App A Custom Staining
	All-porcelain restorations	Ch 3 Dentin Bonding Agents Ch 4 Color Modifiers and Opaquers Ch 8 Porcelain-Full Coverage and Partial Coverage Restorations Ch 12 Esthetic Dentistry and Luting Agents Ch 23 Esthetics and Computer-Aided Design and Computer-Aided Manufacturing (CAD/CAM) Systems Ch App A Custom Staining
	Porcelain laminate veneers	Ch 3 Dentin Bonding Agents Ch 4 Color Modifiers and Opaquers Ch 7 Porcelain Laminate Veneers Restorations Ch 12 Esthetic Dentistry and Luting Agents Ch 23 Esthetics and Computer-Aided Design and Computer-Aided Manufacturing (CAD/CAM) Systems Ch App A Custom Staining
	Bleaching	Ch 13 Bleaching and Related Agents
Discoloration	Direct composite resin veneers	Ch 3 Dentin Bonding Agents Ch 4 Color Modifiers and Opaquers Ch 5 Composite Resin: Fundamentals and Direct Technique Restorations
	Indirect composite resin veneers	Ch 3 Dentin Bonding Agents Ch 4 Color Modifiers and Opaquers Ch 6 Composite Resin: Indirect Technique Restorations

Problem	Solution	Chapter Number and Title
		Color Problems
Discoloration-cont'd	Ceramometal restoration	Ch 9 Ceramometal Full Coverage Restorations Ch 12 Esthetic Dentistry and Luting Agents Ch App A Custom Staining
	All-porcelain restorations	Ch 3 Dentin Bonding Agents Ch 4 Color Modifiers and Opaquers Ch 8 Porcelain-Full Coverage and Partial Coverage Restorations Ch 12 Esthetic Dentistry and Luting Agents Ch 23 Esthetics and Computer-Aided Design and Computer-Aided Manufacturing (CAD/CAM) Systems Ch App A Custom Staining
	Porcelain laminate veneer	Ch 4 Color Modifiers and Opaquers Ch 7 Porcelain Laminate Veneers Restorations Ch 12 Esthetic Dentistry and Luting Agents Ch 23 Esthetics and Computer-Aided Design and Computer-Aided Manufacturing (CAD/CAM) Systems Ch App A Custom Staining
	Direct composite resin veneers	Ch 3 Dentin Bonding Agents Ch 4 Color Modifiers and Opaquers Ch 8 Porcelain-Full Coverage and Partial Coverage Restorations Ch 12 Esthetic Dentistry and Luting Agents Ch 23 Esthetics and Computer-Aided Design and Computer-Aided Manufacturing (CAD/CAM) Systems Ch App A Custom Staining
	Bleaching	Ch 13 Bleaching and Related Agents
	Prophylaxis (extrinsic stains)	Ch 13 Bleaching and Related Agents
Endemic fluorosis	Direct composite resin veneer	Ch 3 Dentin Bonding Agents Ch 4 Color Modifiers and Opaquers Ch 5 Composite Resin: Fundamentals and Direct Technique Restorations
	Indirect composite resin veneer	Ch 3 Dentin Bonding Agents Ch 4 Color Modifiers and Opaquers Ch 6 Composite Resin: Indirect Technique Restorations
	Ceramometal restoration	Ch 9 Ceramometal Full Coverage Restorations Ch 12 Esthetic Dentistry and Luting Agents Ch App A Custom Staining
	All-porcelain restoration	Ch 3 Dentin Bonding Agents Ch 4 Color Modifiers and Opaquers Ch 8 Porcelain-Full Coverage and Partial Coverage Restorations Ch 12 Esthetic Dentistry and Luting Agents Ch 23 Esthetics and Computer-Aided Design and Computer-Aided Manufacturing (CAD/CAM) Systems Ch App A Custom Staining
	Porcelain laminate veneer	Ch 3 Dentin Bonding Agents Ch 4 Color Modifiers and Opaquers Ch 7 Porcelain Laminate Veneers Restorations Ch 12 Esthetic Dentistry and Luting Agents Ch 23 Esthetics and Computer-Aided Design and Computer-Aided Manufacturing (CAD/CAM) Systems Ch App A Custom Staining
	Bleaching	Ch 13 Bleaching and Related Agents
Endodontic discoloration	Direct composite resin veneer	Ch 3 Dentin Bonding Agents Ch 4 Color Modifiers and Opaquers Ch 5 Composite Resin: Fundamentals and Direct Technique Restorations
	Indirect composite resin veneer	Ch 3 Dentin Bonding Agents Ch 4 Color Modifiers and Opaquers Ch 6 Composite Resin: Indirect Technique Restorations

Continued

Problem	Solution	Chapter Number and Title
Color Problems		
Endodontic discoloration-cont'd	Ceramometal restoration	Ch 9 Ceramometal Full Coverage Restorations Ch 12 Esthetic Dentistry and Luting Agents Ch App A Custom Staining
	Direct composite resin veneer	Ch 3 Dentin Bonding Agents Ch 4 Color Modifiers and Opaquers Ch 8 Porcelain-Full Coverage and Partial Coverage Restorations Ch 12 Esthetic Dentistry and Luting Agents Ch 23 Esthetics and Computer-Aided Design and Computer-Aided Manufacturing (CAD/CAM) Systems Ch App A Custom Staining
	All-porcelain restoration	Ch 3 Dentin Bonding Agents Ch 4 Color Modifiers and Opaquers Ch 8 Porcelain-Full Coverage and Partial Coverage Restorations Ch 12 Esthetic Dentistry and Luting Agents Ch 23 Esthetics and Computer-Aided Design and Computer-Aided Manufacturing (CAD/CAM) Systems Ch App A Custom Staining
	Porcelain laminate veneer	Ch 3 Dentin Bonding Agents Ch 4 Color Modifiers and Opaquers Ch 7 Porcelain Laminate Veneers Restorations Ch 12 Esthetic Dentistry and Luting Agents Ch 23 Esthetics and Computer-Aided Design and Computer-Aided Manufacturing (CAD/CAM) Systems Ch App A Custom Staining
	Bleaching	Ch 13 Bleaching and Related Agents
Fluorosis	Direct composite resin veneer	Ch 3 Dentin Bonding Agents Ch 4 Color Modifiers and Opaquers Ch 5 Composite Resin: Fundamentals and Direct Technique Restorations
	Indirect composite resin veneer	Ch 3 Dentin Bonding Agents Ch 4 Color Modifiers and Opaquers Ch 6 Composite Resin: Indirect Technique Restorations
	Ceramometal restoration	Ch 4 Color Modifiers and Opaquers Ch 9 Ceramometal Full Coverage Restorations Ch 12 Esthetic Dentistry and Luting Agents Ch 23 Esthetics and Computer-Aided Design and Computer-Aided Manufacturing (CAD/CAM) Systems Ch App A Custom Staining
	All-porcelain restoration	Ch 3 Dentin Bonding Agents Ch 4 Color Modifiers and Opaquers Ch 8 Porcelain-Full Coverage and Partial Coverage Restorations Ch 12 Esthetic Dentistry and Luting Agents Ch 23 Esthetics and Computer-Aided Design and Computer-Aided Manufacturing (CAD/CAM) Systems Ch App A Custom Staining
	Porcelain laminate veneer	Ch 3 Dentin Bonding Agents Ch 4 Color Modifiers and Opaquers Ch 7 Porcelain Laminate Veneers Restorations Ch 12 Esthetic Dentistry and Luting Agents Ch 23 Esthetics and Computer-Aided Design and Computer-Aided Manufacturing (CAD/CAM) Systems Ch App A Custom Staining
	Bleaching	Ch 13 Bleaching and Related Agents

Problem	Solution	Chapter Number and Title
	Color Problems	
Staining	Direct composite resin veneer	Ch 3 Dentin Bonding Agents Ch 4 Color Modifiers and Opaquers Ch 5 Composite Resin: Fundamentals and Direct Technique Restorations
	Indirect composite resin veneer	Ch 3 Dentin Bonding Agents Ch 4 Color Modifiers and Opaquers Ch 6 Composite Resin: Indirect Technique Restorations
	Ceramometal restoration	Ch 9 Ceramometal Full Coverage Restorations Ch 12 Esthetic Dentistry and Luting Agents Ch App A Custom Staining
	All-porcelain restoration	Ch 3 Dentin Bonding Agents Ch 4 Color Modifiers and Opaquers Ch 8 Porcelain-Full Coverage and Partial Coverage Restorations Ch 12 Esthetic Dentistry and Luting Agents Ch 23 Esthetics and Computer-Aided Design and Computer-Aided Manufacturing (CAD/CAM) Systems Ch App A Custom Staining
	Porcelain laminate veneer	Ch 3 Dentin Bonding Agents Ch 4 Color Modifiers and Opaquers Ch 7 Porcelain Laminate Veneers Restorations Ch 12 Esthetic Dentistry and Luting Agents Ch 23 Esthetics and Computer-Aided Design and Computer-Aided Manufacturing (CAD/CAM) Systems Ch App A Custom Staining
	Bleaching	Ch 13 Bleaching and Related Agents
	Prophylaxis (extrinsic stains)	Ch 13 Bleaching and Related Agents
Tetracycline discoloration	Direct composite resin veneer	Ch 3 Dentin Bonding Agents Ch 4 Color Modifiers and Opaquers Ch 5 Composite Resin: Fundamentals and Direct Technique Restorations
	Indirect composite resin veneer	Ch 3 Dentin Bonding Agents Ch 4 Color Modifiers and Opaquers Ch 6 Composite Resin: Indirect Technique Restorations
	Ceramometal restoration	Ch 9 Ceramometal Full Coverage Restorations Ch 12 Esthetic Dentistry and Luting Agents Ch App A Custom Staining
	All-porcelain restoration	Ch 3 Dentin Bonding Agents Ch 4 Color Modifiers and Opaquers Ch 8 Porcelain-Full Coverage and Partial Coverage Restorations Ch 12 Esthetic Dentistry and Luting Agents Ch 23 Esthetics and Computer-Aided Design and Computer-Aided Manufacturing (CAD/CAM) Systems
	Porcelain laminate veneer	Ch 3 Dentin Bonding Agents Ch 4 Color Modifiers and Opaquers Ch 7 Porcelain Laminate Veneers Restorations Ch 12 Esthetic Dentistry and Luting Agents Ch 23 Esthetics and Computer-Aided Design and Computer-Aided Manufacturing (CAD/CAM) Systems Ch App A Custom Staining
	Bleaching	Ch 13 Bleaching and Related Agents

Continued

Problem	Solution	Chapter Number and Title
Color Problems		
Tooth color—too dark	Direct composite resin veneer	Ch 3 Dentin Bonding Agents Ch 4 Color Modifiers and Opaquers Ch 5 Composite Resin: Fundamentals and Direct Technique Restorations
	Indirect composite resin veneer	Ch 3 Dentin Bonding Agents Ch 4 Color Modifiers and Opaquers Ch 6 Composite Resin: Indirect Technique Restorations
	Ceramometal restoration	Ch 9 Ceramometal Full Coverage Restorations Ch 12 Esthetic Dentistry and Luting Agents Ch App A Custom Staining
	All-porcelain restoration	Ch 3 Dentin Bonding Agents Ch 4 Color Modifiers and Opaquers Ch 8 Porcelain-Full Coverage and Partial Coverage Restorations Ch 12 Esthetic Dentistry and Luting Agents Ch 23 Esthetics and Computer-Aided Design and Computer-Aided Manufacturing (CAD/CAM) Systems Ch App A Custom Staining
	Porcelain laminate veneer	Ch 3 Dentin Bonding Agents Ch 4 Color Modifiers and Opaquers Ch 7 Porcelain Laminate Veneers Restorations Ch 12 Esthetic Dentistry and Luting Agents Ch 23 Esthetics and Computer-Aided Design and Computer-Aided Manufacturing (CAD/CAM) Systems Ch App A Custom Staining
	Bleaching	Ch 13 Bleaching and Related Agents
	Prophylaxis (extrinsic stains)	Ch 13 Bleaching and Related Agents
Tooth color—too light	Direct composite resin veneer	Ch 3 Dentin Bonding Agents Ch 4 Color Modifiers and Opaquers Ch 5 Composite Resin: Fundamentals and Direct Technique Restorations
	Indirect composite resin veneer	Ch 3 Dentin Bonding Agents Ch 4 Color Modifiers and Opaquers Ch 6 Composite Resin: Indirect Technique Restorations
	Ceramometal restoration	Ch 9 Ceramometal Full Coverage Restorations Ch 12 Esthetic Dentistry and Luting Agents Ch App A Custom Staining
	All-porcelain restoration	Ch 3 Dentin Bonding Agents Ch 4 Color Modifiers and Opaquers Ch 8 Porcelain-Full Coverage and Partial Coverage Restorations Ch 12 Esthetic Dentistry and Luting Agents Ch 23 Esthetics and Computer-Aided Design and Computer-Aided Manufacturing (CAD/CAM) Systems Ch App A Custom Staining
	Porcelain laminate veneer	Ch 4 Color Modifiers and Opaquers Ch 7 Porcelain Laminate Veneers Restorations Ch 12 Esthetic Dentistry and Luting Agents Ch 23 Esthetics and Computer-Aided Design and Computer-Aided Manufacturing (CAD/CAM) Systems Ch App A Custom Staining

Problem	Solution	Chapter Number and Title
		Color Problems
Traumatic discoloration	Direct composite resin veneer	Ch 3 Dentin Bonding Agents Ch 4 Color Modifiers and Opaquers Ch 5 Composite Resin: Fundamentals and Direct Technique Restorations
	Indirect composite resin veneer	Ch 3 Dentin Bonding Agents Ch 4 Color Modifiers and Opaquers Ch 6 Composite Resin: Indirect Technique Restorations
	Ceramometal restoration	Ch 9 Ceramometal Full Coverage Restorations Ch 12 Esthetic Dentistry and Luting Agents Ch App A Custom Staining
	All-porcelain restorations	Ch 3 Dentin Bonding Agents Ch 4 Color Modifiers and Opaquers Ch 8 Porcelain-Full Coverage and Partial Coverage Restorations Ch 12 Esthetic Dentistry and Luting Agents Ch 23 Esthetics and Computer-Aided Design and Computer-Aided Manufacturing (CAD/CAM) Systems Ch App A Custom Staining
	Porcelain laminate veneer	Ch 3 Dentin Bonding Agents Ch 4 Color Modifiers and Opaquers Ch 7 Porcelain Laminate Veneers Restorations Ch 12 Esthetic Dentistry and Luting Agents Ch 23 Esthetics and Computer-Aided Design and Computer-Aided Manufacturing (CAD/CAM) Systems Ch App A Custom Staining
	Bleaching	Ch 13 Bleaching and Related Agents
	Domestic violence	Ch 30 Esthetic Dentistry and Domestic Violence
White spots	Direct composite resin restorations	Ch 3 Dentin Bonding Agents Ch 4 Color Modifiers and Opaquers Ch 5 Composite Resin: Fundamentals and Direct Technique Restorations
	Indirect composite resin restorations	Ch 3 Dentin Bonding Agents Ch 4 Color Modifiers and Opaquers Ch 6 Composite Resin: Indirect Technique Restorations
	Ceramometal restoration	Ch 9 Ceramometal Full Coverage Restorations Ch 12 Esthetic Dentistry and Luting Agents Ch App A Custom Staining
	All-porcelain restorations	Ch 3 Dentin Bonding Agents Ch 4 Color Modifiers and Opaquers Ch 8 Porcelain-Full Coverage and Partial Coverage Restorations Ch 12 Esthetic Dentistry and Luting Agents Ch 23 Esthetics and Computer-Aided Design and Computer-Aided Manufacturing (CAD/CAM) Systems Ch App A Custom Staining
	Porcelain laminate veneer	Ch 3 Dentin Bonding Agents Ch 4 Color Modifiers and Opaquers Ch 8 Porcelain-Full Coverage and Partial Coverage Restorations Ch 12 Esthetic Dentistry and Luting Agents Ch 23 Esthetics and Computer-Aided Design and Computer-Aided Manufacturing (CAD/CAM) Systems Ch App A Custom Staining
	Bleaching	Ch 13 Bleaching and Related Agents
	Prophylaxis (extrinsic stains)	Ch 13 Bleaching and Related Agents

Continued

Problem	Solution	Chapter Number and Title
	Color Problems	

Missing Teeth Problems

Problem	Solution	Chapter Number and Title
Migrated teeth—multiple	Direct composite resin veneer	Ch 3 Dentin Bonding Agents Ch 4 Color Modifiers and Opaquers Ch 5 Composite Resin: Fundamentals and Direct Technique Restorations
	Indirect composite resin veneer	Ch 3 Dentin Bonding Agents Ch 4 Color Modifiers and Opaquers Ch 6 Composite Resin: Indirect Technique Restorations
	Ceramometal restoration	Ch 9 Ceramometal Full Coverage Restorations Ch 12 Esthetic Dentistry and Luting Agents Ch App A Custom Staining
	All-porcelain restorations	Ch 3 Dentin Bonding Agents Ch 4 Color Modifiers and Opaquers Ch 8 Porcelain-Full Coverage and Partial Coverage Restorations Ch 12 Esthetic Dentistry and Luting Agents Ch 23 Esthetics and Computer-Aided Design and Computer-Aided Manufacturing (CAD/CAM) Systems
	Porcelain laminate veneer	Ch 3 Dentin Bonding Agents Ch 4 Color Modifiers and Opaquers Ch 7 Porcelain Laminate Veneers Restorations Ch 12 Esthetic Dentistry and Luting Agents Ch 23 Esthetics and Computer-Aided Design and Computer-Aided Manufacturing (CAD/CAM) Systems Ch App A Custom Staining
	Removable prosthesis	Ch 11 Acrylic and Other Resin: Removable Prosthetics
	Implant retained restorations	Ch 17 Esthetics and Implant Prosthetics Ch 12 Esthetic Dentistry and Luting Agents Ch App A Custom Staining
	Orthodontic therapy	Ch 15 Esthetics and Orthodontics
Migrated tooth—single	Direct composite resin restoration	Ch 3 Dentin Bonding Agents Ch 4 Color Modifiers and Opaquers Ch 5 Composite Resin: Fundamentals and Direct Technique Restorations
	Indirect composite resin restoration	Ch 3 Dentin Bonding Agents Ch 4 Color Modifiers and Opaquers Ch 6 Composite Resin: Indirect Technique Restorations
	Ceramometal restoration	Ch 9 Ceramometal Full Coverage Restorations Ch 12 Esthetic Dentistry and Luting Agents Ch App A Custom Staining
	All-porcelain restoration	Ch 3 Dentin Bonding Agents Ch 4 Color Modifiers and Opaquers Ch 8 Porcelain-Full Coverage and Partial Coverage Restorations Ch 12 Esthetic Dentistry and Luting Agents Ch 23 Esthetics and Computer-Aided Design and Computer-Aided Manufacturing (CAD/CAM) Systems Ch App A Custom Staining
	Removable prosthesis	Ch 11 Acrylic and Other Resins: Removable Prosthetics
	Implant retained restorations	Ch 17 Esthetics and Implant Prosthetics Ch 12 Esthetic Dentistry and Luting Agents Ch App A Custom Staining
	Orthodontic therapy	Ch 15 Esthetics and Orthodontics

Color Problems

Problem	Solution	Chapter Number and Title
	Color Problems	
Multiple missing teeth	Ceramometal restoration	Ch 9 Ceramometal Full Coverage Restorations Ch 12 Esthetic Dentistry and Luting Agents Ch App A Custom Staining
	All-porcelain restorations (select cases)	Ch 3 Dentin Bonding Agents Ch 4 Color Modifiers and Opaquers Ch 8 Porcelain-Full Coverage and Partial Coverage Restorations Ch 12 Esthetic Dentistry and Luting Agents Ch 23 Esthetics and Computer-Aided Design and Computer-Aided Manufacturing (CAD/CAM) Systems Ch App A Custom Staining
	Removable prosthesis	Ch 11 Acrylic and Other Resins: Removable Prosthetics
	Implant retained restorations	Ch 17 Esthetics and Implant Prosthetics Ch 12 Esthetic Dentistry and Luting Agents Ch App A Custom Staining
	Domestic violence	Ch 30 Esthetic Dentistry and Domestic Violence
Single missing tooth	Ceramometal restoration	Ch 9 Ceramometal Full Coverage Restorations Ch 12 Esthetic Dentistry and Luting Agents Ch App A Custom Staining
	All-porcelain restorations	Ch 3 Dentin Bonding Agents Ch 4 Color Modifiers and Opaquers Ch 8 Porcelain-Full Coverage and Partial Coverage Restorations Ch 12 Esthetic Dentistry and Luting Agents Ch 23 Esthetics and Computer-Aided Design and Computer-Aided Manufacturing (CAD/CAM) Systems Ch App A Custom Staining
	Removable prosthesis	Ch 11 Acrylic and Other Resins: Removable Prosthetics
	Implant retained restorations	Ch 17 Esthetics and Implant Prosthetics Ch 12 Esthetic Dentistry and Luting Agents Ch App A Custom Staining
	Domestic violence	Ch 30 Esthetic Dentistry and Domestic Violence
Traumatic injury— avulsion	Temporary splinting	Ch 19 Esthetics and Pediatric Dentistry
	Domestic violence	Ch 30 Esthetic Dentistry and Domestic Violence
Caries		
Carious restoration margins	See Repairs	Ch 4 Color Modifiers and Opaquers
Carious tooth	Direct composite resin restoration	Ch 3 Dentin Bonding Agents Ch 4 Color Modifiers and Opaquers Ch 5 Composite Resin: Fundamentals and Direct Technique Restorations
	Indirect composite resin restoration	Ch 3 Dentin Bonding Agents Ch 4 Color Modifiers and Opaquers Ch 6 Composite Resin: Indirect Technique Restorations
	Ceramometal restoration	Ch 9 Ceramometal Full Coverage Restorations Ch 12 Esthetic Dentistry and Luting Agents Ch App A Custom Staining

Continued

Problem	Solution	Chapter Number and Title
Color Problems		
Carious tooth-cont'd	All-porcelain restorations	Ch 3 Dentin Bonding Agents Ch 4 Color Modifiers and Opaquers Ch 8 Porcelain-Full Coverage and Partial Coverage Restorations Ch 12 Esthetic Dentistry and Luting Agents Ch 23 Esthetics and Computer-Aided Design and Computer-Aided Manufacturing (CAD/CAM) Systems
	Porcelain laminate veneer	Ch 3 Dentin Bonding Agents Ch 4 Color Modifiers and Opaquers Ch 7 Porcelain Laminate Veneers Restorations Ch 12 Esthetic Dentistry and Luting Agents Ch 23 Esthetics and Computer-Aided Design and Computer-Aided Manufacturing (CAD/CAM) Systems Ch App A Custom Staining
	Porcelain laminate veneer	Ch 3 Dentin Bonding Agents Ch 4 Color Modifiers and Opaquers Ch 7 Porcelain Laminate Veneers Restorations Ch 12 Esthetic Dentistry and Luting Agents Ch 23 Esthetics and Computer-Aided Design and Computer-Aided Manufacturing (CAD/CAM) Systems Ch App A Custom Staining

Repairs

Problem	Solution	Chapter Number and Title
Acrylic veneer facing—dislodgment	Acrylic veneer repair	Ch 4 Color Modifiers and Opaquers
Carious restoration margins	Gingival grafting (if caused by recession)	Ch 14 Esthetics and Periodontics
Porcelain fractures—ceramometal restoration	See repairs	Ch 4 Color Modifiers and Opaquers
	Evaluate restoration margins and contours	Ch 9 Ceramometal Full Coverage Restorations Ch 12 Esthetic Dentistry and Luting Agents
	Evaluate restoration margins and contours	Ch 8 Porcelain-Full Coverage and Partial Coverage Restorations

Non–Tooth-Related Problems		

Periodontal Problems

Problem	Solution	Chapter Number and Title
Gingival asymmetry	Gingival recontouring—surgical (if necessary)	Ch 14 Esthetics and Periodontics
	Gingival recontouring—laser surgery (if necessary)	Ch 21 Esthetics and Laser Surgery
	Artificial gingiva (pink porcelain)	Ch 3 Dentin Bonding Agents Ch 4 Color Modifiers and Opaquers Ch 6 Composite Resin: Indirect Technique Restorations Ch 7 Porcelain Laminate Veneers Restorations Ch 8 Porcelain-Full Coverage and Partial Coverage Restorations Ch 9 Ceramometal Full Coverage Restorations Ch 12 Esthetic Dentistry and Luting Agents Ch 23 Esthetics and Computer-Aided Design and Computer-Aided Manufacturing (CAD/CAM) Systems Ch App A Custom Staining
	Gingival grafting (if caused by recession)	Ch 14 Esthetics and Periodontics
Gingival hypertrophy	Gingival recontouring—surgical (if necessary)	Ch 14 Esthetics and Periodontics
	Gingival recontouring—laser surgery (if necessary)	Ch 21 Esthetics and Laser Surgery

Problem	Solution	Chapter Number and Title
Non–Tooth-Related Problems		
Gingival inflammation	Evaluate restoration margins and contours	Ch 3 Dentin Bonding Agents Ch 4 Color Modifiers and Opaquers Ch 5 Composite Resin: Fundamentals and Direct Technique Restorations Ch 6 Composite Resin: Indirect Technique Restorations
	Evaluate restoration margins and contours	Ch 9 Ceramometal Full Coverage Restorations Ch 12 Esthetic Dentistry and Luting Agents
	Evaluate restoration margins and contours	Ch 8 Porcelain-Full Coverage and Partial Coverage Restorations
	Evaluate restoration margins and contours	Ch 3 Dentin Bonding Agents Ch 4 Color Modifiers and Opaquers Ch 8 Porcelain-Full Coverage and Partial Coverage Restorations Ch 12 Esthetic Dentistry and Luting Agents Ch 23 Esthetics and Computer-Aided Design and Computer-Aided Manufacturing (CAD/CAM) Systems
	Periodontal therapy	Ch 14 Esthetics and Periodontics
	Oral surgery (possibly with restoration—see Long tooth)	Ch 9 Ceramometal Full Coverage Restorations Ch 12 Esthetic Dentistry and Luting Agents Ch App A Custom Staining
	Evaluate medical status	
Gingival recession	Gingival graft	Ch 14 Esthetics and Periodontics
	Artificial gingiva (pink porcelain)	Ch 3 Dentin Bonding Agents Ch 4 Color Modifiers and Opaquers Ch 6 Composite Resin: Indirect Technique Restorations Ch 7 Porcelain Laminate Veneers Restorations Ch 8 Porcelain-Full Coverage and Partial Coverage Restorations Ch 9 Ceramometal Full Coverage Restorations Ch 12 Esthetic Dentistry and Luting Agents Ch 23 Esthetics and Computer-Aided Design and Computer-Aided Manufacturing (CAD/CAM) Systems Ch App A Custom Staining
	Frenectomy	Ch 21 Esthetics and Laser Surgery
	Gingival recontouring—laser surgery (if necessary)	Ch 21 Esthetics and Laser Surgery
	Oral surgery (possibly with restoration—see Long tooth)	Ch 18 Esthetics and Oral and Maxillofacial Surgery
	Splinting	Ch 14 Esthetics and Periodontics
Dermatologic Problems		
Aging	Dermatologic treatment	Ch 24 Esthetics and Dermatologic Pharmaceuticals
	Restore lip support—direct composite resin restorations	Ch 3 Dentin Bonding Agents Ch 4 Color Modifiers and Opaquers Ch 5 Composite Resin: Fundamentals and Direct Technique Restorations
	Restore lip support—indirect composite resin restorations	Ch 3 Dentin Bonding Agents Ch 4 Color Modifiers and Opaquers Ch 6 Composite Resin: Indirect Technique Restorations
	Restore lip support—ceramometal restorations	Ch 9 Ceramometal Full Coverage Restorations Ch 12 Esthetic Dentistry and Luting Agents Ch App A Custom Staining

Continued

Problem	Solution	Chapter Number and Title
Dermatologic Problems		
Aging-cont'd	Restore lip support—all-porcelain restorations	Ch 3 Dentin Bonding Agents Ch 4 Color Modifiers and Opaquers Ch 8 Porcelain-Full Coverage and Partial Coverage Restorations Ch 12 Esthetic Dentistry and Luting Agents Ch 23 Esthetics and Computer-Aided Design and Computer-Aided Manufacturing (CAD/CAM) Systems
	Restore lip support—porcelain laminate veneers	Ch 3 Dentin Bonding Agents Ch 4 Color Modifiers and Opaquers Ch 7 Porcelain Laminate Veneers Restorations Ch 12 Esthetic Dentistry and Luting Agents Ch 23 Esthetics and Computer-Aided Design and Computer-Aided Manufacturing (CAD/CAM) Systems Ch App A Custom Staining
	Restore lip support—removable prostheses	Ch 12 Acrylic and Other Resins—Removable Prostheses
	Restore lip support—implant retained restorations	Ch 17 Esthetics and Implant Prosthetics Ch 12 Esthetic Dentistry and Luting Agents Ch App A Custom Staining
	Lip augmentation	Ch 18 Esthetics and Oral and Maxillofacial Surgery
	Skin resurfacing	Ch 18 Esthetics and Oral and Maxillofacial Surgery
Scars	Skin resurfacing	Ch 18 Esthetics and Oral and Maxillofacial Surgery
	Cosmetic skin resurfacing	Ch 21 Esthetics and Laser Surgery
	Plastic surgery	Ch 25 Esthetics and Plastic Surgery
	Domestic violence	Ch 30 Esthetic Dentistry and Domestic Violence
Wrinkles	Dermatologic treatment	Ch 24 Esthetics and Dermatologic Pharmaceuticals
	Restore lip support—direct composite resin restorations	Ch 3 Dentin Bonding Agents Ch 4 Color Modifiers and Opaquers Ch 5 Composite Resin: Fundamentals and Direct Technique Restorations
	Restore lip support—indirect composite resin restorations	Ch 3 Dentin Bonding Agents Ch 4 Color Modifiers and Opaquers Ch 6 Composite Resin: Indirect Technique Restorations
	Restore lip support—ceramometal restorations	Ch 9 Ceramometal Full Coverage Restorations Ch 12 Esthetic Dentistry and Luting Agents Ch App A Custom Staining
	Restore lip support—all-porcelain restorations	Ch 3 Dentin Bonding Agents Ch 4 Color Modifiers and Opaquers Ch 8 Porcelain-Full Coverage and Partial Coverage Restorations Ch 12 Esthetic Dentistry and Luting Agents Ch 23 Esthetics and Computer-Aided Design and Computer-Aided Manufacturing (CAD/CAM) Systems
	Restore lip support—porcelain laminate veneers	Ch 3 Dentin Bonding Agents Ch 4 Color Modifiers and Opaquers Ch 7 Porcelain Laminate Veneers Restorations Ch 12 Esthetic Dentistry and Luting Agents Ch 23 Esthetics and Computer-Aided Design and Computer-Aided Manufacturing (CAD/CAM) Systems Ch App A Custom Staining
	Restore lip support—removable prostheses	Ch 12 Acrylic and Other Resins—Removable Prostheses
	Restore lip support—implant retained restorations	Ch 17 Esthetics and Implant Prosthetics Ch 12 Esthetic Dentistry and Luting Agents Ch App A Custom Staining

Problem	Solution	Chapter Number and Title
Dermatologic Problems		
Wrinkles-cont'd	Skin resurfacing	Ch 18 Esthetics and Oral and Maxillofacial Surgery
	Cosmetic skin resurfacing	Ch 21 Esthetics and Laser Surgery
Facial Contours and Skeletal Problems		
Asymmetry	Orthodontic surgery	Ch 15 Esthetics and Orthodontics
	Orthognathic surgery	Ch 18 Esthetics and Oral and Maxillofacial Surgery
	Plastic surgery (severe)	Ch 25 Esthetics and Plastic Surgery
	Domestic violence	Ch 30 Esthetic Dentistry and Domestic Violence
Bimaxillary prognathism/ protrusion	Orthodontic surgery	Ch 15 Esthetics and Orthodontics
	Orthognathic surgery	Ch 18 Esthetics and Oral and Maxillofacial Surgery
	Plastic surgery	Ch 15 Esthetics and Orthodontics
Excessive lip support	Orthodontic surgery	Ch 18 Esthetics and Oral and Maxillofacial Surgery
	Orthognathic surgery	Ch 18 Esthetics and Oral and Maxillofacial Surgery
	Plastic surgery	Ch 25 Esthetics and Plastic Surgery
Facial asymmetry	Orthognathic surgery	Ch 18 Esthetics and Oral and Maxillofacial Surgery
	Plastic surgery	Ch 25 Esthetics and Plastic Surgery
	Domestic violence	Ch 30 Esthetic Dentistry and Domestic Violence
Hypogenia	Orthognathic surgery	Ch 18 Esthetics and Oral and Maxillofacial Surgery
	Plastic surgery	Ch 25 Esthetics and Plastic Surgery
Insufficient lip support	Dermatologic treatment	Ch 24 Esthetics and Dermatologic Pharmaceuticals
	Restore lip support—direct composite resin restorations	Ch 3 Dentin Bonding Agents Ch 4 Color Modifiers and Opaquers Ch 5 Composite Resin: Fundamentals and Direct Technique Restorations
	Restore lip support—indirect composite resin restorations	Ch 3 Dentin Bonding Agents Ch 4 Color Modifiers and Opaquers Ch 6 Composite Resin: Indirect Technique Restorations
	Restore lip support—ceramometal restorations	Ch 9 Ceramometal Full Coverage Restorations Ch 12 Esthetic Dentistry and Luting Agents Ch App A Custom Staining
	Restore lip support—all-porcelain restorations	Ch 3 Dentin Bonding Agents Ch 4 Color Modifiers and Opaquers Ch 8 Porcelain-Full Coverage and Partial Coverage Restorations Ch 12 Esthetic Dentistry and Luting Agents Ch 23 Esthetics and Computer-Aided Design and Computer-Aided Manufacturing (CAD/CAM) Systems Ch App A Custom Staining
	Restore lip support—porcelain laminate veneers	Ch 3 Dentin Bonding Agents Ch 4 Color Modifiers and Opaquers Ch 7 Porcelain Laminate Veneers Restorations Ch 12 Esthetic Dentistry and Luting Agents Ch 23 Esthetics and Computer-Aided Design and Computer-Aided Manufacturing (CAD/CAM) Systems Ch App A Custom Staining

Continued

Problem	Solution	Chapter Number and Title
Facial Contours and Skeletal Problems		
Insufficient lip support-cont'd	Restore lip support—removable prostheses	Ch 12 Acrylic and other resins—removable prostheses
	Restore lip support—implant retained restorations	Ch 17 Esthetics and Implant Prosthetics Ch 12 Esthetic Dentistry and Luting Agents Ch App A Custom Staining
	Orthodontic therapy	Ch 15 Esthetics and Orthodontics
	Orthognathic surgery (severe)	Ch 18 Esthetics and Oral and Maxillofacial Surgery
	Plastic surgery (severe)	Ch 25 Esthetics and Plastic Surgery
Macrogenia problem	Orthognathic surgery	Ch 18 Esthetics and Oral and Maxillofacial Surgery
	Plastic surgery	Ch 25 Esthetics and Plastic Surgery
Mandibular prognathism/ protrusion	Orthodontic therapy	Ch 15 Esthetics and Orthodontics
	Orthognathic surgery	Ch 18 Esthetics and Oral and Maxillofacial Surgery
	Plastic surgery	Ch 25 Esthetics and Plastic Surgery
Mandibular retrognathism/ retrusion	Orthodontic therapy	Ch 15 Esthetics and Orthodontics
	Orthognathic surgery	Ch 18 Esthetics and Oral and Maxillofacial Surgery
	Plastic surgery	Ch 25 Esthetics and Plastic Surgery
Maxillary prognathism/ protrusion	Orthodontic therapy	Ch 15 Esthetics and Orthodontics
	Orthognathic surgery	Ch 18 Esthetics and Oral and Maxillofacial Surgery
	Plastic surgery	Ch 25 Esthetics and Plastic Surgery
Maxillary retrognathism/ retrusion	Orthodontic therapy	Ch 15 Esthetics and Orthodontics
	Orthognathic surgery	Ch 18 Esthetics and Oral and Maxillofacial Surgery
	Plastic surgery	Ch 25 Esthetics and Plastic Surgery
Open bite—mild	Direct composite resin veneers	Ch 3 Dentin Bonding Agents Ch 4 Color Modifiers and Opaquers Ch 5 Composite Resin: Fundamentals and Direct Technique Restorations
	Indirect composite resin restorations	Ch 3 Dentin Bonding Agents Ch 4 Color Modifiers and Opaquers Ch 6 Composite Resin: Indirect Technique Restorations
	Ceramometal—full coverage restorations	Ch 9 Ceramometal Full Coverage Restorations Ch 12 Esthetic Dentistry and Luting Agents Ch App A Custom Staining

Problem	Solution	Chapter Number and Title
Facial Contours and Skeletal Problems		
Facial Contours and Skeletal Problems bite—severe	All-porcelain restorations	Ch 3 Dentin Bonding Agents Ch 4 Color Modifiers and Opaquers Ch 8 Porcelain-Full Coverage and Partial Coverage Restorations Ch 12 Esthetic Dentistry and Luting Agents Ch 23 Esthetics and Computer-Aided Design and Computer-Aided Manufacturing (CAD/CAM) Systems Ch App A Custom Staining
	Porcelain laminate veneers	Ch 3 Dentin Bonding Agents Ch 4 Color Modifiers and Opaquers Ch 7 Porcelain Laminate Veneers Restorations Ch 12 Esthetic Dentistry and Luting Agents Ch 23 Esthetics and Computer-Aided Design and Computer-Aided Manufacturing (CAD/CAM) Systems Ch App A Custom Staining
	Orthodontic therapy	Ch 15 Esthetics and Orthodontics
	Orthognathic surgery	Ch 18 Esthetics and Oral and Maxillofacial Surgery
Prognathism	Orthodontic therapy	Ch 15 Esthetics and Orthodontics
	Orthognathic surgery	Ch 18 Esthetics and Oral and Maxillofacial Surgery
	Plastic surgery	Ch 25 Esthetics and Plastic Surgery
Protrusion	Orthodontic therapy	Ch 15 Esthetics and Orthodontics
	Orthognathic surgery	Ch 18 Esthetics and Oral and Maxillofacial Surgery
	Plastic surgery	Ch 25 Esthetics and Plastic Surgery
Retrognathism	Orthognathic surgery	Ch 18 Esthetics and Oral and Maxillofacial Surgery
	Plastic surgery	Ch 25 Esthetics and Plastic Surgery
Retrusion	Orthodontic therapy	Ch 15 Esthetics and Orthodontics
	Orthognathic surgery	Ch 18 Esthetics and Oral and Maxillofacial Surgery
	Plastic surgery	Ch 25 Esthetics and Plastic Surgery

Part 2

Principles of Esthetics

1

Introduction to Esthetics

Milton B. Asbell

The search for beauty can be traced to the earliest civilizations. Dental art has long been part of the quest to enhance the esthetics of the teeth and mouth. Assyrio-Babylonian cuneiform tablets dating from the dawn of recorded history advise the following:

> "If a man's teeth become yellow . . . thou shalt bray together "salt of Akkad," ammi, lolium, pine-turpine with these, with thy fingers shalt bur his teeth."

Writing in the ninth century BC, the author of the *Song of Solomon* (4:2) offers a poetic description of dental esthetics:

> "Thy teeth are like a flock of well-selected sheep, which are come up from the washing, all of which bear twins, and there is not one among them that is deprived of her young."

Both the Phoenicians (approximately 800 BC) and Etruscans (approximately 900 BC) carefully carved animal tusks to simulate the shape, form, and hue of natural teeth for use as pontics (Fig. 1-1). The Central and South American Mayas (approximately 1000 AD) beautified themselves by filing the incisal edges of their anterior teeth into various shapes and designs (Figs. 1-2 and 1-3). They also placed plugs of iron pyrites, obsidian, and jade into the facial surfaces of the maxillary anterior teeth (Fig. 1-4). This practice was common among both sexes, and tooth mutilation is still practiced in some societies (Figs. 1-5 and 1-6).

During the Roman Empire dental cosmetic treatment was available only to the affluent classes. Oral hygiene was practiced primarily by women for reasons of beauty rather than dental health. Mouthwashes, dentifrices, and toothpicks were common in Roman boudoirs, and when teeth were lost, they were replaced with substitutes of bone or ivory carved to the likeness of the missing ones.

Interest in dental esthetics was virtually absent during the Middle Ages. It was not until the eighteenth century that dentistry was recognized as a separate discipline and its various branches were established. The leader of the movement to modernize and promote dentistry was Pierre Fauchard (1678-1761) of France. He, together with several colleagues, advocated such esthetic practices as proper oral hygiene and the use of gold shell crowns with enamel "veneers." They also introduced a technique for the manufacture of mineral (as opposed to ivory or bone) "incorruptible" teeth for use in dentures. In England *The British Journal* carried the following advertisement (1724):

> "The incomparable powder for cleaning the teeth which has given great satisfaction to most of the nobility and gentry for above these twenty years . . . it, at one using, makes the teeth as white as ivory, and never black or yellow."

ESTHETICS IN THE UNITED STATES

In the colonial United States primitive dental conditions prevailed for almost a century (from roughly 1670 to 1770) until the arrival of "operators for the teeth," dental professionals who had been trained in Europe. They brought with them not only medications for toothache but also prescriptions for toothpowder "to make teeth white" and "attend to your teeth and preserve your health and beauty." They claimed their toothpowder "[prepared] and [fixed] real enameled teeth, the best contrivance yet to substitute the loss of natural ones" (Figs. 1-7 and 1-8). Transplantation of teeth between patients was practiced, with donors being paid for their trouble: "Any person that will dispense of the front teeth, five guineas for each (Fig. 1-9)."

Cosmetic dentistry did not meet with universal acceptance, however. The following is an official edict published by His Britannic Majesty at Perth Amboy, New Jersey:

> "All women of whatever age, rank, profession or degree, whether virgins, maids, or widow, who after this Act shall impose upon, seduce and betray unto matrimony any of His Majesty's subjects by virtue of cosmetics, scents, washes, paints, artificial teeth, false hair or high-heeled shoes, shall incur the penalty of the law in force against witchcraft and like misdemeanors."

Competent dental practitioners could be found in the leading cities of the United States by the early years of the nineteenth century.

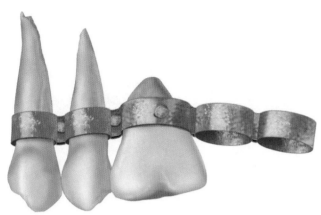

FIGURE 1-1 Representation of an ancient Etruscan appliance, showing gold soldered rings and rivets to hold dental replacements as a bridge. In this specimen there are two natural teeth and one riveted oxtooth. (From Posnick JC: Orthognathic surgery: principles and practice, St. Louis, 2014, Saunders.)

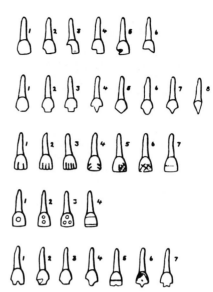

FIGURE 1-3 Various forms of tooth mutilation that were considered beautification techniques. (From Weinberger BW: *An introduction to the history of dentistry*, vol 1, St Louis, 1948, Mosby.)

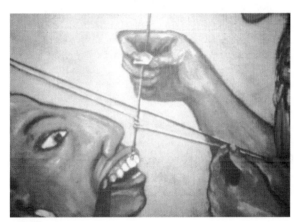

FIGURE 1-2 Ancient painting depicting a probable method of preparing teeth used by the Mayas about 1000 AD. (Courtesy Dr. Pedro Beltranena.)

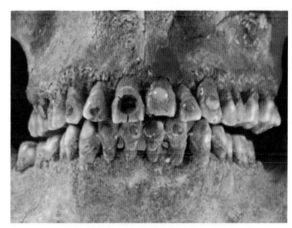

FIGURE 1-4 Mayan specimen dating to approximately 1000 AD showing multiple inlays and turquoise restorations. (Courtesy of the Director of Physical Anthropology, National Institute of Anthropology and History (INAH), Mexico.)

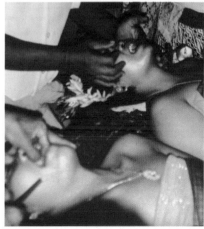

FIGURE 1-5 Photograph taken in 1987 showing traditional filing of the maxillary anterior teeth designed to beautify Polynesian brides.

The introduction of mineral teeth in 1817 was soon followed by the manufacture of porcelain teeth. Dentures were fabricated with a gingival component made of carved ivory or animal bone that was designed for adaptation to ivory or bone bases (Fig. 1-10). These denture bases were common until the 1850s, when various alternative materials were introduced to afford more esthetic results. The technique of mounting artificial teeth on gold or platinum fused with a continuous pink gingival body made of porcelain was patented in the nineteenth century. "Auroplasty", colored gutta-percha, "parkesine" (a celluloid-like material), "cheoplasty" (an alloy of tin, silver, and bismuth), "rose pearl", collodion, pink hecolite, and even tortoise shells were used for esthetic effect in dentistry. Vulcanite was the first universally acceptable denture material. Patented by Nelson Goodyear in 1851, it was made by heating caoutchouc (Indian rubber) with sulphur, resulting in a firm yet flexible material. Vulcanite, which was relatively inexpensive and simple to make, propelled the use of dentures out of the luxury category by allowing for relatively inexpensive and simple fabrication. Synthetic materials such as vinyl acrylic resins, copolymer acrylic resins, and styrene acrylic resins were introduced about 1934.

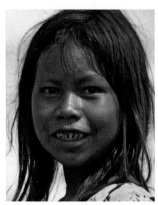

FIGURE 1-6 Ticuana tribal tooth mutilation. (© WOLFGANG KAEHLER.)

1767 November 5.
ROBERT WOOFFENDALE,
SURGEON DENTIST, lately from LONDON, (who wa
inftructed by THOMAS BERDMORE, Efq; Operator fo
the Teeth to his Britannick Majefty):
BEGS leave to inform the Public, that he perform
all operations on the TEETH, GUMS and SOCKETS
ikewife fets in ARTIFICIAL TEETH, fo as to efcap
difcernment and without the leaft inconvenience, a
Mrs. HUNT's, oppofite to where Mr. Roberdeau latel
ived, in Second-ftreet.
N. B. As he intends going to England the latter en
f next week, returns thanks to the public for thei
avours.

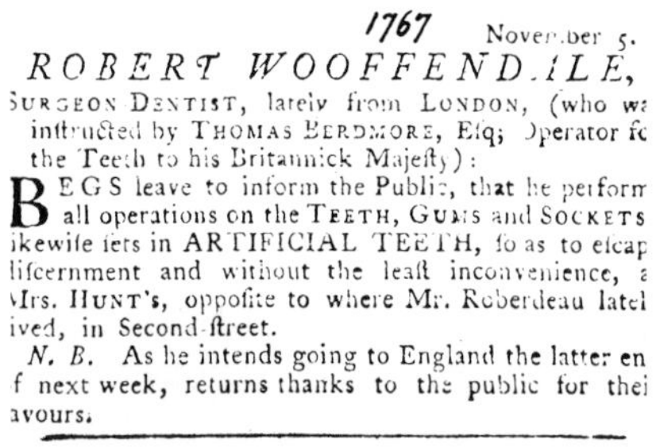

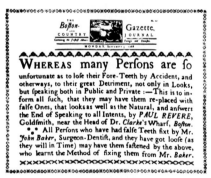

FIGURE 1-7 Colonial United States advertisement that appeared in the Pennsylvania Chronicle and Universal Advocate on November 5, 1767, selling "artificial teeth, so as to escape discernment."

Bofton-Gazette, COUNTRY JOURNAL

WHEREAS many Perfons are fo unfortunate as to lofe their Fore-Teeth by Accident, and otherways, to their great Detriment, not only in Looks, but fpeaking both in Public and Private:—This is to inform all fuch, that they may have them re-placed with falfe Ones, that looks as well as the Natural, and anfwers the End of Speaking to all Intents, by PAUL REVERE, Goldfmith, near the Head of Dr. Clarke's Wharf, Bofton.

All Perfons who have had falfe Teeth fixt by Mr. John Baker, Surgeon-Dentift, and they have got loofe (as they will in Time) may have them faftened by the above, who learnt the Method of fixing them from Mr. Baker.

FIGURE 1-8 Paul Revere's advertisement for his services as a dentist (dated September 5, 1768). (Courtesy of U.S. Library of Congress.)

In the late nineteenth century various techniques used in esthetic fixed prosthodontics were introduced. The open-faced crown was invented around 1880, the interchangeable porcelain facing (a ridged facing that fitted into a grooved pontic) was developed in the 1880s, and the porcelain jacket crown came into vogue in the early 1900s. The three-quarter crown was introduced in 1907.

Practitioners of operative dentistry sought more esthetic material than the gold, lead, tin, and platinum in use in the late nineteenth century. One option was "Hill's Stopping," a mixture of bleached gutta-percha, carbonates of lime and quartz, plastic, bone, and fused glass. Porcelain was another option in restorative

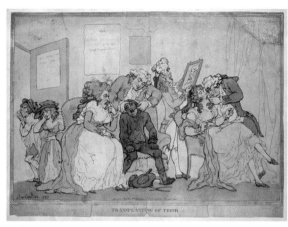

FIGURE 1-9 Eighteenth-century Thomas Rowlanson etching depicting the transplantation of a tooth from a maid to her mistress. (Courtesy Wellcome Library, London.)

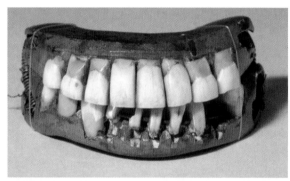

FIGURE 1-10 George Washington's denture. (Copyright 2013 Mount Vernon Ladies' Association.)

material. By 1897 a relatively modern composition of silicate cement was developed. It consisted of powdered aluminum and zinc oxide mixed with phosphoric and hydrofluoric acid. After being briefly abandoned because it was difficult to manage and became brittle, it resurfaced in modified form in 1904 and revolutionized operative dentistry. The inventive combination of acid-soluble glasses blended with a liquid containing phosphoric acid produced dentistry's first truly translucent restorative material. Further modifications continued until 1938, when the American Dental Association (ADA) published its definitive specification of acceptability known as "ADA Specification No. 9." This was the first cosmetic dental material to be accepted by the ADA. However, newer and more exciting innovations were about to arrive.

In the 1930s chemically activated acrylic resins were developed. In the 1940s acrylic-veneer facings came into widespread use. By the 1970s composite resins virtually replaced acrylic resins and silicate cements as "permanent" restorations. Refinements of this basic formula of resin matrix and glass filler are currently in use.

Acid etching, often called *bonding,* radically changed cavity treatment by emphasizing conservation of tooth structure. It also allowed for the numerous veneering techniques introduced in the 1970s. Variations include direct resin veneers, commercially produced acrylic "shells," and laboratory-processed veneers of resin and porcelain.

Research continues. Study groups, societies, journals, and continuing education courses dedicated to the discipline of cosmetic dentistry have proliferated. Undoubtedly, the quest for the elusive ultimate restoration will continue to reveal new vistas in the art and science of esthetic and cosmetic dentistry.

BIBLIOGRAPHY

Asbell MB: *A bibliography of dentistry in America, 1790-1840*, Cherry Hill, NJ, 1973, Sussex House.

Asbell MB: *Dentistry: a historical perspective*, Pittsburgh, PA, 1988, Dorrance & Co.

Bremner MDK: *The story of dentistry*, New York, 1954, Dental Items of Interest.

Foley GPH: *Foley's footnotes: a treasury of dentistry*, Wallingford, PA, 1972, Washington Square East Publishing.

Guerini V: *A history of dentistry from the most ancient times until the end of the eighteenth century*, Philadelphia, 1969, Lea & Febiger.

Herschfeld J. *The progress of esthetic restorations in dentistry*. J Phila Cty Dent Soc. 56(6): 10-13, 1991.

Kanner L: *Folklore of the tooth*, New York, 1934, Macmillan.

Prinz H: *Dental chronology. A record of more important historic events in the evolution of dentistry*, Philadelphia, 1945, Lea & Febiger.

Ring ME: *Dentistry: an illustrated history*, New York, 1985, Harry N. Abrams.

Weinberger BW: *An introduction to the history of dentistry*, vols 1 and 2, St Louis, 1948, Mosby.

2

Fundamentals of Esthetics and Smile Analysis

Kenneth W. Aschheim and Bruce A. Singer

The development of new materials and techniques in dentistry has required the enlightened practitioner to develop new artistic skills. The restorative dentist manipulates light, color, illusion, shape, and form to create an esthetic outcome. Expertise in these areas differentiates the technically proficient dentist from one practicing a higher level of care and artistry.

LIGHT AND SHADOW

Objects cannot be distinguished without light. When lit, most objects (Fig. 2-1) exhibit two dimensions—length and width. True natural light, however, is multidirectional; it reveals texture and throws shadows, adding the lifelike third dimension of depth (Fig. 2-2).

Therefore *the communication of form is by shadow.* A comparison of Figures 2-1 and 2-2 makes this concept apparent. Dental restorations can *mimic* the shadows of adjacent teeth to create a shape that blends with the surrounding tooth forms. Shadow manipulation can make poorly shaped teeth esthetically pleasing.

THE PRINCIPLES OF COLOR

In 1666, Sir Isaac Newton observed that white light passing through a prism divided into an orderly pattern of colors now termed the *spectrum.* He also discovered that these colors produced white light when passed back through the prism, proving that all spectral colors were in the original beam.[1]

Color, as the eye interprets it, is either a result of absorption or reflection. In absorption, a white light is passed through a filter. The colors that pass through the filter and reach the eye are perceived as the color of the filter. In reflection, as with solid objects, the perceived color is the portion of the spectrum that is reflected back to the eye.

Light entering the eye stimulates the photoreceptor rods and cones in the retina. The energy is converted through a photochemical reaction into nerve impulses and carried through the optic nerve into the occipital lobe of the cerebral cortex. The rod cells are responsible for interpreting brightness differences and value. The cone cells function in hue and chroma interpretation. If the light source contains all the colors of the spectrum, a true reading occurs. If the light source is deficient in a certain color, a false reading occurs (see the section on Metamerism). Precise description of these colors and organization of their interrelationships, however, did not occur until 249 years after Newton's work. Robert Louis Stevenson, one of the most concise writers in the English language, demonstrated the problems of describing color: "red—it's not Turkish and it's not Roman and it's not Indian, but it seems to partake of the two last."[2] In 1915, Albert Henry Munsell created an orderly numeric system of color description that is still the standard today. In this system color is divided into three parameters—hue, chroma, and value.[3]

Hue

Hue (Fig. 2-3) is the name of the color. Roy G. Biv (*Red, Orange, Yellow, Green, Blue, Indigo, Violet*) is an acronym for the hues of the spectrum. In the younger permanent dentition, hue tends to be similar throughout the mouth. With aging, variations in hue often occur because of intrinsic and extrinsic staining from restorative materials, foods, beverages, smoking, and other influences.

Chroma

Chroma (Fig. 2-4) is the saturation or intensity of hue; therefore it can only be present with hue. For example, to increase the chroma of a porcelain restoration, more of that hue is added. Chroma is the quality of hue that is most amenable to decrease by bleaching. Almost all hues are amenable to chroma reduction

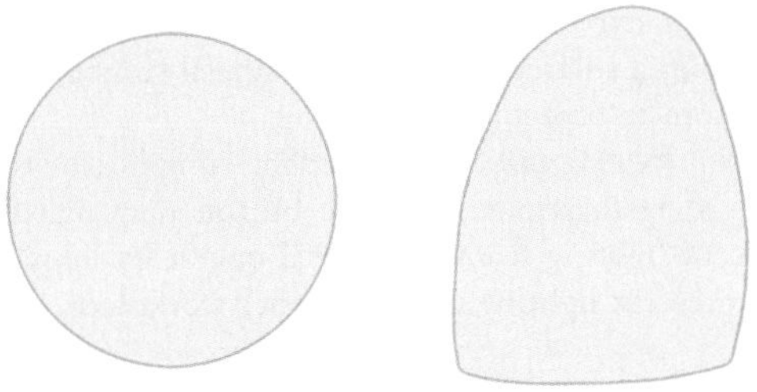

FIGURE 2-1 Omnidirectional lighting throws no shadows. Only length and width are represented.

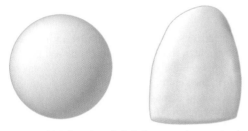

FIGURE 2-2 Unidirectional lighting produces shadows and therefore promotes a feeling of depth—a three dimensional effect.

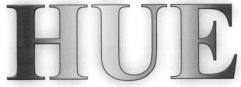

FIGURE 2-3 Hue is the name of the color.

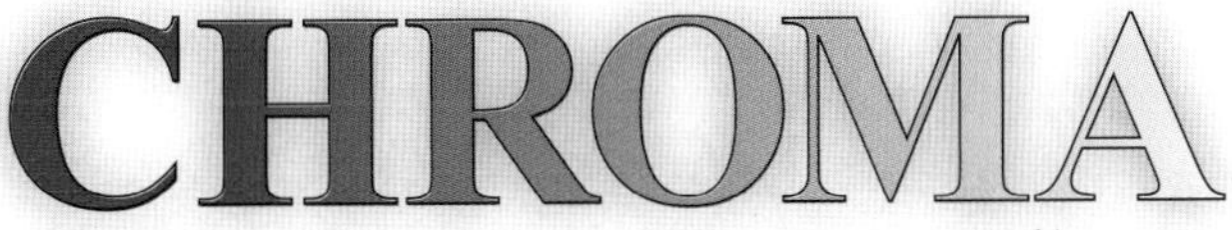

FIGURE 2-4 Chroma is the saturation or amount of hue.

in vital and nonvital bleaching.[4] In general, the chroma of teeth increases with age.

Value

Value (Fig. 2-5) is the relative lightness or darkness of a color. A light tooth has a high value; a dark tooth has a low value. It is not the *quantity* of the "color" gray, but rather the *quality* of brightness on a gray scale.[5] That is, the shade of color (hue plus chroma) either seems light and bright or dark and dim. It is helpful to regard value in this way because the use of value in restorative dentistry does not involve adding gray but rather manipulating colors to increase or decrease amounts of grayness.

CLINICAL TIP

Value is the most important factor in shade matching. If the value blends, small variations in hue and chroma will not be noticeable.[5]

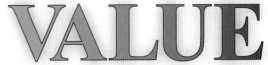

FIGURE 2-5 Value is the brightness of a shade. A low value is darker than a high value.

COLOR (HUE) RELATIONSHIP

The Color Wheel

Hues, as used in dentistry, have a relationship to one another that can be demonstrated on a color wheel. The relationships of primary, secondary, and complementary hues are graphically depicted by the color wheel (Fig. 2-6).

Primary Hues

The primary hues—red, yellow, and blue—form the basis of the dental color system. In dentistry, the metal oxide pigments used in coloring porcelains are limited in forming certain reds; therefore pink is substituted. The primary hues and their relationships to one another form the basic structure of the color wheel.

Secondary Hues

The mixture of any two primary hues forms a secondary hue. When red and blue are mixed they create violet, blue and yellow create green, and yellow and red create orange. Altering the chroma of the primary hues in a mixture changes the hue of the secondary hue produced. Primary and secondary hues can be organized on the color wheel with secondary hues positioned between primary hues.

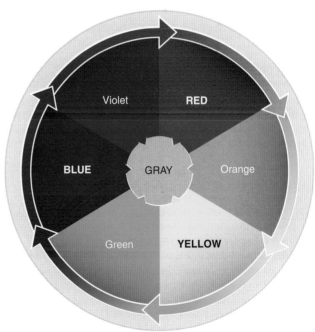

FIGURE 2-6 The color wheel. The primary colors (red, yellow, and blue), mixed two at a time, produce the secondary colors (orange, green, and violet) Opposite colors on the color wheel cancel each other out and produce gray.

Complementary Hues

Colors directly opposite each other on the color wheel are termed *complementary hues.* A peculiarity of this system is that a primary hue is always opposite a secondary hue and vice versa. When a primary hue is mixed with a complementary secondary hue, the effect is to "cancel" out both colors and produce gray. *This is the most important relationship in dental color manipulation.*

CLINICAL TIP

To change hue, lessen chroma, or lower value, place the complementary hue over the color to be modified.

When a portion of a crown is too yellow, lightly washing with violet (the complementary hue of yellow) produces an area that is no longer yellow. The yellow color is canceled out and the area will have an increased grayness (a lower value). This is especially useful if the body color of a crown has been brought too far incisally and if a more incisal color is desired toward the cervical area. If a cervical area is too yellow and a brown color is desired, washing the area with violet cancels the yellow. This is followed by the application of the desired color, in this situation brown.

Complementary hues also exhibit the useful phenomenon of intensification. When complementary hues are placed next to one another, they are each intensified and appear to have a higher chroma. A light orange line on the incisal edge intensifies the blue of an incisal color.

Hue Sensitivity

After 5 seconds of staring at a tooth or shade guide, the human eye accommodates and becomes biased. If an individual stares at any color for longer than 5 seconds and then stares at a white surface or closes his or her eyes, the image appears, but in the complementary hue. This phenomenon, known as *hue sensitivity,* adversely affects shade selection.

CLINICAL TIP

After 5 seconds, look away or stare briefly at a blue surface (such as a patient napkin). This will readapt your vision to the orange-yellow portion of the spectrum, the portion most involved in color matching.

Metamerism

Metamerism is a phenomenon that can cause two color samples to appear as the same hue under one light source, but as dissimilar hues under a different light source.

There is more than one way to produce a color. It can either be pure, or a mixture of two other colors (e.g., pure green versus a mix of blue and yellow). Pure green reflects light in the green band, but the green mixture reflects light in the blue and yellow bands simultaneously. If both colors are exposed to a light with a full color spectrum, they will appear similar. If, however, they are exposed to a light source that does not contain light in the blue band, the two colors will appear dissimilar. True green will still appear green, but the mixture will appear yellow because without a source of light in the blue band the blue component of the mix is not visible.

A spectral curve is a measure of the wavelength of light reflected from a surface. It reveals the actual component colors reflected from an object (Fig. 2-7).[5]

Clinical Relevance. Metamerism complicates the color matching of restorations. A shade button may match under incandescent lighting from the dental operatory lamp but not under fluorescent lighting in the patient's workplace.

CLINICAL TIP

The best approach to color matching is to use three light sources.

A color selection that works well under a variety of lights is preferred to a match that is exact under one source of light but completely wrong under others.[6] Usually three sources of light are available in the dental operatory:
1. Outside daylight through a window
2. Incandescent lighting from the dental operatory lamp
3. Cool white fluorescent lighting from overhead fixtures

Color-corrected fluorescent lamps more closely approximate natural daylight and some practitioners prefer them as the standard in dental operatories. If the entire office is illuminated by color-corrected fluorescent lamp, one room should have cool white fluorescent lighting for comparative shade matching. The color match that appears best in these three lights is usually preferable.

CLINICAL TIP

Some patients spend a great deal of time in one lighting situation. This should be taken into consideration during shade selection.

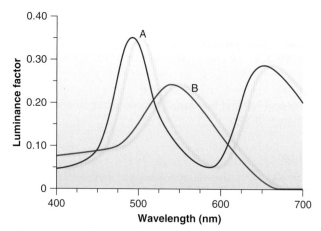

FIGURE 2-7 The spectral curves of two metameric green surfaces that appear identical but exhibit different reflection properties. Surface B reflects light in the green wavelengths and, thus, appears green. Surface A, on the other hand, reflects both cyan and yellow light, which also results in the perception of a green surface. As long as all the required wavelengths of light are present, these two metameric pairs look identical. If, however, the incident light is deficient in either the yellow or cyan, Surface A will not appear green and the colors will not match. (Adapted from Preston JD, Bergen SF: *Color science and dental art: a self-teaching program,* St Louis, 1980, Mosby.)

Opacity

An opaque material does not permit any light to pass through. It reflects all the light that is directed onto it.

Clinical Relevance. A porcelain-fused-to-metal restoration must have a layer of opaque porcelain applied to the metal substructure to prevent the color of the metal from appearing through the translucent body and incisal porcelains. Improper tooth reduction results in two unacceptable results:

1. An ideally contoured restoration with minimal porcelain thickness and too much opaque porcelain, resulting in a "chalky" appearance
2. A bulky, poorly contoured restoration with ideal porcelain thickness

Tooth reduction must be sufficient to allow enough room for an adequate bulk of porcelain (Fig. 2-8).

> ### CLINICAL TIP
>
> The usual areas of underpreparation are the cervical one third and, if a second plane of reduction is not placed, the incisofacial aspect of the preparation.

Translucency

Translucent materials allow some light to pass through them. Only some of the light is absorbed. Translucency provides realism to a dental restoration.

Depth

In restorative dentistry, depth is a spatial concept of color blending combining the concepts of opacity and translucency. In the natural dentition, light passes through the translucent enamel and is reflected out from the depths of the relatively opaque dentin.

White porcelain colorants used in color modification are opaque. Gray porcelain colorants are a mixture of black and white. A tooth restoration with a white opaque colorant on the surface appears artificial because it lacks the quality of depth that would be seen if the opaque layer were placed *beneath* a translucent layer of porcelain. Similarly a bright restoration (high value) in need of graying (a decrease in value) would

appear falsely opaque if it were simply painted gray. Adding a complementary hue, however, both decreases the value and adds to the translucency. If characterization is added to porcelain to represent white hypoplastic spots or gray amalgam stains, white or gray colorant can be used, but translucency will be reduced in these areas.

Depth may be problematic if translucent composite resins are used to restore Class III or IV cavities that extend completely from facial to lingual surfaces. The restoration may appear gray or overly translucent. However, if a more opaque composite resin is placed on the lingual portion of the restoration and then overlaid with a translucent resin, a natural illusion of depth results.

Shade Progression. The maxillary anterior teeth and premolars are not uniform in shade.[7] The lateral incisors are similar in hue to the central incisors but are slightly lower in value. The canines are also lower in value than the incisors but also exhibit greater chroma saturation. The premolars have values similar to the lateral incisors.[7]

Fluorescence

Fluorescence occurs when a material absorbs short wavelength light (usually near ultraviolet) and reemits light of longer wavelength (usually visible light).[8] Because of its higher organic content, dentin is the primary source of fluorescence in human teeth. Fluorescence reduces chroma and raises value without effecting translucency.[9] Fluorescent porcelains mimic dentin resulting in brighter and more vital, life-like restorations.[8]

Opalescence

Opalescence occurs when a material appears as one color when light is reflected off its surface and a different color when light is transmitted through it.[10] Opalescence mimics enamel and is highly wavelength dependent. Opalescent materials such as hydroxyapatite act like a prism and tend to refract shorter wavelengths (violet) more than longer wavelengths (red and yellow).[6] Therefore, enamel will transilluminate red and yellow light but scatter violet and blue light within its body. This has the effect of causing the incisal enamel to appear bluish (and translucent) as well as producing optical depth.[11]

Bleached Teeth. Tooth bleaching dehydrates enamel and sometimes dentin, and sometimes removes pigmented organic material from between the hydroxyapatite crystals. Bleaching changes the hue, chroma, and value of a tooth, resulting in a brighter appearance.[12] Whitening resulting from dehydration is temporary and reverses upon tooth rehydration. Removal of pigment, if it occurs at all, is permanent, although restaining may occur in the future. The degree of "rebound" shortly following bleaching depends on the amount of dehydration and subsequent rehydration that occurs. After bleaching, shade matching should be delayed for at least 1 month.[8]

THE PRINCIPLES OF FORM

Perception

Unconscious perceptions about color, size, shape, age, and gender are based on certain natural biases indigenous to an individual's cultural background. Perceptual biases can be divided into two types: cultural and artistic.

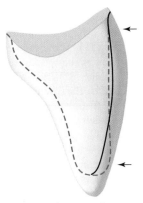

FIGURE 2-8 The arrows indicate underprepared areas in a full crown. Underpreparation results in opaque areas in the finished restoration. The correct preparation is illustrated by the solid line.

Cultural Biases

Cultural biases are naturally occurring environmental observations about the world.. We perceive (and believe) that darker, heavily worn, highly stained, longer teeth belong to an older person because we know that teeth naturally darken, wear, and stain in grooves and along the cervical area with age, and that they lengthen because of gingival recession. We perceive (and believe) rounded, smooth-flowing forms are feminine, whereas harsher, more angular forms are masculine.

Masculine and Feminine. Culturally defined masculine qualities may enhance the appearance of a woman. (Many feminine fashions include a modification of a shirt and tie.) However, usually these masculine nuances appear best on a woman with stereotypically feminine features. Square, angular anterior teeth, therefore, may be desirable on what some might term a a more "feminine" woman, but on other women this tooth shape may not be as flattering. In Western culture, contrast evokes a certain allure. With no contrast, the allure is gone.

The Golden Proportion. Western civilization has drawn the conclusion that for objects to be proportional to one another the ratio of 1:1.618 is esthetically pleasing. Much has been hypothesized from this ratio, from the mathematical relationship of the chambers of the nautilus shell to facial proportions. As a rule, if the *apparent* (see the section on The Law of the Face) size of each tooth, as observed from the frontal view, is 60% of the size of the tooth anterior to it, the relationship is considered esthetically pleasing. That is, if proportionately the *apparent* width of the central incisor is 1.608, the lateral incisor and canine should be 1.0 and 0.608, respectively.[13] This "golden proportion" occurs in 80% of the population.[14]

Artistic Biases

Artistic biases are inherent in the perception of form. The most important of these is the perception that light approaches and dark recedes; this is the *principle of illumination.*[15] The light areas in Figure 2-2 appear to be positioned forward, whereas the darker areas appear to recede. This produces the illusion of a third dimension (depth) despite the two-dimensional nature (length and width) of the printed page. This bias applies to clothing, cosmetics, and teeth. The purpose of cosmetic "makeup" is to enhance facial contours (Fig. 2-9).

The second artistic bias of great importance in dentistry is the use of horizontal and vertical lines. A horizontal line causes an object to *appear* wider, whereas a vertical line causes an object to *appear* longer (Fig. 2-10). This can be termed the *principle of line.*

These cultural and artistic biases are so entrenched in our subconscious thought that they are unavoidable and automatic. Artistic manipulation of these biases allows the esthetic dentist to fool the eye of the observer when fabricating artificial esthetic restorations.

Illusion

Illusion is the art of changing perception to cause an object to appear different than it actually is. Teeth can be made to appear wider, narrower, smaller, larger, shorter, longer, older, younger, masculine, or feminine. An understanding of the basic principles of perception and their use in controlling illusion must precede their use.

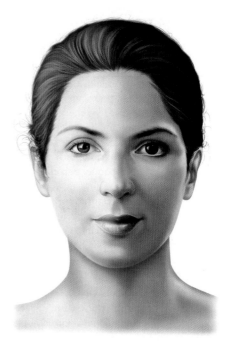

FIGURE 2-9 The principle of illumination: Light approaches and dark recedes. The illusion of contour is produced as cosmetic makeup is applied to the face.

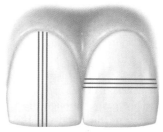

FIGURE 2-10 The principle of line: Horizontal lines created by cervical staining, texturing, white hypoplastic lines, and straight incisal edges create the illusion of width; vertical lines created by narrowing the face of the tooth, carving the incisal edges to slope cervically, and deepening the incisal embrasures create the illusion of length.

Computerized Digital Shade Technology

The electronic dental color-measuring device has recently been introduced into the dental armamentarium (e.g., VITA Easyshade Compact, Vident, Inc., Fig. 2-11). These devices use a digital spectrophotometer that measures the spectral reflectance or spectral transmittance of a specimen.[16] White light from a tungsten-filament bulb is dispersed by the spectrophotometer into a wavelength of between 5 and 20 nm,[17] which is directed at a specimen. The amount of light reflected from the specimen is measured for each wavelength in the visible spectrum and is correlated to popular dental shade guides. Some devices include software (e.g., VITA ShadeAssist software, Vident, Inc.; Fig. 2-12) that can read and record the information measured by the device.

They are unaffected by metamerism and have shown great reproducibility and accuracy.[17-20] Because the cost of these instruments inevitably decrease over time, they may become commonplace in clinical dental shade management.

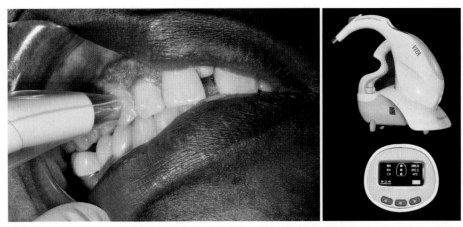

FIGURE 2-11 VITA Easyshade Compact.

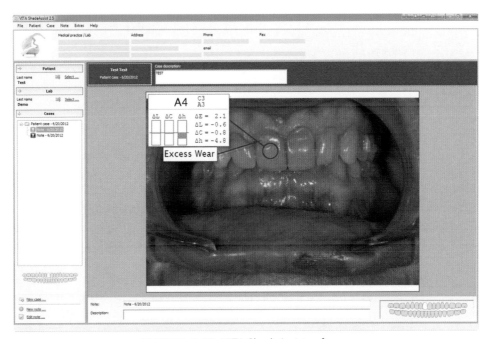

FIGURE 2-12 VITA ShadeAssist software.

USING THE PRINCIPLES OF PERCEPTION TO CONTROL ILLUSION

Principle of Illumination

The principle of illumination can be manipulated by the dentist to change the apparent size and shape of a tooth through illusion. This bias is the key to *The Law of the Face*.

The Law of the Face

The law of the face is the most important single concept in shaping dental restorations. Understanding this concept and its interplay with the concept of light and dark enables the esthetic dentist to shape all esthetic restorations correctly.

The *face* of a tooth is the area on the facial surface of anterior and posterior teeth that is bounded by the transitional line angles as viewed from the facial (buccal) aspect (Fig. 2-13A). The transitional line angles mark the transition from the facial surface to the mesial, cervical, distal, and incisal surfaces. The tooth surface slopes lingually toward the mesial and distal approximating surfaces and toward the cervical root surface from these line angles. Often no transitional line angle appears on the incisal portion of the facial surface; in this situation, the face is bounded by the incisal edge or the occlusal tip. Shadows created as light strikes the facial surface of the tooth begin at the transitional line angles. *These shadows delineate the boundaries of the face.*

The apparent face of a tooth is the portion that is visible to the viewer from any single view. The perimeter of the apparent face is dictated by the position of the viewer relative to the tooth. For example, from the frontal view, the entire incisor faces are visible, but usually only the mesial half of the faces of the maxillary canines is visible from this angle (Fig. 2-13B).

The law of the face states that to make dissimilar teeth appear similar, the dentist should make the apparent faces equal (see Figs. 2-13 A, B and C).

Creating equal apparent faces in two dissimilar adjacent teeth produces dissimilar areas outside the transitional line angles (i.e., outside the faces). These dissimilarities are esthetically acceptable because they are essentially invisible; the similar apparent faces of the teeth catch the light and appear to protrude, whereas the dissimilar areas are in shadow and appear to recede (Fig. 2-13D). Through cultural biases, we are conditioned to expect the faces of contralateral teeth to be equal even though exposed roots may be unequal in length. The six teeth in Figure 2-13 are dissimilar. Shaping the maxillary right central incisor, lateral incisor, and canine so that their apparent faces equal those of the maxillary left central incisor, lateral incisor, and canine produces the illusion that these teeth are equal.

CLINICAL TIP

Equal apparent faces can be most effectively created by shaping the facial surface to reposition the transitional line angles. This creates an appropriate shadow.

When the transitional line angle cannot be repositioned on a ceramic restoration, the artistic principle of illumination can be employed. A portion of the tooth can be stained darker to create the illusion that the transitional line angle has been moved and that the portion of the tooth is receding. In reality, the tooth contour remains unchanged (Fig. 2-13E).

Only the "apparent face" should be manipulated, not the actual face. This becomes particularly significant in posterior regions where the apparent face significantly differs from the actual face (see the section on Canines and The Law of the Face).

Alteration of the Face—Incisors

For clarity, the tooth to be mimicked is referred to as the *guide tooth* and the tooth to be altered as the *related tooth*.

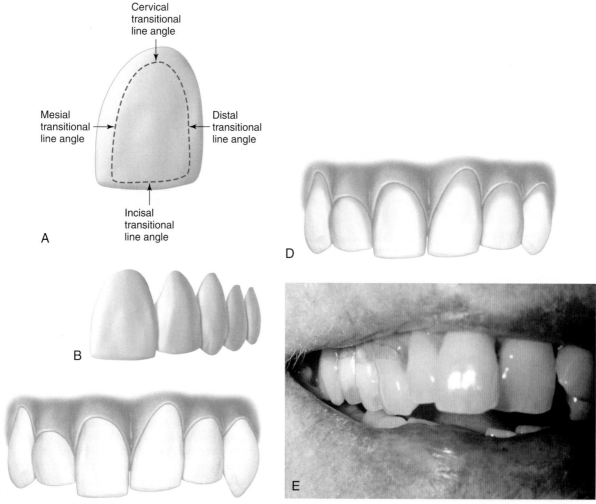

FIGURE 2-13 A, The face of the tooth is bound by the transitional line angles. **B,** From a frontal view the canine displays only the mesial portion of the tooth up to and including the midfacial ridge. **C,** Teeth with numerous disharmonious esthetic problems. **D,** Selective grinding of the incisal edges, moving the labial prominence of the left canine mesially and altering the transitional line angles to make the apparent faces equal, creates an illusion of harmony. **E,** The porcelain-fused-to-metal crown restoring the maxillary right second premolar has been darkened at the gingival third to create the illusion of a discolored restoration The root surface appears to recede because it has a lower (darker) value.

Armamentarium.

+ Basic "Alteration of the Face" Setup
  + Pencil
  + Greenstones (porcelain)
  + Multifluted carbides or finishing diamonds (tooth structure, composite resin)
  + Aluminum oxide disks in varying coarseness, 4 grits are preferred (i.e., Sof-Flex, 3M Inc.) (tooth structure, acrylic, composite resin)
  + Diamond disks (porcelain modification)
  + Porcelain stains

Clinical Technique.

1. Outline the face of the guide tooth with a pencil.
2. Examine the related tooth from the incisal angle to determine the buccolingual dimensions.
3. If sufficient tooth structure (or restorative material) is available, flatten the facial surface to the same level of protrusion as the guide tooth using greenstones, multifluted carbides, finishing diamonds, or coarse disks.
4. Using a pencil, draw a mirror image of the face of the guide tooth onto the related tooth.
5. Carve back toward the proximal surfaces from the boundaries of the face using greenstones, multifluted carbides, finishing diamonds, and coarse disks followed by diamond disks and successively finer aluminum oxide disks. If this is not possible, shade the restorative material a darker color in the areas lateral to the face (pencil lines). Surface staining can be employed on porcelain. A resin with a lower value or increased chroma should be used on composite resin.

Canines and the Law of the Face

The concept of the apparent face becomes more important when dealing with teeth posterior to the incisor teeth. From a frontal view only a portion of the canine and posterior teeth are visible (see Fig. 2-12). In the frontal view, the canine face is bounded by the mesial transitional line angle, the cervical transitional line angle, and the midfacial ridge. Usually the distal half of the tooth is not visible from a frontal view. The left and right side views cannot be seen simultaneously and are of secondary importance. Four steps are required to blend a poorly shaped canine into a smile.

Alteration of the Face—Canines

For clarity, the tooth to be mimicked is referred to as the *guide tooth* and the tooth to be altered as the *related tooth*.

Armamentarium.

+ Basic "Alteration of the Face" Setup (see the preceding)

Clinical Technique.

1. Using the frontal view, outline the apparent face of the guide tooth (the contralateral canine) with a pencil (Fig. 2-14*A*).
2. Again looking from the front, draw a mirror image of the apparent face of the guide tooth onto the related canine with a pencil.
3. Using these lines, move the midfacial ridge of the related tooth either mesially or distally to approximate the amount of tooth structure shown on the guide canine. Because only the area mesial to this ridge is seen from the frontal view, the viewer extrapolates the full size of the tooth as twice that size (Fig. 2-14*B*).
4. From the side view, if the mesial half of the related tooth has been made smaller by the mesial movement of the midfacial ridge, make the distal half of the face equal by locating the distal transitional line angle in a symmetric position to

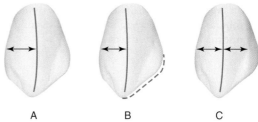

FIGURE 2-14 From a frontal view the canine appears too wide. Several steps are required to create the illusion of a narrower tooth. **A,** Preoperative view of the canine with the width delineated by an arrow. **B,** The midlabial ridge is moved mesially, creating the illusion of a narrower tooth. The incisal tip is also moved mesially by removing tooth structure from the distal aspect of the incisal edge. **C,** The distal transitional line angle is moved mesially until the distal face is equal to the mesial face. The canine now appears narrower from both the frontal and side views.

the mesial transitional line angle. This is done by carving the tooth structure back toward the lingual area from the distal transitional line angle (Fig. 2-14*C*).

Principle of Line

Horizontal lines—in the form of cervical staining, texturing, white hypoplastic lines, or long, straight incisal edges—create the illusion of width. Widening the face also produces an illusion of width (Fig. 2-15).

Vertical lines in the form of accentuated developmental grooves, hypoplastic lines, and vertical texturing accentuate height (see Fig. 2-15*B*). Incisal edges of anterior teeth carved to slope cervically toward the distal area with larger incisal embrasures and narrower (mesiodistally) incisal edges create an illusion of increased height. Narrowing the face also creates this illusion (see Fig. 2-19). These same concepts apply for clothing and makeup. Individuals wearing clothing with vertical lines appear thinner. Conversely, horizontal stripes accentuate width (see Fig. 2-15*A*). To "lengthen" and "slim" the nose with cosmetics, a light highlighter

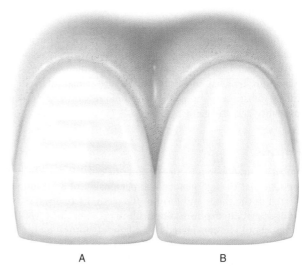

FIGURE 2-15 The principle of line can be used to create the illusion of a shorter **(A)** or longer **(B)** tooth. Stain lines, texturing, and modification of the face and incisal edge all contribute to the illusion.

is applied in a vertical line down the center bridge of the nose. Then a darker contour shade of makeup is applied on each side of the nose to cause that area to appear to recede.[21]

Age

The Western negative cultural bias toward age is a sensitive issue for patients seeking esthetic care and must be considered.

Older Teeth. See Figure 2-16A. Older teeth have the following characteristics:

They are smoother.
They are darker (i.e., not as bright, lower value).
They have a higher saturation (higher chroma).
They are shorter incisally (less tooth shows when the patient is smiling).
They are longer gingivally (although they may be shorter incisally).
They exhibit more wear, even on incisal edges with small incisal embrasures.
They have wider, more open gingival embrasures.
They are more characterized.
The amount of incisal display of the maxillary central incisors diminishes with age, whereas the amount of incisal display of the mandibular central incisors increases.[22]
The mandibular incisors exhibit flat broad incisal edges, which show a dentin core.

Younger Teeth. See Figure 2-16B. Younger teeth have the following characteristics:

They are more textured.
They are lighter (i.e., brighter, higher value).
They have a lower saturation (lower chroma).
They have a gingival margin at approximately the cementoenamel junction.
They have incisal edges that make the laterals appear shorter than the incisors or canines.
They have significant incisal embrasures.
They have small gingival embrasures.
They have light characterization, often with white hypoplastic lines or spots.

Clinically, the ultimate esthetic goal is to fabricate prostheses which appear natural. (This should elicit a third-party response of, "What beautiful teeth you have," rather than an observer noticing an artificial substitution.) Beautiful natural teeth or artificial substitutes should be harmonious with the patient's personality, age, and gender.

Gender

Lombardi[8] described a theory of anterior esthetics in which he proposed that the age, gender, and personality of a person was reflected in the shape and form of the teeth. Factually, the concept of sexual dimorphism is difficult to prove or disprove. This concept should be considered in the light of cultural bias.

Feminine Teeth. Feminine teeth are more rounded, both on the incisal edges and at the transitional line angles. The incisal embrasures therefore are more pronounced. The incisal edges are more translucent and white hypoplastic striations may be used to give the illusion of delicacy (Fig. 2-17A).

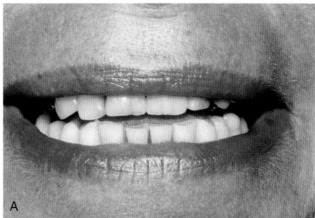

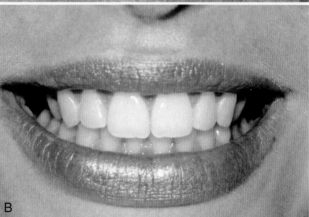

FIGURE 2-16 A, Older teeth are smoother, darker, shorter, have worn incisal edges, and are more characterized. **B,** Younger teeth are brighter and more textured, have lower chroma, and have gingival margins at the cementoenamel junction. They have pronounced incisal embrasures, small gingival embrasures, and are only lightly characterized. Lateral incisors are shorter than the central incisors and the canines. These feminine-looking teeth are more rounded at the transitional line angles and have pronounced incisal embrasures.

The translucency on the incisal edges appears as a gray line in the incisal one eighth of the facial surface paralleling the incisal edge with a white hypoplastic rim on the edge.

Masculine Teeth. Masculine teeth are more angular and rugged. In older men, chroma is greater and body color often extends to the incisal edges. The incisal embrasures are more squared and not as pronounced. Characterization is often stronger, incorporating darker craze lines (Fig. 2-17B).

Cultural and artistic biases are central to understanding dental esthetics. They must be thoroughly understood so that the dentist can use these biases artistically to create illusions to satisfy the esthetic demands of the patient. Only then can the technically proficient dentist rise to the level of an artist, providing a higher level of care.

TOOTH BIOMETRICS

A smile is defined as a pleased, kind, or amused facial expression, typically with the corners of the mouth turned up and the front teeth exposed.[23] It is this amount of tooth exposure that is defined by the smile line. The smile line refers to an imaginary line connecting the incisal edges of the maxillary anterior teeth,

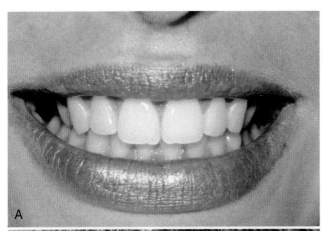

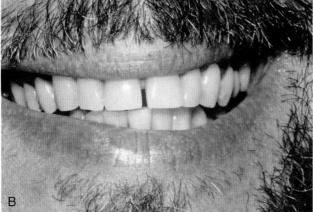

FIGURE 2-17 A, Feminine-looking teeth are more rounded and translucent, giving an appearance of delicacy. **B,** Masculine-looking teeth are more angular and have a higher chroma, square incisal edges, and darker craze lines.

and typically follows the border of the lower lip.[24] Tooth size and shape vary, although there are limitations. Geometric morphometric analyses of teeth objectively define norms for the size and shape of human teeth.[25] Restorations fabricated outside of these parameters appear unnatural.

Analysis of the patient smile is vital in determining the degree of required treatment, particularly as it relates to the gingival extent of the dental restorations. The science of esthetics has repeatedly confirmed the validity of the relationship between the golden proportions[26] and "beauty."[26] In addition, other biometric values that are highly relevant have been described.

Facial Midline

The facial midline is the critical starting point in dental esthetics.[27] Most patients exhibit facial asymmetries; therefore the midline is determined by the line between the nasion, the point on the skull corresponding to the middle of the nasofrontal suture, to the base of the philtrum, which is referred to as *cupid's bow*. This line determines the position of the facial midline and is used as the reference for the midline between the maxillary central incisors.[27] If the incisal midline cannot coincide with the facial midline, then the midlines should be made parallel. Nonparallel (canted) midlines can be highly unesthetic and should be avoided.[28] Ideally the maxillary and mandibular central incisor midlines should align; however, the mandibular midline is not as crucial.[28]

Maxillary Lip Line

The position of the lip and the mandibular range of motion during function are critical components in determining the extent of visibility of tooth and gingival structures and are sometimes referred to as the *labial display*. The lip line, which refers to the inferior border of the maxillary lip, should not be confused with the smile line (Table 2-1).[10] The extent of treatment is often determined by the degree of visibility of the intraoral structures

CLINICAL TIP

The true lip position may be deceptive. Patients with unattractive smiles often habitually adapt a high lip line position, which is significantly less revealing of tooth structure than is anatomically possible. After and esthetic rehabilitation, the high lip line may significantly elevate, because the patient's psychological barriers to full smiling have dissipated.

High Maxillary Lip Line. A lip line is considered high if it displays more than 3-4 mm of gingiva.[10] This can present the most challenging esthetic treatment scenario. Every feature of each individual tooth or restoration will be prominently displayed. Loss of any portion of the interproximal papilla will result in a clearly evident "black triangle." The minutest area of gingival recession will reveal an exposed restoration margin. This is the most difficult situation to treat because typically, the attached gingiva and the alveolar mucosa are visible during function. Rehabilitation of both hard and soft tissue may be required.

Standard Maxillary Lip Line. The standard maxillary lip line is the most common anatomic configuration and occurs when between 75% and 100% of the each tooth in the labial display is exposed. Typically the inferior border of the maxillary lip is positioned within 2 mm of the most apical extent of tooth structure.[10] Some or all of the treatment challenges that present during treatment of a high lip line are also evident when treating patients with a standard lip line.

CLINICAL TIP

In most situations, the lip line is acceptable if it is within a range of 2 mm apical to the height of the gingiva on the maxillary centrals.

Low Maxillary Lip Line. A low lip line displays less than 75% of each tooth in the labial display teeth.[29] These are the easiest situations to treat because supragingival restoration margins may be acceptable and interproximal papilla considerations may not be displayed during function.

CLINICAL TIP

Despite the fact that less than 75% of the tooth is displayed, it is important to manage a patient's expectations concerning the cosmetic outcomes before treatment begins. Many patients expect the same outcome as in the high maxillary lip line situation despite the fact that little of the tooth is visible during function.

Table 2-1 Smile Lines

	Amount of Cervico-Incisal Length of the Maxillary Anterior Teeth Revealed	Frequency in Population	
High Maxillary Lip Line	>100%	29%	
Standard Maxillary Lip Line	75%-100%	56%	
Low Maxillary Lip Line	<75%	15%	

Data from Dong J, Jin T, Cho H, et al: The Esthetics of the Smile: A Review of Some Recent Studies, *Int J Prosthodont* 12(1):9-19, 1999.

CLINICAL TIP

Evaluate critically the true position of the lip during maximum smiling (the high lip line) before planning supragingival finishing lines. The true lip position may be deceptive. Patients with unattractive smiles often habitually adapt a high lip line position, which is significantly less revealing of tooth structure than is anatomically possible. After porcelain laminate veneers are placed, the high lip line may significantly elevate, because the patient's psychologic barriers to full smiling have dissipated.

Maxillary Lip Curvature

The curvature of the maxillary lip contributes to the degree of display of the anterior and posterior gingiva (Table 2-2).

Upward Maxillary Lip Curvature. A maxillary lip that curves upward (i.e., in which the corners of the lip are superior to than the center),[30] tends to display more of the posterior gingiva than other types of lip curvature. This must be addressed during treatment planning and treatment.

Straight Maxillary Lip. A straight maxillary lip, is one in which the corner of the mouth and the center of the mandibular border of the maxillary lip are on a straight line.[30] It tends to expose a similar degree of anterior and posterior gingiva. The degree of restorative difficulty varies.

Downward Maxillary Lip Curvature. Downward maxillary lip curvature is one in which the corners of the lip are inferior to the center. It tends to display less of the posterior gingiva than other types of lip curvature.

Smile Line

The smile line refers to the line of the inferior border of the lips compared with a reference line drawn between the pupils of the eyes. Ideally the two lines should be parallel and the incisal plane should also be parallel to this line; however, sometimes the eyes are positioned on differing planes. The preferred metric would be the creation of an incisal plane perpendicular to the facial midline.

Parallelism of the Maxillary Anterior Incisal Curve with the Smile Line

Differences in parallelism of the maxillary anterior incisal curve relate to both sexual bias as well as age bias. Parallel and straight smiles are considered more esthetic than a reverse smile (Table 2-3).[30]

Relationship Between the Maxillary Anterior Teeth and the Lower Lip

The relationship between the maxillary anterior teeth and the lower lip controls the degree of exposure of the incisal edges of the maxillary incisors (Table 2-4).

The Number of Teeth Displayed in the Smile

The number of teeth displayed in the smile determines the extent, parameters, and difficulty of the restorative rehabilitation (Table 2-5).

Table 2-2 Maxillary Lip Curvature

	Curvature	Frequency in Population	
Upward	The corner of the mouth is higher than the center of the lower border of the maxillary lip.	12%	
Straight	The corner of the mouth and the center of the lower border of the maxillary lip are on a straight line.	45%	
Downward	The corner of the mouth is lower than the center of the lower border of the maxillary lip.	43%	

Data from Dong J, Jin T, Cho H, et al: The Esthetics of the Smile: A Review of Some Recent Studies, *Int J Prosthodont* 12(1):9-19, 1999.

Table 2-3 Parallelism of the Maxillary Anterior Incisal Curve with the Smile Line

	Curvature	Frequency in Population	
Parallel (Concave)	The incisal edges of the maxillary anterior teeth are parallel to the maxillary border of the lower lip.	60%	
Straight	The incisal edges of the maxillary anterior teeth are in a straight line	34%	
Reverse (Convex)	The incisal edges of the maxillary anterior teeth curved in reverse to the maxillary border of the lower lip	25%	

Data from Dong J, Jin T, Cho H, et al: The Esthetics of the Smile: A Review of Some Recent Studies, *Int J Prosthodont* 12(1):9-19, 1999.

Table 2-4 Relationship Between the Maxillary Anterior Teeth and the Lower Lip

	Incisal Tooth Exposure	Frequency in Population	
Slightly Covered	The incisal edges of the maxillary anterior teeth were slightly covered by the lower lip	10%	
Touching	The incisal edges of the maxillary anterior teeth just touched the lower lip.	36%	
Not Touching	The incisal edges of the maxillary anterior teeth did not touch the lower lip.	54%	

Data from Dong J, Jin T, Cho H, et al: The Esthetics of the Smile: A Review of Some Recent Studies, *Int J Prosthodont* 12(1):9-19, 1999.

Incisal Embrasures

The incisal embrasure is defined as the space existing on the incisal aspect of the interproximal contact area between adjacent anterior teeth. Both the size and volume of the incisal embrasures progressively increase posteriorly from the midline (Fig. 2-18).

Incisal Length

The ideal length of the maxillary centrals incisors is influenced by the smile line and incisal reveal as well as physiological norms. Numerous norms for the length of the central incisors include:

1. 1/16th of the facial length[10]
2. 5:4 or 75% to 80% of the incisor width[10]
3. 10 to 11 mm[10]
4. Phonetic analysis of the anterior teeth with a minimum facial reveal of 2 to 4 mm based on the "*m*" sound rest position[31]
5. Phonetic analysis of the anterior teeth with a complete maxillary incisal "fill" during maximal extension of the lips as measured by the "*e*" sound[32]
6. Maximal incisal edge position as measured but minimal impingement of the vermillion border of the mandibular lip during the formation of the "*f*" and "*v*" sound[13]

7. An average incisal display of 1.91 mm for males and 3.40 mm in females, which changes with age (see the section on Older Teeth)[12]
8. The height of the occlusal plane[10]

Depending on the etiology of the discrepancy, corrective cosmetic surgical crown lengthening and/or the restorative procedures can be performed.

Anterior Contact Area

The contact area is the area between two adjacent teeth that lies between the gingival and incisal embrasures. The area is sometimes referred to as the *connector space*; however, the connector space is technically a larger broader area that is defined as the zone in which two adjacent teeth *visually appear* to touch, whereas the contact point is the area in which the teeth actually touch.[27] Ideal esthetic results can be achieved when the connector space area is 50% between the central incisors, 50/40% between the central and lateral incisors, and 40/30% between the lateral incisors and canines (Fig. 2-19).[33]

Gingival Zenith

The gingival zenith is the most apical area of the clinical crown, and its shape and location is determined by the anatomy of the

Table 2-5 **The Number of Teeth Displayed in the Smile**

		Number of Teeth Displayed	Frequency in Population	
3	6	Displayed teeth includes the canine region	≈1%	
4	8	Displayed teeth includes the first premolar region	≈19%	
5	10	Displayed teeth includes the second premolar region	57%	
6	>10	Displayed teeth includes the first molar or second molar region	≈22%	

Data from Dong J, Jin T, Cho H, et al: The Esthetics of the Smile: A Review of Some Recent Studies, *Int J Prosthodont* 12(1):9-19, 1999.

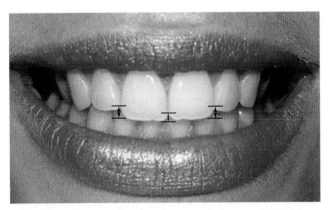

FIGURE 2-18 Incisal embrasures size increases as you move posteriorly.

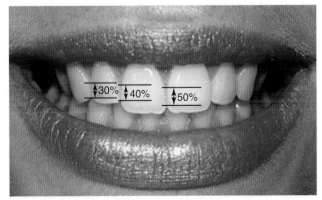

FIGURE 2-19 The percent of anterior contact area decreases as you move posteriorly.

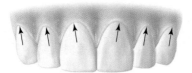

FIGURE 2-20 Gingival zenith.

tooth and the gingival architecture.[9] It is typically located at the junction of the middle and the distal third of the facial aspect of a tooth although lateral incisors exhibit more variability and may display a midline zenith (Fig. 2-20). Manipulation of the gingival zenith usually requires modification of the gingival tissue and may require alveolar bone surgery.[34]

Axial Inclinations

Frontal View. The axial inclination of a tooth is measured from the mesiodistal center of the incisal edge to the gingival zenith. It tends to become more pronounced distally, thus the lateral incisors have a greater axial inclination than the central incisors and the canines a greater inclination than the lateral incisors. The maxillary central incisor incisoapical inclination in the sagittal plane is approximately 22 degrees from a line drawn between the most anterior point of the maxilla (point A) to nasion, a depressed point midway directly between the eyes just superior to the bridge of the nose.[35] The posterior teeth exhibit axial inclination similar to the canine. Ideally, contralateral incisors should have identical distal inclinations.[36]

Lateral View. The facial surface of the maxillary teeth should be perpendicular to the occlusal plane, which allows for optimal reflection of light from the teeth and enhances the smile. The mandibular central incisors should have an inclination of about 25 degrees when compared with the line between the nasion and the most anterior point of the mandible in the sagittal plane.[36]

Because the inclination of the anterior teeth can affect the appearance of the external facial structures, it is important to analyze these changes with transitional restorations to be certain that the results will be esthetically pleasing.

LABORATORY COMMUNICATIONS

Many practical methods are available to enhance communication with the dental laboratory. Shape and texture can be communicated by intraoral photographs or slides. The desired form also may be conveyed with digital photography (see Chapter 22). Shape is perhaps best communicated three dimensionally. Preoperative study casts, wax-ups for development of the provisional phase, and casts of provisional restorations are helpful. Casts of the seated bisque bake allow the technician to see the relation of tooth shape to the soft tissue.

Desired color can be communicated by demonstration, electronic shade guide (see section Computerized Digital Shade Technology) or written prescription. Custom-colored shade tabs sent to the laboratory as a three-dimensional prescription are most effective. They can be shaded with the same materials used in chairside dental porcelain staining with the only modification being the use of a product such as one of the Ceramco stain and glaze sets (Dentsply International, York, PA) as a liquid medium (see Appendix A). The same technique can be used to communicate definitive coloring when the treatment is at the bisque bake stage.

CONCLUSION

The development of new materials and techniques in dentistry has required the enlightened practitioner to develop new artistic skills. The restorative dentist manipulates light, color, illusion, shape, and form to create an esthetic outcome. Expertise in these areas differentiates the technically proficient dentist from one practicing a higher level of care and artistry.

BIBLIOGRAPHY

Adams A: *Artificial-light photography*, Hastings-on-Hudson, NY, 1968, Morgan and Morgan.

Agoston GA: *Color theory and its application in art and design*, New York, 1979, Springer-Verlag.

Appleby DS, Craig C: Subtleties of contour: a system for recognition and correction, *Compend Contin Ed* 7:109, 1986.

Beder OE: Esthetics—an enigma, *J Prosthet Dent* 25:588, 1971.

Bergen SF, McCasland J: Dental operatory lighting and tooth color discrimination, *JADA* 94:130, 1977.

Ceramco stain system manual, East Windsor, 1977, Johnson and Johnson.

Culpepper WD: A comparative study of shade-matching procedures, *J Prosthet Dent* 24:166, 1970.

Culpepper WD: Esthetic factors in anterior tooth restoration, *J Prosthet Dent* 30:576, 1973.

De Van M: Methods of procedure in a diagnostic service to the edentulous patient, *JADA* 29:1981, 1942.

Edwards B: *Drawing on the artist within: a guide to innovation, invention, imagination, and creativity*, New York, 1986, Simon & Schuster.

Edwards B: *Drawing on the artist within: an inspirational and practical guide to increasing your creative powers*, New York, 1986, Simon & Schuster.

Edwards B: *Drawing on the right side of the brain: a course in enhancing creativity and artistic confidence*, New York, 1979, St. Martin's Press.

Feigenbaum N, Mopper KW: *A complete guide to dental bonding*, East Windsor, 1984, Johnson and Johnson.

Friedman M: Staining and shade control of dental ceramics. Part I, *Quintessence Dent Technol*. 1981. Oct;5(9):883-5.

Friedman M: Staining and shade control of dental ceramics. Part II, *Quintessence Dent Technol*. 1981. Nov-Dec;5(10):987-92.

Friedman M: Staining and shade control of dental ceramics. Part III, *Quintessence Dent Technol*. 1982. Jan;6(1):49-57.

Frush JP, Fisher RD: The age factor in dentogenics, *J Prosthet Dent* 7:5, 1957.

Frush JP, Fisher RD: Dentogenics: its practical application, *J Prosthet Dent* 9:914, 1959.

Frush JP, Fisher RD: The dysesthetic interpretation of the dentogenic concept, *J Prosthet Dent* 8:558, 1958.

Frush JP, Fisher RD: How dentogenic restorations interpret the sex factor, *J Prosthet Dent* 6:160, 1956.

Frush JP, Fisher RD: How dentogenics interprets the personality factor, *J Prosthet Dent* 6:441, 1956.

Frush JP, Fisher RD: Introduction to dentogenic restorations, *J Prosthet Dent* 5:586, 1955.

Garber DA, Goldstein RE, Feinman RA: *Porcelain laminate veneers*, Chicago, 1988, Quintessence.

Goldstein RE: *Change your smile*, Chicago, 1987, Quintessence.

Goldstein RE: *Esthetics in dentistry*, Philadelphia, 1976, Lippincott.

Held R: *Readings from Scientific American—image, object, and illusion*, San Francisco, 1974, Freeman.

Light and film, New York, 1970, Time-Life Books.

Pincus CL: Cosmetics—the psychologic fourth dimension in full mouth rehabilitation, *Dent Clin North Am*, March 1967.

Rickets RM: The golden divider, *J Clin Orthop* 15:752, 1981.

Rogers LR: *Sculpture*, Toronto, 1969, Oxford University Press.

Sorensen JA, Torres TJ: Improved color matching of metal-ceramic restorations. Part I. A systematic method for shade determination, *J Prosthet Dent* 58:133, 1987.

Sorensen JA, Torres TJ: Improved color matching of metal-ceramic restorations. Part II. Procedures for visual communication, *J Prosthet Dent* 58:669, 1987.

Sorensen JA, Torres TJ: Improved color matching of metal-ceramic restorations. Part III. Innovations in porcelain application, *J Prosthet Dent* 59:1, 1988.

Sproull RC: Color matching in dentistry. Part I. The three-dimensional nature of color, *J Prosthet Dent* 29:416, 1973.

Sproull RC: Color matching in dentistry. Part II. Practical applications of the organization of color, *J Prosthet Dent* 29:556, 1973.

Swedlund C: *Photography*, New York, 1974, Holt, Rinehart and Winston.

REFERENCES

1. Waltke R: *Color in the human dentition*, New Rochelle, NY, 1977, Jelenko.
2. Clark EB: Tooth color selection, *JADA* 1065, 1933.
3. Munsell AH: *A grammar of color*, New York, 1969, Van Nostrand Reinhold.
4. Feinman RA, Goldstein RE, Garber DA: *Bleaching teeth*, Chicago, 1987, Quintessence.
5. Preston JD, Bergen SF: *Color science and dental art: a self-teaching program*, St Louis, 1980, Mosby.

6. Sproull RC: Color matching in dentistry. Part III. Color control, *J Prosthet Dent* 31:146, 1974.
7. Goodkind RJ, Schwabacher WB: Use of a fiber-optic colorimeter for in vivo measurements of 2,830 anterior teeth, *J Prosthet Dent* 58:535, 1987.
8. Fondriest J: Shade matching in restorative dentistry: the science and strategies, *Int J Periodont Restor Dent* 23(5):467, 2003.
9. McLaren E: The 3D-master shade-matching system and the skeleton buildup technique: science meets art and intuition, *Quintessence Dent Technol* 22:55, 1999.
10. Sundar V, Amber PL: Opals in nature, *J Dent Technol* 16:15, 1999.
11. Garber DA, Adar P, Goldstein RE, Salama H: The quest for the all-ceramic restoration, *Quintessence Dent Technol* 23:27, 2000.
12. Cornell D, Winter R: Manipulating light with the refractive index of an all-ceramic material, *Pract Periodontics Aesthet Dent* 11:913, 1999.
13. Sproull RC: Color matching in dentistry. Part III. Color control, *J Prosthet Dent* 31:146, 1974.
14. Feigenbaum NL: Aspects of aesthetic smile design, *Pract Periodontics Aesthet Dent* 3(3):9, 1991.
15. Lombardi RE: Visual perception and denture esthetics, *J Prosthet Dent* 29:363, 1973.
16. Seungyee K-P, Brewer JD, Davis EL, Wee AG: Reliability and accuracy of four dental shade-matching devices, *J Prosthet Dent* 101(3):193, 2009.
17. Berns RS: *Billmeyer and Saltzman's principles of color technology*, ed 3, New York, 2000, Wiley.
18. Paravina RD, Powers JM: *Esthetic color training in dentistry*, St Louis, 2004, Elsevier.
19. Lehmann KM, Igiel C, Schmidtmann I, Scheller H: Four color-measuring devices compared with a spectrophotometric reference system, *J Dent* 38(suppl 2):e65, 2010.
20. Lagouvardos PE, Fougia AG, Diamantopoulou SA: Repeatability and interdevice reliability of two portable color selection devices in matching and measuring tooth color, *J Prosthet Dent* 101(1):40, 2009.
21. Jackson C: *Color me beautiful makeup book*, New York, 1988, Ballantine.
22. Vig RG, Brundo GC: The kinetics of anterior tooth display, *J Prosthet Dent* 39:502, 1972.
23. Oxford Dictionaries: http://oxforddictionaries.com/definition/smile. Accessed May 7, 2012.
24. Blitz N, Steel C, Willhite C: *Diagnosis and treatment evaluation in cosmetic dentistry: a guide to accreditation criteria*, Madison, WI, 2001, American Academy of Cosmetic Dentistry.
25. Kato A, Kouchi M, Mochimaru M, Isomura A, Ohno N: A geometric morphometric analysis of the crown form of the maxillary central incisor in humans, *Dent Anthropol* 24(1):1, 2011.
26. Snow SR: Esthetic smile analysis for maxillary anterior tooth width: the golden percentage, *J Esthet Dent* 11(4):177, 1999.
27. Morley J, Eubank J: Macroesthetic elements of smile design, *J Am Dent Assoc* 132(1):39, 2001.
28. Johnston CD, Burden DJ, Stevenson MR: The influence of dental midline discrepancies on dental attractiveness ratings, *Eur J Orthod* 21:517, 1999.
29. Tjan AHL, Miller GD, Josephine GP: Some esthetic factors in a smile, *J Prosthet Dent* 51(1):24, 1984.
30. Dong JK, Rashid RG, Rosenstiel S: Smile arcs of Caucasian and Korean youth, *Int J Prosthodont* 22(3):290, 2009.
31. Calamia JR, Levine JB, Lipp M, Cisneros G, Wolff MS: Smile design and treatment planning with the help of a comprehensive esthetic evaluation form, *Dent Clin North Am* 55(2):187, 2011.
32. Morley J, Eubank J: Macroesthetic elements of smile design, *J Am Dent Assoc* 132(1):39, 2001.
33. Raj V et al: The apparent contact dimension and covariates among orthodontically treated and nontreated subjects, *J Esthet Restor Dent* 21:96, 2009.
34. Davis NC: Smile design, *Dent Clin North Am* 51(2) 299, 2007.
35. Tarnow DP, Chu SJ, Kim J: *Aesthetic restorative dentistry: principles and practice*, Mahwah, NJ, 2008, Montage Media.
36. Lombardi RE: The principles of visual perception and their clinical application to denture esthetics, *J Prosthet Dent* 29:358, 1973.

Part 3

Esthetic Materials
and Techniques

3

Dentin Bonding Agents

Mark E. Jensen

The search for ideal dental adhesives is probably as old as dentistry itself. Significant advances in adhesive dentistry have steadily progressed over the past four decades. The bonding of bis-GMA resin to etched enamel[1] introduced esthetic restorations without the need for mechanical retention form. An obvious goal was to develop an adhesive material that bonds to dentin with a strength at least equal to that of resin bonded to etched enamel. Creating this strong bond is extremely difficult because dentin is only about 50% inorganic by volume compared with the approximately 98% mineral content of enamel. The remaining volume of dentin is primarily water and collagen. In addition, a freshly prepared dentin surface is physically altered by instrumentation during operative procedures (smear layer) (Fig. 3-1).

This mechanically altered surface is relatively homogeneous with occluded dentinal tubular openings. Achieving a biocompatible bond to moist dentin while preventing bacterial invasion is critical.

HISTORIC PERSPECTIVE

Seven and possibly eight distinct generations of dentin bonding agents have evolved. The first generation was developed in the late 1950s and early 1960s and was composed of polyurethanes, cyanoacrylates, glycerophosphoric acid dimethacrylate, and NPG-GMA (N-phenyl glycine and glycidalmethacrylate). All these materials were disappointing clinical failures. In vitro shear bond strengths were only approximately 10 to 20 kg/cm[2]. Nearly two decades later, second-generation dentin bonding materials were introduced (Scotchbond, Dentin Bonding Agent, Creation Bonding Agent, Dentin-Adhesit, Bondlite, and Prisma Universal Bond). Most were halophosphorus esters of bis-GMA that were designed to adhere to the mineral portion of the dentin as a phosphate-calcium bond. In vitro bond strengths of these materials were reported to be 30 to 90 kg/cm.[2,3] The bond, however, was hydrolyzed over time in the oral environment, which contributed to their poor clinical success.[3-7]

The third-generation dentin bonding agents flooded the market in the early 1980s. Bowen et al.[4] introduced a novel oxalate dentin bonding system in 1982. Originally this system was cumbersome and unpredictable, but it demonstrated a marked improvement, with bond strengths of 100 to 150 kg/cm[2]. The acidified ferric oxalate in this system was believed to be a source of marginal discoloration, and the complicated series of reagents made the system clinically cumbersome. Bond strengths improved, with modifications close to that of composite resin bonded to etched enamel at 200 to 220 kg/cm[2]. Nevertheless, clinical success was not satisfactory.

Fourth-generation dentin bonding agents are probably the closest to an ideal dentin bond. The effect on the pulp of conditioning the dentinal surface was long an issue.[5,6]

Clinical procedures were simplified by the simultaneous etching of the enamel surface and conditioning of the dentin. This "total etch technique" improved the bond strength to dentin as well.[7]

Fifth-generation bonding agents are essentially a modification of the fourth generation materials. They are self-priming "one-bottle" systems allowing faster and easier clinical application.[8] The self-etching bonding systems demonstrate some chemical bonding but they do not show enough improvement to surpass those of the bond created when etch-and-rinse systems with phosphoric acid etched enamel are used.[9]

In the late 1990s, sixth-generation "self-etching" primers were introduced. These bonding adhesives incorporated an acidic primer that eliminated a separate acid-etching step.[10] Some systems require mixing the primer with an adhesive before placement, whereas others require a separate adhesive to be placed over previously applied primer. Although they reduced the incidence of posttreatment sensitivity[11] their bond strengths are lower than those of previous fourth- and fifth-generations systems.[12]

Introduced in late 2002, seventh-generation "all-in-one" systems combine materials for etching, priming, and bonding in a single solution. Studies show that these agents exhibit bond strengths and margin sealing equal to sixth-generation systems.[13] All-in-one bonding solutions are available in bottles and unit doses.

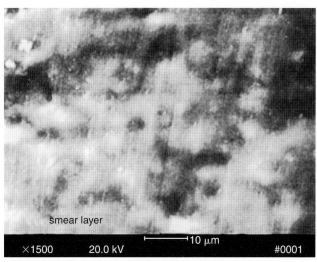

FIGURE 3-1 Scanning electron micrograph of dentin surface with "smear-layer" produced from cavity preparation.

In 2010, VOCO America introduced VOCO, Futurabond DC, a nano-reinforced, self-cured, light-cured, and dual-cured one-step, self-etch adhesive in a single-dose delivery system that they have designated as an eighth generation system.[14] With a manufacturer's reported adhesive strength of more than 30 MPa to both dentin and enamel when used with light-cured composite resins, Futurabond DC exhibits bond strengths similar to those of fourth- and fifth-generation adhesives.[15]

IDEAL CHARACTERISTICS OF A DENTIN BONDING AGENT

The ideal dentin bonding agent should achieve the following:
1. Bond to dentin with a strength equal to or greater than that of a composite resin bonded to etched enamel.
2. Rapidly (within a few minutes) attain maximum bond strength to permit finishing and polishing procedures and postoperative patient functioning within a reasonable time frame.
3. Be biocompatible and nonirritating to the pulp.
4. Prevent microleakage.
5. Exhibit long-term stability in the oral environment.
6. Be easy to apply and clinically forgiving.

Despite dramatic improvements in dentin bonding agents, clinical techniques are still confusing, even though research and product information on the subject have dramatically increased. An electronic Medline search using the phrase "dentin adhesive" as of July 2012, lists more than 50 publication abstracts. A Google web search using the keywords "dentin" and "adhesive" produced more than 24,900 scholarly works and 322,000 web search results with up-to-date research, discussion groups, and promotional information.[16]

PRODUCT SELECTION

Sufficient laboratory and animal data to predict clinical performance of dentin bonding agents are currently lacking. In addition, no large-scale controlled clinical trials comparing the performance of these materials in humans have been done. The most important long-term data include only 100 restorations, but demonstrated a 93% success rate for the three-step bonding approach over a 12-year period.[16] This study implies the validity of the three-step approach. Fortunately, however, some progress has been made in attempting to support scientifically the clinical choice between bonding agents. The American Dental Association (ADA) Acceptance Program was extended for professional products that included "Dentin and Enamel Adhesive Materials;" however, this Acceptance Program was discontinued in 2007. The ADA Standards Committee on Dental Products (SCDP) develops standards for dental materials, but standards are still pending for dentin bonding agents. However, the Acceptance Program with guidelines for materials that treat hypersensitivity is still current, and two dentin bonding materials are listed by the ADA (Table 3-1). Even though the Acceptance Program for dentin and enamel adhesive materials was eliminated, the ADA lists current products in the dentin bonding category, as shown in Table 3-2.

AVAILABLE DENTIN BONDING PRODUCTS

Dentin bonding agents are available in both multicomponent (see Table 3-1) and single-component systems. Multicomponent systems are the most reliable at the present time, but require more time and steps to complete. The single-component systems are a simplification of the wet-bonding process and are easier to use, but they produce less reliable results.

Table 3-1 Desensitizing Agents

Product	Vendor	Information	Specifications
Microprime B	Danville Materials Inc	Microprime B with benzethonium chloride and HEMA, is a formulation that will not burn soft tissues. Reliably eliminate postoperative sensitivity with superior antimicrobial qualities. Use with all total-etch, cements, amalgam and on cervical erosions.	• Eliminate postoperative sensitivity • Jumbo 10 mL • Value priced • Does not burn soft tissues • 3-yr shelf life
G5 All Purpose Desensitizer	Clinician's Choice Dental Products Inc	G5 helps solve the problem of postoperative sensitivity in a single step. G5 contains 5% glutaraldehyde and 35% HEMA to decrease in sensitivity without affecting bond strength and help prevent bacterial growth in tooth/restoration interface.	None

Data from ADA Dental Product Guide. http://www.ada.org/productguide/c/19/Bonding-Agents. Accessed October 2013.

Table 3-2 Bonding Agents

Product	Vendor	Information	Specifications
ACE ALL-BOND SE	BISCO Dental Products	ACE ALL-BOND SE is a self-etching bonding agent that combines etching, priming, and bonding in a dual-chamber cartridge dispensing system.	• Self-etch adhesive bonds to self- and dual-cured materials • No postoperative sensitivity • Low film thickness • Can be used for indirect applications • Packaged for the convenient and easy ACE dispenser
ACE ALL-BOND TE	BISCO Dental Products	ACE ALL-BOND TE is a single drop universal dental adhesive dispensing system that lets you prime and bond in one application. ALL-BOND TE is based on proven ALL-BOND 3 technology. It is an ethanol-based, dual-cured, total-etch adhesive system that combines outstanding performance, versatility, and durability for all dental applications.	• Compatible with light-, self-, and dual-cured materials • Bonds to all substrates • Dual-cured with one-drop dispensing • Cross-linking monomers eliminate need for additional bonding resin • Packaged for the convenient and easy ACE dispenser
Adper Easy Bond Self-Etch Adhesive	3M ESPE	Adper Easy Bond Self-Etch Adhesive is a one-bottle, one-coat solution. For those who prefer using a total etch adhesive, a new "selective etch" technique allows dental professionals to etch cut and uncut enamel surfaces.	• 35-second placement time • Unit-dose delivery available • Refrigeration not required
Adper Single Bond Plus Adhesive	3M ESPE	Adper Single Bond Plus Adhesive incorporates a nanofiller technology that contributes to high dentin bond strength performance. The nanoparticles will not clump or settle, so no shaking is required before use. The adhesive is available in a convenient, transparent bottle or an easy-to-use unit-dose delivery system.	• Unit-dose or squeeze bottle
ALL-BOND 2	BISCO Dental Products	ALL-BOND 2, the original three-step adhesive, is still unsurpassed in its comprehensive ability to bond to a multitude of substrates. ALL-BOND 2 has a dual-cured primer for higher conversion rates, and contains BISCO's own patented hydrophilic monomer (BPDM).	• Compatible with light-, self-, and dual-cured materials • Dual-cured material designed for all bonding procedures • Proven clinically in more than 200 research articles • More than 19 years of proven efficacy • Can be used for bonding amalgams
ALL-BOND 3	BISCO Dental Products	ALL-BOND 3 micro-mechanically bonds to all substrates, is used for all bonding procedures and is compatible with light-, dual-, and self-cured materials. The ALL-BOND 3 system offers increased hydrophobicity for a long-lasting adhesive bond. The HEMA-free, radiopaque ALL-BOND 3 resin reduces the chance of misdiagnosing caries.	• Compatible with light-, self-, and dual-cured materials • One to two coats of parts A and B are required • Ethanol-based = less technique sensitivity • HEMA free = hydrophobic bonding to prevent degradation
ALL-BOND UNIVERSAL	BISCO Dental Products	BISCO's ALL-BOND UNIVERSAL is a single-bottle bonding agent that combines self- and total-etch bonding, plus the resin layer and an activator into one universal bottle. As a universal adhesive, it is designed to work with light-, dual-, and self-cured composite resin and cement materials for all direct and indirect procedures.	• Total- or self-etch • Direct or Indirect • No activator—single bottle system • Universal compatibility • All procedures
BeautiBond	Shofu Dental Corporation	New seventh-generation bonding agent has an exclusive chemistry with unique dual adhesive monomers that deliver equal bond strength to enamel and dentin.	• Bond strengths comparable to leading multicomponent brands • Single coat for shorter working time • Efficient 30 second application • 5 μm film thickness • HEMA-free

Table 3-2 **Bonding Agents—cont'd**

Product	Vendor	Information	Specifications
Bond-1 SF Solvent Free SE Adhesive	Pentron Clinical	Bond-1 SF Solvent-Free SE Adhesive is a light-cure, one-coat, self-etch adhesive that is truly in a league of its own! Bond-1 SF forms an interactive bond between the minerals of the tooth structure and the resins of the bonding agent, without the use of acetone, water, or alcohol, providing a superior bond to both dentin and enamel.	
Clearfil SE Bond	Kuraray America, Inc.	Kuraray, after inventing the self-etching technique with CLEARFIL LINER BOND 2 in 1993, has surpassed their universally accepted total-etch technology with a new product—a new-generation self-etching primer and bonding system called CLEARFIL SE BOND. CLEARFIL SE BOND is a simplified, light-cure bonding system containing a water-based primer.	• Secure, fast, and easy to use • High bond strength • Water-based, self-etch primer
Clearfil SE Protect	Kuraray America, Inc.	CLEARFIL SE PROTECT provides the same defining properties that have made CLEARFIL SE BOND the market leader plus two other clinically significant technologies— fluoride release and newly developed MDPB monomer.	• High bond strength • Fluoride-releasing properties • Low postoperative sensitivity • Fast and simple procedure
Futurabond DC	VOCO America, Inc.	Self-etch dual-cured bonding agent for all light-, dual-, and self-cured resin materials. Futurabond DC is unique in that it is reinforced with nano-particles, which increases the bond values and marginal integrity. It is moisture tolerant, needs no refrigeration, and gets more than 30 MPa to dentin and enamel with light-cured composite resins.	• Easy/fast application • Nearly no postoperative sensitivity • Bond strength of 30 MPa to dentin and enamel • Perfect chemistry each use with the single-dose packaging
G-ænial Bond	GC America, Inc.	G-ænial Bond is a one-step, self-etch, seventh-generation bonding agent. Its improved design, HEMA-free formulation, improved bond strengths and easy application make it the bonding agent of choice. Designed specifically for "selective etching" technique to give the professional the maximum advantages.	• Seventh-generation one-step self-etch bonding agent • Easy application—30 seconds from application to finish • Long-lasting, durable restorations. Easy to clean up excess. • Composite resin not slippery when placed • Available in kits, refills, and combination of G-ænial Flowables
G-BOND	GC America, Inc.	G-BOND is a revolutionary seventh-generation (single component) adhesive that takes the guesswork out of bonding. The unique combination of phosphoric acid ester monomer and 4-MET adhesive technology creates superior etch and adhesion to enamel in addition to providing chemical and mechanical seal to dentin—referred to as the Nano Interaction Zone.	• Seventh-generation bonding adhesive • Single component • Etch, desensitize, prime, and bond in as little as 20 seconds • Not technique sensitive like other "all in one" systems • No postoperative sensitivity. Fast and easy application
ONE-STEP	BISCO Dental Products	ONE-STEP is a light-cured, single component adhesive that, unlike others, bonds to a multitude of dental substrates, including self- and dual-cured materials. Its proprietary chemistry makes it an exceptional adhesive for metal bonding, including implant abutments	• Compatible with light-, self-, and dual-cured materials • One-bottle total-etch adhesive • Low film thickness (approx. 10 μm) • Great for metal bonding, including implant abutments
Oxford Bond SE	Oxford Scientific Dental	A self-etch bonding agent that is dual-curing without the need for a separate activator. Rated + + + + by the Dental Advisor. Available in 2 × 5 mL bottles or 0.15 mL Single Mix units.	
Prelude SE	Danville Materials, Inc.	Prelude is a fast and reliable self-etch light-cured adhesive. It offers full strength even to uncut enamel. Two-bottle system for maximum reliability. Fast and simple to use with only one 10-second application per bottle.	• High bond strengths • Bonds even to uncut enamel • 5 μ film thickness • 10-second primer and adhesive • Link converts to dual cure

Continued

Table 3-2 Bonding Agents—cont'd

Product	Vendor	Information	Specifications
Prime & Bond NT Nano-Technology Light Cured Dental Adhesive	DENTSPLY Caulk	Prime & Bond NT Total Etch Adhesive is based on 16+ years of trusted, clinically proved PENTA (dipentaerythritol penta acrylate monophosphate) resin technology and can be used in virtually all restorative bonding procedures. Exclusive nanofillers ensure marginal integrity and exhibit deep penetration into tubules and horizontal interconnects.	• Proven long-term results • Low film thickness • High bond strength values to enamel and dentin • Simple to use one-bottle system
SELECT HV ETCH	BISCO Dental Products	New SELECT HV ETCH is a 35% high viscosity phosphoric acid etchant containing benzalkonium chloride, designed for the "selective etch" or "hybrid" technique—etching enamel margins without etching dentin. It can also be used for everyday total-etch restorative procedures. SELECT HV ETCH is formulated for optimized handling and accuracy.	• Thixotropic • Blue in color for easy visualization and contrast • Washes off easily without leaving residue • Bulk syringe dispensing
Surpass Self Etch Adhesive System	Apex Dental Materials Inc	Combining proven self-etching technologies with a new primer/bonding resin approach, SURPASS offers high shear strengths while eliminating sensitivity in one simple technique.	• Dentin bond strengths >MPa • Enamel bond strengths >50 MPa • Film thickness 10 to 12 microns • Postoperative sensitivity: zero
Xeno IV One Component Light Cured Self-Etching Dental Adhesive	DENTSPLY Caulk	Xeno IV self-etching dental adhesive is a trusted, proven PENTA (dipentaerythritol penta acrylate monophosphate) resin technology—just like Prime & Bond NT. Strength and durability are exceptional, creating a superb seal. Independent testing has demonstrated Xeno IV to have one of the highest bond strengths of any self-etch dual-cure adhesives.	• Chemistry based on class leading Prime & Bond NT • One-bottle, one-brush application • No overdrying of dentin
XP Bond Universal Total Etch Adhesive	DENTSPLY Caulk	XP Bond Total Etch Adhesive has wide wet-to-dry prep tolerance making Dentsply's most forgiving bonding agent. XP Bond offers substantially smaller nanofiller particles meaning a more densely packed bonding matrix. Usable as a light cure, self-, and dual-cure adhesive.	• Wide wet-to-dry prep tolerance • Tertiary-butanol solvent improves handling • Self-cure for PFM and endo canal applications • Simple to use one-bottle system
Z-PRIME Plus	BISCO Dental Products	Z-PRIME Plus is a single-component priming agent used to enhance adhesion between indirect restorative materials and composite resin cements. Z-PRIME Plus significantly enhances bond strengths to Zirconia.	• Unparalleled bond strengths • Bonds to zirconia, alumina, and metal substrates • Compatible with light- and dual-cured resin luting cements • Single bottle delivery

Data from ADA Dental Product Guide. http://www.ada.org/productguide/c/19/Bonding-Agents. Accessed October 2013.

Indications

Products listed by the ADA can be expected to perform well in the "saucer-shaped" Class V preparations that have been evaluated. However, including mechanical retention even in these situations is prudent.[16,17] Mechanical retention can be achieved with small rotary instruments in conventional preparations with converging cavity walls, retention "dimples" or "cuts," or air abrasive units that can be carefully manipulated to provide undercut areas. Most clinical data about dentin bonding agents refer to these minor operative dental procedures.[16] A dentin bonding agent is also indicated on all exposed dentin whenever a composite resin material will be used for adhesion to the tooth structure. To avoid future leakage at the enamel interfaces, it is recommended that the enamel be etched with orthophosphoric acid gel limited to the enamel surface. Self-etching dentin adhesives do not etch the enamel to the same pattern, and it is not clear that the self-etch approach provides long-term success without discoloration or loss of bond.[16] In extremely deep preparations in which the dentin tubular diameters are large and the vital pulp tissue is less than 1.0 mm from the surface, it is prudent to use a resin-ionomer. When cavosurface margins are on

dentin or cementum, achieving the best possible bond is particularly important to reduce, if not eliminate, microleakage, thereby reducing the effects of pulpal irritation, postoperative sensitivity, marginal discoloration, and recurrent caries.

Indications for clinical applications of dentin bonding agents are as follows:

1. All direct composite resin restorations—anterior and posterior
2. Indirect (as well as direct/indirect) composite resin restorations—laboratory processed inlays/onlays and veneers
3. Indirect ceramic restorations and alloys that are to be resin-bonded—inlays/onlays
4. Amalgam restorations—if isolation can be achieved so that the bonding process is not contaminated; all dentin bonding systems can be used to bond amalgam to the prepared tooth
5. Post and core restorations (composite resin, ceramic and amalgam) of endodontically treated teeth—both prefabricated and indirect
6. Retrograde fillings after apicoectomy—when isolation is possible; both composite resin and amalgam can be used for the retrograde filling material

7. Fixed prostheses (precious alloy, nonprecious alloy, resin-bonded prostheses, composite resin prosthesis, fiber-reinforced composite resin prosthesis [Targis-Vectris or Sculpture Fibercore] and all ceramic prostheses and laminate veneers)
8. Desensitization of exposed dentin

THEORY AND PRACTICE OF BONDING TO DENTIN

Attempts to bond to the smear layer (a mechanically altered layer of tooth structure that coats the surface of the prepared dentin surface, occluding the dentinal tubules, after rotary instrument preparation) were doomed to failure because this layer is itself only weakly attached to the dentin (Fig. 3-2A).

The total etch technique has proved to produce a stronger bond. Enamel and dentin are etched concomitantly. The etching process removes the smear layer completely and demineralizes the surface of the dentin to a depth of approximately 5 to 10 microns, creating collagen "scaffolding" with wide-open tubules. The deeper mineralized dentin has an irregular hydroxyapatite surface. The key to bonding is the infiltration of this collagen matrix and tubules through the mineralized layer of dentin (Fig. 3-2B).

Except for nonvital teeth, dentin is moist with tubular fluid. After the etching acid is rinsed away, bonding must be performed on a "wet" dentin surface. If the dentin is overdried the collagen will collapse, producing an inadequate bond.

CLINICAL TIP

Even nonvital dentin is moist in the oral environment and should not be completely desiccated or an inadequate bond will result. Both nonvital and vital dentin should be treated with wet bonding.

The priming agent (or bonding resin itself, in the situation of "single-bottle" agents) must be somewhat hydrophilic, or have an affinity for water. These resin materials are actually hydrophobic but can be considered to be more hydrophilic than previous materials. The primer or bonding resin infiltrates the moist collagen and penetrates the tubules to the peritubular area, which was demineralized in the etching process (Fig. 3-2C).

Bonding is believed to be primarily a micromechanical interlocking of resin into the mineral portion or the dentin. Recent evidence indicates that bonding agents also form covalent bonds with the molecular structure of the collagen.[17]

Some of the earliest dentin bonding agents to have hydrophilic components were those containing 4-META. The somewhat hydrophilic material allowed bonding resin to penetrate the moist collagen surface and flow into the "wet" tubules, creating a real hybrid or transition layer. This transition layer can be seen in both transmission electron micrograph (TEM) (Fig. 3-3A) and scanning electron microscopy (SEM) (Fig. 3-3B) of a 4-META/MMA-TBB–containing product (Amalgambond Plus, Parkell, Inc.). The creation of transition layers, or hybrid layers, of dentin and bonding agent can be seen in the SEM for both the multicomponent (Scotchbond Multi-Purpose Plus, 3M ESPE; Fig. 3-3C) and "single-bottle" materials (Single Bond, 3M ESPE) (Fig. 3-3D).

A recent study indicates that in vitro and in vivo dentin bond strengths may be comparable.[18] Another study indicates that coronal and apical dentin adhesion is high but cervical root dentin bond strengths are significantly lower.[19] Other work shows bond strengths vary considerably depending on the depth of the dentin; bonding to deep dentin is significantly weaker than superficial dentin.[20] Similarly, differences have been found with deciduous dentin.[21-23] The latter study suggests that less etching time is appropriate for deciduous dentin. Other applications

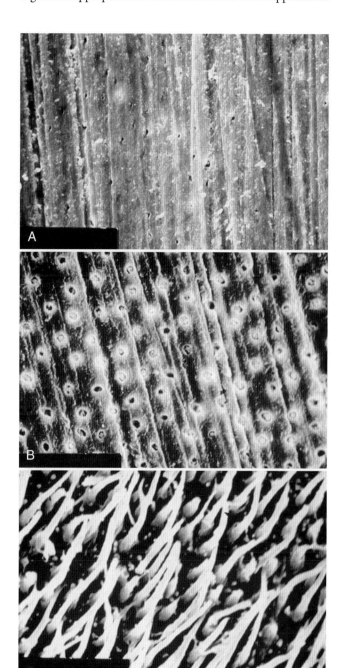

FIGURE 3-2 A, Scanning electron micrograph of dentin with smear layer before bonding. Note that areas of dentin tubules are barely visible. **B,** Scanning electron micrograph after application of primer (Syntac), showing that resin has penetrated smear layer and formed a hybrid surface. **C,** Scanning electron micrograph of dentin bonded composite restoration after demineralization with acid to remove dentin. Note tubular extensions of resin that penetrated into the opened dentinal tubules to the irregular hydroxyapatite surface, thus creating a bond. (**A** and **B,** Courtesy Ivoclar Vivadent, Amherst, NY. **C,** Courtesy Dr. Nelson J. Gendusa, Parkell, Inc., Edgewood, NY.)

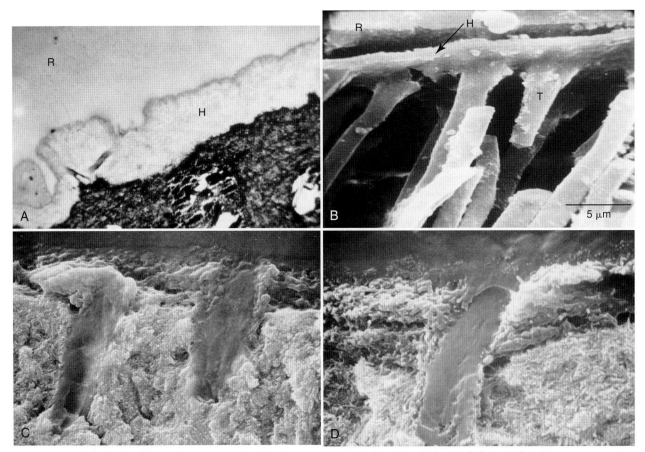

FIGURE 3-3 A, Transmission electron micrograph of Amalgambond Plus (Parkell, Inc.) showing resin (R), layer of bonding agent/tooth structure, hybrid (H) layer, and hydroxyapatite crystals in the undercalcified dentin below. **B,** Scanning electron micrograph of Amalgambond Plus specimen showing resin (R), hybrid layer of bonding material/tooth component (H), and tubular extensions (T) of bonding material. **C,** Scanning electron micrograph of multicomponent bonding agent (Scotchbond Multi-Purpose Plus) after total-etch of dentin. Scotchbond Multi-Purpose Plus provides a reliable bond to etched dentin by using a primer with an activating component of ethanol-based solution of sulfinic acid salt plus a photoinitiator. The adhesive component consists of an adhesive of bis-GMA and HEMA with a photoinitiator and a catalyst component of bis-GMA with a peroxide chemical initiator. **D** SEM of single-component bonding agent "one-bottle" approach (Single Bond Plus, 3M ESPE) showing interface between resin and etched dentin. The bonding agent is composed of bis-GMA, HEMA, ethanol, water, diacrylates, photoinitiator, methacrylate functional copolymer of polyacrylic acid, and polyitaconic acids. (**B,** Courtesy Dr. Nelson J. Gendusa, Parkell, Inc., Edgewood, NY. **C** and **D,** Courtesy Dr. Robert L. Erickson, Creighton University, Omaha, NE.)

include successful retrograde fillings,[24,25] amalgam to dentin bonding,[26] use with post and cores,[27,28] and use with all types of indirect restorations luted with composite resin cements.

GENERAL CONSIDERATIONS AND PROCEDURES

Cavity preparation, basing (to achieve a protective layer when the preparation is 0.5 mm or less from the pulp) to eliminate resin penetration to the pulp, and composite restorative material placement are generally identical for all dentin bonding agents and involve three essential steps.

Clean the Preparation

The tooth surfaces must be clean (use of cavity cleansers and disinfectants is encouraged) and remain completely noncontaminated during the procedure, or clinical failure is to be expected. Isolation is absolutely necessary. Should contamination occur at any step, the entire process must be repeated, beginning with the thorough surface cleansing achieved with a prophylaxis brush or cup and pumice. Pumice used with a cup or brush removes the contaminated resin, leaving a clean dentin surface.

Etch the Tooth Surface

The manufacturers' suggested etching gel always should be used. Generally, etching gel is 30% to 40% orthophosphoric acid (some evidence indicates that greater than 37% acid denatures the collagen). The etchant should be applied to both enamel and dentin and allowed to remain for only 15 seconds. The gel must then be thoroughly rinsed away with the air/water spray. A thorough rinse with a water stream alone is satisfactory but must be complete and not abbreviated so that no acid gel remains on the treated surface.

Excess water can be evacuated, or the preparation can be blotted dry, without air drying. Small sponges or applicator tips can be used to remove excess water, leaving the surface moist but not soaking wet. If an air syringe is used to the point of complete dryness, it should be followed with a water-saturated small sponge or nonlinting applicator tip applied to the dry surface to remoisten the dentin. An air spray can be used to gently remove the pooled water, but care must be taken to leave a moist surface.

Apply Dentin Bonding Agent

A dentin bonding agent (either primer/bonding resin or primer followed by bonding resin) is applied. Primers from single-bottle as well as multicomponent systems are essentially applied in the same way. Protocols from the specific manufacturer should be followed, but application generally involves applying the primer or resin with a brush or applicator tip continuously for 15 to 20 seconds. A scrubbing action is not warranted, but gentle agitation or light rubbing seems to facilitate the infiltration of the agent into the etched dentin surface. About 5 to 10 seconds of a gentle stream of air after the resin has been applied evaporates the solvent (either acetone or ethanol-based systems).

CLINICAL TIP

Do not blast the surface with air. Proceed gently without using maximum air pressure. The step is designed to simply vaporize the solvent without blowing the primer or resin off the tooth surface. Generally, single-bottle techniques require at least two applications, and evidence indicates that several more may facilitate higher bond strength.

CLINICAL TIP

The dentin surface must appear very shiny after the last coat of material has been applied. If this shiny appearance is not evident, the dentin is not sealed and another coat must be applied.

Single-bottle agents should be light-cured for 10 to 20 seconds. The dentin surface should appear uniformly shiny with a complete coat of bonding resin; otherwise additional coats should be applied to achieve this appearance. When the single-bottle agents are used with indirect restorations, pooling of resin in any line angles or on any surfaces must be eliminated. Improper pooling will prevent the indirect restoration from seating properly. An applicator tip can be drawn across the surface to prevent pooling, or excess adhesive can be blotted away. Use of the air syringe to thin the resin is not advised because overdrying (instead of solvent evaporation) may occur. Air drying with a gentle stream from the air-syringe must be carried out with great caution to prevent desiccation. If the single-bottle agent is properly applied and light-cured on the tooth, the indirect restoration can be completely seated because the bonding layer is thin enough to leave the surface essentially unaltered.

Multicomponent systems, in general, cannot be light-cured on the tooth when using an indirect restorative technique because a much thicker layer is present and the restoration will not completely seat. The multicomponent dentin bonding agents must be light-cured with the luting resin after seating the restoration to prevent incomplete seating of the restoration.

CLINICAL PROCEDURES

Procedures for the fourth and fifth generations of dentin bonding agents are quite similar. The following step-by-step procedure outlines the clinical application of a multicomponent bonding agent that has received full acceptance by the ADA.

Clinical Technique for Multicomponent Bonding Agents

Example Product	Composition
Primer	25% Tetraethylene glycol dimethacrylate
	4% Maleic acid
	71% Acetone and water
Adhesive	35% Polyethylene glycol dimethacrylate
	5% Glutaraldehyde
	60% Water
	60% bis-GMA
Light-cured bonding resin	40% triethylene glycol dimethacrylate

Armamentarium.
+ Standard Dental Setup
    + Explorer
    + Mouth mirror
    + Periodontal probe
    + Suitable anesthesia
    + Rubber dam setup
    + High-speed handpiece and burs
+ Low-speed handpiece, burs, mandrel, and polishing disks
+ Light-curing resin-ionomer base or Dycal if needed for deep areas
+ Etching gel—orthophosphoric acid
+ Dental bonding primer (e.g., All Bond 2 Primer A)
+ Dental bonding adhesive (e.g., All Bond 2 B)
+ Composite resin of choice (see Chapter 5)

Clinical Technique.
1. Examine the area to determine the extent of carious lesion and evaluate periodontal health (Fig. 3-4*A*).
2. Administer appropriate anesthesia if necessary.
3. Isolate the lesion with rubber dam. Nonlatex dams are preferred because of increasing concerns about latex allergies.

CLINICAL TIP

If a rubber dam will not be used, the preparation to be bonded must have adequate isolation or the denting bonding approach cannot be used successfully. Retraction cords can be packed, or troughing with a carbon dioxide laser can be used to gain an isolated field in which to operate successfully (see Chapter 21).

4. Clean the tooth surface with a nonfluoridated flour of pumice for adequate shade visualization and promotion of a surface free of plaque, debris, and calculus (see Figs. 3-4*B* and 3-9).
5. Prepare the cavity in a conventional manner with high-speed air turbine and appropriate burs (Fig. 3-4*C*).
6. Use a low-speed air turbine and round burs to remove all decay.

CLINICAL TIP

Caries detection dyes are appropriate to use, especially in areas in which visualization is difficult, such as tunnel preparations. Continue until all dentin is noncarious.

7. Use burs to place slots, cuts, or retention points for mechanical retention (Fig. 3-4D).

   Use of nonretentive saucer-shaped designs is not advised unless the entire restoration margins are in enamel. An enamel bevel is also advisable.

8. In deep cavity preparations (within approximately 0.5 mm of the pulp), place an acid-resistant calcium hydroxide base or resin-ionomer base to protect the pulpal tissues. This based area should be kept to a minimum to expose an adequate amount of exposed dentin for bonding (Fig. 3-4E).

9. Place orthophosphoric etching gel (total etch technique) over entire cavity preparation for 15 seconds (Fig. 3-4F).

10. Wash the etching gel away with an air/water spray for 20 seconds (Fig. 3-4G).

See the preceding section on the application of dentin bonding agents.

11. Ensure dentin is moist (not soaking wet) by blotting it dry with a sponge, dry applicator, or cotton pellet.

CLINICAL TIP

Do not air dry. An alternative approach is to briefly air dry the surfaces to visualize the frosty appearance of the etched enamel and immediately reapply water on a sponge or applicator to remoisten the dentin. To ensure the moistness of the dentin surface, extreme care must be taken if an air stream is used.

12. Mix one drop each of Primer A and B according to the manufacturer's instructions and apply the primer to all surfaces with a brush or small applicator, adding more primer during the process for 20 seconds (Fig. 3-4H). Use a gentle agitating action. Do not use a forceful scrubbing action!

13. Gently evaporate the solvents with a very light stream of air.

14. Apply the primer over the entire preparation for a second time. A gentle stream of air should be used to evaporate the solvents for 15 seconds.

15. Apply a thin layer of bonding resin (Heliobond Ivoclar Vivadent), and remove excess with sponge or applicator (Fig. 3-4I). If this is a filled adhesive and does not require an additional layer of resin, then light cure as indicated in following step.

CLINICAL TIP

Do not blow the resin away with an air spray. Use a small sponge, applicator, or even an endodontic paper point to remove excess resin.

16. Photocure the resin with a light-curing unit for 15 to 20 seconds (Fig. 3-4J).

CLINICAL TIP

Be sure to maintain a daily or weekly schedule that is comfortable for adequate testing of the photo-curing unit with a radiometer to ensure adequate intensity of light output. Each time a new lamp is installed it should be tested as well. Radiometers include the Curing Radiometer (Demetron LED Radiometer/Kerr Corp.), (EFOS), Coltolux Light Meter (Coltene/Whaledent), and the built-in testing unit in the XL-3000 photo-curing unit (3M ESPE).

17. Restore the cavity preparation with your choice of composite resin restorative materials (Fig. 3-4K).

18. Finish and polish the restoration with carbide burs and polishing disks.

19. An additional layer of resin may be applied and photocured to "heal" surface cracks produced during finishing and polishing and possible microscopic marginal discrepancies that may later show marginal staining. Other resins are manufactured specifically for this purpose; however, most new "filled" bonding agents can be used instead.

Clinical Technique for Single-Bottle Bonding Agents

Example Product	**Single Bond (3M ESPE)**
Composition	bis-GMA
	Hydroxyethyl methacrylate
	Ethanol
	Water
	Diacrylates
	Photoinitiator
	Methacrylate functional copolymer of polyacrylic and polyitaconic acid (polyalkenoic acid)
Light-cured bonding resin	60% bis-GMA 40% triethylene glycol dimethacrylate

Armamentarium. The same as for multicomponent systems except with substitution of appropriate single-bonding system.
Clinical Technique.

1. Examine the area to determine the extent of the carious lesion and evaluate periodontal health (Fig. 3-5A).

2. Administer local anesthetic as necessary.

3. Isolate the lesion with a rubber dam. A nonlatex dam is preferred because of increasing concerns about latex allergies.

CLINICAL TIP

If a rubber dam will not be used, the preparation to be bonded must have adequate isolation or the denting bonding approach cannot be used successfully. Retraction cords can be packed, or troughing with a carbon dioxide laser (see Chapter 22) can be used to gain an isolated field in which to operate successfully.

4. Clean the tooth surface with nonfluoridated pumice.

5. Prepare the cavity in a conventional manner with high-speed air turbine and appropriate burs.

6. Use a low-speed air turbine and round burs to remove all decay.

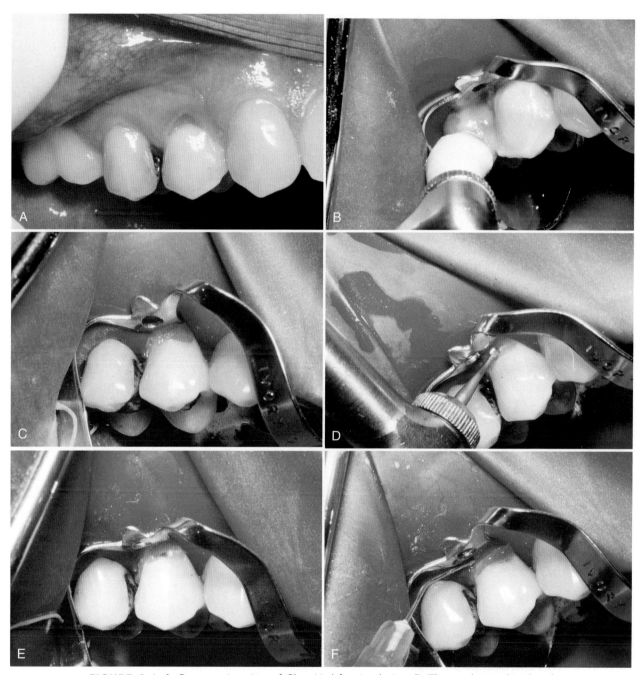

FIGURE 3-4 A, Preoperative view of Class V abfraction lesion. **B,** The tooth is isolated and cleaned with plain nonfluoridated pumice. **C,** The tooth is prepared with high-speed air turbine. **D,** A low-speed air turbine is used to completely remove the caries and place mechanical retention such as slots, grooves, or dimples. **E,** A resin-ionomer base/liner or acid-resistant calcium hydroxide liner is placed in extremely deep areas. **F,** To achieve a total etch, orthophosphoric acid gel is placed on the entire preparation for 15 seconds.

Continued

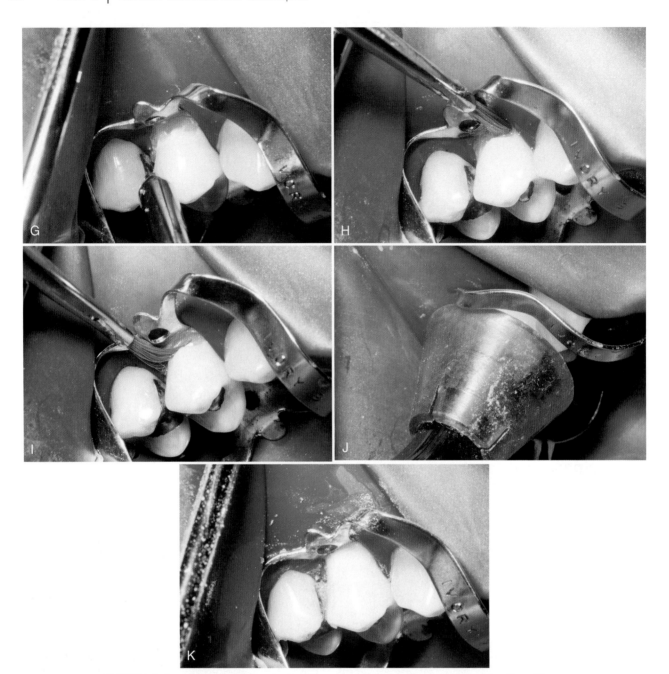

FIGURE 3-4, cont'd G, The etched cavity preparation is thoroughly washed for 15 to 20 seconds. **H,** The dentin primer is applied to all surfaces with a brush, using a gentle agitation action. Multiple applications of the primer ensure that the tooth has been amply primed. A gentle stream of air is used to evaporate the solvent. **I,** A thin layer of bonding resin is applied with a brush. Excess resin is removed with an applicator or paper point. The resin must not be blown too thin. **J,** The bonding agent is photocured for 15 to 20 seconds. **K,** The chosen composite resin restorative material is applied in increments and finished with carbide burs, followed by polishing disks. A final glaze of bonding resin may be applied to seal the marginal microgaps and cracks that may remain after finishing.

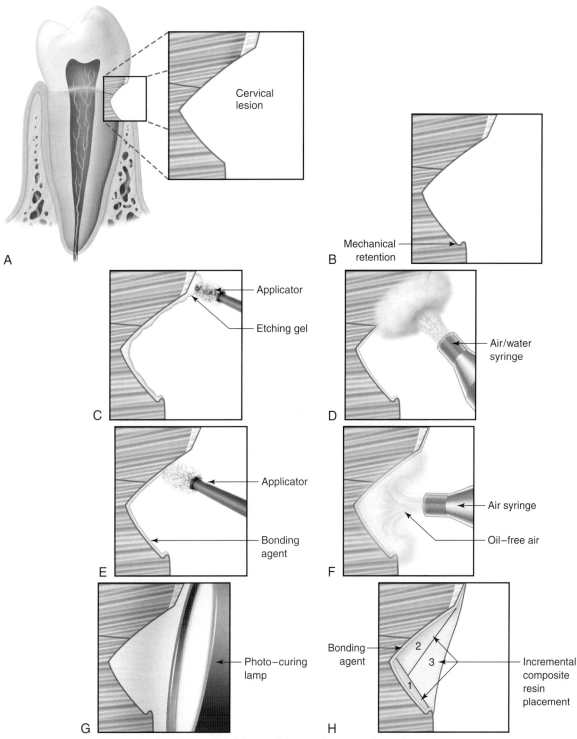

FIGURE 3-5 **A,** Tooth with cervical abfraction/abrasion lesion involving dentin/cementum at the gingival cavosurface margin. **B,** After preparation, which maximizes mechanical retention, the pulp is protected by placing a resin-ionomer liner or acid-resistant calcium hydroxide liner in deep areas of preparation. **C,** The etching gel is placed over the entire surface of the cavity preparation and onto a portion of the unprepared enamel for 15 to 20 seconds. The clinician should ensure that no voids caused by air bubbles exist. **D,** The etching gel is thoroughly washed off with the water syringe. The preparation is blotted with a dry applicator to leave moist (not dripping wet) dentin or dried briefly with air, with moisture reapplied with a damp applicator. **E,** Single-component bonding agent is applied with a brush to the entire cavity preparation for 20 seconds with a gentle agitation action. **F,** The solvent evaporates from the bonding agent with application of gentle air. The surface should appear shiny at this point. If not, the agent should be applied a second time. **G,** The bonding agent is light-cured for 10 seconds. **H,** The cavity is restored with the chosen composite resin material using the incremental placement technique to minimize the effects of polymerization shrinkage.

7. Use burs to place slots, cuts, or retention points for mechanical retention. Use of nonretentive saucer-shaped designs is not advised. An enamel bevel is advisable (Fig. 3-5*B*).
8. Place orthophosphoric etching gel (total etch technique) over entire cavity preparation for 15 to 20 seconds (Fig. 3-5*C*).
9. Wash the etching gel away with an air/water spray for 20 seconds (Fig. 3-5*D*).

See the preceding section on the application of dentin bonding.

10. Assure moist (not soaking wet) dentin by blotting dry with a sponge dry applicator or cotton pellet.

11. Apply single-bottle bonding agent (e.g., Single Bond, 3M ESPE) with enough material to keep the cavity preparation saturated with adhesive for 20 seconds (according to manufacturer's instructions) (Fig. 3-5*E*).

12. Gently evaporate the solvents with a very light stream of air for 5 to 10 seconds (Fig. 3-5*F*).
13. Light-cure the bonding agents for 10 seconds (Fig. 3-5*G*).

14. Place the composite resin restoration in increments to reduce the effects of polymerization shrinkage (Fig. 3-5*H*). Some manufacturers recommend a second application, which requires repeating steps 12 through 14.
15. Finish and polish the restoration with carbide burs and polishing disks.
16. An additional layer of resin may be applied and photo-cured to "heal" surface cracks produced during finishing, polishing, and possible microscopic marginal discrepancies that may later show marginal staining. Other resins are

manufactured specifically for this purpose; however, most new "filled" bonding agents can be used instead.

CONCLUSION

Dentin bonding agents have dramatically improved in recent years. The major breakthrough has been the "total etch" technique, in which the smear layer is removed simultaneously with the enamel etching. The primers and bonding agents of multicomponent systems and combined primer/agent of one-bottle systems provide a dramatic bond to both the collagen and etched hydroxyapatite of the dentin. Although dentin bonding agents are not yet considered "ideal" materials, they are certainly close. Hopefully more controlled clinical trials will be forthcoming, allowing choices of material and technique to be made on a sound scientific basis.

REFERENCES

1. Buonocore MG, Wileman W, Brudevold F: Simple methods of increasing adhesion of acrylic filling materials to enamel surfaces, *J Dent Res* 34(6):849, 1955.
2. Asmussen E: Clinical relevance of physical, chemical and bonding properties of composite resins, *Oper Dent* 10:61, 1985.
3. Fan PL: Dentin bonding systems: an update, *J Am Dent Assoc* 114:91, 1987.
4. Bowen RL, Cobb EN, Rapson JE: Adhesive bonding of various materials to hard tooth tissues: improvement in bond strength to dentin, *J Dent Res* 61:1070, 1982.
5. Cox CF: Evaluation and treatment of bacterial microleakage, *Am J Dent* 7(5):293, 1994.
6. Goracci G, Mori G, Bazzucchi M: Marginal seal and biocompatibility of a fourth-generation bonding agent, *Dent Mater* 11(6):343, 1995.
7. Kanca J 3rd: Resin bonding to wet substrate. I. Bonding to dentin, *Quintessence Int* 23(1):39, 1992.
8. Ferrari M, Goracci G, Garcia-Godoy F: Bonding mechanism of three "one-bottle" systems to conditioned and unconditioned enamel and dentin, *Am J Dent* 10(5):224, 1997.
9. Erickson RL, Barkmeier WW, Latta MA: The role of etching in bonding to enamel: a comparison of self-etching and etch-and-rinse adhesive systems, *Dent Mater* 25(11):1459, 2009.
10. Nazarian A: *The progression of dental adhesives*, http://www.aranazariandds.com/pdf/dental_adhesives.pdf. Accessed October 28, 2013.
11. Miller MB: Self-etching adhesives; solving the sensitivity conundrum, *Pract Proced Aesthet Dent* 14:406, 2002.
12. Van Meerbeek B, Inoue S, Pedigao J, et al: In Summitt JB, Robbins JW, Schwartz RS, editors: *Fundamentals of operative dentistry: contemporary approach*, ed 2, Carol Stream, IL, 2001, Quintessence Publishing, pp 194-214.
13. Farah JW, Powers JM, eds. 6th- and 7th-generation bonding agents. *Dental Advisor*. 23(8):5, 2006.
14. Kakar S, Goswami M, Kanase A: Dentin bonding agents, I: Complete classification—a review, *World J Dent* 2(4):367, 2011.
15. Google Web search. keywords "dentin" and "adhesive." Accessed July 29, 2012.
16. Wilder AD Jr, Swift EJ Jr, Heymann HO, Ritter AV, Sturdevant JR, Bayne SC: A 12-year clinical evaluation of a three-step dentin adhesive in noncarious cervical lesions, *J Am Dent Assoc* 140(5):526, 2009.
17. Xu J, Stangel I, Butler IS, Gilson DF: An FT-Raman spectroscopic investigation of dentin and collagen surfaces modified by 2-hydroxyethylmethacrylate, *J Dent Res* 76(1):596, 1997.
18. Mason PN, Ferrari M, Cagidiaco MC, Davidson CL: Shear bond strength of four dentinal adhesives applied in vivo and in vitro, *J Dent* 24(3):217, 1996.
19. Yoshiyama M, Carvalho RM, Sano H, Horner JA, Brewer PD, Pashley DH: Regional bond strengths of resins to human root dentine, *J Dent* 24(6):435, 1996.
20. Tam LE, Yim D: Effect of dentine depth on the fracture toughness of dentine-composite adhesive surfaces, *J Dent* 25(3-4):339, 1997.
21. Royse MC, Ott NW, Mathieu GP: Dentin adhesive superior to copal varnish in preventing microleakage in primary teeth, *Pediatr Dent* 18(7):440, 1996.
22. de Araujo FB, Garcia-Godoy F, Issáo M: A comparison of three resin bonding agents to primary tooth dentin, *Pediatr Dent* 19(4):253, 1997.
23. Nör JE, Feigal RJ, Dennison JB, Edwards CA: Dentin bonding: SEM comparison of the dentin surface in primary and permanent teeth, *Pediatr Dent* 19(4):246, 1997.
24. Jou YT, Pertl C: Is there a best retrograde filling material? *Dent Clin North Am* 41(3):555, 1997.
25. Rud J, Rud V, Munksgaard EC: Retrograde root filling with dentin-bonded modified resin composites, *J Endod* 22(9):477, 1996.
26. Hasegawa T, Retief DH: Shear-bond strengths of two commercially available dentine-amalgam bonding agents, *J Dent* 24(6):449, 1996.
27. Mendoza DB et al: Root reinforcement with a resin-bonded pre-formed post, *J Prosthet Dent* 78:410, 1997.
28. Christensen GJ: Posts and cores: state of the art, *J Am Dent Assoc* 129:96, 1998.

Color Modifiers and Opaquers

Jerry B. Black and Richard D. Trushkowsky

The introduction of the acid-etch technique in 1955[1] and the bis-GMA resin by Bowen in 1962[2] set the stage for a new era in dentistry. As the chairside or direct bonding technique gained impetus, many dentists were lacking in a basic knowledge of dental anatomy, a subject that had traditionally been relegated to the laboratory technician. In addition to a focus on external anatomic features, dentists began to appreciate internal anatomy and the individual roles that enamel and dentin play in the determination of tooth color. The facial enamel could be visualized as a translucent window through which light could pass and reflect off the dentin background. The direct bonded veneer became, in a sense, the anatomic equivalent of the facial enamel. The challenge to reproduce normal shades stimulated interest in the components of color: hue, chroma, and value.

Enamel reduction and the desire for reversibility were debated subjects in the early days of direct enamel bonding. It became obvious that, to prevent overcontouring, enamel reduction was often necessary to provide space for color modifiers, opaquers, and the veneer resin. At least one study showed that even minimal enamel reduction resulted in a significant increase in the shear bond strength between etched enamel and composite resin.[3]

In cases involving intrinsically stained teeth, efforts are concentrated on opaquing or masking the dark background. In 1982 Black[4] described a definitive technique that included enamel reduction and masking of severe tetracycline stain in the fabrication of direct bonded composite resin veneers. Color modifiers and opaquers helped create highly esthetic and realistic restorations.

HISTORY

The first color modifiers (Estilux Color, Heraeus Kulzer, Inc. were introduced in 1982. These low-chroma, tooth-colored tints expanded the possibilities for shade matching, characterization, and opaquing. Two years later, high-chroma color modifiers were introduced by Heraeus Kulzer, Inc. (Durafill Color) and Den-Mat Corp. (Rembrandt). When diluted with low-viscosity bonding resins, these color modifiers allowed unlimited variation of chroma and more flexibility.

In 1984 Cosmedent, Inc. introduced its Creative Color and Renamel opaquing system.

In 1987 Heraeus Kulzer, Inc., USA introduced Durafill Color VS, a series of highly pigmented Vita opaque shades. When coordinated with corresponding Vita composite resin, these provide a high degree of color predictability in the composite resin veneer. Bisco, Inc. introduced Biscolor color modifiers. These were highly pigmented, heavy filled (50%) microfilled liquids available in eight shades. Heraeus Kulzer, Inc. introduced "Effect" color. These were intense opaque color modifiers that were used to mask dark stains and characterize composite resins.

The need for intense metal opaquers prompted the introduction of many products, including Heliocolor Opaque (Ivoclar Vivadent), Prisma Metal Opaque (Dentsply Caulk), Panavia (J. Morita USA, Inc.), and C & B Metabond (Parkell, Inc.).

CHEMISTRY

Most of the visible light-polymerized color modifiers contain metal oxide pigments suspended in a low viscosity bis-GMA resin or a mixture of bis-GMA and urethane dimethylacrylate resins. Moderate opaquers such as Durafill VS (Heraeus Kulzer, Inc.) contain 20% to 30% microfilled pigmented bis-GMA resin by weight. IPS Empress Direct Color (Ivoclar Vivadent) contains seven selected shades for the creation of natural-looking characterizations. Their fillers have been adjusted to ensure optimum translucency. It contains bis-GMA, urethane dimethacrylate, and triethylene glycol dimethacrylate.

IPS Empress Direct Opaque (Ivoclar Vivadent), a light-curing opaquing agent, masks stained and discolored teeth, exposed metal surfaces, and core build-ups.[5] Its high filler content exhibits physical properties similar to conventional flowable composite resin and can be applied in thin layers.[5]

Metal opaques, such as C & B Metabond II (Parkell, Inc.), are reported to chemically bond resin opaquers to nickel-chromium alloys and to amalgam. The bond is mediated through a 4-methacryloxy-ethyl trimellitate anhydride component. Panavia 21, based on 10-methacryloyloxydecyl dihydrogen phosphate technology, provides chemical adhesion to nonprecious alloys, tinplated noble alloys, porcelain, tooth enamel, and unetched dentin. Because the long-term strength of these adhesive formulations is unknown, wherever possible mechanical retention should be used in addition to chemical adhesion.

GENERAL CONSIDERATIONS

Color modifiers can be mixed with composite resins to change their shades; however, this procedure can result in the following:
1. Incorporation of air, which may result in surface porosity
2. Decreased filler loading
3. Increased curing times because of the pigments in the modifiers

The introduction of composite resins in an extended range of shades, including Vita shades, makes the admixing of color modifiers with composite resins seldom necessary.

The color characteristic of a natural tooth is the result of the subtle interplay of light reflected from the underlying dentin through the relatively translucent enamel. This phenomenon is simulated through the creative use of opaquers and color modifiers that are subsequently overlaid with a relatively translucent composite resin. The main advantages of opaquers are that they produce opacity by blocking light transmission and are useful to increase the value (brightness) and mask dark stains and metal. Tints are used to help increase the hue and chroma of the restoration. They also decrease value, allow the transmission of light, and create more translucency in the final restoration. Tints can also be used to mimic pit and fissure staining and recreate craze lines, check lines, maverick colors, and cervical chroma.

> ### CLINICAL TIP
>
> The rough enamel surface created by diamond burs should be smoothed with fine diamond burs or flexible disks before placing an opaquer. This allows the opaquer to flow evenly over the prepared surface and results in a uniform background.

> ### CLINICAL TIP
>
> Always mask out in very thin layers and be certain to observe the required curing time for each layer. Thicker layers result in incomplete curing and uneven layers caused by pooling of the material. Opaquers and tints are particularly subject to wear and therefore should not be placed relatively on the surface of the restoration. They should be overlaid with a layer of hybrid or microhybrid composite resin of at least 0.3mm.[6]

INDICATIONS FOR COLOR MODIFIERS

The most frequently used color modifiers are pink, white, gray, yellow, yellow-brown, blue, and red. Table 4-1 provides the visual effects of available color modifiers.

> ### CLINICAL TIP
>
> Because most color modifiers have high chromas, they must be diluted with a low-viscosity resin before use.

Table 4-1 Visual Effects of Color Modifiers

Color	Indications
Yellow-orange	Creates illusion of narrowness Simulates craze lines
Yellow-brown	Masks blue tetracycline stains
Blue, gray, violet	Simulates translucency Decreases value or brightness
White	Increases the brightness of any color modifier Simulates craze lines Simulates enamel hypocalcifications; white spots Masks yellow spots
Red, pink	Simulates gingival tones Enhances vitality Masks blue tetracycline stains

Yellow and Yellow-Brown

Yellow and yellow-brown shades are most often used in the cervical third of the crown (Fig. 4-1). Sometimes they are used along proximal surfaces to create the illusion of narrowness (see Chapter 2).

They can also be used to simulate craze lines. Because yellow is the complementary color of violet, it is effective in neutralizing and masking blue-gray tetracycline stains (see Chapter 2). Yellow can also be used in combination with white to mask brown tetracycline stains.

Blue, Gray, or Violet

Blue, gray, or violet shades are used on the incisal third of the tooth to simulate translucency (compare Fig. 4-2). They can also be used to reduce value (brightness).

White

White is used to increase the value (brightness) of any color modifier. It can be effectively used to simulate craze lines and enamel hypocalcifications (Fig. 4-3) and to mask yellow stains (Fig. 4-4).

Red or Pink

Red or pink simulates gingival tones, enhances vitality, and can neutralize blue tetracycline stains (see Chapter 2).

CLASS III AND CLASS IV RESTORATIONS

Truly "invisible" Class III and Class IV restorations are possible only through proper cavity preparation in conjunction with proper color matching (Fig. 4-5). Blending the color of the restorative resin into the color of the tooth is essential. Color modifiers are indispensable in fine tuning the definitive color.

In Class III or Class IV cavity preparations involving a through-and-through loss of both the facial and lingual enamel, the definitive restoration can exhibit undesirable "shine-through" (Fig. 4-5C).

This shine-through occurs because the missing lingual tooth structure is replaced by a composite resin that is more translucent

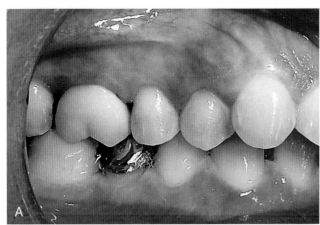

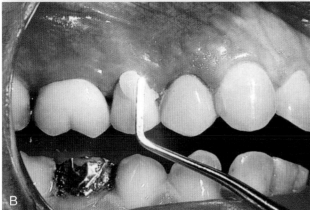

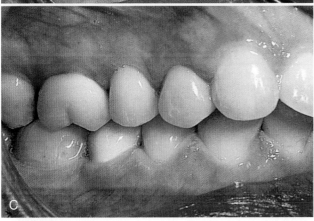

FIGURE 4-1 A, Preparation of the maxillary right first and second premolars for direct bonded veneers. **B,** The color of the cervical third of the veneers must harmonize with the adjacent teeth. A diluted yellow-brown color modifier was placed on the cervical third and overlaid with shade A-3 composite. **C,** Color harmony from the maxillary right first molar to the maxillary right canine has been established.

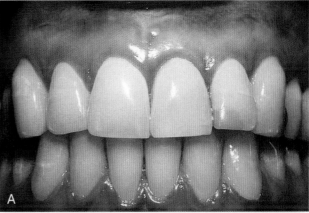

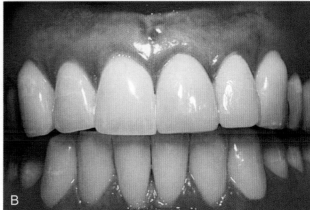

FIGURE 4-2 A, Intrinsic yellow discoloration of maxillary left central incisor. **B,** White color modifier was used to mask the yellow background, and blue color modifier was added to the incisor to simulate translucency.

than the original dentin. The result is a visible outline of the restoration. Shine-through can be prevented by careful cavity preparation, the judicious use of color modifiers and opaquers, and a "sandwich" of various types of composite resins.

Armamentarium.

- Standard Composite Resin Restoration dental setup
  - Rubber dam
  - Cotton rolls
    - Explorer
    - High-speed handpiece
    - Low-speed handpiece
    - Mouth mirror
    - Periodontal probe
    - 2 × 2 gauze
  - Mylar matrix strips
  - Wooden or plastic wedge (optional)
  - Assorted round carbide dental burs
  - Flame-shaped, tapered, and ovoid coarse diamonds for cavity preparations.
  - Oil-free pumice
  - Rubber prophy cup
  - Cavity liner (optional)
  - Acid etchant
  - Bonding agent of choice (see Chapter 3)
  - Composite resin placement instruments (e.g., 8A, Hu-Friedy Mfg. Co., LLC; #8, Brasseler USA; IPC-I, Premier Dental Products, Inc.; Goldstein Series 1-4 and mini 1 and 3, Hu-Friedy Mfg. Co.)
  - Hybrid composite resin of choice (see Chapter 5)
  - Microfilled composite resin of choice (see Chapter 5)
  - Diamond finishing burs (e.g., ET-9-Carbide - Diamond and ET-OSI ovoid carbide burs; Brasseler USA OR Carbide Flame H246-009 - Premier Dental Products)
    - For microfilled composite resins, low-speed, water-cooled diamond burs are best for trimming and finishing. For

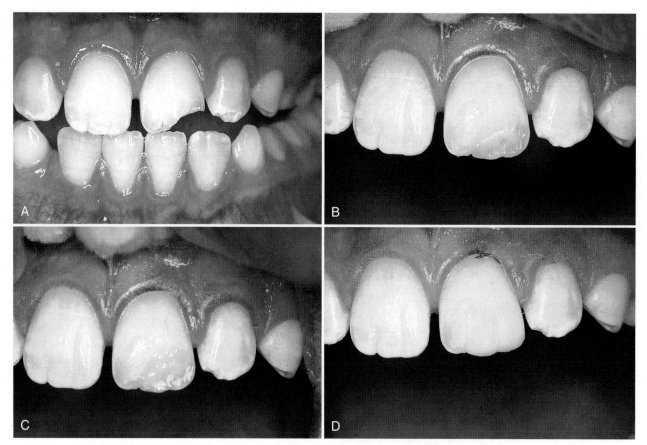

FIGURE 4-3 A, Fractured distoincisal angle. Adjacent teeth have white hypoplastic enamel areas. **B,** A layer of Multifill VS (Heraeus Kulzer, Inc.) is placed on the lingual wall and polymerized. **C,** Creative Color white is added to simulate the hypoplastic areas. **D,** The completed restoration. (Courtesy Dr. William Mopper, Glenview, IL.)

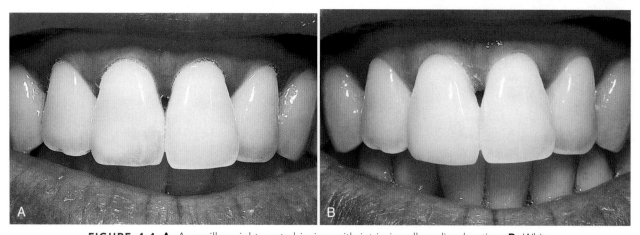

FIGURE 4-4 A, A maxillary right central incisor with intrinsic yellow discoloration. **B,** White color modifier is used to mask the yellow background.

small-particle hybrid composite resins, high-speed tungsten carbide burs and low-speed, water-cooled diamond burs are recommended.
- 12-fluted carbide finishing burs (e.g., ET-9-Carbide and ET-OSI ovoid carbide burs; Brasseler USA OR 2015153 (Fine) - Premier Dental Products)
- Finishing and polishing disks (e.g., Sof-Lex, 3M ESPE; Super Snaps, Shofu Dental Corp.; or Flexi-Discs, Cosmedent, Inc.)

- Finishing and polishing strips
  - Metal backed (e.g., Compo Strips, Premier Dental Products, Inc.) or plastic backed (e.g., Soft Lex, 3M ESPE; Flexi Strips, Cosmedent, Inc.; Jiffy diamond strips, Brassler USA)
- Polishing Kit (EP200 Esthetic Polishing Kit, Brassler USA)
- Rubber wheels, cups, and points containing abrasives
  - Medium-grit rubber wheels for prepolishing (e.g., Burlew, Jelenko), or complete systems (e.g., CompoMaster/

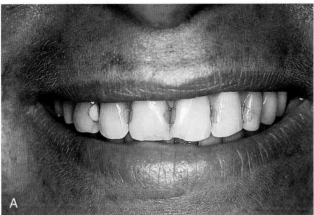

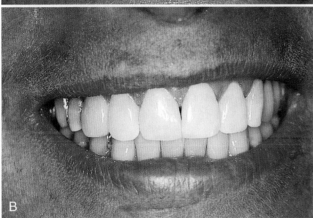

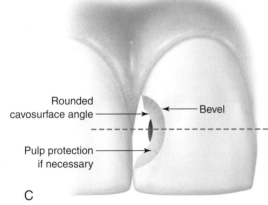

FIGURE 4-5 A, Preoperative view of discolored Class III composite resin restorations. (Courtesy Dr. William Mopper.) **B,** Postoperative view of invisible restoration. (Courtesy Dr. William Mopper.) **C,** Typical Class III preparation with a through-and-through loss of both the facial and lingual enamel. The line denotes the cross-section area of subsequent drawings.

CompoMaster Coarse Polishers, Shofu Dental Corp.; OR Astropol , Ivoclar Vivadent; ET Illustra Composite Polishers, Brasseler USA; Venus Supra Polishing System Heraeus Kulzer Inc., USA; Top Finisher System, Cosmedent, Inc.; Enhance Finishing System L.D. Caulk Co.
+ Composite resin polishing paste (containing aluminum oxide)
+ Dry felt wheel (Felt Wheel Keystone, Inc.)
+ Padded discs (e.g., Flexi Buffs, Cosmedent, Inc.)
+ Color modifiers and opaquers

+ Color modifiers: yellow, yellow-brown, white, blue, gray, violet (e.g., Effect Color Heraeus Composite Tints and Opaquers, Heraeus Kulzer, Inc.; Creative Color, Cosmedent Inc.; Kolor + Plus Kerr Corp; Artiste Maverick Tints, Pentron Clinical Technology; Bisco's Characterization Tints, Bisco, Inc.

Clinical Technique.
1. Administer anesthetic (optional).
2. Cleanse the tooth and neighboring teeth with pumice.
3. Determine the appropriate shade while the teeth are wet with saliva.
4. Isolate the lesion with a rubber dam.
5. Prepare the cavity in a conventional manner (Fig. 4-6A).
6. Round the cavosurface angle and place a long bevel to create an invisible transition from resin to tooth (Fig. 4-6B).

CLINICAL TIP

If the enamel is very translucent, create a longer and deeper bevel. If the tooth is more opaque, the bevel can be shorter and less pronounced.

7. Place a pulp protection as necessary. Place dentin-bonding agent according to the manufacturer's instructions.

CLINICAL TIP

Avoid the use of opaque lining materials beneath very translucent enamel. They interfere with the transmission of light through the enamel into the underlying tooth structure or composite resin.

8. To prevent "shine-through," place a more opaque hybrid composite resin in the lingual portion of the preparation.
9. Build up the resin to the level of the original dentoenamel junction.
10. If necessary, place custom tinting resins over this layer and blend the background color of the resin with the color of the tooth (Fig. 4-6C).

CLINICAL TIP

Always apply color modifiers in very thin layers and be certain to observe the required curing time for each layer. Thicker layers result in incomplete curing and uneven layers caused by pooling of the material.

CLINICAL TIP

Chroma (intensity) must be appropriately diluted with a bonding resin to create a tooth-colored hue.

CLINICAL TIP

Place custom tints, such as gray, blue, or violet, to simulate incisal translucency in Class IV restorations. Place yellow or yellow-brown custom tints for fine tuning the background color. Place white for increasing value (Fig. 4-6).

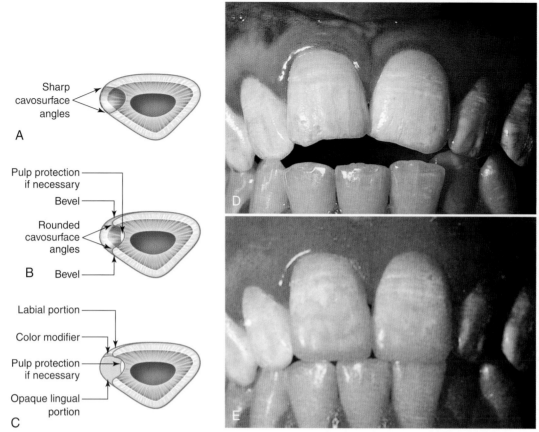

FIGURE 4-6 A, The cavity is prepared in a conventional manner. **B,** The cavosurface angle is rounded, and a long bevel is placed to facilitate an invisible transition from resin to tooth. **C,** An opaque composite resin is placed on the lingual portion of the restoration. This step is followed by placement of color modifiers or opaquers (if necessary) and completed with a facial veneer of a microfilled, microhybrid, or nano composite resin. **D,** Maxillary central incisors in open-occlusion relationship. **E,** A lingual wall of Multifill VS was first created. Durafill VS (white) was then used to simulate white hypoplastic enamel areas. A Multifill VS (incisal) overlay on the facial surface completed the restoration.

11. To complete the restoration, fill the remaining facial portion with a translucent microfilled composite resin.
12. Contour the restoration.
13. Prepolish the restoration with rubber wheels or cups.
14. Smooth with a microfine diamond in a low-speed handpiece with water cooling.
15. Polish with disks or strips.

CLINICAL TIP

An excellent definitive high gloss can be obtained by using a dry felt wheel or padded disk without paste on the dry composite resin surface.

DIASTEMA CLOSURES

A microfilled composite resin is the material of choice for diastema closure because of its excellent polishability and enamel-like luster (Figs. 4-7A and B). If the diastema is very large, the lingual surface of the esthetic resin could be subjected to high functional stress in patients with heavy centric contacts. In these situations, the dentist may elect to use a hybrid composite resin for the entire restoration or a hybrid on the lingual portion overlaid on the facial surface with a microfilled composite resin. Shine-through is usually not a problem in diastema closure because of the labiolingual thickness of the add-on composite resin in the body area of the clinical crown. In many situations some translucency is desirable because the composite resin thins out at the incisal edge. If shine-through is a problem, follow the procedure described for the Class III and Class IV restorations.

DIRECT FACIAL VENEERS

Direct composite resin veneers can be divided into two types: Those that require incisal lengthening and those that do not. If tooth length is to be maintained, place an opaque or color-modifying layer underneath a microfilled layer (Fig. 4-8A). If incisal lengthening is required, materials are used in the following order, from lingual to facial (Fig. 4-8B):
1. Opaquer
2. Hybrid or small-particle composite resin
3. Color modifiers
4. Microfilled composite resins

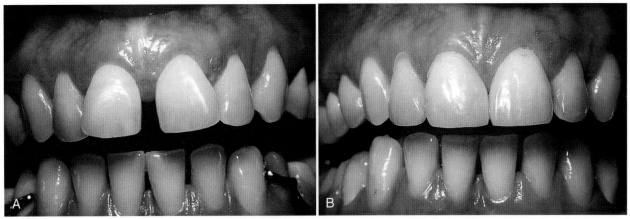

FIGURE 4-7 A, Malposed maxillary right and left central incisors with a 2-mm diastema. **B,** The distal surface was recontoured, and a mesial partial composite resin veneer was placed. Usually a matching composite resin shade can be blended into the tooth without the need for color modifiers.

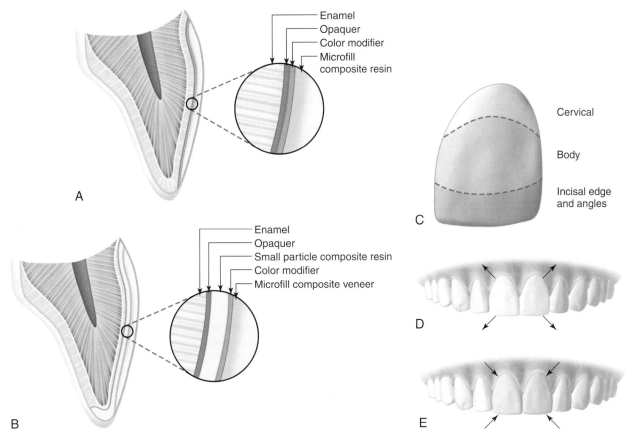

FIGURE 4-8 A, Cross-sectional view of a direct facial veneer when incisal lengthening was not required. **B,** Cross-sectional view of a direct facial veneer when incisal lengthening was required. **C,** The three zones of the clinical crown. **D,** Use of a color modifier with a high value (usually white) can make teeth appear larger and more prominent in the arch. **E,** Use of a color modifier with a low value (usually gray) can make teeth look less prominent in the arch.

The shades and distribution of color modifiers are related to the three zones of the clinical crown. Each of the zones may require a different combination of colors according to the individual requirements of the tooth to be restored (Fig. 4-8C). A color modifier with a high value (usually white), can make teeth appear larger and more prominent in the arch (Fig. 4-8D). A gray tint lowers value, which creates a less prominent appearance (Fig. 4-8E).

In addition, teeth can be made to appear narrow by staining the interproximal surfaces yellow-brown or orange. As a result, the central aspect appears relatively lighter, that is, has a higher value (Fig. 4-9A).

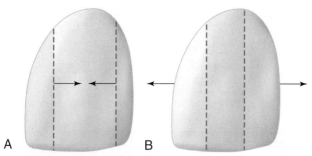

FIGURE 4-9 A, Teeth can be made to appear narrow by staining the interproximal surfaces yellow-brown or orange. **B,** Teeth can be made to appear wider by staining the central vertical axis yellow-brown or orange.

See Chapter 2) Staining the central vertical axis of the crown makes the lateral aspects appear lighter, and therefore the entire crown appears wider (Fig. 4-9*B*).

Armamentarium. Use the same dental setup as for Class III and Class IV composite resin restorations with the following exceptions:

- Assorted diamond burs for the preparation, such as 850-014, 6850-016, 8392-016, 8392-016EF, and Nixon II Kit (Brasseler USA)
- Retraction cord
  - Ultrapak No. 0 (Ultradent Products, Inc.)
  - Gingibraid No. 0 (Van R Products, Inc.)
- Mylar strips (optional) (e.g. Mylar Matrix Strips, Palmero Sales Co. Inc.)
- Wooden or clear plastic wedges (optional) (e.g., Cure-Thru Reflective Curing Wedges, Premier Dental Products)
- Color modifiers and opaquers
  - Color modifiers: yellow, yellow-brown, white, blue, gray, violet (e.g., Effect Color Heraeus Composite Tints and Opaquers, Heraeus Kulzer, Inc. USA; Creative Color, Cosmedent Inc.; Kolor + Plus Kerr Manufacturing Co.; Artiste Maverick Tints, Pentron Clinical Technology; Bisco's Characterization Tints, Bisco Inc
- Artist's brushes (e.g., Composite Brushes for Restorative Dentistry, Cosmedent)
  Clinical Technique.
1. Administer anesthetic (optional).
2. Cleanse the tooth and neighboring teeth with pumice.
3. Determine the appropriate shade while the teeth are wet with saliva.
4. Isolate the area to maintain a dry field.

> ### *CLINICAL TIP*
>
> A rubber dam is not recommended for direct facial veneers, because the creative (artistic) nature of the work requires an unobstructed view of the patient to harmonize tooth color and form with the patient's face. Moisture can usually be controlled with cotton rolls, cheek retractors, and retraction cord.

5. Prepare the teeth (Fig. 4-10*A*). The need for enamel reduction depends upon the reason for veneering.
   a. If the reason for veneering is to close diastemata and change the length of teeth with a blending shade of composite resin, minimal or no enamel reduction is necessary.
   b. If the reason for veneering is to effect a color change, enamel reduction is usually necessary to create space for color modifiers and veneer resins. In most situations, reduce the enamel by 0.3 mm in the gingival third, and by 0.5 mm in the body area. Depth-cutting diamonds (Nixon II Kit, Brasseler USA) can be used to establish appropriate levels of enamel reduction. (If the intrinsic discoloration is severe, as in the situation of tetracycline stain, reduce the enamel by 0.5 mm in the gingival third and by 1.0 mm in the body.) The gingival margin must be subgingival for major color changes. In all other situations the gingival margin should be supragingival if possible.
6. Place the opaquers and color modifiers (Figs. 4-10*B* and C).
7. Finish and polish (see the section on Class III and Class IV restorations).

> ### *CLINICAL TIP*
>
> It is usually better to complete one veneer at a time, including final polishing (Fig. 4-10*D*). This practice allows for precise evaluation of the definitive color and prevents bonding through the contact area. Unpolymerized resin from the adjacent veneer will not bond readily to the highly polished resin surface of the finished veneer.

8. To minimize the possibility of chipping, eliminate all premature centric contacts and all interferences in facial excursive movements. Provide for canine guidance whenever possible.

REPAIR OF ACRYLIC VENEER CROWNS

Partial or total separation of the acrylic veneer from an otherwise serviceable crown or fixed partial denture is common. Composite resin can be used to restore the veneer; however, an adequate layer of opaquer is necessary to conceal the metal (Fig. 4-11*A*). Both mechanical and chemical retention assist in preventing dislodgment of the restorative material.

Armamentarium. Use the same dental setup as for Class III and Class IV composite resin restorations with the following exceptions:

- Small round or inverted cone high-speed tungsten carbide burs for providing mechanical retention (e.g., No. 1 round or 33½ inverted cone bur, Operative Carbide Burs, Midwest)
- Metal coupling agent (e.g., C & B Metabond, Parkell, Inc., GC METALPRIMER II, GC America) ALLOY PRIMER, Kuraray Dental Z-PRIME Plus Bisco Scotchbond Universal Adhesive 3M ESPE
- Intraoral air abrasion unit (e.g., Microetcher ERC Sand Blaster Danville Engineering) (optional)
- Aluminum oxide—50 Micron (Danville Materials Abrasive and Polishing Material) (optional)
- Bonding resin of choice
- Composite resin of choice
- Composite resin instruments (same as those listed under Direct Labial Veneers)
- Composite resin color opaquer of choice
- Composite resin color modifiers of choice
  Clinical Technique.
1. Cleanse the tooth and neighboring teeth with pumice.
2. Determine the appropriate shade while the teeth are wet with saliva.

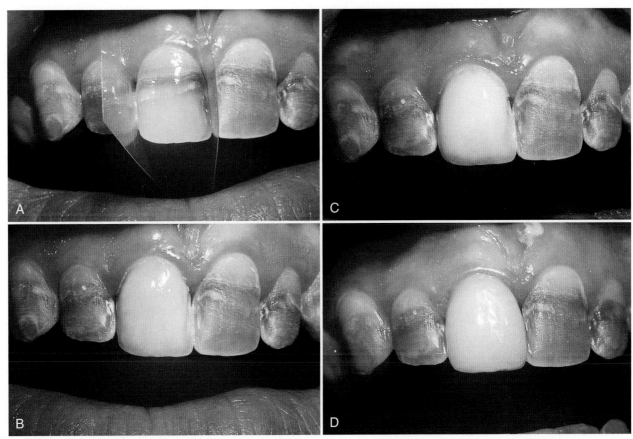

FIGURE 4-10 A, Preparation of severe tetracycline stained teeth for direct bonded facial veneers. The maxillary right central incisor has been etched and composite bond placed and polymerized. **B,** A complementary color (yellow) was placed to neutralize the blue-gray tetracycline stain. **C,** Estilux Color (white) was placed over the yellow to create a normal dentin background color. **D,** A-1 Composite was used to complete the veneer.

3. Using a water-cooled, high-speed, small, round, or inverted cone bur, remove any remaining acrylic.
4. Place retention cuts around the entire peripheral margin. Place four to six retention holes in the metal, penetrating through the metal and into the dentin (Fig. 4-11*B*). Coupling agents may preclude the need for penetration into dentin.

5. For all remaining steps, maintain a dry operating field. Air abrade the metal with 50-micron aluminum oxide.

6. Treat and coat the exposed metal surface with a coupling agent and opaquer, according to the manufacturer's recommendation (Fig. 4-11*C*).
7. Place a color modifier (if necessary) to adjust the background color (Fig. 4-11*D*).

8. Apply the composite resin in increments (Fig. 4-11*E*).
9. Finish and polish (Figs. 4-11*F* and *G*).

PORCELAIN REPAIRS

Repair of Fractured Porcelain with No Exposed Metal

Recent advances in silane coupling agents and opaquers and color modifiers have allowed for the repair of porcelain fractures of ceramometal restorations.

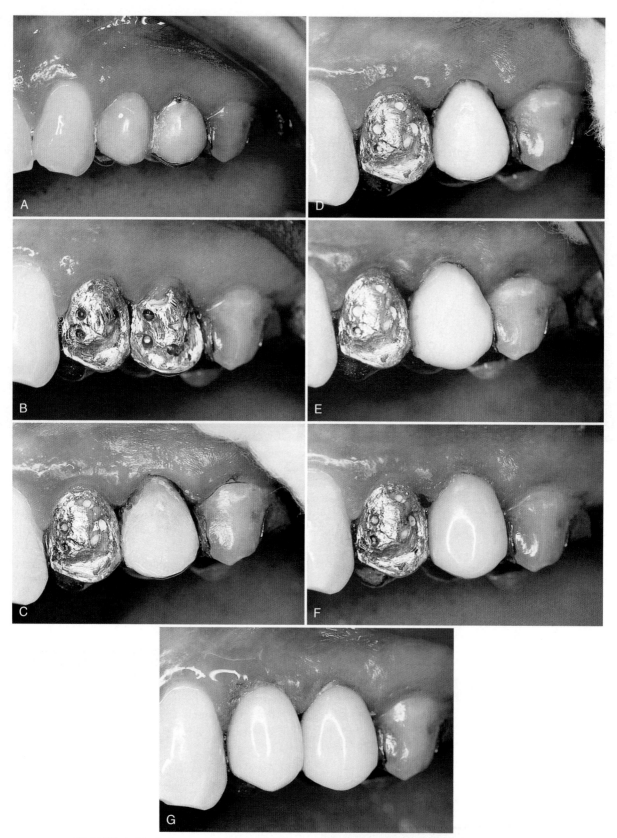

FIGURE 4-11 A, Preoperative view of defective acrylic veneer gold crowns with an inadequate opaquer. The gold can be seen through the composite resin. **B,** Retention holes are placed through the metal into dentin. **C,** After treatment with a metal bonding agent, a layer of opaquer is placed. **D,** Color modifiers are placed over the opaque resin. **E,** Incremental layers of composite resin are added. **F,** Postoperative view of the repair. **G,** Postoperative view of the repair of the adjacent tooth. (All views courtesy Dr. William Mopper.)

Armamentarium. Use the same dental setup as for Class III and Class IV composite resin restorations with the following exceptions:

- Intraoral air abrasion unit (e.g., Microetcher ERC Sand Blaster Danville Engineering) (optional)
- Aluminum oxide—50 Micron (Danville Materials Abrasive and Polishing Material) (optional)
- Hydrofluoric acid etching gel
- Rubber dam or dam replacement (e.g., OpalDam, Ultradent)
- Acid neutralizing barrier (Etch Arrest, Ultradent) (optional)
- Silane (e.g., Monobond Plus. Ivoclar Vivadent)
- Bonding resin of choice (Clearfil SE Bond Primer and Clearfil Porcelain bond can be used with Clearfil SE Bond resin without using hydrofluoric acid, Kuraray Dental)
- Composite resin of choice
- Composite resin instruments (same as those listed under Direct Labial Veneers)
- Color modifiers of choice
  Clinical Technique.
1. Cleanse the tooth and neighboring teeth with pumice. Determine the appropriate shade while the teeth are wet with saliva.
2. Using water-cooled, high-speed coarse diamonds, remove any loose porcelain and place a broad 2-mm bevel in the porcelain around the fracture site. Featheredge the porcelain peripheral to the bevel.

CLINICAL TIP

Featheredging beyond the beveled porcelain facilitates the blending of the resin into the porcelain.

3. For all of the remaining steps, maintain a dry operating field.
4. Etch the prepared porcelain with 9.5 % hydrofluoric acid gel for 90 seconds (or according to the manufacturer's instructions). Alternatively, the prepared porcelain can be air abraded with 50-micron aluminum oxide.

CLINICAL TIP

Although hydrofluoric acid for dental use is buffered, it should be handled with care. When applying it to teeth, take precautions to avoid contact with skin and mucosal surfaces (e.g., use a rubber dam or protective gel).

5. Apply silane to the prepared porcelain.
6. Let dry according to manufacturer's instructions.
7. Apply bonding resin; gently remove excess with an air syringe and polymerize.
8. Apply the composite resin in increments.
9. Apply color modifiers (if necessary).

CLINICAL TIP

Always apply color modifiers in very thin layers and be certain to observe the required curing time for each layer. Thicker layers result in incomplete curing and uneven layers caused by pooling of the material.

10. Complete the application of composite resin.
11. Finish and polish.

Repair of Fractured Porcelain with Exposed Metal

The use of metal bonding agents (Table 4-2) has greatly enhanced the ability to repair porcelain that has fractured and exposed metal (Figs. 4-12A and B).

Armamentarium. Use the same dental setup as used for Class III and Class IV composite resin restorations (see Chapter 5), but also needed are the following:

- Small round or inverted cone high-speed tungsten carbide burs for providing mechanical retention (e.g., No. 1 round or 33½ inverted cone bur, Operative Carbide Burs, Midwest)

Table 4-2 Metal Bonding Agents

Product	Manufacturer
C & B Metabond	Parkell, Inc.
Panavia 21 (nonprecious only)	J. Morita USA, Inc.
Alloy Primer	Kuraray Dental
Metal Primer II	GC America
Z Prime	Bisco, Inc.

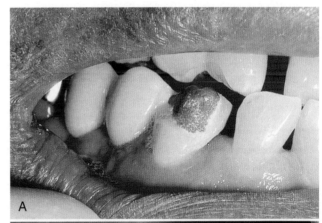
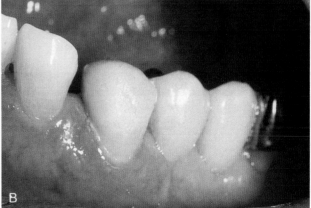

FIGURE 4-12 A, Fractured porcelain veneers with exposed metal. The metal was roughened with a coarse diamond. The porcelain was beveled, featheredged, and etched and silane was applied. **B,** The completed repair.

- Metal opaquer of choice (e.g., Creative Color Pink Opaque, Cosmedent, Inc., Panavia 21, Kuraray Dental)
- Light-polymerize resin dam material (e.g., Ginga-Guard, Cosmedent)
- Intraoral air abrasion unit (e.g., Microetcher ERC Sand Blaster Danville Engineering) (optional)
- Aluminum oxide—50 Micron (Danville Materials Abrasive and Polishing Material) (optional)
- Porcelain primer (e.g., Rely X Ceramic Primer 3M ESPE Dental Products)
- Metal primer (e.g., Metal Primer II, GC America, Inc.)
- Bonding agent (see Chapter 3)
Clinical Technique.
1. Cleanse the tooth and neighboring teeth with pumice.
2. Determine the appropriate shade while the teeth are wet with saliva.
3. Using water-cooled, high-speed diamonds, remove any loose porcelain and place a broad 2-mm bevel in the porcelain around the fracture site. Featheredge the porcelain peripheral to the bevel.

CLINICAL TIP

Featheredging beyond the bevel porcelain will facilitate the blending of the resin into the porcelain.

4. Retention can be accomplished in one of two ways:
   a. Place retentive holes through the metal.
   b. Use a coarse diamond or a microetcher to roughen the metal surface and remove the oxide layer.
5. For all remaining steps maintain a dry operating field.
6. Etch the prepared porcelain with 9.5 % hydrofluoric acid according to the manufacturer's instructions). Alternatively, the prepared porcelain can be air abraded with 50 micron aluminum oxide.

CLINICAL TIP

Although hydrofluoric acid for dental use is buffered, handle it with care. When applying it to teeth, take precautions to avoid contact with skin and mucosal surfaces (e.g., use a rubber dam or protective gel).

7. Apply silane to the prepared porcelain.
8. Let dry according to manufacturer's instructions.
9. Apply a thin layer of the metal opaquer of choice.

CLINICAL TIP

Panavia 21 will not set in the presence of oxygen. Cover the Panavia with Oxyguard for 2 to 3 minutes, then rinse off the Oxyguard and dry.

CLINICAL TIP

It is not necessary to apply a bonding resin between the metal opaquer and the composite resin.

10. Incrementally apply the composite resin of choice.
11. Apply color modifiers (if necessary).

CLINICAL TIP

Always apply color modifiers in very thin layers and be certain to observe the required curing time for each layer. Thicker layers result in incomplete curing and uneven layers caused by pooling of the material.

12. Complete the application of the composite resin.
13. Finish and polish.

REPAIR OF CERAMOMETAL MARGINS

Cervical Addition to Exposed Metal Crown Margins or Restorations of Recurrent Caries Around Ceramometal Margins

Restorations of ceramometal margins are especially complex because of the necessity for bonding to cementum, dentin, metal, and porcelain (Fig. 4-13A). The clinician should be aware of the importance of following the proper sequence in the use of the material, because the materials have specific chemistries or formulations for specific functions.

Armamentarium. Use the armamentarium listed for Repair of Acrylic Veneer Crowns, Porcelain Repairs, and Repair of Fractured Porcelain with Exposed Metal, but also needed are the following:
- Dentin bonding agent (see Chapter 3)
- Metal opaquer of choice (e.g., Creative Color Pink Opaque, Cosmedent, Panavia 21, Kuraray Dental)
Clinical Technique.

CLINICAL TIP

It is often difficult to place a rubber dam on these types of restorations (Fig. 4-13B). Take extra care to maintain a dry field and avoid contact with skin and mucosal surfaces.

1. Cleanse the tooth and neighboring teeth with pumice.
2. Determine the appropriate shade while the teeth are wet with saliva.
3. Prepare the tooth. Remove the metal collar to greatly simplify the restoration. Hold a coarse diamond at an angle to the crown and tooth, create a long bevel on the adjacent portion of the porcelain, and remove the metal collar. The crown margin should be located at a cervical level (Fig. 4-13C). Featheredge the incisal porcelain and bevel the gingival margin (Fig. 4-13D). A retention groove can be optionally placed in the gingival wall (Fig. 4-13E).

CLINICAL TIP

Featheredging beyond the beveled porcelain facilitates the blending of the resin into the porcelain.

4. For all remaining steps, maintain a dry operating field.
5. Sandblast or etch the prepared porcelain with hydrofluoric acid gel according to the manufacturer's instructions.

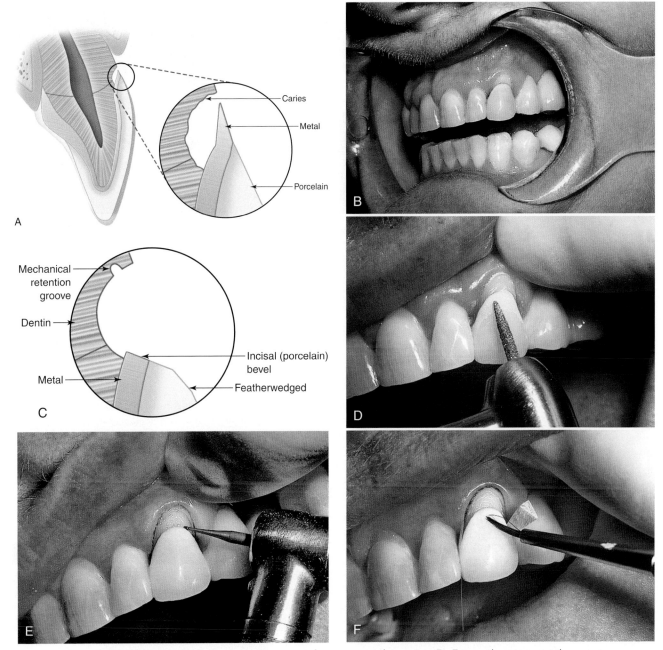

FIGURE 4-13 A, Recurrent caries around ceramometal margins. **B,** Exposed ceramometal crown margin with class V caries. **C,** The prepared tooth after removal of the metal collar and placement of a long bevel and featheredge on the porcelain. A retention groove can be optionally placed in the gingival floor. **D,** A bevel and featheredge were placed on porcelain. **E,** Class V preparation and caries removal. Note retraction cord in place. **F,** Silane was applied to the etched porcelain.

Continued

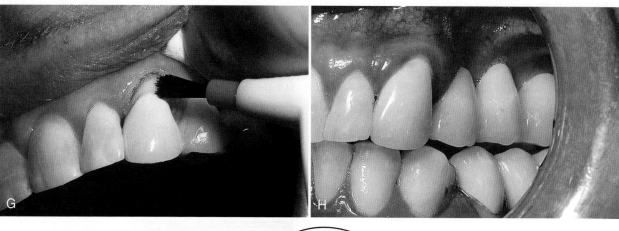

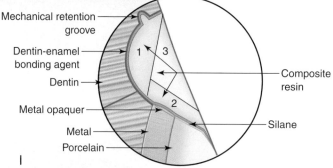

FIGURE 4-13, cont'd G, Application of bonding resin. **H,** The completed restoration with Durafill VS A-30. **I,** The completed restoration showing metal opaquer, silanated porcelain, dentin bonding agent, and incremental placement of composite resin.

CLINICAL TIP

Although hydrofluoric acid for dental use is buffered, it should be handled with care. When applying it to teeth, take precautions to avoid contact with skin and mucosal surfaces (e.g., use a rubber dam or protective gel).

6. Rinse and dry thoroughly.
7. Apply silane to the prepared porcelain (Fig. 4-13F).
8. Let dry according to the manufacturer's instructions.
9. If a large amount of metal is exposed, apply the metal opaquer of choice in thin layers.

CLINICAL TIP

Panavia 21 will not set in the presence of oxygen. Cover the Panavia with Oxyguard for 2 to 3 minutes, then rinse off the Oxyguard and dry.

10. If exposed dentin remains, apply a dentin bonding agent to the exposed dentin and enamel only (Fig. 4-13G).
11. Incrementally apply the composite resin of choice (Fig. 4-13H).

CLINICAL TIP

In general, more opaque composite resins are needed in the cervical area (e.g., Cervical Opaque Composite Shade BO [brown] or YO [yellow], Heraeus Kulzer, Inc., USA).

12. Apply color modifiers (if necessary).
13. Complete the application of composite resin.
14. Finish and polish (Fig. 4-13I).

CLINICAL TIP

Always apply color modifiers in very thin layers and be certain to observe the required curing time for each layer. Thicker layers result in incomplete curing and uneven layers caused by pooling of the material.

CONCLUSION

Composite resins have vastly increased the range of options available to the dentist. The use of color modifiers and opaquers along with agents capable of bonding to porcelain or metal, have allowed the dentist to not only create an "invisible filling" but also greatly improve the esthetics of the patient's existing dentition.

REFERENCES

1. Buonocore MG: A simple method of increasing the adhesion of acrylic filling materials to enamel surfaces, *J Dent Res* 34:849, 1955.
2. Bowen RL: Dental filling material comprising vinyl silane treated fused silica and a binder consisting of a reaction product of bisphenol and glycidyl acrylate, US Patent 3,006,112 (1962).
3. Schneider RM, Messer LB, Douglas WH: The effect of enamel surface reduction in vitro on the bonding of composite resin to permanent human enamel, *J Dent Res* 60:895, 1981.
4. Black JB: Esthetic restoration of tetracycline stained teeth, *J Am Dent Assoc* 104:846, 1982.
5. Ivoclar Vivadent Corporate: *IPS Empress Direct Color and Opaque.* http://www.ivoclar-vivadent.com/en/press/2011/ips-empress-direct-color-and-opaque. Accessed Dec 2012.
6. Felippe LA, Monteiro S Jr, Baratieri LN: Caldeira de Andrada MA, Ritter AV, *J Esthet Restor Dent* 15(6):327-336, 2003.

Composite Resin: Fundamentals and Direct Technique Restorations

Richard D. Trushkowsky

In 1955, Michael Buonocore published the first paper in the *Journal of Dental Research* describing the technique of placing an unfilled resin (Serviton) on the facial surface of incisor teeth after conditioning with two different types of acid. Conditioning with phosphoric acid resulted in a hundredfold increase in retention of the none adhesive resin to the facial surface compared with the control.[1] In 1950 a Swiss chemist named Osaka Hagger developed the first enamel and dentin bonding agent based on glycerophosphoric acid dimethacrylate.[2] In addition, Buonocore devised a phosphate-based adhesive resin in an attempt to bond composite resins to dentin.[3] However, bond strengths were only 2 to 3 MPa, whereas the bond strengths obtained with acid-etched enamel were 15 to 20 MPa. Rafael Bowen obtained the first clinically significant bond strengths in the early 1980s. He obtained measured bond strengths to dentin of 14 MPa.[4] The ability to bond reliably to dentin and enamel, in addition to the development of composite resins, led to a new era in restorative dentistry.

HISTORY

In 1938, Castan, who was working for DeTrey-Zurich, invented the epoxy resins that are the basis for current composite resins. S.A. Leader introduced an incremental layering technique involving an auto-polymerized acrylic resin in Britain in 1948, and light-curing catalysts based on alpha-diketone amines were invented by ICI in Britain.[2] Acrylic filling materials containing aluminosilicate glass filler were formulated in the 1950s. The silicate glass was precoated with polymer (or primed with silane). Although this process improved the material's physical properties, the materials were still hard to manipulate. In 1962, Raphael Bowen synthesized a new resin, a dimethacrylate

(2,2-bis-[4{2-hydroxy-3-methacryloxypropyloxy-phenyl}]-propane, referred to as *bis-GMA*).[5] Bis-GMA is a reaction product of bisphenol A and a glycidyl methacrylate.

Bis-GMA was only originally available in a chemically polymerized system as a powder-liquid or paste-paste formulation. Ultraviolet (UV)-polymerized resins were developed in 1972. This form of curing allowed adequate working time because the setting time was under the control of the clinician. Light-activated composite resins were reported by Michael Buonocore in 1970 and introduced by L.D. Caulk in 1971. Visible light-polymerized systems have exponentially increased composite resin use and improved on problems inherent in UV systems. Composite resins have undergone continuous development, but they still remain similar to the original formulation by Bowen.[6] Nevertheless, many improvements have been made in the resin and filler compositions. Previously a general trend had been to reduce filler particle size and optimize its distribution, which improves the physical properties. More recently changes have been concentrated on the polymeric matrix of the material to create materials with decreased polymerization shrinkage, reduce polymerization stress and create materials that are self-adhesive to tooth structure.[7-9] Another aspect that has been addressed is the degree of conversion. Bis-GMA/TEGDMA only exhibits a 60% conversion, leaving more than 15% as free monomer. This jeopardizes biocompatibility and both physical and mechanical properties of the composite resin material.[10] The replacement of bisphenol A diglycidil methacrylate (Bis-GMA) or triethylene glycol dimethacrylate (TEGDMA) with urethane dimethacrylate (UDMA) resulted in materials like Venus Diamond and Venus Pearl (Heraus Kulzer, Inc.) (which has UDMA and TCD-urethane) having a high diametral tensile strength (DTS) . In addition to a higher

DTS, the solubility decreases because of higher conversion. Long-term water sorption is also lower. However, Schmidt and Ilie[11] found, despite some improvements in macromechanical properties such as DTS, that micromechanical properties such as hardness value (HV) and creep were affected negatively for nanohybrid composite resin such as Venus Diamond and N'Durance (Septodont).[12] Ilie and Hickel found nano-hybrids have good flexural values (FVs), excellent DTS but poor flexural modulus (FM). The decrease in particle size was needed for improved esthetics but the increased surface area to volume ratio of fillers in nanocomposite resins results in increased water uptake and degradation of the filler/matrix interface reducing mechanical properties.

BASIC CHEMISTRY

Composite resin literally means "of distinct phases."[5] Composite resins have four main components: (1) a matrix (resin) phase (dimethacrylate resin or polymerizable resin), (2) polymerization initiators (activated either chemically or by visible light), (3) a dispersed phase of filler and tints, and (4) a coupling phase that results in the adherence of the matrix to the filler particles (e.g., silanes). The matrix (resin) phase consists of polymerizable monomers that are changed from a liquid phase to a highly cross-linked polymer upon exposure to visible light, and the creation of free radicals resulting in polymerization. The fillers increase the modulus and radiopacity, modify thermal expansion, and reduce polymerization shrinkage as a result of reducing the volume of resin.[13] The filler-resin interface allows the joining of the polymerizable matrix to the filler particles. A diluent (e.g., triethylene glycol dimethacrylate, or TEG-DMA) is often added to control viscosity to make the polymerized resin more flexible and less brittle.[14]

In 1974, another difunctional resin, urethane dimethacrylate was introduced. (Note: A difunctional molecule has two reactive groups for polymerization.) Its low viscosity allows an increase in filler loading without the need for the addition of low molecular weight monomers to lower viscosity. However, urethane dimethacrylate is more brittle and undergoes more polymerization shrinkage than bis-GMA.[5]

In 2007, 3M ESPE introduced Filtek Silorane to reduce polymerization shrinkage without reducing physical and handling properties. Unlike previous composite resins that rely upon radical polymerization of methacrylates and acrylates Filtek Silorane restorative uses a new ring opening silorane chemistry. Siloranes are a combination of siloxane (known for their hydrophilicity) and oxiranes (known for their low shrinkage and stability). Polymerization of this material occurs via a cationic ring-opening reaction, which results in a lower polymerization contraction. This counteracts the loss of space when chemical bonds are formed. In addition to shrinkage, polymerization stress can be detrimental to the longevity of the restoration. Polymerization stress is created when composite resins are polymerized in the bonded state and the polymerization shrinkage develops forces on the cavity walls. Polymerization stress is determined by the following: polymerization shrinkage, the internal flow of the material, and the polymerization speed. Fast curing rates do not allow enough time for viscous flow, and the elastic modulus acquisition in composites occurs rapidly.[13]

Initiators in the system are camphorquinone (matches conventional light sources), iodonium salts and electronic donors serve to generate cationic species that initiate the ring-opening process. The three-component initiating system must generate sufficient cationic species to start the polymerization process. However, the system required a new adhesive because the silorane resin is more hydrophobic than conventional methacrylate resins, which results in less water uptake. The adhesive is designed as a two-step process with the adhesive self-etch primer hydrophilic and the adhesive bond optimized for wetting and adhering to the hydrophobic posterior restorative.[12]

Another light activated low-shrink composite resin (N'Durance, Septodont) contains monomer resulting from dimer acid. The dimer acid derivative monomers create homopolymers with high conversion, low shrinkage, and a high degree of hydrophobicity. A new filler system consists of two types of nanofillers (silica and ytterbium fluoride) and conventional barium glass.[9]

Initiators are also added to produce the free radicals necessary for polymerization. Heat-activated systems split benzoyl peroxide to form free radicals. In chemically activated systems, benzoyl peroxide is split by a tertiary aromatic amine (acting as an electron donor) into free radicals. UV light-activated systems use a 365-nm UV light source to split benzoin methyl ether into free radicals without tertiary amines. Visible light-polymerized systems use a 468 ± 20 nm light source to excite camphor quinones or other diketones to react with an aliphatic amine to start a free radical reaction. This amine is more color stable than the aromatic amine in chemically polymerized composite resins.

Chemical activation results in the least uniform curing of the resin systems. Air incorporation during mixing weakens the resin because oxygen inhibits polymerization. Mixing also causes voids, which may result in increased surface roughness and long-term discoloration.

The dispersed phase, or inorganic filler component, is responsible for the improved physical properties; the fracture resistance, wear resistance, polymerization shrinkage, water sorption, and coefficient of thermal expansion improve as the amount of filler in the composite resin increases. Common filler particles include quartz, lithium, aluminum silicate, borosilicate, barium, and other glasses. These particles range in size from 0.5 to 10 μm.

In the definitive or coupling phase, the properties of a composite resin improve as the attraction of the filler to the resin matrix increases. The adhesion between resin and filler transfers stress between both components. Silanes, which are bipolar molecules, are often used to bring the two phases together. Theoretically silanes chemically bridge the matrix and filler stages. Unfortunately, silanes have a tendency to dimerize or trimerize, forming acrylate moieties that do not function as a coupling agents.[15] Long-term hydrolysis may reverse this coupling by allowing water to penetrate the resin matrix.

PARTICLE SIZE

The type and size of the filler particles used in a composite resin affect its handling properties and longevity. Composite resins originally contained very large particles (15-100 μm). Quartz was the most commonly used filler in the first generation of composite resins. It has excellent esthetics and durability, but its lack of radiopacity is a distinct drawback, especially for posterior resins.[5] It is also difficult to obtain a smooth surface with quartz because polishing causes exposure of the large, irregular particles, and plucking these filler particles from the surface causes increased roughness and staining. In addition, masticatory stress is transferred through these filler particles to the resin matrix, causing microcracks in the resin matrix.[16] The sizes of the particles in macrofilled composite resins have been reduced to about 1 to 5 μm (small particles). Heavy-metal glasses such as strontium and barium are smaller, radiopaque, easier to grind, and softer, resulting in improved polishability and decreased roughness and staining.

Microfilled resins were developed in the late 1970s to improve polishability. They are produced from silicon dioxide ash (fumed silica) or by adding colloidal sodium silicate to water and hydrochloric acid (colloidal silica). Microfills can either be homogeneous (i.e., formed by adding the microfiller directly to the resin) or heterogeneous (i.e., formed by compressing the microfiller into clumps and adding the clumps to heated resin). These prepolymerized resin filler blocks are ground and added to unpolymerized resin, which also contains microfiller. Microfills contain submicroscopic silica particles about 0.04 in size. The filler concentration is usually 35% by weight. They polish extremely well and maintain the polish over time. However, they are weaker than hybrids, have increased water sorption, are not radiopaque and exhibit reduced fracture toughness. They are usually best suited for Class III and Class V restorations.

Hybrid composite resins combine particles of different sizes; small particles (0.6-5 mm) and 0.04 mm microfillers are added to the resin matrix. The shape of the filler particle determines its properties. Irregularly shaped particles cause stress concentration at the area where the particle is angled.[14] Spherical particles distribute stress between the filler and the matrix more uniformly. Manufacturers have also introduced microhybrid composite resins with particles ranging from 0.02 to 1 μm to improve polishability and strength. However, these restorations do not maintain their polish over time. Nanocomposite resins are composed of two varieties of nanofillers, nanomeric particles, and nanoclusters. The nanomeric particles consist of monodispersed discrete nonaggregated and nonagglomerated nanosized silica particles that are 20 nm and 75 nm in diameter.[17]

Radiopacity is desirable in Class II and Class III restorations. However, this can be detrimental when veneering the facial area of a tooth; radiographic contrast is reduced, making caries detection more difficult. Different composite resins have different degrees of fill and radiopacity and different shades. Hybrid composite resins and microfilled resin placement both have advantages and disadvantages. Hybrid composite resin is less technique sensitive than microfilled resin and shrinks less on polymerization. Therefore less microleakage would occur at the gingival margin of Class II or Class III restorations if the shrinkage and strength of the dentin bonding were the only considerations. Paradoxically, several in vitro studies have shown that microfilled resins can produce a better seal than hybrid composite resins.[18,19]

The microfiller particles in the resin matrix may increase the stress-bearing capacity and reduce microcrack propagation. Increased filler loading by weight also increases physical properties. The addition of microfiller particles allows the production of a relatively smooth surface. This, combined with high translucency, allows the use of a hybrid resin in critical esthetic areas.

In an attempt to overcome the disadvantages of self-polymerized glass ionomers, new generations of the materials have been developed. The new materials are hybrids of conventional glass ionomer cements and visible light-activated resin. The term *resin-modified glass ionomer* refers to materials that are set with an acid-base reaction in addition to photochemical polymerization. Materials that contain glass ionomer ingredients but do not exhibit an acid-base reaction are called *polyacid-modified resin composite resins*, or *compomers*. The compomers have a relatively high bond strength and fluoride release. Because their modulus of elasticity is close to that of tooth structure, the strain capacity of the restoration is increased and its deformation under a load is prevented, preserving adhesion at the margins of the restoration. The strength of compomers is higher than that of resin-modified glass ionomers but lower than composite resins. Flowable composite resins, or new, low-viscosity resin composite resin materials have also been introduced. However, their mechanical properties are about 60% to 90% as strong as those of conventional composite resins. Flowable composite resins are created by retaining the same size of traditional hybrid composite resins but reducing the filler content and increasing the resin, thereby reducing the viscosity of the mixture. Flowable composite resins are very useful for minimally invasive techniques, especially those used in conjunction with air abrasion. Some clinicians have recommended their use under Class I and Class II composite resins to achieve an initial seal and, as a result of their reduced modulus of elasticity, to reduce strain in the definitive restoration. The physical properties of currently available materials vary widely. However, some flowable materials have a filler content approaching that of conventional composite resins.[20]

Recently there has been an introduction of self-adhesive flowable composite resins Vertise Flow (Kerr Corp.) and Fusio Liquid Dentin (Pentron Clinical). Both systems are derived from traditional methacrylate products and also contain acidic monomers that are incorporated in self-etching bonding agents. However, phosphoric acid etching was required to achieve higher bond strength to enamel. Torii et al. demonstrated that self-etching adhesives are not capable of decalcifying the enamel prism core and enamel adhesion is adversely affected.[21]

GENERAL CONSIDERATIONS: ACID ETCHING

Mature enamel contains 96% to 97% inorganic material (mainly hydroxyapatite) by weight. The rest is mainly water (≈4%) and organic material or collagen (≈1%). The enamel's surface is usually covered by an organic pellicle,[22] which makes bonding difficult because of its low reactivity.[23] Etching enamel with phosphoric acid raises the critical surface tension and increases the bonding area and roughness, allowing the hydrophobic resins to penetrate the porosities of the dry etched enamel.[24] Some important acid etching considerations include the following:

1. Liquid acid etchants must be applied repeatedly because they have a tendency to dry on the tooth surface. Gel etchants can be left in place for the required time.
2. The top layer of fluoride-rich enamel is removed with a diamond bur, and pumice is used to remove plaque. A commercial prophylaxis paste can be used if it does not contain oils or is water soluble. Fluoridated water can be used for rinsing.[25,26]
3. Rubber dam isolation or other precautions are necessary to minimize gingival fluid contamination or ambient moisture.
4. Etchants should be applied for 15 seconds. If this does not produce a frosted appearance on the enamel after washing

and drying, etch repeatedly in 15-second increments until the frosted appearance is obtained. Recent studies have shown that shorter etching times produce the same or greater adhesive strength than the originally suggested 60 seconds.[27]

In addition, morphologic studies have shown significant differences in etching results based on the viscosity of the etchant.[28,29] A liquid or a thin gel produced a more even etch pattern than a thick gel. In addition, the thin gel seemed to have the best defined etch pattern. Etching for too long produces insoluble reaction products and a weak bond.[5] A selective etch can be achieved with a high viscosity phosphoric acid product Select HV Etch (Bisco, Inc.).

5. Some reports have stated that agitation with a soft brush may alter the etching pattern.[29] Mechanical agitation of the etching agent allows fresh acid to be in constant contact with the enamel,[30] which increases the amount of enamel that is dissolved.[31] The agitation of etchant may also aid in removing residual precipitates.[32] Other studies have concluded that agitation has no effect on the outcome of the etch.[33]

6. Shiny areas that appear after etching indicate the presence of old composite resins. The resins can be removed with a diamond bur and etched again to obtain the appropriate frosted surface.

7. An effective bond between composite resin and etched enamel can be achieved with a short rinse of the etchant from the etched enamel surface. Studies have concluded a 2- to 5-second rinse per tooth surface should sufficiently cleanse gel-etched enamel, resulting in adequate shear bond strength.[33] Rinsing for 1 second from a smooth enamel surface resulted in essentially no microleakage.[34-36]

8. Bleaching teeth before bonding may adversely affect bond strengths and result in increased microleakage. Hydrogen peroxide may denature proteins in the organic components of dentin and enamel. The presence of oxygen, a breakdown product of hydrogen peroxide has been associated with the reduction in bond strength. Oxygen can inhibit the curing of composite resins and reduce adhesion. The oxygen remains trapped in the porous enamel. Dentin traps oxygen longer than enamel because it is more porous. Waiting 1 to 2 weeks after bleaching allows tensile bond strengths to return to a value comparable to that of unbleached dentin.[27] Saliva, with its high remineralization capacity, may increase remineralization of bleached enamel.[37] Peroxide is an oxidant and may react with the highly organic smear layer and interfere with bonding and hybrid layer formation. Surface porosity and formation of precipitates increase as bleaching time increases. Bleaching may also increase the microleakage of previously placed composite resin. The leakage appears to be specific to the cementum-dentin margin[36,38-40]and is not reversed after subsequent exposure to saliva. Water-clearing solvents such as acetone and ethanol-based adhesive systems can reverse the effects of bleaching on bond strengths.[40]

ENAMEL AND ENAMEL-DENTIN BONDING

Currently, dental adhesives are categorized according to their bonding regimens, etch and rinse with two or three steps and self-etching systems with one or two steps. Bonding agents are unfilled or lightly filled composite resins that improve the bond between a viscous composite resin and the microporosities

created in the etched enamel. Application of a bonding agent reduces microleakage. Dentin-enamel bonding agents are more hydrophilic and can strengthen the bond between composite resin and dentin.

Etching enamel surfaces with phosphoric acid results in a superficial etched zone and underlying qualitative and quantitative porous zone.[41] The depth of the etched zone and the amount of the surface enamel removed during this etching procedure depend on the acid concentration, duration of the etching process, and the chemical composition of the etchant.[3] Adhesion to dentin is more of a challenge. Previous dentin bonding systems did not yield high bond strengths in the laboratory or prevent microleakage. Newer dentin-enamel adhesive systems use a phosphoric acid to condition the dentin, and then the primer resins in acetone, alcohol, or aqueous solution are placed on the dentin and allowed to diffuse into the few micrometers of tissue rendered porous by acid conditioning. This will result in the formation of a hybrid zone.[42]

Hybridization created by resin interdiffusion into open dentin tubules seems to be a requirement for adequate bonding. The hybrid layer acts as a stress absorber against polymerization shrinkage.[42]

The physical integrity of collagen is a key factor in bonding to dentin. The phosphoric acid used during the removal of the smear layer denatures the exposed collagen. The degree of denaturation depends on the phosphoric acid concentration and exposure time. The demineralized and denatured collagen fibers collapse easily during air drying and lose their permeability to resin monomers. Effective priming is needed to reexpand the collapsed collagen network and allow permeation of bonding monomers.[43] In addition, acid-denatured collagen fibers are susceptible to hydrolysis unless they are sufficiently enveloped by the primer. Reexpanding the collagen fibers is accomplished by strict adherence to the manufacturer's instructions during this critical stage. Exposed collagen fibrils created by incomplete resin infiltration may undergo denaturation, creep[44] or cyclic fatigue rupture[45] after extended function. The resulting denuded collagen matrices are filled with water that allows the hydrolysis of resin matrices by esterases and collagen by means of endogenous and exogenous collagenolytic ennzymes.[46]

Optimal bond strength is derived from the complete resin's diffusion into the chemically altered dentin. Moisture plays a significant role in achieving optimal bond strength for some of the resins in fourth-generation dentin bonding.[47-49]

The most effective solvent systems incorporate water, which reexpands collapsed fibrils. The water in the adhesive may simultaneously expand the collagen fibrils and allow better resin infiltration.[43] Bonding to dry dentin reduces potential bond strengths because of collagen collapse. Increased microleakage occurs in cervical areas because the bond between the composite resin and cervical dentin or cementum is much weaker than the bond to the occlusal enamel.[50,51]

Brushing on only a thin layer of bonding agent may be better than air drying, which can incorporate air into the composite resin and inhibit curing. Air drying from a triple syringe can also incorporate moisture into the preparation (see Chapter 3).

CLINICAL TIP

Dry with a syringe that is not connected to a water line or with a hair dryer to prevent moisture contamination.

Unfortunately, the bond to dentin is not as durable as the bond to enamel because dentin bonding relies on the diverse nature of dentin with hydroxyapatite in a network of collagen.[51] The interface between the dental substrate and the adhesive depends on two relatively recent approaches: two-step etch-and-rinse or self-etch. However, placing all the adhesive components in one bottle required increased acidity and more hydrophilicity. The pulpal tissue also provides outward pressure through fluid-filled tubules making the dentin surface moist and rendered it hydrophilic. However, because of the hydrophilicity of the dentin surface created by these bonding agents, fluid is moved from the tubules toward the bonded interface creating two disadvantages.[52,53] One disadvantage is a result of water attraction. It is difficult to evaporate all the water in all-in-one adhesives and water rapidly diffuses back from the bonded dentin into the adhesive resin. The water plasticizes polymers and lowers their mechanical properties. Water trees can form despite the addition of hydrophobic dimethylacrylates as the hydrophilic monomers cluster together to form hydrophilic domains. Staining can also be a problem.[54]

POLYMERIZATION SHRINKAGE

The polymerization reaction consists of three stages: (1) initiation, (2) propagation, and (3) termination. Initiation occurs when the camphorquinones are promoted to a free radical state. When the free radical camphorquinone reacts with a monomer molecule, it forms a bond that converts the monomer to a free radical state. Propagation occurs when this camphorquinone-monomer-free radical complex reacts with another monomer and converts it into another free radical. This chain reaction terminates when two free radical complexes react with each other to form a stable bond. Ideally, the termination should not occur too quickly so that the free radical complex can react with many monomers, thus creating longer, more flexible polymer chains. If termination occurs too rapidly, the chains are too short (and therefore less flexible). Reducing the number of available free radicals can minimize early termination of the reaction. This makes it more likely that the free radicals will react with a monomer and increase chain length rather than react with other free radicals and terminate the polymerization reaction.

A major drawback of using composite resin as a direct restorative material is polymerization shrinkage. Linear polymerization shrinkage (i.e., a straight-line measurement of shrinkage) is approximately 0.4% to 1.6%.[55] Commercial materials contract by 2% to 5% by volume during setting. Volumetric shrinkage is related to the density of the material—the higher the filler content by weight, the less volumetric shrinkage. Volumetric shrinkage is determined by placing a sample in a liquid (usually water or mercury) and measuring the displacement before and after the reaction. Cracks in enamel margins caused by polymerization shrinkage have been reported.[42] Polymerization shrinkage may cause marginal gaps, promoting postoperative sensitivity, marginal staining, and recurrent caries. Composite resin shrinkage is dictated by the volume fraction (the relative amounts of filler and resin material) of the polymerized resin, its composition and the completeness of the curing reaction.

Several techniques to overcome this problem include the use of self-polymerized materials or glass ionomers that have slower setting rates than light-polymerized composite resins.[56,57]

Application of an intermediate layer of a low-viscosity resin or a resin-modified glass ionomer cement between the dentin and the restoration has been shown to relieve polymerization stress by 20% to 50%.[45,58] A gradual transition in modulus of elasticity from dentin through the bonded interface to the restoration resin appears to be desirable. Bulk placement may result in less shrinkage, but if the surfaces remain bonded the resin composite resin has internal stress that can be alleviated by initial flow. The total shrinkage and its stress field are a result of the combined effect of the contraction of all the incremental layers and the deformation of the surrounding tooth structure of the definitive restoration. When the restoration is in full contact with the cavity, the polymerization contraction of each individual filling increment will cause some deformation of the cavity, forcing the cavity wall inward and downward and decreasing the cavity volume.[59]

Polymerization shrinkage has been periodically reduced by introducing changes in chemistry and composition.[60] However, elastic modulus, post-gel shrinkage, filling and curing protocol, cavity shape, and remaining tooth structure need to be considered in calculating shrinkage stress.[61] The introduction of low-shrinking composite resins has modified composite resin placement techniques. Incremental layering may no longer be necessary, offering the advantage of bulk placement, which would streamline composite resin placement. However, a recent study demonstrated incremental placement of composite resin still may be beneficial as higher bond strengths were achieved because there was more free surface (reduced C-factor), creating less stress on the bond.

In addition, greater exposure to light not attenuated by material thickness resulted in a higher degree of conversion, which allowed better adaptation of the composite resin and reduced microleakage even with low-shrinkage composite resins.

A higher degree of conversion of composite resin will provide increased toughness (the resistance to fracture from impact) and greater biocompatibility as less monomer is released. The newer materials have provided a higher degree of conversion but with minimum contraction stress. In addition, adequate conversion at the floor of the preparation must be accomplished. Nanohybrid composite resins based on new Nano-Dimer Technology has shown reduced shrinkage stress from 2.3% to 1.5% on average for conventional composite resins and shrinkage stress of N'Durance (Septodont) was reduced from 2.5% to 1.1% with an increase of approximately 27% of the conversion of the N'Durance monomer to a polymer. This is owing to a lack of BIS-GMA. A series of high molecular weight monomers with different functional groups were manipulated to create dimers that decreased initial double-bond concentration to reduced volume shrinkage. The dimers are created from a core configuration built on hydrogenated dimer acid. The dimers produce a polymer with high flexibility and decreased modulus of elasticity.[62] In addition there was a 27% increase of monomer conversion.[9] N'Durance shows a 75% conversion of monomers to polymers compared with that of Bis-GMA. The material also has low water absorption and minimal solubility, making it very color stable and exhibiting minimal staining. The wear rate is similar to enamel.[63]

DENTIN BONDING AND POLYMERIZATION SHRINKAGE

The placement of bonded composite resins into cavity preparations leads to a competition between polymerization contraction forces and the bond to tooth structure. If the lesion is completely surrounded by enamel (Fig. 5-1A), the stress is relieved by detachment of composite resin from the dentin; however, marginal integrity in enamel is maintained. If the lesion is completely contained within the root surface (Fig. 5-1B) and polymerization shrinkage forces exceed the instantaneous strength of the dentin bonding agent, the restoration may leak and will most likely dislodge. The most common clinical situation involves a restoration that is bonded to enamel incisally and to the root structure at the gingival margin (Fig. 5-1C).

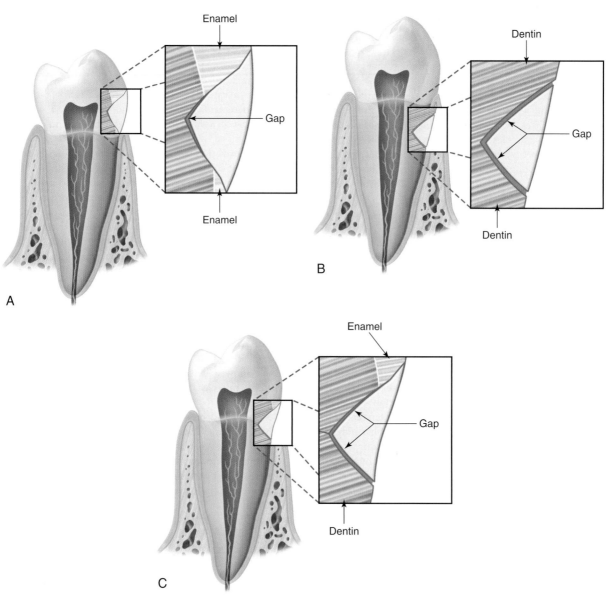

FIGURE 5-1 A, In a restoration completely surrounded by enamel, polymerization contraction causes composite resin to detach from the dentin. Although a gap may form under the restorations, the marginal integrity in the enamel is maintained. If the dentin bonding agent could be formulated to be as strong as an enamel bonding agent, the composite resin could break away from the enamel or cause the enamel rods to pull out. If the enamel and dentin bonds hold, they could place the tooth and resin under tremendous stress. **B,** If the restoration is completely contained within the root surface and polymerization shrinkage forces exceed the instantaneous strength of the dentin bonding agent, a gap may form around the entire restoration, possibly leading to leakage and restoration failure. **C,** The most commonly seen clinical situation: a restoration bonded to enamel incisally and to the root at the gingival margin. If the dentin bond is not instantaneous and is not stronger than the composite resin shrinkage, a contraction gap forms at the gingival margin, resulting in restoration failure. (Modified from Davidson CL, Kemp-Shulte CM: Shortcomings of composite resins in Class V restorations, *J Esthet Dent* 1:1, 1989.)

If the dentin bond is not instantaneous and not stronger than the composite resin shrinkage, a contraction gap forms at the gingival margin and the restoration will probably leak at that location. The amount of stress development can be controlled to some extent by the configuration factor (or *C-factor*—the ratio of bound to unbound surfaces of adhesive restorations); the use of bases; the size, shape, and position of increments placed in the cavity; and the type of resin curing (i.e., light polymerized or chemically polymerized). Studies have found no significant difference in marginal integrity using a self-polymerized composite resin (P-10) and a light-polymerized composite resin (Z-100).[64] Ideally, the C-factor should be kept as low as possible by the use of chemically polymerized resin and low-modulus liners.[65] Reestablishment of marginal seals may occur as a result of gradual expansion of the composite resin as a result of water sorption; however, this depends on the configuration of the cavity and the resin volume. Polymerization is rapid, whereas this process is slower and allows bacterial invasion to occur. Water sorption may cause erosion of the filler and matrix, possibly resulting in a reduction in strength stiffness and wear resistance.[66]

A linear relationship between light intensity and polymerization contraction has been demonstrated. Reduced rates of polymerization during the maturation of the bond between the tooth structure and the composite resin may allow for increased flow of material and less stress formation, which may disrupt the bond between the tooth and restoration.[67-71] Some reports state that even thin layers of composite resin, such as those produced under porcelain inlays, can produce shrinkage stress that challenges the dentin fond.[72]

LINERS AND BASES

Traditionally, liners and bases have been used under restorations. However, new developments in liners and bases and an increased understanding of pulp biology have changed the indications for use of these materials.

The current generation of dentin bonding agents has significantly reduced the need for protective liners and bases. However, despite dramatic improvements since their introduction, modern dentin bonding agents leak immediately when bonded to superficial dentin. Nearly all dentin bonding agents show significant loss of bond strength when bonding to deep rather than superficial dentin.[73,74] This difference is a result of the amount of intertubular and peritubular dentin found at different dentinal depths. Deep dentin has more peritubular dentin and more surface moisture.

In some specific instances, placement of a liner may be warranted. Calcium hydroxide is still useful for direct pulp capping as a stimulus for reparative dentin formation, despite its inability to provide a permanent seal against bacterial invasion. This inability to form a permanent seal may be caused by tunnel defects that form in reparative dentin and the eventual dissolution of the calcium hydroxide after long-term placement.[75,76] Tunnels in a dentin- bridge are inactive vascular channels that were once active. The number and sizes of vessels injured by exposure determine the number of tunnels formed during the healing process.

CLINICAL TIP

After any pulpal exposure the preparation should be disinfected with Concepsis (Ultradent) and then dried. Alternatively, 2.625% sodium hypochlorite can be applied and then rinsed off with water. (Sodium hypochlorite also helps create hemostasis.) An adequate amount of calcium hydroxide to cover the exposure should be applied, and then a small amount of light-polymerized resin-modified glass ionomer should be used to cover the calcium hydroxide, creating a bacterial barrier.[77,78]

CLINICAL TIP

Alternatively, TheraCal (Bisco, Inc.) a light-polymerized, resin-modified calcium silicate filled base/liner could be placed. The calcium release and alkaline pH promotes sealing of the pulp, hydroxyapatite formation, and secondary fixed partial denture formation. Another material, Biodentine (Septodont), a bioactive cement with dentin-like properties, also can be used as a pulp-capping material. The material consists of a powder in a capsule and a liquid in a pipette. The powder consists of tricalcium and dicalcium silicate (the principal component of portland cement), calcium carbonate, and zirconium oxide as contrast medium. The liquid consists of calcium chloride in aqueous solution and polycarboxylate. The powder and liquid are triturated for 30 seconds and set in 12 minutes.

The preparation is then etched and primed and adhesive is applied.

CLINICAL TIP

The use of any calcium hydroxide should be kept to a minimum because it dissolves over time, resulting in an unsupported restoration.[79]

Light-polymerized glass ionomers are useful as liners because of their good compressive strength, adhesiveness to dentin, and ability to release fluoride and chemically bond to the composite resin restoration. Glass ionomers are useful for eliminating undercuts and developing the ideal thickness for indirect ceramic restorations. They are also useful, as indicated in the previous Clinical Tip, as part of the direct pulp-capping process. In deep-cavity preparations, placement of glass ionomers reduces the bulk of composite resin, resulting in less stress. The release of fluoride may reduce instances of recurrent caries.[80,81]

CLINICAL TIP

Placing resin ionomers, such as Vitrebond (3M ESPE), or Fuji Liner LC (GC America, Inc.) in the gingival portion of Class II, Class III, and Class V composite resin restorations (the "open-sandwich" technique) may be a practical method of reducing microleakage, especially apical to the cementum-enamel junction.

CLINICAL TIP

If postoperative sensitivity is anticipated because of the preparation depth, a glass ionomer, light-polymerized resin-modified glass ionomer, or resin ionomer can be used as a dentin replacement. The material should be built up to resemble the form of an "ideal" cavity preparation. Gluma Desensitizer PowerGel or Calm-It (Dentsply Caulk) desensitizers can also be used to reduce or eliminate hypersensitivity because these Glutaraldehyde-based products react with plasma protein in dentinal fluids to block the dentinal tubules.[83] The evaluation of dentinal tubule occlusion by desensitizing agents: a real-time measurement of dentinal fluid flow rate and scanning electron microscopy.

Marginal Bevels

Enamel margins of composite resin restoration are beveled in most situations. Beveling enamel provides an increased surface area for etching, resulting in increased retention and reduced microleakage. The beveling exposes the ends of enamel rods, which is optimal for acid etching.[82] Bevels should be prepared with a medium grit diamond bur.

Beveling provides a gradual transition between the composite resin restoration and the tooth. Bevels of 45 degrees and 1 to 2 mm wide are used in facial areas, whereas a smaller (0.5-mm) bevel is used in other areas. (A wider bevel is placed on the facial surface to achieve better blending in the esthetic zone.)

Bevels (on the occlusal surface) should be avoided in Class I and Class II restorations because thin composite resin margins are subject to fracturing. Widening the preparation to allow a bevel may extend the restoration into areas of occlusal function and possibly increase wear.

Areas at the cervical margin with only a thin layer of enamel should not be beveled because thin areas of enamel may be removed. It is always desirable to terminate the restoration on enamel rather than cementum or dentin.[50,84]

FINISHING

Finishing involves margination, contouring, and polishing. The primary goals are good contour, occlusion, smoothness, and appropriate embrasure form.[5]

> ### CLINICAL TIP
>
> Adequate contouring of a restoration before polymerization is essential for minimizing finishing time and reducing damage to the composite resin. (Finishing procedures can cause microcracks.) Damage to the composite resin results in a higher wear rate, an increased fracture rate, and a greater tendency for opening of margins.

The bonding agent should cover all etched enamel surfaces. Etched enamel that is not covered with resin may take as long as 2 to 3 months to remineralize, leaving the tooth surface vulnerable to discoloration. Running a composite resin knife, a number 12 Bard Parker blade, or a gold foil finishing instrument from the enamel to the composite resin will remove all unattached bonding agent. (These instruments are also excellent for removing small proximal overhangs in Class II restorations before finishing with aluminum oxide strips [see Fig. 5-5D].) This will leave a small step, which can be finished with composite resin finishing diamonds or disks. The restoration can have a lifelike appearance. Finishing burs, diamonds, rubber points, and disks can be used to create lobes, ridges, and surface texture. To produce a textured surface, a slight excess of composite resin is left after finishing. A micron diamond can be used to produce the desired texture. A polishing cup and polishing paste are then used to bring out the luster, although care should be taken not to destroy the created texture.

The restoration is smoothed with discs or rubber polishing instruments for the anterior surface and points, cups, and brushes for the posterior surface. Metal or plastic finishing strips can be used interproximally. Some controversy surrounds whether burs or diamonds are best for finishing composite resins. Diamonds are usually preferred because finishing burs are more damaging to the surface, causing more plucking of filler particles. These defects result in staining or loss of surface luster. Micron diamonds at slow speeds (with water spray to prevent clogging of the diamonds) can be used for excess removal and contouring and to provide a smooth surface with minimal resin damage. A variety of shapes, sizes, and degrees of fineness are available. White and green stones can loosen the fillers from the resin matrix and need to be used with copious amounts of water to prevent heat buildup.

POLISHING

Achievement and maintenance of a smooth surface on a restoration will improve esthetics and in addition reduce plaque and stain formation.[85]

Several studies have suggested certain techniques may be suitable for specific materials.[86] Differences in surface smoothness has been demonstrated using identical finishing systems with different composite resins.[87]

Microfilled composite resins can be polished with disks. The tooth surface should be wet when using coarse disks and dry when using superfine disks. The heat from the dry disk procedure produces a durable, highly polymerized smear layer of resin over the microfill. However, aggressive use of disks may destroy the previously created texture. A composite resin polishing paste (Prisma Gloss, Dentsply Caulk; Enamelize, Cosmedent, Inc.; HiLuster PLUS Polishing System, Kerr Corp.) can be used if necessary for 15 to 30 seconds using a rubber cup moistened with water. Small particle hybrids are polished with fine diamonds, flexible disks, and a very fine polishing paste (e.g., Luminescence, Premier, or Nano/Microhybrid Diamond Polishing, Cosmedent, Inc.).

> ### CLINICAL TIP
>
> Surface-penetrating sealants (e.g., Fortify, Bisco, Inc.; Optiguard, Kerr Corp.) can be used to repair surface defects created during finishing, which improves the wear of posterior composite resins and decreases microleakage around Class V composite resins.[88] In addition, the composite resin that is closest to the light is often the most polymerized and therefore the hardest part of the restoration. Because this layer is removed with occlusal adjustment and polishing, placement of the sealant and postcuring are necessary.[89-91]

> ### CLINICAL TIP
>
> It is impossible to overcure a composite resin. An additional 60-second polymerization is recommended if the tooth is dark or a dark shade of composite resin is used. The additional polymerization is most beneficial after the restoration is finished to its definitive form.

TECHNIQUES AND MATERIALS

Class I Composite Resin Restorations

Armamentarium.

* Standard Dental Setup
  * Explorer
  * Mouth mirror
  * Cotton forceps
  * Anesthesia (if necessary)
  * Rubber dam setup
  * High-speed handpiece
  * Slow-speed handpiece
* Burs: carbide (e.g., #557, #330, #4, S.S. White Technologies, Inc.)
* Diamond: coarse and medium grit (e.g., Brassler USA, Axis Dental, Premier Dental Products, Inc., Komet USA)
* 37% phosphoric acid
* Placement and carving instruments (e.g., instruments by Hu-Friedy Mfg., Co; Cosmedent, Inc.; Coltene/Whaledent, Inc.; Premier Dental Products, Inc.; Almore International)
* Suitable liner (if necessary) (e.g., Vitrebond Plus, 3M ESPE, Vivaglass Liner, Ivoclar Vivadent; Fuji Lining LC, GC America Inc., Ionosit, DMG America)
* Suitable base (if necessary) (e.g., Vitromer Cement, 3M ESPE, Fuji II LC, GC America, Inc.)
* Articulating paper or wax (e.g., Bausch BK 01, Bausch, Inc.; Accufilm II, Parkell, Inc.)
* Radiopaque composite resin or microfilled resin designed for posterior use (e.g., Surefil, Caulk/Dentsply; Z-100, Paradigm Nano Hybrid, Filtek Supreme Ultra Nano composite resin, 3M EPSE; Herculite XRV Microhybrid, Herculite Ultra Nanohybrid, Kerr Corp.; Heliomolar and Tetric N-Ceram, Ivoclar Vivadent)
* Oil-free pumice (Moyco Technologies, Inc.)
* Cavity disinfectant (e.g., Tubulicid Red, Temrex Corp.; Consepsis, Ultradent, Inc.)
* Composite resin placement syringe (e.g., Centrix Syringe, Centrix, Inc.)
* Glycerin gel (e.g., Liquid Strip, Ivoclar/Vivadent, Inc.)
* Finishing instruments (e.g., Esthetic Trimming Kit, Brasseler, USA; Raptor System, Bisco, Inc.; Two Striper MPS Kit, Premier Dental Products, Inc.)
* Polishing instruments (D*Fine, Clinicians Choice; Diacomp II, Brasseler; Flexi [points, cups, and wheels], Cosmedent, Inc.; Composite resin Technique Kit, Shofu, Inc.; Diagloss, Axis Dental; Composite Resin Polishing System, Komet USA)
* Polishing paste materials (e.g., Luminescence, Premier Dental Products, Inc., Prisma Gloss, Dentsply Caulk, Inc.; Diamond Polishing Paste, Shofu, Dental Corp.)

Clinical Technique.

1. Cleanse the tooth with pumice.
2. Evaluate the shade of the tooth before isolation (from the middle third of tooth).
3. Use articulating paper to determine the location of occlusal contacts so that they can be avoided, if possible, during preparation.

> **CLINICAL TIP**
>
> If the occlusal surface is intact, fabricate a registration of the occlusal surface with a clear polyvinyl siloxane bite registration material (e.g., Memosil, Heraeus Kulzer, Inc.; Sharp Parkell, Inc.) or a thermoplastic button (Advantage Dental Products). (This step decreases the need for subsequent carving and occlusal adjustment.)[91]

4. Administer local anesthetic if necessary.
5. Isolate the area with a rubber dam.

> **CLINICAL TIP**
>
> The preparation does not have to be extended to dentin for retention.

6. Place an appropriate liner or base if necessary. See section on Liners and Bases in this chapter.

> **CLINICAL TIP**
>
> See the Clinical Tip concerning pulpal exposure and alternative treatments in the section Liners and Bases.

> **CLINICAL TIP**
>
> The use of any calcium hydroxide should be kept to a minimum because it dissolves over time, resulting in an unsupported restoration.[79]

> **CLINICAL TIP**
>
> See the Clinical Tip concerning postoperative sensitivity in the section Class I Composite Resin Restorations.

7. Etch the enamel for 15 seconds and the dentin for 10 seconds. See the section on Acid Etching.
8. Wash with water and/or water/air spray for a minimum of 10 seconds for gel or liquid etchants. See the section on Acid Etching.
9. Air dry the enamel and blot the dentin, leaving it slightly moist. The cavity preparation can be disinfected with a cavity disinfectant and the excess blown off and blotted with a cotton pellet. However, in some systems the smear layer is not removed but only modified, and bond strengths may decrease as a result of disinfection.[92,93]
10. Repeat the procedure if the enamel does not have a frosted white appearance after air drying. If the dentin is dry, moisten the dentin again with a cotton pellet moistened with water.
11. Place the dentin-enamel bonding agent according to the manufacturer's instructions.
12. With a syringe, place an increment of a dentin shade posterior composite resin against the pulpal floor and against one of the buccal cusps. Light polymerize for 40 seconds through the cusp. Build up the other buccal cusp and subsequently the lingual cusps in a similar manner. This creates appropriate fissure position and depth.

> **CLINICAL TIP**
>
> When composite resin is initially polymerized with an attenuated light, a better interface between the composite resin and tooth surface is created. Curing through the tooth

structure provides the light attenuation. Because polymerization shrinkage occurs toward the bonded surface, curing through the tooth may allow the composite resin to better adapt. See the complete discussion on this topic in the conclusion of this chapter.

13. Place tints and opaques to achieve a natural appearance. Place brown and ochre tints into pits and fissure and white or colored opaques at the crest of triangular ridges (e.g., Kolor+, Kerr Corp.; Creative Color, Cosmedent, Inc.).
14. Place a layer of an enamel/incisal composite resin to build up the definitive contour. This anatomic layering technique reduces stress within the adhesive interface.
15. Place glycerin to reduce the air-inhibited layer. Light polymerize for 40 seconds.

16. Finish the restoration. See the section on Finishing.[95]
17. Polish the restoration. See the section on Polishing.
18. Sealant and postcuring procedures are the following:
    a. Rinse off polishing debris with water; air dry.
    b. Etch for 15 seconds.
    c. Rinse with water for a minimum of 10 seconds.
    d. Air dry the surface. (If the surface is not enamel, leave it moist.)
    e. Apply sealant (e.g., Fortify, Bisco, Inc., Optiguard, Kerr Corp., PermSeal, Ultradent Products, Inc.)
    f. Air thin.
    g. Light polymerize for 40 seconds.

Class II Composite Resin Restorations

Improved clinical performance has been a result of more durable dentin bonding[96-98] and improvement in composite resins.[99-101] However, despite these resin improvements, composite resins remain technique sensitive.[102] Failures often involve inadequate proximal contours and contacts, microleakage, secondary caries, postoperative sensitivity, occlusal wear, marginal degradation, and bulk fracture of the material.[103]

Occlusal Wear. In the 1960s, high wear rates made the composite resins unacceptable for restoring occlusal surfaces.[104] However, recent formulations have reduced the wear rate for many materials to 7 to 10 μm per year. The composite resins have been made radiopaque, allowing the detection of excess material and recurrent decay.[105] The addition of ytterbium trifluoride provides an element of fluoride release (e.g., Heliomolar).

Postoperative Sensitivity. Postoperative sensitivity was initially attributed to inadvertent acid etching of the dentin.[106] However, recent research has shown that pulp inflammation is primarily caused by bacterial microleakage resulting from a breakdown of marginal integrity of the restoration.[107]

Light-polymerized composite resins are generally used for posterior restorations because they are more resistant to occlusal wear. Unlike chemically polymerized resins, which contract toward the geometric center (Fig. 5-2A), light-polymerized resins shrink toward the light source (Fig. 5-2B).

The portion of the composite resin closest in proximity to the light hardens first, pulling the composite resin away from the gingival margin. However, it is now believed composite resins polymerize toward the bonded surface (see the discussion [Versluis] in the conclusion at the end of this chapter). This process results in leakage, especially if the restoration terminates on dentin or cementum.[108-111]

When present, cervical enamel bonds poorly compared with occlusal enamel. Sometimes enamel prisms can actually be torn during shrinkage toward the occlusal surface.

Incremental curing reduces but does not eliminate the gingival shrinkage (Fig. 5-2C). A plastic wedge acting as a fiberoptic guide can further reduce the gap[112] (Fig. 5-2D), especially in combination with incremental placement of resins[113] (Fig. 5-2E,F). However, the plastic wedges do not adapt to varying tooth morphology and may loosen during manipulations of the restorative material. There is a difference in opinion as to whether or not wedges with a reflecting core

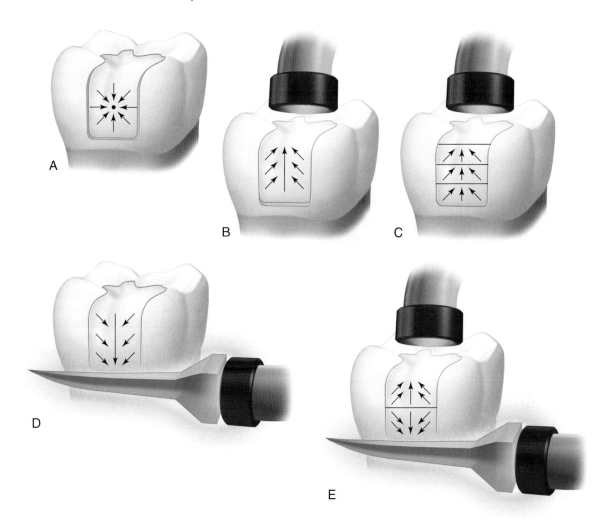

FIGURE 5-2 A, Chemically polymerized composite resin shrinks toward the geometric center of the mass. This may only occur if the composite is not bonded. It is believe that composites shrink toward the adhesively bound surfaces.[59] This process leaves a small contraction gap at the gingival margin. The composite resin is strongly bonded to enamel on the buccal and lingual walls, preventing the formation of gaps at these walls; however, stresses may be set up in the tooth and the composite resin. **B,** Photopolymerized composite resin shrinks toward the light source because the composite resin closest to the light hardens first. This pulls the softer composite resin from the gingival areas, creating a gap. The mass of composite resin being pulled to the occlusal area is twice that found in chemically polymerized resins; therefore the gingival contraction gap is roughly twice as large. Studies show that composites shrinks toward the adhesively bound surfaces.[59] However, if the contraction is toward bound surfaces and not toward the light, this would not occur. **C,** Incremental curing reduces but does not completely eliminate the gingival contraction gap. **D,** A plastic wedge, which acts as a fiberoptic extension, can pull the composite resin gingivally to minimize gap formation. **E,** Although not ideal, this incremental technique should reduce the gingival contraction gap and the stress better than a two-increment technique involving only occlusal curing. The first layer is placed and photopolymerized through the plastic wedge. A second layer is placed and polymerized occlusally. Two improvements could be made in the most gingival increment. First, regardless of tooth color, a light-color resin should be used to ensure additional curing depth. Second, before adding the definitive increment, a second, occlusal polymerization of the first increment should be performed to ensure complete hardening of the mass. (Modified from Lutz F et al: Improved proximal margin adaptation of Class II composite resin restorations, *Quintessence Int* 17:659, 1986.)

Continued

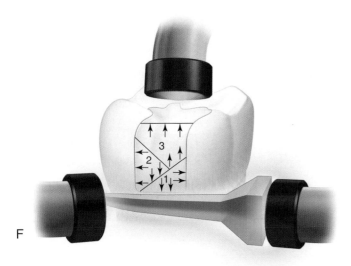

FIGURE 5-2, cont'd F, A technique that takes advantage of composite resin contraction and uses only one 11- to 13-mm polymerized light tip. The first increment can be pulled lingually and gingivally (via the light-reflecting wedge directing light at a 90-degree angle to the light tip) before an additional occlusal polymerization. The second increment is pulled buccally and gingivally before it too receives an additional occlusal polymerization. The definitive increment is hardened occlusally after placing a ball of prepolymerized composite to act as an internal wedge. Additional occlusal increments may be necessary in large teeth. This design also minimizes pulling together of the cusps.

are more effective in producing better polymerization than clear wedges. It has been stated that light reflecting wedges with a reflecting core to be more effective in producing better polymerization than clear wedges.[114]

Cure-Thru Wedges, Premier Dental Products, Inc. or (Cure Through G-Wedge, Garrison Dental Solutions) reversed the shrinkage vectors 180 degrees (by directing them toward the enamel margins).[115] Use of retention cuts has been recommended to reduce gingival margin microleakage.[115] However, this cuts were no benefit with an incremental technique. In general the clinician should minimize the size of the cavity preparation so that only carious areas are encompassed. Extension of the gingival floor or embrasure area or extension into other cuts on the occlusal surface is unwarranted. The pulpal floor need only be as deep as the dimension of the lesion because composite resin has a relatively low elastic modulus, and incorporation of the energy-absorbing properties of dentin is not needed.[116] Evidence suggests that shrinkage can pull cusps together, creating postoperative sensitivity. If this occurs, bisecting the restoration (from mesial to distal) to the occlusal floor permits the cusps to spring back and eliminates the sensitivity.

> **CLINICAL TIP**
>
> Placing a sectional matrix decreases sensitivity because an overly tightened circumferential matrix can pull the cusps together (i.e., Contact Matrix System, Danville Materials, and Composi-Tight 3D, Garrison Dental Solutions; V3 Ring [Narrow and Universal], Triodent Ltd.).

Research suggests that a layering procedure can minimize cusp contraction. Buildup of individual cusps prevents the cusps

from being pulled together. Although many clinicians advocate a layering buildup of the composite resin to minimize the amount of polymerization shrinkage and reduce the possibility of enamel fracturing, several studies advocate bulk placement of composite resin in Class II preparations.[117, 118] Two of these studies used a dual-polymerized material (Marathon, Den-Mat Corp). It was theorized that shrinkage occurs toward the center of its mass, and the slightly warmer surface of the tooth may initiate polymerization at the junction between the wall of the preparation and the composite resin.[119,120] However, further research is necessary to validate this concept.

The advent of bulk placement is evidenced by the recent introduction of several new materials such as Quixx (which is very translucent) and Surefil SDR flow (Dentsply/Caulk),[121,122] Venus Bulk Fill (Heraeus Kulzer), SonicFill (Kerr Corp.), X-tra fil (Voco GmbH), Tetric Evoceram bulk fill (Ivoclar/Vivadent), and Filtek Bulk Fill Flowable Restorative (3M ESPE).

SureFil stress decreasing resin (SDR) achieves stress reduction by inserting a polymerization modulator into the polymerizable resin. This has been found to act in conjunction with the camphoquinone photoinitiator to slow modulus development. This results in less stress but no decrease in polymerization rate or conversion. There is more linear/branching chain propagation and minimal cross-linking creating a decreased rate of modulus development.

One of the controversies surrounding the bulk fill technique is the depth of polymerization (DOC). It has been suggested that changing the definition of DOC may be appropriate by taking into account the transition between glassy and rubbery states of the resin matrix.[123] The authors felt that current methods such as microhardness, degree of conversion, and scraping methods do not detect this transition and may have the consequence of overestimation of the DOC. If the organic matrix is not vitrified but exists in a gel state, flow will lead to reduced stress on the existing tooth structure. The depth of polymerization may not properly evaluate the quality of the polymerization and the degree of cross-linking has to be considered.[123] In addition, Flury et al. demonstrated the current ISO 4049 method overestimated DOC as compared with DOC as extrapolated from Vickers hardness.[124] Frauscher and Ilie found "curing time" and "material" demonstrated the greatest effect on depth of polymerization (DOC) with newer materials such as N'Durance and Venus Diamond, showing the lowest decrease of conversion with increased depth and the best DOC.[125]

Tight Proximal Contacts. Placement of the posterior composite resins depends on the matrix for correct interproximal contour. Unlike an amalgam restoration, a circumferential band is not necessary and a contoured segmental matrix may be preferred. In a mesial-occlusal-distal (MOD) composite resin restoration, the wedge and matrix initially should be placed on the distal side only, which displaces the tooth slightly in a mesial direction. (Placing a wedge and matrix simultaneously on the mesial surface would interfere with and prevent some of this mesial displacement and increase the chance of an open, or "light," contact.) Similarly, when the mesial surface is filled, no wedge or matrix should be present at the distal surface.

> **CLINICAL TIP**
>
> A small, egg-shape ball of prepolymerized composite resin (shaped and polymerized on the finger) can be wedged into unpolymerized composite resin (at increment 3) against the

axial wall and the band. The composite resin ball acts as an additional wedge,[126-129] placing pressure from within on the axial wall and the matrix. A plugger is used to exert active downward pressure and expose increment 3 (unpolymerized) to the curing light. The mesial box is restored in a similar manner, with the composite resins joined at the occlusal area.

CLINICAL TIP

When new composite resin is added within 5 minutes of placement of uncontaminated polymerized composite resin, chemical adhesion is as strong as it would be if the two resins had been placed simultaneously.[130,131]

Strengthening Cusps. A dentist may think that a strong dentin-enamel bond and high composite resin tensile strength can tie the buccal and lingual cusps together to strengthen the tooth. However, research on this topic is equivocal. One study has shown that this method causes less reinforcement because of thermal cycling.[132]

Contact Forming Devices. Various devices and instruments have been manufactured to aid in achieving a tight contact (e.g., Contact Pro 2, CEJ Dental, Inc.; Belvedere Contact Former, American Eagle Dental Instruments; Composite resin Contact Instrument, Premier; Light-Tip, Denbur;[133-135] Trimax, AdDent, Inc., PerForm Proximal Contact Instrument, Garrison Dental Solutions). These instruments are made of a wide variety of materials and shapes, and they all have a range of advantages and disadvantages.

Most of the instruments reduce the bulk of composite resin, thereby reducing polymerization shrinkage. They also expedite contact formation. However, the contact formed is not always at the correct height, dimension, and position.[126,127] Devices such as the Light Tip permit curing at the critical gingival area.[136]

Multiple-Step Buildup Technique.
Armamentarium.
Use the same dental setup as for Class I restorations with the following exceptions:
- Mylar matrix strip (possibly the contoured variety), a sectional matrix and Bitine ring, or a retainerless matrix system (e.g., AutoMatrix II, L.D. Caulk; ReelMatrix, Garrison) that can be preloaded with a wide variety of bands (pediatric, metal, combination, and transparent; e.g., Slick Bands Tofflemire matrices, G-Wedge, or Composi-Tight 3D Clear Sectional Matrix System, Garrison Dental Solutions)
- Light-reflecting wedge (Cure-Thru, Premier Dental Products, Cure Through Wedge Wands. Garrison Dental Co.; Luciwedge, Coltene/Whaledent) or a contoured Sycamore Wedge (Premier)
- Radiopaque composite resin or microfilled resin designed for posterior use (e.g., Heliomolar RO, Tetric Evo Ceram, Tetric EvoCeram Bulk Fill Ivoclar/Vivadent, Inc.; Surefil, Caulk/Dentsply, Inc.; Herculite XRV, SonicFill Kerr Corp., Clearfil Majesty Posterior Kuraray Venus Heraeeus-Kulzer, Inc.; Filtek P60, Filtek P250, Fitek Supreme Ultra, 3M ESPE)
Clinical Technique.
1. Determine the appropriate shade of the tooth while it is wet with saliva.
2. Cleanse the tooth with pumice and clean the proximal surface with a strip where necessary.

3. Before cavity preparation, use articulating paper to ensure that the cavity design avoids including occlusal contacts where possible.

CLINICAL TIP

See the ClinicalTip concerning the fabrication of a registration of the occlusal surface with a clear polyvinyl siloxane bite registration material in the section Class I Composite Resin Restorations.

4. Administer appropriate anesthesia if necessary.
5. Place a rubber dam. When warranted, the preparation may be *entirely* based in enamel, because extension into dentin for retention is not necessary.
6. Place appropriate liner and base if necessary. (See section on Liners and Bases.)

The preparation is then etched and primed and adhesive is applied.

CLINICAL TIP

See the Clinical Tipconcerning pulpal exposure and alternative treatments in the section on Liners and Bases.

CLINICAL TIP

The use of any calcium hydroxide should be kept to a minimum because it dissolves over time, resulting in an unsupported restoration.[79]

CLINICAL TIP

See the Clinical Tip concerning postoperative sensitivity in the section Class I Composite Resin Restorations.

7. Etch the enamel for 15 seconds and the dentin for 10 seconds. See the section on Acid Etching.
8. Wash with water and/or water/air spray for a minimum of 10 seconds for gel or liquid etchants. (See the section on Acid Etching.)
9. Air dry the enamel and blot the dentin, leaving it slightly moist. The cavity preparation can be disinfected with a cavity disinfectant and the excess blown off and blotted with a cotton pellet. However, in some systems the smear layer is not removed but only modified, and bond strengths may decrease during disinfection.[77,78]
10. Repeat the procedure if the enamel does not have a frosted white appearance after air drying. If the dentin is dry, moisten the dentin again with a cotton pellet moistened with water.
11. Place selected matrix, retainer, and wedge.
12. Place the appropriate dentin-enamel bonding agent.
13. A thin layer of a flowable composite resin (e.g., Tetric Flow, Ivoclar/Vivadent; Flow-It, Jeneric-Pentron) can be placed at the gingival margin and all axial walls, which allows curing of the initial thin layer of composite resin to seal these critical areas. However, research has not demonstrated any reduced microleakage.[137,138]

14. Depending on the composite resin used, the subsequent step may vary. Materials such as Surefil are recommended for bulk placement if the curing depth is not greater than 5 mm. Other materials may require a layered buildup of the composite resin in 2-mm increments.

15. An alternative is to use the "snowplow" technique. Place a flowable resin (Filtek Bulk Fill) into the apical third of the proximal box but do not light polymerize. Inject a conventional composite resin (Filtek Supreme Plus) into the flowable composite resin under pressure and without creating any bubbles. Remove the excess composite resin, contour the material, and light-polymerize.[138]

> ### CLINICAL TIP
> If the first two layers are not visible in the facial display, use a light-color resin to ensure more complete light penetration and subsequent polymerization.

> ### CLINICAL TIP
> Place an incremental layer of composite resin on the lingual wall; it should not touch the buccal wall (see Fig. 5-2F). Use bonding agent, rather than alcohol, to prevent the composite resin from sticking to the plastic instrument. See the Clinical Tip on bonding resin and alcohol in the section on Class I Composite Resin Restorations.

> ### CLINICAL TIP
> Place the composite resin with a Centrix-type syringe (see Fig. 5-5A). See the Clinical Tip on Centrix syringes in the section on Class I Composite Resin Restorations.

16. Polymerize from the lingual direction for 60 seconds if a 2-mm layer of composite resin is the initial increment. During bulk placement, polymerize proximally for 60 seconds if the areas (buccal and lingual surfaces) are accessible to the light, and then polymerize the occlusal surface for 60 seconds.

> ### CLINICAL TIP
> Use an 11- to 13-mm angle-tip light to ensure that the light exposes the lingual surface and the wedge (if a light conducting wedge is used), which optimizes light direction vectors and polymerization (see arrows in Fig. 5-2E).

17. Polymerize from the occlusal direction for 60 seconds for incremental placement.
18. Remove the wedge and place it buccally.
19. Place a second layer of composite resin on the buccal wall. It should not touch the lingual wall.
20. Polymerize from the buccal direction for 60 seconds.
21. Polymerize from the occlusal direction for 60 seconds.
22. Shape a small piece of posterior composite resin into an egg-shaped ball on a gloved finger and polymerize the resin.

> ### CLINICAL TIP
> Wash and dry your gloves before beginning this procedure so that no powder remains on the surface.

23. Place the resin into the proximal box, and push the ball into the polymerized resin so that it contacts the axial wall and the Mylar strip. This forms an internal wedge to further tighten the contact with the adjacent tooth. Remove the excess composite resin with an interproximal carver. See section on finishing in this chapter.
    Alternative method: If a contact-forming instrument is used, the proximal box is filled and the instrument inserted and torqued toward the adjacent tooth (Fig. 5-3). An interproximal carver is used to remove the excess material. The composite resin is then light polymerized and the remainder of the box filled.
24. Polymerize from the occlusal direction for 60 seconds.
25. Add additional increments as necessary. The shade of these increments should blend with the surrounding tooth structure. The definitive increment should be a translucent layer (enamel replacement).

> ### CLINICAL TIP
> The previously fabricated occlusal registration can be used at this time. It is pressed back into position, and the resin is light polymerized for 60 seconds from the occlusal direction. Occlusal adjustments are minimal when this technique is used.

> ### CLINICAL TIP
> In a mesial-occlusal-distal preparation, fill the distal portion first and place the Mylar or metal strip and wedge in the distal area only. It is usually not necessary for the matrix to encircle the tooth; the absence of the band and wedge in the mesial area ensures tighter distal contact. Remove the distal matrix and repeat the process in the mesial area.

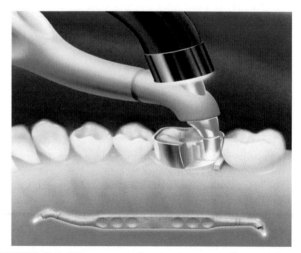

FIGURE 5-3 Trimax contact forming instrument (*bottom*). Trimax instrument in position (*top*). The light from the curing unit is transmitted through the adjustible light conducting tip into the composite resin. (Courtesy AdDent, Inc., Danbury, CT.)

26. Adjust the occlusion and contour the restoration See the section on finishing.
27. Polish the restoration. See the section on Polishing.
28. Sealant and postcuring procedures are the following:
    a. Rinse off polishing debris with water; air dry.
    b. Etch for 15 seconds.
    c. Rinse with water for a minimum of 10 seconds.
    d. Air dry the surface. (If the surface is not enamel, leave it moist.)
    e. Apply sealant (e.g., Fortify, Bisco, Inc.; Optiguard, Kerr Corp.).
    f. Air thin.
    g. Light polymerize for 40 seconds.

> **CLINICAL TIP**
>
> Although not mandatory, sealing can increase wear and stain resistance. Sealants should be polymerized in 40-second increments.

> **CLINICAL TIP**
>
> See the Clinical Tip concerning the composite resin closest to the light in the section Class I Composite Resin Restorations.

Class III Composite Resin Restorations

Class III restorations include the simple two-surface lingual approach situation and the three-surface facial approach situation. The three-surface through-and-through preparation presents shade matching and blending challenges because of darkness "show through" from the back of the mouth. A radiopaque composite resin material should be used to aid in the detection of recurrent decay.

Armamentarium. Use the same dental setup as for Class I restorations with the following exceptions:

- Conventional Mylar strip, stop strips (Mylar anterior bands with an integrated stopper to secure the matrix band between adjacent teeth; Premier Dental Products, Inc.)
- Strip aids (Premier, Inc.)
- Wedges (desirable if near the gingiva; Premier, Inc.)
- Hybrid composite resin (e.g., Renamel, Cosmedent Inc.; Z-100, 3M, Inc.; TPH Spectrum, Caulk/Dentsply, Inc.; Tetric, Ivoclar Vivadent)
- Microfilled composite resin (e.g., Silux Plus, 3M ESPE; Durafill Heraeus, Kulzer, Inc.; Renamel, Cosmedent, Inc.; Epic-TMPT, Parkell, Inc.)
Clinical Technique.
1. Pumice the tooth and clean the proximal surface with a strip where necessary.
2. Determine the appropriate shade of the tooth while it is wet with saliva.
3. Apply appropriate anesthesia if necessary.
4. Place a rubber dam.
5. Determine the direction of access depending on the extent of decay, and prepare the tooth as conservatively as possible.
6. Place appropriate liner or base if necessary. See the section on Liners and Bases.

> **CLINICAL TIP**
>
> See the Clinical Tip concerning pulpal exposure and alternative treatments in the Section Liners and Bases.

> **CLINICAL TIP**
>
> The use of any calcium hydroxide should be kept to a minimum because it dissolves over time, resulting in an unsupported restoration.[79]

> **CLINICAL TIP**
>
> See the Clinical Tip concerning postoperative sensitivity in the section Class I Composite Resin Restorations.

7. Place a bevel of 1 to 2 mm on all visible margins with a medium grit diamond to aid in creating an invisible restoration (Fig. 5-4A).
8. Place 0.5-mm bevels on nonvisible margins except in areas that are in occlusion. No bevel is necessary on cementum.
9. Place appropriate liner and base if applicable (Fig. 5-4B). See the section on Liner and Bases.
10. Etch the preparation with 37% phosphoric acid several millimeters past the bevel for 15 seconds (Fig. 5-4C). Protect the adjacent teeth with a Mylar strip.
11. Wash with water and/or water/air spray for a minimum of 10 seconds for gel or liquid etchants. See the section on Acid Etching.
12. Air dry the enamel and blot the dentin, leaving it slightly moist. The cavity preparation can be disinfected with a cavity disinfectant and the excess blown off and blotted

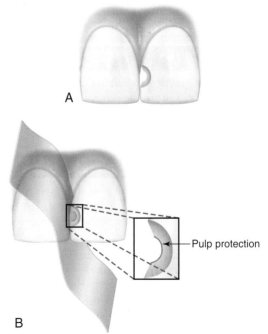

FIGURE 5-4 A, Because the lesion is completely surrounded by enamel, the definitive preparation does not require an undercut. Note the bevel around the entire preparation. **B,** A Mylar strip is placed, and calcium hydroxide or a glass ionomer cement or both can be placed if necessary.

Continued

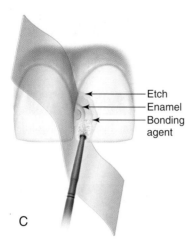

C

FIGURE 5-4, cont'd C, A brush being used to apply acid etchant to enamel and dentin followed by a wash, dry, and the use of a different brush for the application of an enamel dentin bonding agent. The gel etchant can also be applied with a syringe and needle.

with a cotton pellet. However, in some systems the smear layer is not removed but is only modified, and bond strengths may decrease during disinfection.[92,93]

13. Repeat the procedure if the enamel does not have a frosted white appearance after air drying. If the dentin is dry, moisten the dentin again with a cotton pellet moistened with water.

14. Place the primers and adhesive resin according to the manufacturer's directions and light polymerize for 20 seconds.

Placing the Restorative Material. The cavity can be filled in one or two increments, depending on its size and configuration.

Type I Class III Restorations: Lingual Access Only.

1. Place the Mylar strip interproximally and inject hybrid composite resin (dentin replacement).

CLINICAL TIP

Use bonding agent rather than alcohol to prevent the composite resin from sticking to the plastic instrument. See the Clinical Tip on bonding resin and alcohol in the section on Class I Composite Resin Restorations.

CLINICAL TIP

Place the composite resin with a Centrix-type syringe (Fig. 5-5A). See the Clinical Tip on Centrix syringes in the section on Class I composite resin restorations.

---

2. Overfill the cavity slightly and pull the Mylar strip to the facial to properly adapt the composite resin.

3. Wrap the strip around the proximal surface, keeping it tightly adapted at the gingival margin. (A wedge can be used to stabilize the strip or minimize excess, but this may also cause gingival bleeding.)

4. Hold one finger on the facial side of the Mylar strip and compress the strip. The strip will "bow out" to contact the adjacent tooth.

5. Polymerize from the facial direction for 60 seconds. The facial area therefore is fully cured, whereas the lingual area is partially cured (see Fig. 5-5A).

6. Remove the gloved finger from the Mylar strip and cure from the lingual direction for 60 seconds (Fig. 5-5B).

7. Contour and finish the restoration (Fig. 5C-F). See the section on Finishing.

8. Polish the restoration. See the section on Polishing Considerations.

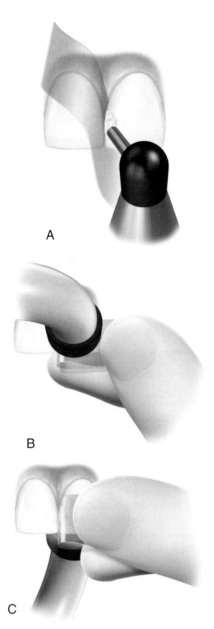

A

B

C

FIGURE 5-5 A, Application of the composite resin with a syringe minimizes "pullback," which often occurs when hand-held instruments are used. **B,** The Mylar strip is pulled tightly with finger pressure to minimize subsequent finishing. Placement of a wedge to reduce gingival composite resin excess is optional. Note that the index finger exerts facial pressure against the Mylar strip. In addition to reducing composite resin excess, the facial direction of force moves the central incisors slightly facially during the polymerization. When the pressure is released, the tooth springs back, which can partially compensate for the thickness of the Mylar strip and ensure a tight contact area. **C,** After 60 seconds of facial curing, the lingual resin has partially hardened. A 60-second lingual polymerization completes the process.

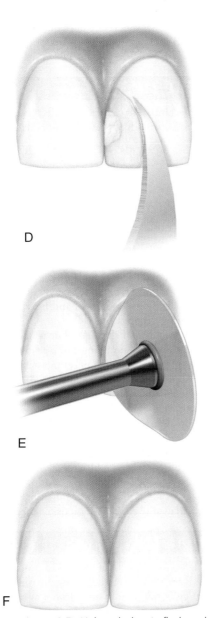

D

E

F

FIGURE 5-5, cont'd D, Unbonded resin flash and small resin overhangs are removed with a Bard-Parker blade or composite resin knife before the definitive polishing. The hand-held instrument is always moved from the tooth to the composite resin. **E,** Shaping and polishing can be done with diamonds, burs, disks, or rubber wheels. This step is followed by application of composite resin polishing paste using a prophy cup or felt wheel. **F,** The finished restoration.

9. Sealant and postcuring procedures are the following:
    a. Rinse off polishing debris with water; air dry.
    b. Etch for 15 seconds.
    c. Rinse with water for a minimum of 10 seconds.
    d. Air dry the surface. (If the surface is not enamel, leave it moist.)
    e. Apply sealant (e.g., Fortify, Bisco, Inc.; Optiguard, Kerr Corp.).
    f. Air thin.
    g. Light polymerize the facial and lingual surfaces for 60 seconds each.

> ### CLINICAL TIP
>
> See the Clinical Tip concerning composite resin closest to the light in the section Class I Composite Resin Restorations.

> ### CLINICAL TIP
>
> Because a Class III restoration is usually not in a high-stress area, the facial and lingual portions can be restored with a microfiller. Optimal results can be achieved using a sandwich technique. A microfil is used on the facial and lingual surfaces, and a tooth-colored, opaque, or hybrid composite resin in between. The microfils are easier to polish, they retain a smooth surface, and they maintain their luster over a long period. However, either a microfil or hybrid can be used alone effectively.

Type 2 Class III Restorations: Facial Access. A microfil composite resin or a combination of hybrid resin overlayed with a microfil composite resin can be used.
1. Place the Mylar strip interproximally and inject the hybrid or microfilled composite resin.
2. Pull the Mylar strip to the lingual and adapt it to the lingual surface.
3. Place your thumb on the lingual surface and forefinger on the facial surface. Bow the matrix toward the adjacent tooth. If using only one increment, allow sufficient excess to cover the facial bevel. If a combination of hybrid and microfil are used, inject the hybrid and then the microfil.
4. Light polymerize.
5. Use a small amount of opaque to cover the demarcation between the tooth structure and resin.
6. A translucent microfil can be placed as the last layer (enamel).
Type 3 Class III Restoration: Through-and-Through.
1. Place a Mylar strip interproximally and hold it against the lingual surface. Inject either an opaque microfil or a hybrid resin (dentin replacement).
2. Place a translucent microfil or hybrid from the facial direction over the previously placed polymerized resin and slightly overfill.
3. Wrap the strip around the tooth, making sure it is adapting to the gingival margin.
4. Squeeze with your thumb and forefinger and polymerize for 40 seconds facially and lingually. (The lingual material can also be placed separately to fill the lingual half to two thirds of the preparation. It is then light polymerized for 40 seconds.) The enamel replacement material and opaque can be placed if necessary so that no demarcation is created between the restoration and tooth structure. Contour with an interproximal carver to the proper anatomic form. A sable hair brush can be used to blend the material with the adjacent tooth structure.[138]

Class IV Composite Resin Restorations

Class IV restorations involve the facial, incisal, and lingual surfaces. Polymerization shrinkage is not a problem because no area of the restoration is enclosed. Hybrid composite resins are ideal because they have superior physical properties and can be overlaid to achieve esthetically pleasing results.

Porcelain laminate veneers, full-coverage porcelain, or cera-mometal crowns should be considered for patients with heavy bruxism or lack of adequate enamel for retention. Hybrid composite resin can be used to build up mandibular anterior surfaces if the occlusion is favorable.

Most hybrids can be polished to an acceptable level. However, hybrids do not maintain their luster, and the surface will need periodic renewal and polishing. However, some of the new nano-filled composite resins do maintain their luster to a greater degree. The hybrid composite resins are used as dentin replacements because of their opacity, which prevents darkness "show through" from the posterior of the oral cavity.

Occlusal adjustment or cosmetic recontouring, which creates adequate clearance for the composite resin's thickness, may be required before placement of the restoration.

Single-Step Buildup Technique. The Class IV single-step technique is similar to the Class III single-step technique. See the preceding section for a complete discussion of the limitations of this technique. This technique includes the use of opaque to limit the gray "show through" from the mouth's posterior and the addition of tints and color modifiers.

Armamentarium. Use the same dental setup as for the Class III multiple-step technique with the following exceptions:

- Putty matrix (e.g., Sil-Tech Plus Putty; Ivoclar Vivadent), clear crown or incisal matrix CoForm (Premier), Directa (JS Dental)

Clinical Technique. Use the same clinical technique as described in the Class III single-step buildup technique; an incisal matrix or a clear crown form can also be used to aid in the buildup of the incisal corner.

Multiple-Step Buildup Technique.

Armamentarium. Use the same dental setup as for Class I restorations with the following exceptions:

- Conventional Mylar strip, stop strips (Mylar anterior bands with an integrated stopper to secure the matrix band between adjacent teeth; Premier, Inc.)
- Putty matrix (e.g., Sil-Tech Plus Putty; Ivoclar Vivadent)
- Posterior, small-particle, hybrid composite resin
- Optional microfil composite resin (e.g., Silux Plus, 3M, Inc.; Durafill, Kulzer Inc.; Renamel, Cosmedent, Inc.)

Clinical Technique.

1. Pumice the teeth and clean the proximal surface with a strip where necessary.
2. Determine the appropriate shade of the tooth while it is wet with saliva.
3. Administer appropriate anesthesia if necessary.
4. Place a rubber dam.

The use of any calcium hydroxide should be kept to a minimum because it dissolves over time, resulting in an unsupported restoration.[79]

5. Place the liner or base where appropriate (Fig. 5-6A). See the section on Liners and Bases.
6. Place a 2- to 3-mm long chamfer about 0.3 mm deep around the entire margin. Place a scalloped bevel on the esthetic areas of the chamfer to help disguise the margins. Bevel the gingival margin only if beveling does not entirely remove the enamel. Avoid placing the lingual chamfer under an occlusal load (Fig. 5-6B).

Cavity disinfectants may adversely affect bond strength. Verify compatibility with the disinfectant and bonding agent manufacturers.

7. Etch the enamel and dentin for 15 seconds. See the section on Acid Etching.
8. Wash with water and/or water/air spray for a minimum of 10 seconds for gel or liquid etchants. See the section on Acid Etching.
9. Air dry the enamel and blot the dentin, leaving it slightly moist. The cavity preparation can be disinfected with a cavity disinfectant and the excess blown off and blotted with a cotton pellet. However, in some systems the smear layer is not removed but only modified, and bond strengths may decrease during disinfection.[92,93]
10. Repeat the procedure if the enamel does not have a frosted white appearance after air drying. If the dentin is dry, moisten the dentin again with a cotton pellet moistened with water.
11. Place the appropriate dentin-enamel bonding agent.
12. To eliminate lingual finishing, closely adapt the Mylar strip to the tooth with a gloved finger.
13. Place the posterior, small-particle, hybrid composite resin against the Mylar strip. If a translucent incisal area is desired, this layer can be built up with a translucent hybrid material. Place a dentin shade and add internal stain and opaque if necessary to duplicate the internal coloring of the adjacent tooth. Place an amount that leaves sufficient room for a continuous overlay of microfilled composite resin (Fig. 5-6C).

Use bonding agent rather than alcohol to prevent the composite resin from sticking to the plastic instrument. See the Clinical Tip on bonding resin and alcohol in the section on Class I Composite Resin Restorations.

14. Polymerize the composite resin from the facial surface and then the lingual surface to form a lingual wall (Fig. 5-6D).

Place the composite resin with a Centrix-type syringe (see Fig. 5-5A). See the Clinical Tip on Centrix syringes in the section on Class I Composite Resin Restorations.

15. Place the microfilled composite resin over the previously placed hybrid composite resin (Fig. 5-6E). The microfilled composite resin may consist of a body shade and a definitive, clear translucent incisal shade.
16. Shape the composite resin as much as possible with a sable hairbrush.
17. Polymerize the microfilled composite resin from the lingual direction (Fig. 5-6F) and then from the facial and incisal directions (Fig. 5-6G).
18. Create the definitive texture and contour and then finish (Fig. 5-6H,I). See the section on Finishing.

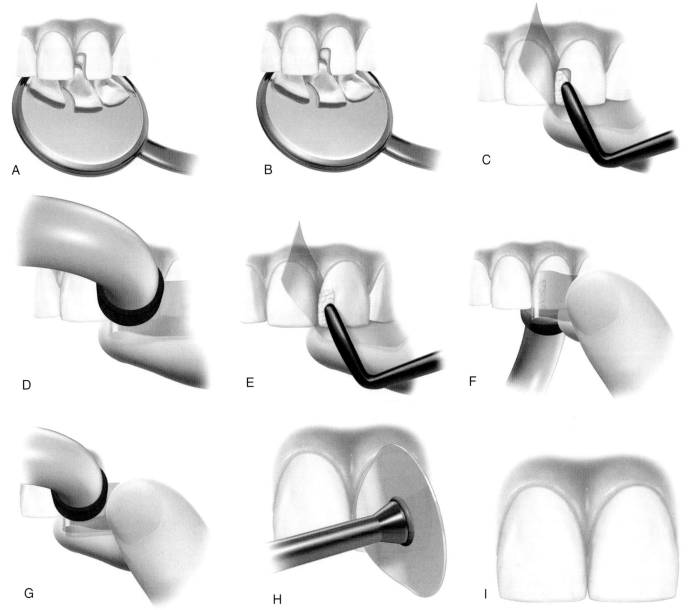

FIGURE 5-6 A, Calcium hydroxide should be placed only in areas close to the pulp and is followed by the placement of a radiopaque resin-modified glass ionomer base in the area immediately surrounding the exposure. This step seals the area, and a "total etch" process is used to seal the remaining tooth structure. Etch the preparation slightly beyond the chamfer. Wash, dry, and paint bonding agent beyond the area of the etch. **B,** A chamfer bevel has been placed completely around the border of the restoration. Should the fracture extend to the root surface, a bevel is not placed at the gingiva, but a gingival retention groove is placed to aid retention and minimize microleakage. **C,** Pack a small increment of hybrid resin against the lingual Mylar matrix (wedging is optional), and support with the finger. This increment can be placed with the plastic instrument or a syringe. **D,** The increment is polymerized from the facial aspect first, followed by the lingual. Pressure from the finger against the Mylar matrix can ensure good adaptation and can minimize lingual finishing. **E,** A second increment can be packed against the hardened lingual wall. The increment can be made of either a hybrid or microfilled resin. If necessary a layer of tint or opaque can be sandwiched between these two layers. **F,** The second increment should be polymerized from the lingual aspect. Wrapping the matrix band around the facial surface is optional but usually minimizes the amount of finishing and provides a realistic curve of composite resin around the interproximofacial areas. **G,** The facial and incisal aspects should then be polymerized again. The Mylar strip is removed and the occlusion adjusted. Because the surface next to the light is the hardest, it is sometimes removed during occlusion adjustment and a definitive, additional polymerization is advisable. **H,** Facial flash is removed with a Bard-Parker blade or composite resin knife in an enamel-to-composite resin direction. Creation of developmental cuts or texturing is best accomplished with micron diamonds or knife-edge disks. Finishing is accomplished with burs, diamonds, disks, and rubber cusps. Definitive polishing can be accomplished with a composite resin polishing paste. **I,** The definitive restoration.

19. Polish the restoration. See the section on Polishing.
20. Sealant and postcuring procedures are the following:
    a. Rinse off polishing debris with water; air dry.
    b. Etch for 15 seconds.
    c. Rinse with water for a minimum of 10 seconds.
    d. Air dry the surface. (If the surface is not enamel, leave it moist.)
    e. Apply sealant (e.g., Fortify, Bisco, Inc.; Optiguard, Kerr Corp.).
    f. Air thin.
    g. Light polymerize the facial and lingual surfaces for 60 seconds each.

> **CLINICAL TIP**
>
> See the Clinical Tip concerning composite resin closest to the light in the section Class I Composite Resin Restorations.

Class V Composite Resin Restorations

Single-Step Buildup Technique. The Class V single-step technique is similar to the Class III single-step technique. This technique is recommended for preparations in which the margins are entirely in enamel. A finite element stress analysis of three filling techniques by Winkler et al.[140] concluded that bulk filling is indicated in restorations that are sufficiently shallow to be polymerized to their full depth. The highest stress levels developed during the curing process, and bulk filling resulted in the lowest maximum normal transient stress compared with three horizontal increments and three wedge-shaped increments.

Armamentarium. Use the same dental setup as for the Class V multiple-step buildup technique with the following exception:
- Class V cervical matrix (i.e., Cure-Thru, Premier Dental Products, Co.)

Clinical Technique. Use the same clinical technique as that described for the Class V multiple-step buildup technique, except place all the composite resin in a single increment. Apply pressure with a cervical matrix and polymerize the composite resin, or shape and sculpt the composite resin with an interproximal carver before curing.

Multiple-Step Buildup Technique.

Armamentarium. Use the same dental setup as for Class I restorations. However a microfilled resin may be preferable because its high modulus of elasticity permits flexing of the restoration, and its high polishability permits excellent soft tissue response.[141] A flowable microfil that allows appropriate contour may be ideal for this procedure (e.g., Renamel Flowable Microfill, Cosmedent, Inc.). The tooth can be isolated with a rubber dam and a #212 rubber dam clamp or retraction cord and cotton rolls.

Clinical Technique.
1. Pumice the teeth and clean the involved proximal surface with a sand paper strip.
2. Determine the shade of the tooth while it is wet.
3. Administer appropriate anesthesia if necessary.
4. Place a rubber dam or retraction cord and cotton rolls if adequate isolation can be achieved.

> **CLINICAL TIP**
>
> See the Clinical Tip concerning pulpal exposure and alternative treatments in the Section Liners and Bases.

> **CLINICAL TIP**
>
> The use of any calcium hydroxide should be kept to a minimum because it dissolves over time, resulting in an unsupported restoration.[79]

> **CLINICAL TIP**
>
> See Clinical Tip concerning postoperative sensitivity in the section Class I Composite Resin Restorations.

5. Place appropriate liner and base if indicated. See the section on Liners and Bases.
6. Place bevels with a medium grit diamond bur around the border if the restoration has borders made entirely of enamel. In esthetic areas, 1- to 2-mm bevel should be placed; however, the gingival margin should not be beveled if the enamel margin is thin. Beveling permits a gradual transition from the composite resin to the enamel.
7. Place a retention groove at the gingival margin if the Class V restoration ends on the root surface, and use a low-modulus material to ensure retention in the event that the dentin bonding fails. Beveling the gingival margin on cementum is usually undesirable.
8. Etch the enamel and dentin for 15 seconds. See the section on Acid Etching.
9. Wash with water and/or water/air spray for a minimum of 10 seconds for gel or liquid etchants. See the section on Acid Etching.
10. Air dry the enamel and blot the dentin, leaving it slightly moist. The cavity preparation can be disinfected with a cavity disinfectant and the excess blown off and blotted with a cotton pellet. However, in some systems the smear layer is not removed but only modified, and bond strengths may decrease during disinfection.[74,75]
11. Repeat the procedure if the enamel does not have a frosted white appearance after air drying. If the dentin is dry, moisten the dentin again with a cotton pellet moistened with water.
12. Place the appropriate dentin-enamel bonding agent.
13. If the restoration is large, place the composite resin in increments that will minimize stress in the restoration and gap formation from polymerization shrinkage. Place an initial pie-shaped increment entirely on the root surface (Fig. 5-7). The bonding agent and composite resin must fill the cervical retention groove if one is deemed necessary.

> **CLINICAL TIP**
>
> Use bonding agent rather than alcohol to prevent the composite resin from sticking to the plastic instrument. See the Clinical Tip on bonding resin and alcohol in the section on Class I Composite Resin Restorations.

> **CLINICAL TIP**
>
> Place the composite resin with a Centrix-type syringe (see Fig. 5-5A). See the Clinical Tip on Centrix syringes in the section on Class I Composite Resin Restorations.

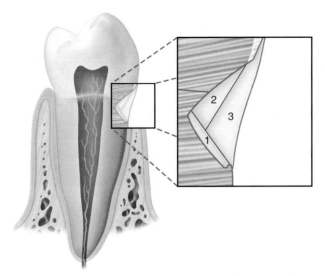

FIGURE 5-7 If the preparation extends onto the root surface, a gingival groove is placed to aid in retention should the dentin bond fail. The clinical situation dictates the necessity of the groove. Heavy occlusal forces and lack of enamel at the gingival margin make groove placement advisable. Neither the first nor the second layer touches the bonded enamel; therefore polymerization shrinkage does not place the enamel bond in competition with the dentin bond. Furthermore, use of increments ensures better light penetration and less shrinkage. The definitive increment, which should also be the thinnest, covers the entire preparation to eliminate a layering effect. The definitive increment is the enamel replacement. A thinner layer shrinks less, thus helping to maintain marginal integrity.

14. Place a second increment on the occlusal enamel bevel; extend it to the axial wall and polymerize.
15. Add a third layer to build the tooth form. This layer can be translucent so that it is similar to the enamel layer.
16. Continue adding and polymerizing composite resin as necessary until the restoration is slightly overfilled.
17. Place a previously fabricated matrix to decrease the amount of excess material. Use an interproximal carver to remove excess composite resin.
18. Contour and finish the restoration. See the section on Finishing.
19. Polish the restoration. See section on Polishing.
20. Sealant and postcuring procedures are the following:
    a. Rinse off polishing debris with water; air dry.
    b. Etch for 15 seconds
    c. Rinse with water for a minimum of 10 seconds.
    d. Air dry the surface.
    e. Apply sealant (e.g., Fortify, Bisco, Inc.; Optiguard, Kerr Corp.).
    f. Air thin.
    g. Light polymerize for 40 seconds.

CLINICAL TIP

See the Clinical Tip concerning composite resin closest to the light in the section Class I Composite Resin Restorations.

CLINICAL CASES

Composite Resin Facial Class IV

A 25-year-old female patient presented with the right lateral primary canine present and with the permanent canine absent (Fig. 5-8A).

The left permanent canine presented with a large incisal embrasure on the mesial that made it appear excessively pointed. The patient desired to improve her smile without any costly or invasive treatment. After discussing alternatives with the patient, direct bonding was used to modify the unesthetic anterior teeth. A wax-up and subsequent in vivo preview using Luxatemp demonstrated the definitive result. An occlusal putty surgical guide was fabricated from the wax-up and used as a guide to create the enamel lingual shelf (Fig. 5-8B).

Dentin shades were used to create internal dentin lobes and overlaid with a definitive translucent enamel layer to create the appearance of a permanent canine composite resin. The incisal edges of the right lateral incisor, left lateral incisor, and left permanent canine were modified with composite resin. Surface irregularities were added with a fine micron diamond after the initial finishing and polishing. An aluminum oxide polishing paste and buffing wheel with water were used to obtain luster while maintaining the original contour and texture. The definitive result (Fig. 5-8C) permitted the patient to smile with bilateral symmetry.

Class II Posterior Composite Resin

A 27-year-old patient presented with and old MO amalgam in tooth #18 with recurrent decay. The patient requested a tooth colored restoration and a Micro-Hybrid composite was placed as the definitive restoration (Fig. 5-9).

Class II Posterior Composite Resin

A 16-year-old male patient presented with extensive decay on tooth #30. The large size of the lesion was such that an indirect restoration would have been preferable, but financial constraints and concerns about the long-term vitality of the tooth resulted in placement of a direct composite resin. The extensive distal-occlusal-lingual composite resin restored the original anatomic structure and helped strengthen the remaining tooth structure (Fig. 5-10).

Class IV Composite Resin

An 11-year-old female patient presented with the chipped maxillary left central incisor incurred during gymnastics (Fig. 5-11A). The incisal edge was repaired with a microhybrid composite and white opaque to match the adjacent central incisor (Fig. 5-11B).

Class V

A 55-year-old male presented sensitivity in the maxillary right quadrant and desired to mask dark roots. A micro-hybrid composite resin in conjunction was used to restore eliminate the sensitivity and cover the roots. The Blue View Cervical Matrice was used to help shape the composite and reduce excess (Figs. 5-12).

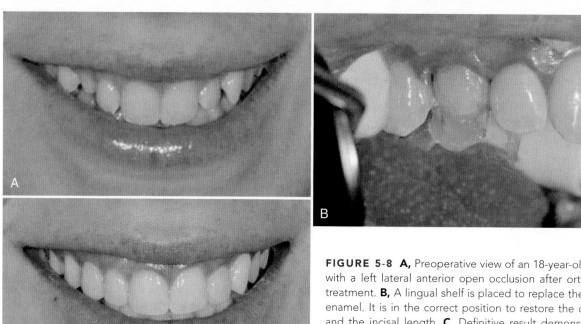

FIGURE 5-8 A, Preoperative view of an 18-year-old female with a left lateral anterior open occlusion after orthodontic treatment. **B,** A lingual shelf is placed to replace the missing enamel. It is in the correct position to restore the occlusion and the incisal length. **C,** Definitive result demonstrate the maxillary deciduous canine now appears to be the permanent canine. The upper left lateral and canine have their incisal embrassures modified and now the incisors parallel the lower lip. (Courtesy of Aikaterini Samandara Thessaloniki, Greece.)

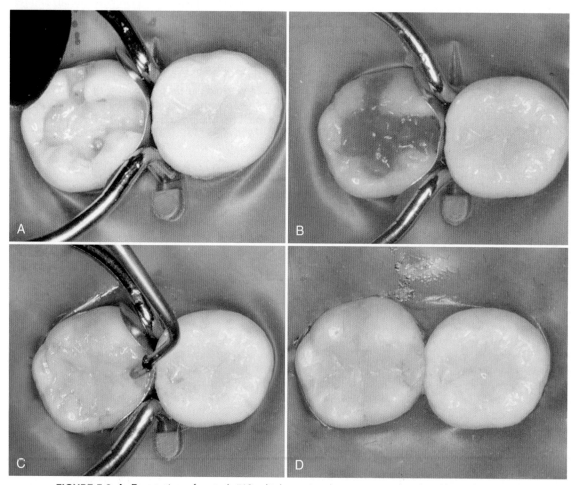

FIGURE 5-9 A, Excavation of a tooth #18, which previously was restored with a Class II amalgam restoration. The tooth was isolated with rubber dam, a Garrison sectional retainer band, and a FlexiWedge (Common Sense Dental). **B,** The tooth is etched. **C,** A variety of composite instruments (P1 plugger and OptraSculpt [Ivoclar Vivadent], XTS Composite Instruments [Hu Friedy], and Dental Composite Instruments [Cosmedent, Inc.]) can be used to sculpt appropriate occlusal anatomy. **D,** Postoperative view of the definitive restoration demonstrating reproduction of the appropriate occlusal anatomy.

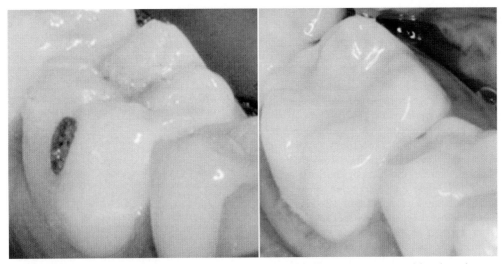

FIGURE 5-10 Preopertative and postoperative view of tooth #30 in a 16-year-old male with an extensive distal-occlusal-buccal composite resin restoring the tooth to function.

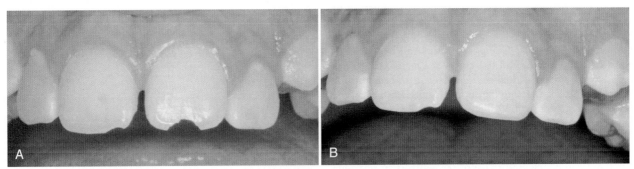

FIGURE 5-11 A, Tooth #9 with incisal chip on a young patient. **B,** Tooth #9 incisal edge restored with white opacities similar to #8.

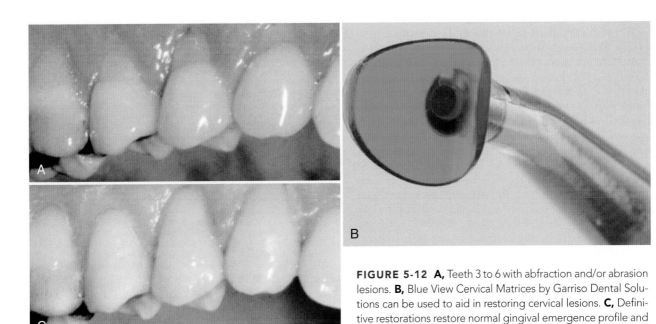

FIGURE 5-12 A, Teeth 3 to 6 with abfraction and/or abrasion lesions. **B,** Blue View Cervical Matrices by Garriso Dental Solutions can be used to aid in restoring cervical lesions. **C,** Definitive restorations restore normal gingival emergence profile and eliminate sensitivity.

CONCLUSION

The indications for composite resins are constantly increasing. The advances in dentin bonding and numerous improvements in resin and filler composition have fueled this expansion. Composite resins have improved handling, superior esthetics, reduced wear, reduced shrinkage, reduced internal stress and satisfactory long-term clinical performance.

However, selecting an appropriate resin-based composite resin for a restoration depends on the requirements for that clinical situation. Mechanical properties include strength, fracture toughness, surface hardness, modulus of elasticity, wear, water sorption and solubility, polymerization shrinkage, fatigue and degradation, radiopacity, and ease of detection during removal. Required biologic properties are biocompatibility, absence of postoperative pain or hypersensitivity, absence of cracks, or fracture formation and caries inhibition. Aesthetics considerations include color match and stability, translucency, the variety of shades, polishability, maintenance of gloss, marginal, or surface staining resistance, and maintenance of anatomic form.[12]

Light-activated resins rely on adequate light intensity to polymerize sufficiently.[142] Light passing through composite resins is absorbed and scattered, resulting in attenuation of the intensity and reduction of the light polymerization effectiveness. Sufficient light is critical now with bulk placement of composite resinresins.[143] Composite resins can be placed in bulk if adequate curing can be achieved, a factor that varies depending on the individual composite resin and cavity configuration. Factors affecting depth of polymerization include filler type, size, and loading; light transmission attenuation; type, thickness, and shade of the restorative resin; exposure time and distance from the light source; and light intensity.[144] A study by Vargas et al.[145] indicated that hybrid resins polymerize more completely and to a greater depth than microfils with any light source. In addition, many of the current restorative techniques are based on the theory that composite resins shrink toward the light. However, studies concluded that composite resins do not shrink toward light, and the direction of shrinkage is predominantly determined by cavity shape and bond quality.[146] In addition, "effective shrinkage" of restrained composite resins is different from that of "free composite resins." None of the currently available direct restorative materials can fill the requirements of a perfect restorative material. However, composite resin can provide high-quality restorations in the anterior area and are usually amalgam alternatives for small posterior restorations (depending on the occlusion and enamel availability). Enamel remaining at the gingival margin and rubber dam isolation are preferred. Arch position is also important because molars wear more than premolars as a result of increased forces. An initial restoration can be made with direct composite resin to reduce the amount of tooth structure removed. Replacement of an amalgam may require an inlay or onlay depending on the buccal-lingual dimensions of the restoration. Nanocomposite resins or modified resins such as silicon compounds, orthospirocarbonates, ormocers, and epoxides may comprise the material of the future.[147] Despite all the improvements, undesirable problems still exist; marginal discrepancies,[148,149] marginal staining, white lines around the restoration, cusp fractures, microleakage,[150] secondary caries, and postoperative sensitivity still occur.[12]

REFERENCES

1. Buonocore MG: A simple method of increasing the adhesion of acrylic filling materials to enamel surfaces, *J Dent Res* 34(6):849, 1955.
2. Roulet J-F: Adhesive techniques: the standard for the restoration of anterior teeth. In Degrange M, Roulet J-F, eds. *Minimally invasive restorations with bonding*, Carol Stream, IL, 1997, Quintessence Publishing.
3. Brudevold F, Buonocore M, Wileman W: A report on a composite resin capable of bonding to human dentin surfaces, *J Dent Res* 35(6):846, 1956.
4. Bowen RL, Cobb EN, Rapson JE: Adhesive bonding of various materials to hard tooth tissues: improvement in bond strength to dentin, *J Dent Res* 61(9):1070, 1982.
5. Albers HF: *Tooth-colored restoratives: an introductory text for selecting, placing and finishing direct systems*, 8th ed, Santa Rosa, CA, 1996, Alto Books.
6. Dietschi D, Dietschi J-M: Current developments in composite resin materials and techniques, *Pract Periodontics Aesthet Dent* 8(7):603, 1996.
7. Chen M-H: Update on dental nanocomposite resins, *J Dent Res* 89:549, 2010.
8. Jandt KD, Sigusch BW: Future perspectives of resin-based dental materials, *Dent Mater* 25(8):1001, 2009.
9. Bracho-Troconis C, Trujillo-Lemon M, Boulden J, Wong N, Wall K, Esquibel K: Characterization of N'Durance: a nanohybrid composite resin based on new nano-dimer technology, *Compend Contin Educ Dent* 31(spec 2):5, 2010.
10. Lu H, Trujillo-Lemon M, Ge J, Stansbury J: Dental resins based on dimer acid dimethacrylates: a route to high conversion with low polymerization shrinkage. *Compend Contin Educ Dent* 31(spec 2):1, 2010.
11. Schmidt C, Ilie N: The effect of aging on the mechanical properties of nanohybrid composite resins based on new monomer formulations, *Clin Oral Invest* 17(1):251, 2013.
12. Ilie N, Hickel R: Resin composite resin restorative materials, *Aust Dent J* 56(suppl 1): 59, 2011.
13. Cramer NB, Stansbury JW, Bowman CN: Recent advances and developments in composite resin dental restorative materials, *J Dent Res* 90(4):402, 2011.
14. Crispin B: *Contemporary esthetic dentistry*, Hanover Park, IL, 1994, Quintessence Publishing.
15. Bayne SC: Dental biomaterials: where are we and where are we going? *J Dent Educ* 69(5):571, 2005.
16. Leinfelder KF: Posterior composites: state-of-the-art clinical applications, *Dent Clin North Am* 137:411-418, 1993.
17. Margeas R: Composite resin: a versatile, multi-purpose restorative material, *Compend Contin Educ Dent* 33(1):42, 2012.
18. Davidson CL, de Gee AJ: Relaxation of polymerization contraction stresses by flow in dental composite resins, *J Dent Res* 63(2):146, 1984.
19. Davidson CL, Kemp-Scholte CM: Shortcomings of composite resins in Class V restorations, *J Esthet Dent* 1(1):1, 1989.
20. Pick B, Pelka M, Belli R, Braga RR, Lohbauer U: Tailoring of physical properties in highly filled experimental nanohybrid resin composites, *Dent Mater* 27(7):664, 2011.
21. Torii Y, Itou K, Hikasa R, Iwata S, Nishitani Y: Enamel bond strength and morphology of resin-enamel interface created by acid etching system with or without moisture and self-etching priming system, *J Oral Rehabil* 29(6):528, 2002.
22. Mjor IA, Fejerskov O, eds: *Human oral embryology and histology*, Copenhagen, 1986, Munksgaard International Publishers.
23. Stanford JW: Bonding of restorative materials to dentine, *Int Dent J* 35(2):133, 1985.
24. Jendresen MD, Glantz PO: Clinical adhesiveness of selected dental materials: an in-vivo study, *Acta Odontol Scand* 39(1):39, 1981.
25. Buonocore MG: Retrospections on bonding, *Dent Clin North Am* 25(2):243, 1981.
26. Rowland GF, Yates JL, Hembree JH Jr, McKnight JP: The influence of topical stannous fluoride application on the tensile strength of pit and fissure sealants, *J Pedod* 4(1):9, 1979.
27. Barkmeier WW, Shaffer SE, Gwinnett AJ: Effects of 15 versus 60 second enamel acid conditioning on adhesion and morphology, *Oper Dent* 11(3):111, 1986.
28. Garcia-Godoy F, Gwinnett AJ: Penetration of acid solution and gel in occlusal fissures, *J Am Dent Assoc* 114(6):809, 1987.
29. Baharav H, Cardash HS, Pilo R, Helft M: The efficiency of liquid and gel acid etchants, *J Prosthet Dent* 60(5):545, 1988.
30. Baharav H, Cardash HS, Helft M, Langsam J: The continuing brushing acid-etch technique, *J Prosthet Dent* 57:147, 1987.
31. Mixson JM, Eick JD, Tira DE, Moore DL: The effects of variable wash times and techniques on enamel-composite resin bond strength, *Quintessence Int* 19(4):279, 1988.
32. Bates D, Retief DH, Jamison HC, Denys FR: Effects of acid etch parameters on enamel topography and composite resin-enamel bond strength, *Pediatr Dent* 4(2):106, 1982.
33. Mixson JM, Eick JD, Tira DE, Moore DL: The effects of rinse volumes and air water pressure on enamel-composite resin bond strengths, *J Prosthet Dent* 62(5):522, 1989.
34. Summit JB, Chan DC, Dutton FB, Burgess JO: Effect of rinse time on microleakage between composite resin and etched enamel, *Oper Dent* 18(1):37, 1993.
35. Holtan JR, Nystrom GP, Phelps RA, Anderson TB, Becker WS: Influence of different etchants and etching times on shear bond strength, *Oper Dent* 20(3):94, 1995.
36. Schulein TM, Chan DC, Reinhardt JW: Rinsing times for a gel etchant related to enamel/composite resin bond strength, *Gen Dent* 34(4):296, 1986.
37. Smidt A, Weller D, Roman I, et al: Effects of bleaching agents on microhardness and surface morphology of tooth enamel, *Am J Dent* 11:83, 1998.
38. Titley KC, Torneck CD, Smith DC, Adibfar A: Adhesion of composite resin to bleached and unbleached bovine material [published correction appears in *J Dent Res* 68(2): inside back cover, 1989.]. *J Dent Res* 67(12):1523, 1988.
39. Rotstein I, Lehr Z, Gedalia I: Effect of bleaching agents on inorganic components of human dentin and cementum, *J Endod* 18(6):290-293, 1992.
40. Swift EJ Jr, Perdigão J: Effects of bleaching on teeth and restorations, *Compend Contin Educ Dent* 19(8):815, 1998.

41. Silverstone LM, Dogon IL, eds: Proceedings of International Symposium on the Acid Etch Technique. St Paul, MN, 1991, North Central Publishing.
42. Nakabayashi N: Resin reinforced dentin due to infiltration of monomers into the dentin at the adhesive interface, *J Dent Mater* 1:78, 1982.
43. Langer A, Ilie N: Dentin infiltration ability of different classes of adhesive systems, *Clin Oral Invest* 17(1):205, 2013.
44. Pashley DH, Agee KA, Wataha JC, et al: Viscoelastic properties of demineralized dentin matrix, *Dent Mater* 19(8):700, 2003.
45. Fung DT, Wang VM, Laudier DM, et al: Subrupture tendon fatigue damage, *J Orthop Res* 27(2):264, 2009.
46. Sano H, Takatsu T, Ciucchi B, Russell CM, Pashley DH: Tensile properties of resin-infiltrated demineralized human dentin, *J Dent Res* 74(4):1093, 1995.
47. Gwinnett AJ, Matsui A: A study of enamel adhesives: the physical relationship between enamel and adhesive, *Arch Oral Biol* 12(12):1615, 1967.
48. Swift E Jr, Triolo PT Jr: Bond strength of Scotchbond Multi-Purpose to moist dentin and enamel, *Am J Dent* 5(6):318, 1992.
49. Gwinnett AJ: Moist versus dry dentin: its effect on shear bond strength, *Am J Dent* 5(3):127, 1992.
50. Jensen ME, Chan DCN: Polymerization shrinkage and microleakage. In Vanherle G, Smith DC, editors:. International Symposium on Posterior Composite Resin Dental Restorative Materials. Amsterdam, the Netherlands, 1985, Peter Szulc Publishing.
51. Crim GA, Mattingly SL: Microleakage and the Class V composite cavosurface, *ASDC J Dent Child* 47(5):333, 1980.
52. Loguercio AD, Moura SK, Pellizzaro A, et al: Durability of enamel bonding using two-step self-etching systems on ground and unground enamel, *Oper Dent* 33(1):79, 2008.
53. Van Meerbeek B, de Munck J, Yoshida Y, et al: Buonocore memorial lecture. Adhesion to enamel and dentin: status and future challenges, *Oper Dent* 28(3):215, 2003.
54. Van Meerbeek B, Yoshihara K, Yoshida Y, Mine A, De Munck J, Van Landuyt KL: State of the art of self-etch adhesives, *Dent Mater* 27(1):17, 2011.
55. Shigehiga I: Posterior restorations: ceramics or composite resins. In Nakajima H, Tani Y, editors: Transactions: Third International Congress on Dental Materials, Sheraton Waikiki, Hawaii, November 4-8, 1998. Lake Oswego, OR, 1997, Academy of Dental Materials Inc.
56. Davidson CL, deGee AJ. Relaxation of polymerization contraction stresses by flow in dental composite resins, *J Dent Res* 63:146, 1984.
57. Trushkowsky RD, Gwinnett AJ: Microleakage of Class V composite resin sandwich, and resin-modified glass ionomers, *Am J Dent* 9:96, 1996.
58. Kemp-Scholte CM, Davidson CL: Marginal integrity related to bond strength and strain capacity of composite resin restorative systems, *J Prosthet Dent* 64:658, 1990.
59. Versluis A, Douglas WH, Cross M, Sakaguchi RL: Does an incremental filling technique reduce polymerization shrinkage stress? *J Dent Res* 75(3):871, 1996.
60. Braga RR, Ferracane JL: Alternatives in polymerization contraction stress management, *Crit Rev Oral Biol Med* 15(3):176, 2004.
61. Tantbirojn D, Pfeifer CS, Braga RR, Versluis A: Do low-shrink composite resins reduce polymerization shrinkage effects? *J Dent Res* 90(5):596, 2011.
62. Ilie N, Rencz A, Hickel R: Investigations towards nano-hybrid resin-based composites, *Clin Oral Invest* 17(1):185, 2013.
63. Burgess J, Cakir D: Comparative properties of low-shrinkage composite resins, *Compend Contin Educ Dent* 31(spec 2):10, 2010.
64. Browning WD, Halter TK: Microleakage in self-cured and light-cured posterior composite resins, *J Dent Res* 1367, 1998.
65. Fan PL, Edahl A, Leung RL, Stanford JW: Alternative interpretations of water sorption values of composite resins, *J Dent Res* 64(1):78, 1985.
66. Söderholm KJ, Zigan M, Ragan M, Fischlschweiger W, Bergman M: Hydrolytic degradation of dental composite resin, *J Dent Res* 63(10):1248, 1984.
67. Bouschlicher MR, Vargas MA, Boyer DB: Effect of composite resin type, light intensity, configuration factor and laser polymerization on polymerization contraction forces, *Am J Dent* 10(2):88, 1997.
68. Goracci G, Mori G, de'Martinis LC: Curing light intensity and marginal leakage of composite resin restorations, *Quintessence Int* 27(5):355, 1996.
69. Curtis JW Jr: Curing efficiency of the turbo tip, *Gen Dent* 43:428, 1995.
70. Newcomb J et al: Self start polymerization using VLC or argon lasers, *J Dent Res* 77:1396, 1998.
71. Degues M et al: Marginal adaptation in Class V composite resin restorations with four curing units, *J Dent Res* 77:1395, 1998.
72. Feilzer AJ, De Gee AJ, Davidson CL: Setting stress in composite resin in relation to configuration of the restoration, *J Dent Res* 66(11):1636, 1987.
73. Strydom C, Retief DH, Russell CM, Denys FR: Laboratory evaluation of the Gluma 3-step bonding system, *Am J Dent* 8(2):93, 1995.
74. Tao L, Tagami J, Pashley DH: Pulpal pressure and bond strengths of Superbond and Gluma, *Am J Dent* 4(2):73, 1991.
75. Cox CF, Sübay RK, Ostro E, Suzuki S, Suzuki SH: Tunnel defects in dentin bridges: their formation following direct pulp capping, *Oper Dent* 21(1):4, 1996.
76. Cox CF, Suzuki S: Re-evaluating pulp protection: calcium hydroxide vs cohesive hybridization, *J Am Dent Assoc* 125(7):823, 1994.
77. Hilton TJ: Cavity sealers, liners and bases: current philosophies and indications for use, *Oper Dent* 21(4):134, 1996.
78. Pameijer CH, Stanley HR: The disastrous effects of the "total etch" technique in vital pulp capping in primates, *Am J Dent* 11:545, 1998.
79. Leinfelder KF, O'Neal SJ, Mueninghoff LA: Use of Ca(OH)$_2$ for measuring microleakage, *Dent Mater* 2(3):121, 1986.
80. Miller MB, Castellanos IR, Vargas MA, Denehy GE: Effect of restorative materials on microleakage of Class II composites, *J Esthet Dent* 8(3):107, 1996.
81. Aboushala A, Kugel G, Hurley E: Class II composite resin restoration using glass ionomer liners: microleakage studies, *J Clin Pediatr Dent* 21:67, 1996.
82. Speiser AM, Kahn M: The etched butt-joint margin, *ASDC J Dent Child* 44(1):42, 1977.
83. Kim SY, Kim EJ, Kim DS, Lee IB. The evaluation of dentinal tubule occlusion by desensitizing, *Oper Dent* 38(4):419-28, 2013.
84. Yazici AR, Baseren M, Dayangaç B: The effect of flowable resin composite on microleakage in class V cavities, *Oper Dent* 28(1):42-6, 2003.
85. Strassler HE, Bauman G: Current concepts in polishing composite resins, *Pract Periodontics Aesthet Dent* 5(3 suppl 1):12, 1993.
86. Boghosian AA, Randolph RG, Jekkals VJ: Rotary finishing of microfilled and small-particle hybrid composite resins, *J Am Dent Assoc* 115(2):299, 1987.
87. Stoddard JW, Johnson GH: An evaluation of polishing agents for composite resins. *J Prosthet Dent* 65(4):491, 1991.
88. Ratanapridakul K, Leinfelder KF, Thomas J: Effect of finishing on in vivo wear rate of posterior composite resin [published correction appears in *J Am Dent Assoc* 118(5):524, 1989], *J Am Dent Assoc* 118(3):333, 1989.
89. Kawai K, Leinfelder KF: Effect of surface-penetrating sealant on composite wear, *Dent Mater* 9(2):108, 1993.
90. Dickinson GL, Leinfelder KF: Assessing the long-term effect of a surface penetrating sealant, *J Am Dent Assoc* 124(7):68, 1993.
91. Trushkowsky RD: Use of a clear matrix to minimize finishing of a posterior composite resin, *Am J Dent* 10(2):111, 1997.
92. Gwinnett AJ: Effect of cavity disinfection on bond strength to dentin, *J Esthet Dent* 4(suppl):11, 1992.
93. Meiers JC, Shook LW: Effects of disinfectants on the bond strength of composite to dentin, *Am J Dent* 9(1):11, 1996.
94. Fahl NF Jr. Tetric Ceram: direct posterior composite resin restorations—a great idea, *AACD J* 8, 1997.
95. Dietchi D: Anatomical application of a new direct Ceromer, *Signature* 4(1):8, 1997.
96. Gwinnett AJ: Bonding basics: what every clinician should know, *Esthet Dent Update* 5:35, 1994.
97. Leinfelder K: Dentin adhesives: the newest generation, *Esthet Dent Update* 5:50, 1994.
98. Cox CI, Suzuki S: Biological update of Ca(OH)$_2$ bases, liners and new adhesive systems, *Esthet Dent Update* 5:29, 1994.
99. Suzuki S, Leinfelder K: An in vitro evaluation of a copolymerizable type of micro-filled composite resin, *Quintessence Int* 25(1):59, 1994.
100. Eick JD, Robinson SJ, Byerley TJ, Chappelow CC: Adhesives and nonshrinking dental resins of the future, *Quintessence Int* 24(9):632, 1993.
101. Leinfelder KF, Lyles MB, Ritsco RG: A new polymer rigid material, *J Calif Dent Assoc* 24(9):78, 1996.
102. Leinfelder K: After amalgam what? Other materials fall short, *J Am Dent Assoc* 125(5):586, 1994.
103. Jordan RE, Suzuki M: Posterior composite restorations: where and how they work best, *J Am Dent Assoc* 122(11):30, 1991.
104. Eames WB, Strain JD, Weitman RT, Williams AK: Clinical comparison of composite, amalgam, and silicate restorations, *J Am Dent Assoc* 89(5):1111, 1974.
105. Leinfelder K: Posterior composite resins: the materials and their clinical performance, *J Am Dent Assoc* 126(5):663, 1995.
106. Eick JD, Welch FH: Dentin adhesives: do they protect the dentin from acid etching? *Quintessence Int* 17(9):533, 1986.
107. Suzuki S, Cox CF: Cohesive bonding between dental clinicians and researchers. In Shimono M, Maeda T, Suda H, Takahashi K, editors: *Dentin/Pulp Complex: Proceedings of the International Conference on Dentin/Pulp Complex 1995 and the International Meeting on Clinical Topics of Dentin/Pulp Complex.* Hanover Park IL, 1997, Quintessence Publishing.
108. Vanherle G, Smith DC, editors: International Symposium on Posterior Composite Resin Dental Restorative Materials. Amsterdam, the Netherlands, 1985, Peter Szulc Publishing.
109. Karaman E, Ozgunaltay G: Polymerization shrinkage of different types of composite resins and microleakage with and without liner in class II cavities. *Oper Dent* 39(3):325-31, 2014.
110. Gross JD, Retief DH, Bradley EL: Microleakage of posterior composite restorations, *Dent Mater* 1(1):7, 1985.
111. Lui JL, Masutani S, Setcos JC, Lutz F, Swartz ML, Phillips RW: Margin quality and microleakage of Class II composite resin restorations [published correction appears in *J Am Dent Assoc* 114(3):294, 1987], *J Am Dent Assoc* 114(1):49, 1987.
112. Lutz F, Krejci I, Luescher B, Oldenburg TR: Improved proximal margin adaptation of Class II composite resin restorations by use of light-reflecting wedges, *Quintessence Int* 17(10):659, 1986.
113. Koenigsberg S, Fuks A, Grajower R: The effect of three filling techniques on marginal leakage around class II composite resin restorations in vitro, *Quintessence Int* 20(2):117, 1989.
114. Barkmeier WW, Cooley RL: Curing ability of plastic wedges, *J Esthet Dent* 1:51, 1989.
115. de Goes MF, Rubbi E, Baffa O, Panzeri H: Optical transmittance of reflecting wedges, *Am J Dent* 5(2):78, 1992.
116. Ben-Amar A, Liberman R, Nordenberg D, Metzger Z: The effect of retention grooves on gingival marginal microleakage in Class II posterior composite resin restorations, *J Oral Rehabil* 15(4):325, 1988.
117. Leinfelder KFI: A conservative approach to placing posterior composite resin restorations, *J Am Dent Assoc* 127:743, 1996.
118. Scherer W, Leinfelder KF: Bulk placement of composite resin in Class II preparations, *Esthet Dent Update* 7:28, 1996.
119. Godder B, Settembrini L, Zhukovsky L: Direct shrinkage composite placement, *Gen Dent* 43(5):444, 1995.

120. Versluis A: Does an incremental filling technique reduce shrinkage stress? *J Dent Res* 75:871, 1996.

121. Jackson RD: Placing posterior composites: increasing efficiency, *Dent Today* 30(4):126, 2011.

122. Burgess JO, Cakir D: Material selection for direct posterior restoratives [continuing education article and test]. PennWell Publications. http://www.ineedce.com/courses/2067/PDF/1108cei_dentsply_Restoratives.pdf. Published September 2011. Accessed November 5, 2013.

123. Leprince JG, Leveque P, Nysten B, Gallez B, Devaux J, Leloup G: New insight into the "depth of cure" of dimethacrylate-based dental composite, *Dent Mater* 28(5):512, 2012.

124. Flury S, Hayoz S, Peutzfeldt A, Hüsler J, Lussi A: Depth of cure of resin composites: is the ISO 4049 method suitable for bulk fill materials? *Dent Mater* 28(5):521, 2012.

125. Frauscher KE, Ilie N: Depth of cure and mechanical properties of nano-hybrid resin-based composites with novel and conventional matrix formulation, *Clin Oral Invest* 16(5):1425, 2012.

126. Trushkowsky RD: A panoramic overview of Class II posterior composite resin placement techniques, *Dent Today* 14(9):60, 1995.

127. Trushkowsky RD: A panoramic overview of Class II posterior composite resin placement techniques: part II, *Dent Today* 14(10):74, 1995.

128. Feinman RA: Class II composite resin restorations using the prepolymerized ball technique, *Pract Periodontics Aesthet Dent* 5(3 suppl 1):5, 1993.

129. Feinman RA: The plunging ball technique: Class II direct composite resins, *Pract Periodontics Aesthet Dent* 4(5):43, 1992.

130. Bouschlicher MR, Reinhardt JW, Vargas MA: Surface treatment techniques for resin composite repair, *Am J Dent* 10(6):279, 1997.

131. Boyer DB: Buildup and repair of light cured composite resins: bond strength, *J Dent Res* 63(10):1241-1244, 1984.

132. Eakle WS: Effects of thermal cycling on fracture strengths of microleakage in teeth restored with bonded composite resin, *Dent Mater* 2(3):114, 1986.

133. Donly KJ, Wild TW, Bowen RL, Jensen ME: An in vitro investigation of the effects of glass inserts on the effective composite resin polymerization shrinkage, *J Dent Res* 68(8):1234, 1989.

134. Eichmiller FC: Clinical use of beta-quartz glass-ceramic inserts, *Compendium* 13(7):568, 570, 1992.

135. Ericson D, Derand T: Reduction of cervical gaps in Class II composite resin restorations, *J Prosthet Dent* 70:219, 1993.

136. Ericson D, Dérand T: Increase of in vitro curing depth of Class II composite resin restorations, *J Prosthet Dent* 70(3):219, 1993.

137. Walshaw PR, McComb D: Microleakage in Class 2 composite resins with low-modulus intermediate materials, *J Dent Res* 77(spec issue):131, 1998.

138. Murray A, Bergeron C, Qian F, Nessler R, Vargas M: Insertion technique and marginal adaptation of class II composite resin restorations, *J Dent Res* 90(spec issue A):Abstract 3206, 2011.

139. Miller MB: Class III composite restorations, *Dent Today* 16(12):58, 1997.

140. Winkler MM, Katona TR, Paydar NH: Finite element analysis of three filling techniques for Class V light-cured composite restorations, *J Dent Res* 75(7):1477, 1996.

141. Prati C, Chersoni S, Cretti L, Mongiorgi R: Marginal morphology of Class V composite restorations, *Am J Dent* 10(5):231, 1997.

142. Rueggeberg FA, Caughman WF, Curtis JW Jr, Davis HC: Factors affecting cure at depths within light-activated resin composite, *Am J Dent* 6(2):91, 1993.

143. Rueggeberg FA, Craig RG: Correlation of parameters used to estimate monomer conversion in a light-cured composite, *J Dent Res* 67(6):932, 1998.

144. Bayne SC, Heymann HO, Swift EJ Jr: Update on dental composite restorations, *J Am Dent Assoc* 125(6):687, 1994.

145. Vargas MA, Cobb DS, Schmit JL: Polymerization of composite resins: argon laser vs conventional light, *Oper Dent* 23(2):87, 1998.

146. Versluis A, Tantbirojn D, Douglas WH: Do dental composites always shrink toward the light? *J Dent Res* 77(6):1435, 1998.

147. Hickel R, Dasch W, Janda R, Tyas M, Anusavice K: New direct restorative materials: FDI Commission Project, *Int Dent J* 48(1):3, 1998.

148. Irie M, Suzuki K, Watts DC: Marginal gap formation of light activated restorative materials: effects of immediate setting shrinkage and bond strength, *Dent Mater* 18:203, 2002.

149. Ferracane JL: Buonocore Lecture. Placing dental composites—a stressful experience, *Oper Dent* 33(3):247, 2008.

150. Ferracane JL, Mitchem JC: Relationship between composite contraction stress and leakage in Class V cavities, *Am J Dent* 16(4):239, 2003.

Composite Resin: Indirect Technique Restorations

Ross Nash and Richard D. Trushkowsky

BASIC CONCEPTS

In some situations indirect composite resin restorations offer distinct advantages over direct composite resin restorations.

When a composite resin is polymerized, polymerization shrinkage occurs in the resin matrix. With the direct technique, such shrinkage can cause a marginal gap where the bond strength is the weakest, such as at the dentin-composite resin interface. When composite resin is polymerized in the laboratory by light, heat, or other methods, the shrinkage occurs before the restoration is bonded into place, thus only a thin layer of luting composite resin is subject to shrinkage at the tooth-restoration interface. This results in less marginal gap, which reduces the likelihood of marginal leakage, sensitivity, recurrent decay, and staining. In addition, studies have shown that some laboratory techniques (such as those that use pressure or vacuum plus heat or light catalysts and those that use heat processing after or simultaneously with light) produce a greater degree of polymerization than that achieved with light alone.[1-4] Thus the physical properties of tensile strength and hardness may be improved, providing for longer lasting and stronger restorations.[5]

Indirect techniques allow the dentist to incorporate the skills of the cosmetic dental laboratory technician. The rapid advances in composite resin technology have produced materials that can rival the beauty of porcelain, and solve some of the problems associated with this time-proven material. For example, porcelain is harder than tooth structure and can cause it to wear during function. Composite resin does not cause accelerated wear of opposing natural tooth structure. Also, after porcelain has been bonded into place, it is difficult to return the surface to the original luster after an adjustment. Composite resin can be adjusted and repolished easily. Laboratory-processed composite resin can be repaired with light-cured composite resin.

Compared with other techniques, indirect techniques may allow better control over interproximal contours and contacts; and, although meticulous attention to detail is important, indirect composite resin procedures may be less technique sensitive than direct ones.

BASIC CHEMISTRY

All composite resins are composed of filler particles in a resin matrix. The filler particles may range in size from 0.04 μm to over 100 μm. They provide the strength, and the resin matrix binds them together and bonds them to the tooth structure. The filler material may be very small silica particles, as in microfilled composite resins, or larger quartz or glass particles, as in small particle composite resin and hybrid composite resins. The resin matrix may be composed of bisphenol A diglycidyl ether methacrylate resin (introduced by Ray Bowen in 1962), urethane dimethacrylate, or similar polymers. Many combinations of resin and filler particles have been tried. In general, the higher the filler content (expressed as a percentage of weight), the greater the strength, and the smaller the filler particles, the greater the surface polishability.[6,7]

COMPOSITE RESIN SYSTEMS

Three types of composite resin material are available for use in indirect techniques: microfilled composite resins, small particle composite resins, and hybrid composite resins (Table 6-1). All show excellent wear resistance, but small particle composite resins and hybrid composite resins can be etched to produce micromechanical retention. They also can be silanated to enhance the bond strength. None of the current systems has proved superior to the others, and all produce good results when used properly.

In the mid 1990s a new category of processed composite resin was introduced. Polymer-glass, polymer-ceramic, and

Table 6-1 **Composite Resin Systems**

Name	Manufacturer	Composite type	Resin type	Curing method	Type of fabrication	Use
Sinfony	3M ESPE	Ultra-fine particle hybrid composite	Mixture of aliphatic and cycloaliphatic monomers	Light	Indirect	Crowns, inlays, onlays, laminate veneers, veneers on metal substructure, glass-fiber reinforced bridges
Gradia	GC America, Inc.	Micro-fine, ceramic/pre-polymer filler	Urethane dimethacrylate	Light	Indirect	Crowns, inlays, onlays, laminate veneers, veneers on metal substructure, glass-fiber reinforced bridges
Tescera ATL	Bisco, Inc.	Microhybrid		Heat, light and pressure under water	Indirect	Crowns, inlays, onlays, laminate veneers, veneers on metal substructure, glass-fiber reinforced bridges
Ceramage	Shofu Dental Corp.	Zirconium silicate micro ceramic PFS (Progressive Fine Structure)	UDMA resin	Light	Indirect	Crowns, inlays, onlays, laminate veneers, veneers on metal substructure, glass-fiber reinforced bridges

cercomer (ceramic-optimized polymer) are all terms used to describe these materials. In reality, they are all composite resins with improved properties. Several systems also have incorporated fiber reinforcement to allow fabrication of metal-free fixed partial dentures.

Premise Indirect

Premise Indirect (Kerr Corp.) dual cure indirect polymer-ceramic is a low-wear, high-strength microhybrid for inlays, onlays, anterior veneers, implants, full coverage crowns, metal-free fixed partial dentures, long-term provisional restorations, or splints. The opalescence of Premise Indirect is reported to achieve optimal shade matching capabilities. Trimodal curing (light, heat, and pressure) achieves over 98% material conversion as compared to 60% to 70% achieved with light-cure only materials. The material is a combination of large prepolymerized filler particles, 0.4 micron structural filler, and small silica nanoparticles that allow higher filler loading, improved physical properties, optimized handling, higher surface gloss, and reduced polymerization shrinkage. The coefficient of thermal expansion is similar to natural dentin and the wear rate over a 5 year period was similar to that of tooth structure. A reinforcing fiber material of woven polyethylene braids coated with a reactive monomeric solution that allows the product (Connect, Kerr Corp.) to be bonded to a resin based crown and fixed partial denture substructure by the application of heat is recommended for use in metal-free fixed partial dentures made with Premise Indirect.

Sinfony

Sinfony (3M ESPE), an ultrafine particle composite resin (or ultrafine particle hybrid composite resin) contains two kinds of filler: macrofiller (strontium aluminum borosilicate glass with a mean particle diameter of 0.5 to 0.7 μm; 40% by wt.) and microfiller (pyrogenic silica; 5% by wt.), which can flow into the gaps between the macrofiller particles. The Sinfony monomer system contains no Bis-GMA or TEGDMA. It is used as an indirect laboratory composite resin that combines strength, beauty, and versatility.

Indirect restorations created from Sinfony indirect laboratory composite resin offer excellent esthetics, translucency, natural vitality, amber opalescent effect, and fluorescence. Composite resin is excellent for inlays/onlays, veneers, and full crowns. A completely new feature is the addition of a special glass ionomer (5% by wt.), which influences the surface potential of Sinfony so that plaque accumulation is minimized. At the same time this additive does not change the other favorable composite resin properties including color and acid stability.

GC Gradia (GC America)

GC Gradia (GC America Inc.) is a light-cured high strength microhybrid (Microfill reinforced composite [MFR] formulation) that can be used for inlays/onlays, veneers. and crowns. GC Gradia couples a microfine ceramic/prepolymer filler with a urethane dimethacrylate matrix to produce a superior ceramic composite resin with exceptionally high strength, wear resistance, and superior polishability. GRADIA is biocompatible and kind to opposing teeth with excellent polishability, high wear resistance, but kind to the opposing dentition. The Foundation Opaque and Opaque shades can be used to mask discoloration effectively. Polymerization doesn't affect color so that the lab technician can visualize the definitive restoration. The system consists of a variety of opaques, intensive colors, enamel shades and translucent materials so that the restorations can be built up like porcelain. In addition to tooth colored composite resins, GC Gradia Gum provides a variety of natural gingival shades with good adaptation to the GC Gradia composite resin system. It is also a microfilled composite resin with high strength and wear resistance. Oxygen also plays an important role in the apparent translucency or opacity of the polymerized resin restoration. Oxygen also plays an important role in the apparent translucency or opacity of the polymerized resin restoration. Removing all of the air causes the restoration to become considerably more translucent.

TESCERA ATL

TESCERA ATL (Bisco, Inc.) is a dual-cured microhybrid composite resin that is provided in every Classic Vita shade. The incremental layers are condensed with pressure and then polymerized to prevent delamination and keep the restoration free of voids. Final polymerization occurs in an oxygen-free environment to achieve a high-gloss–free surface to reduce staining. Tescera Opaceous Dentin composite resins emulate the most dense and most opaque area of the tooth; it will also reflect light resulting in optimal aesthetics. Tescera Opaceous Dentin composite resins emulate the most dense and most opaque area of the tooth; it will also reflect light resulting in optimal aesthetics. TESCERA U-BEAM is a U-shaped, unidirectional, prestressed, quartz fiber reinforced beam for fixed partial dentures. It is resistant to twisting and flexing because of its I-beam effect.

Rods: Unidirectional, pretensed quartz fiber reinforcement bars are used for posterior and anterior fixed partial dentures

Signum Heraeus Kulzer

Signum ceramic is a glass-ceramic composite resin with microfine filler particles, which was specifically developed for the requirements of metal-free restorations; its particularly high intrinsic durability (E-modulus) makes the restoration more durable, even if high levels of stress are encountered.

Ceramage Shofu

Ceramage is a zirconium silicate integrated indirect restorative for both anterior and posterior regions. A progressive fine structure filling of more than 73% plus an organic polymer matrix delivers superior flexural strength, elasticity, and excellent polishability. It has flexural and compressive strength beyond 140 MPa, excellent abrasion resistance of opposing dentition, transmission and diffusion of light with a refractive index similar to natural teeth, and superior color stability over 5 years.

ANTERIOR COMPOSITE RESIN LAMINATE VENEERS

Many composite resins wear much like natural tooth structure and do not cause iatrogenic wear of the opposing dentition. Indirect composite resin laminate veneers are the treatment of choice in many situations:

- Darkly stained teeth. Indirect composite resin can cover dark color without opaquing agents while retaining a vital appearance.
- Conservation of tooth structure. Tooth preparation for composite resin laminate veneers can be more conservative than that for porcelain alternatives because composite resin does not require 0.5 mm thickness, as does porcelain. Composite resin can be much thinner in spots and still function well.
- Fabrication alternatives. Indirect composite resin laminate veneers can be fabricated either in the office or in the dental laboratory. They can be polymerized or processed. They can be made of microfilled, small particle, or hybrid composite resin. The glass in the small particle or hybrid composite resin can be etched with hydrofluoric acid, which provides micromechanical retention rivaling that of etched porcelain.
- Chairside repairs. These restorations can be repaired at the chairside with light-cured composite resins.

The technique described below is for a light-cured hybrid composite resin that is heat tempered, etched with 10% hydrofluoric acid gel, and treated with silane. The silane chemically bonds to the remaining glass particles and then to the luting composite resin, which is used to attach the laminate veneer to the etched enamel surface of the tooth. (Note that techniques may vary among manufacturers.)

Armamentarium.
- Mirror
- Explorer
- Metal "plastic" instrument (e.g., Hu-Friedy, Inc.)
- #12 surgical blade
- Bard parker handle
- Anterior scaler (U-15 Towner, Hu-Friedy, Inc.)
- Medium grit flame or chamfer diamond bur
- Vinyl polysiloxane impression material
- Irreversible hydrocolloid impression material
- Maxillary and mandibular full arch impression trays
- Die stone
- Hybrid composite resin
- Light-cured or dual-cured luting composite resin (see Chapter 12)
- Toaster oven or Coltene oven
- 12- and 30-fluted carbide finishing burs (e.g., ET Esthetic Trimming, Brasseler USA)
- Fine finishing diamond burs (e.g., ET Esthetic Trimming, Brasseler USA)
- Rubber composite resin polishing cups (see Chapter 5)
- Composite resin finishing disks (see Chapter 5)
- Composite resin polishing paste (see Chapter 5)
- 10% hydrofluoric gel
- 37% phosphoric acid gel(see Chapter 5)
- Dentin-enamel bonding resin (see Chapter 3)
- Silane coupling agent
- Intraoral light-curing unit (e.g., Demi Plus LED Dental Curing Light, Kerr Corp.)
- Oil-free pumice

Clinical Technique.
1. Clean the tooth and the neighboring teeth with pumice.
2. Select the desired shades of composite resin while the teeth are wet with saliva.
3. Determine the desired alignment of the teeth.
4. Prepare the eight maxillary anterior teeth by removing small amounts of enamel with a medium grit flame or chamfer diamond bur. If only minimum preparation is necessary to improve alignment and increase facial contour, remove only 0.25 to 0.50 mm of enamel from the facial area and none from the incisal area (Fig. 6-1A). If incisal reduction is necessary, remove 1 to 1.5 mm (Fig. 6-1B).

CLINICAL TIP

Preparation dimensions may vary depending on the manufacturer's recommendations and the amount of desired color change.

CLINICAL TIP

Preparation dimensions may vary depending on the manufacturer's recommendations and the amount of desired color change.

5. Make a full arch impression of the prepared teeth with a vinyl polysiloxane impression material. No retraction cord is needed because the margins are placed at the gingival crest.
6. Make a full arch irreversible hydrocolloid opposing impression.
7. Place a provisional restoration if needed (see Chapter 7)

8. Pour stone casts of both the prepared and the opposing arches. Laminate veneers can be fabricated on the stone cast by using a separating medium or on a flexible cast as described below.

9. After the stone is fully set, soak the cast of the prepared arch in water for 10 minutes and make an irreversible hydrocolloid impression of the cast.

CLINICAL TIP

Soaking the stone in water before making the irreversible hydrocolloid impression prevents the irreversible hydrocolloid from adhering to the stone.

10. Inject a vinyl polysiloxane impression material (medium to heavy viscosity) into the irreversible hydrocolloid impression and form a flexible cast (Fig. 6-1C). This technique was first developed by Dr. K. Michael Rhyne for use in indirect composite resin inlay fabrication.

CLINICAL TIP

A flexible working cast does not require a separating medium, nor is it susceptible to breakage. The chance of chipping the restoration upon removal from the working cast is slight.

11. On the flexible cast, fabricate composite resin veneers using a technique similar to that described for direct intraoral application (Fig. 6-1D).

CLINICAL TIP

To achieve a vital, natural appearance, apply layers of dentin, enamel, and incisal shades and polymerize each layer for 40 seconds (Fig. 6-1E).

12. Remove the laminate veneers from the flexible cast.

13. Contour and polish the laminate veneers using 12- and 30-fluted finishing carbide burs in a high-speed handpiece or porcelain contouring and polishing wheels on a lathe.

CLINICAL TIP

Fabricating every other laminate veneer to completion before fabricating the adjacent laminate veneer allows for good interproximal contours and contacts.

14. Place the laminate veneers on the original stone cast to check the fit and margins; adjust further if necessary (Fig. 6-1F).

15. Heat treat the laminate veneers in boiling water or a heat device, such as the Coltene unit, for 10 minutes to achieve the heat-curing benefits.

16. Acid etch the lingual side of the laminate veneers with 10% hydrofluoric acid gel for 30 seconds (Fig. 6-1G) or lightly sandblast with a microetcher or air abrasion unit and rinse thoroughly.

CLINICAL TIP

Handle hydrofluoric acid carefully because it is caustic.

17. Evaluate the internal surfaces of the laminate veneers to ensure that an etched surface has been achieved (Fig. 6-1H).

18. Clean the teeth with No. 4 fine pumice in a prophylaxis cup, rinse, and dry with water-free and oil-free air.

CLINICAL TIP

At the delivery appointment, use cheek and lip retractors to isolate the teeth. With this technique no cotton rolls or rubber dam is needed.

19. Clean the teeth with No. 4 fine pumice in a prophylaxis cup, rinse, and dry with water-free and oil-free air.

20. Use 37% phosphoric acid for 15 seconds to etch the enamel and remove the smear layer from any exposed dentin surface of the first central incisor (Fig. 6-1I).

21. Rinse thoroughly.

22. Leave the tooth surface slightly moist for wet bonding.

23. Using a brush, apply silane coupling agent to the internal surface of the laminate veneers and air dry.

CLINICAL TIP

Silane is generally indicated for hybrid, microhybrid, and nanohybrid composite resins and generally contraindicated for microfilled composite resins. Check the manufacturer's recommendation.

24. Liberally coat the etched surfaces with a hydrophilic primer from a fourth generation dentin and enamel bonding agent (Fig. 6-1J) and dry the primer with oil-free and water-free air until the surface appears glossy without being wet. This indicates that the "hybrid" layer has been established in the dentin and the enamel is thoroughly coated with the resin in the primer.

25. Paint a thin layer of bonding resin onto the internal surface of the laminate veneers.

26. Apply a luting composite resin to the internal surface of one of the laminate veneers. Place the laminate veneer on the prepared tooth and remove excess luting composite resin with a brush dipped in bonding agent (Fig. 6-1K).

27. Polymerize for 40 seconds on the facial and lingual surfaces of the tooth (Fig. 6-1L).

28. Remove excess polymerized luting composite resin with a #12 surgical blade or a scaler (Fig. 6-1M).

29. Place the other laminate veneers in the same fashion.

30. Finish the margins with 12- and 30-fluted carbide finishing burs, fine diamonds, rubber polishing cups, finishing disks, or other composite resin finishing techniques (Fig. 6-1N-P).

PREFABRICATED COMPOSITE RESIN LAMINATE VENEERS

Componeers (Coltene Whaledent)

Componeers direct composite resin laminate veneers are polymerized, prefabricated composite resin enamel shells made of a nanohybrid composite resin in order to combine the advantages of direct composite resin with laboratory fabricated laminate veneers. The laminate veneers are 0.3 mm in thickness so that

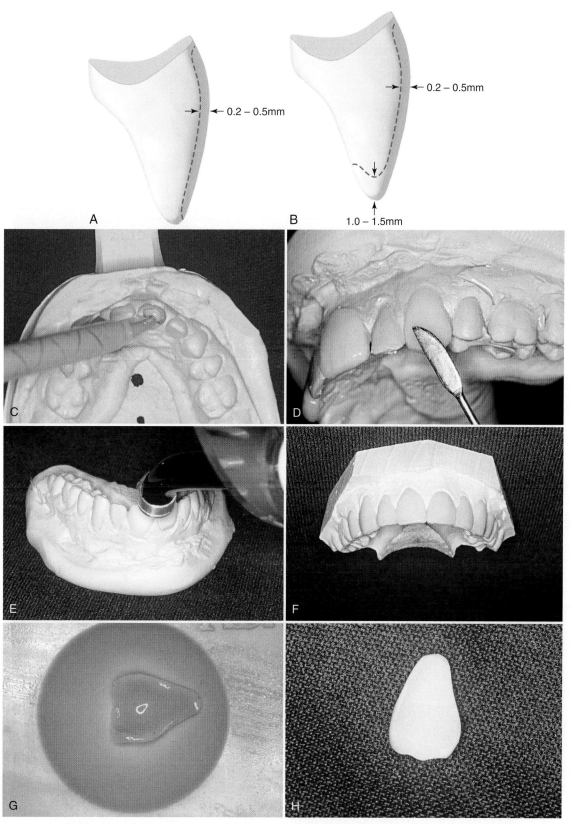

FIGURE 6-1 A, Anterior preparation without incisal reduction. Preparation dimensions may vary (see Clinical Tip). **B,** Anterior preparation with incisal reduction. Preparation dimensions may vary (see Clinical Tip). **C,** Vinyl polysiloxane is injected into an irreversible hydrocolloid impression of a stone cast of prepared teeth. **D,** On the flexible cast, fabricate composite resin veneers using a technique similar to that described for direct intraoral application. **E,** Composite resin veneer is polymerized. **F,** Eight indirect composite resin laminate veneers on a stone cast. **G,** Hydrofluoric acid gel (10%) is applied for 30 seconds. **H,** Etched internal surface of the hybrid composite resin laminate veneer.

Continued

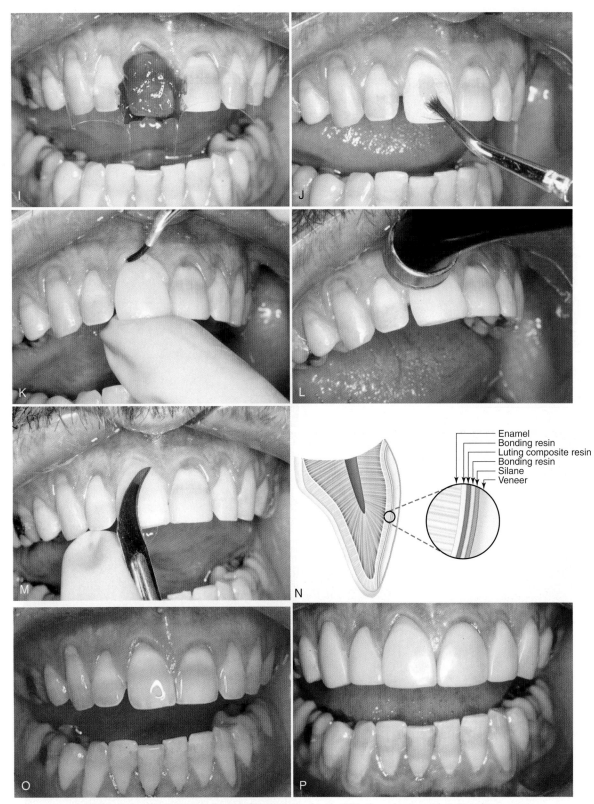

FIGURE 6-1, cont'd I, Enamel surface is etched with 37% phosphoric acid. **J,** Bonding resin is applied to the etched enamel. **K,** Excess luting composite resin is removed with a brush dipped in bonding agent. **L,** Luting composite resin is polymerized. **M,** Excess polymerized luting composite resin is removed with a #12 surgical blade. **N,** Final anterior restoration with various layers displayed. Silanation may be contraindicated. Refer to the manufacturer's recommendations. **O,** Preoperative view of tetracycline-stained teeth. **P,** Postoperative view of eight indirect composite resin laminate veneers.

minimal preparation is usually required. They are available in different sizes and are then directly customized by the clinician at the time of placement. They possess a microretentive inner surface to increase wettability and allow a more durable bond. No special conditioning is necessary. No impressions or the use of a dental laboratory are required.

Armamentarium.

+ Standard prefabricated composite resin laminate veneer setup
    + Mirror
    + Explorer
    + Metal "plastic" instrument (e.g., Hu-Friedy, Inc.)
    + #12 surgical blade
    + Bard parker handle
    + Anterior scaler (U-15 Towner/, Hu-Friedy, Inc.)
    + Medium grit flame or chamfer diamond bur (Brasseler USA)
    + 12- and 30-fluted carbide finishing burs (e.g., ET Esthetic Trimming—Brasseler USA)
    + Fine finishing diamond burs (e.g., ET Esthetic Trimming—Brasseler USA)
    + Rubber composite resin polishing cups (see Chapter 5)
    + Composite resin finishing disks (see Chapter 5)
    + Composite resin polishing paste (see Chapter 5)
    + Intraoral light-curing unit (e.g., Demi Plus LED Dental Curing Light, Kerr Inc.)
    + Oil-free pumice
+ Componeers Accessory Set/(Coltene Whaledent) includes
    + MBS modeling instrument
    + Etchant Gel S
    + One coat Bond
    + Synergy D6/Synergy D6 Flow/Synergy D6 connect
    + Holder
    + Holder caps (black)
    + Placer (white)
    + Placer adapter (white)
    + Placer adapter (red)
    + Application needles
    + Brush holder (black)
    + Brushes
    + Shade guide Componeer Synergy D6
    + Componeer Contour guide

Clinical Technique.

1. The correct componeer shade and size are selected with the template provided. The Componeer Contour guide (a blue transparent guide) aid in selection of the correct tooth shape. Thirty different shapes with 6 sizes per shape.
2. The teeth are then prepared as needed for the Componeer laminate veneer. Usually minimal preparation is needed. The Componeer Modeling Instrument MB5 is sharp and can be used to remove excess composite resin.
3. Bonding resin of choice is placed on the tooth and then the Componeer Holder (a specially designed tweezers to aid in shape correction of the Componeer as well as placement of the bond) is used for reshaping as required and placement of the bonding resin. The interchangeable holder caps protect the Componeer. Conventional microhybrid composite resin and polymerized.
4. Place the Compomer cement on the tooth (Fig. 6-2A)
5. The Componeer placer is used to align and position the laminate veneers (Fig. 6-2B and C). The Componeer Casting Instrument MB5 is sharp and can be used to remove excess composite resin.

6. The Componeer is light cured as per manufacturer's guidelines (Fig. 6-2D).
7. The Componeer is trimmed with carbide finishing burs (Fig. 6-2E) and excess cement is removed with finishing strips (Fig. 6-2F).
8. The laminate veneers are polished (Fig 6-2G).

Edelweiss Composite Laminate Veneers (Ultradent Products Inc.)

Edelweiss Composite Laminate Veneers (Ultradent Products, Inc.) are composite resin laminate veneers which are laser sintered so that the laser particles are fused together to provide a high gloss, uniform surface, and a thermally tempered base. The laminate veneer filler ratio is 82% by weight and 65% by volume. The variation of inorganic filler particle is between 0.02 and 0.03 μm.

Armamentarium.

+ Standard prefabricated composite resin laminate veneer setup
+ Edelweiss composite laminate veneers kit

Clinical Technique.

1. Clean each tooth, including the mesial and distal aspects, with Consepsis Scrub or a fluoride-free flour of pumice.
2. Placing the transparent laminate veneer sizing guide over the teeth, select the size. Slight adjustments to the shape of the laminate veneer can be made with a rough disk at slow speed.
3. Determine the shade on a moist, non-dehydrated tooth using natural daylight conditions.
4. Isolate the treatment area with a rubber dam, if possible.
5. Prepare the tooth surface with as minimal an amount of reduction as possible. Use retraction cord and hemostatic agents where needed to control tissue, bleeding, and moisture.
6. Clean each tooth again, including the mesial and distal aspects, with Consepsis Scrub or a fluoride-free flour of pumice.
7. Securely place a thin, transparent matrix band or Teflon tape interproximally.

Pretreatment of the Enamel Shell.

1. Using a rough surface disk at low speed with no water, adjust the fit of the laminate veneer.
2. To improve adhesion, the internal surface may be roughened by micro abrading with 25 or 50 μm aluminum oxide or a diamond bur.
3. Apply 37% phosphoric acid for 5 seconds, rinse, and dry to cleanse the surface.
4. Brush a coat of bonding agent onto the prepared surface.
5. Blow air using half pressure to thin and remove solvents. The surface will appear shiny.
6. Polymerize for 10 seconds with a curing light. For lights with outputs less than 600mW/cm^2, polymerize for 20 seconds or for lights with output greater than 600mW/cm^2, polymerize for 10 seconds.

Pretreatment of the Prepared Teeth.

1. Apply 37% phosphoric acid to the tooth surface for 20 seconds, rinse thoroughly for 5 seconds and dry lightly leaving the surface slightly damp.
2. Place a puddle coat of bonding agent with a microbrush onto the prepared surface and gently agitate for 10 seconds.
3. Thin/dry for 10 seconds using quarter to half pressure. The surface will appear slightly shiny.
4. Polymerize for 10 seconds with a curing light. For lights with output less than 600mW/cm^2, polymerize for 20 seconds or for lights with output greater than 600mW/cm^2, polymerize for 10 seconds.

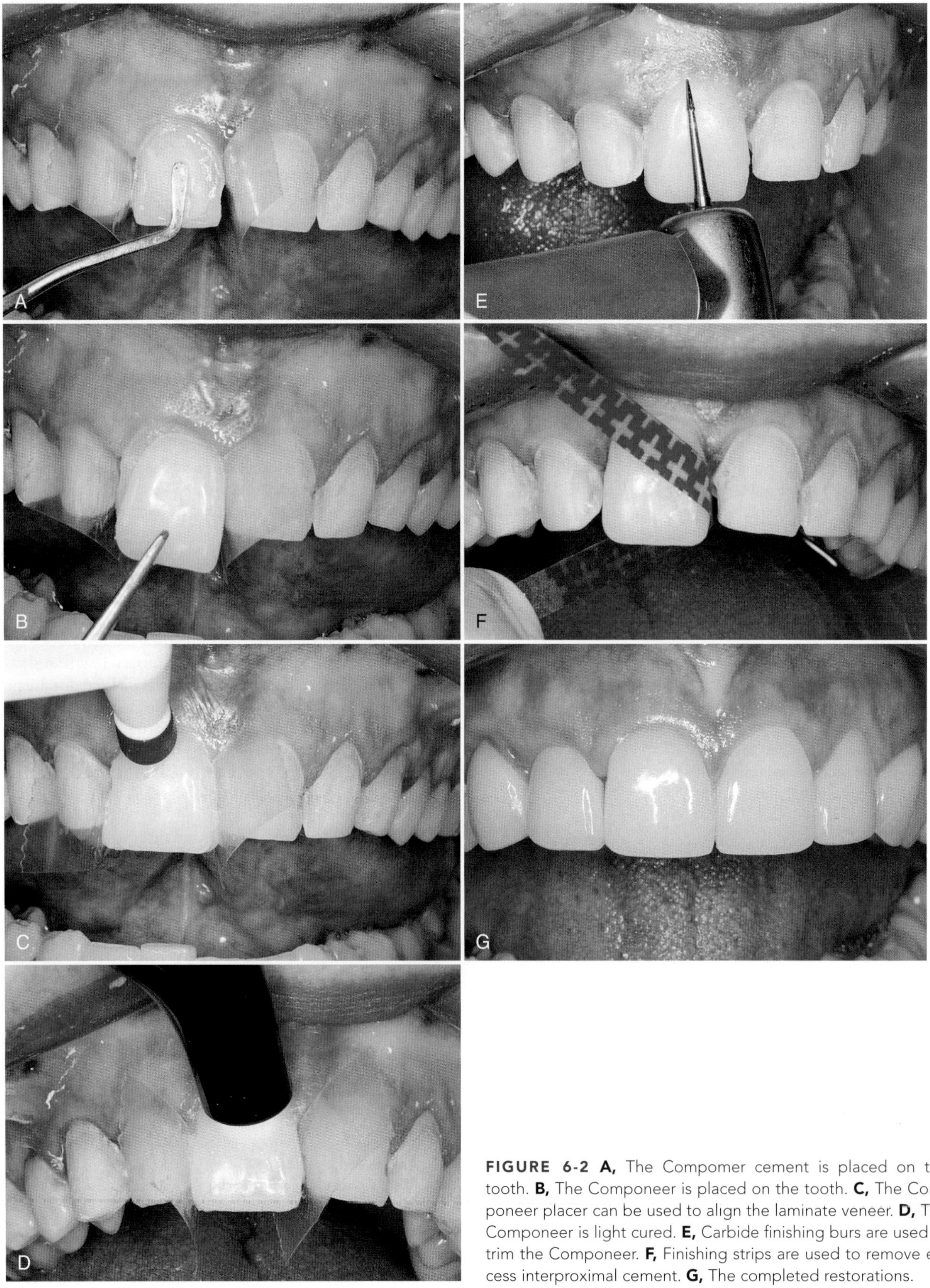

FIGURE 6-2 A, The Compomer cement is placed on the tooth. **B,** The Componeer is placed on the tooth. **C,** The Componeer placer can be used to align the laminate veneer. **D,** The Componeer is light cured. **E,** Carbide finishing burs are used to trim the Componeer. **F,** Finishing strips are used to remove excess interproximal cement. **G,** The completed restorations.

5. Amelogen Plus (Ultradent) can be used as it flows under pressure. Conventional laminate veneer cements are not recommended.

POSTERIOR INLAYS AND ONLAYS

Composite resin inlays and onlays are an excellent choice for teeth with wide proximal occlusal cavities[8]:

- Esthetic considerations. A bonded restoration can provide esthetics and function of high quality and may be a long-lasting alternative to full coverage or the porcelain or direct composite resins counterparts.
- Structural considerations. A bonded restoration returns nearly all the original strength to the tooth and holds the remaining tooth structure together.[9]
- Abrasion considerations. Because some composite resins have been shown to wear at about the same rate as natural tooth structure, they are an excellent choice of material for restorative purposes. However, newer ceramic materials such as E Max (Ivoclar Vivadent) are a viable alternative.
- Conservation of tooth structure. Onlay preparations have the advantage of requiring the removal of less tooth structure than for a full crown.
- Supragingival margins. Onlay preparations have supragingival margins and therefore infringe less on the periodontal apparatus than restorations with subgingival margins.
- Chairside repairs. These restorations can be repaired at the chairside with light-cured composite resins.

With the advent of strong bonding agents and appropriate restorative materials, indirect composite resins can provide long-lasting alternatives to full crowns or conventional cast onlays.

Direct/Indirect Technique: Fabrication

Armamentarium. The armamentarium is the same as that listed for anterior laminate veneers.

Clinical Technique.

1. The preparation is similar to that for a gold inlay or onlay; however, the divergent walls must have rounded angles and no sharp corners (Fig. 6-3A).

> ### CLINICAL TIP
> No retentive cuts or parallel walls are needed, because the restoration will be bonded into place (Fig. 6-3B).

2. Provide at least 1.5 mm of clearance on the prepared occlusal surface.
3. No bevels are needed, and slightly tapering or butt joint margins should be used.
4. Areas prepared closer than 0.5 mm to the pulp should be lined with calcium hydroxide, and undercuts should be filled with an appropriate liner or base.

> ### CLINICAL TIP
> Do not use solutions containing eugenol, which can interfere with the chemistry of the resins.

> ### CLINICAL TIP
> Undercuts in the preparation make removal impossible; carefully inspect the preparation before placing composite resin and block out or remove undercuts.

5. Apply a separating medium or glycerin to the entire tooth.
6. Place a light-cured hybrid composite resin directly into the prepared tooth using normal direct placement technique.
7. Remove the restoration from the tooth using a large spoon or other instrument.
8. Heat treat the inlay or onlay.
9. Place the inlay or onlay according to the placement technique described later.

Indirect Technique: Flexible Cast Fabrication

A completely indirect technique that can be performed in one appointment and that does not require a provisional restoration can be accomplished using a flexible cast technique.

Armamentarium. The armamentarium is the same as that listed for anterior laminate veneers.

Clinical Technique.

1. The first four steps are identical to those given in the preceding section on direct/indirect technique.
2. Make an irreversible hydrocolloid impression that captures all of the margins of the preparation.
3. Inject a firm-setting vinyl polysiloxane impression material into the irreversible hydrocolloid impression to form a flexible cast (Fig. 6-3C).
4. Fabricate a composite resin inlay using light-cured hybrid composite resin (Fig. 6-3D).
5. Heat treat the restoration.
6. Place the inlay or onlay according to the placement technique described below (Fig. 6-3E).

Indirect Technique: Laboratory Fabrication

Composite resin inlays and onlays can be fabricated by the laboratory technician The preparation is identical to those described in the first four steps in the earlier section on direct/indirect technique. If desired, immediate dentin sealing can be incorporated prior to provisionalization to minimize or eliminate sensitivity. An impression is made with an impression material which would be suitable for any laboratory fabricated single tooth restoration. A provisional restoration must then be fabricated and placed until the definitive restoration is placed during a subsequent office visit.

Dentin Sealing Before Impressioning (Optional).
Bisco Pro V.
Armamentarium.
- Oil-free pumice
- Cavity cleanser
- Bonding Agent (ex ALL-BOND SE or All Bond 3 (Bisco, Inc.)
- Provisional Restorative system (ex PRO-V COAT, PRO-V FILL, PRO-V FLO, Bisco, Inc.)
- Mirror
- Explorer
- Metal "plastic" instrument (e.g., Hu-Friedy, Inc.)

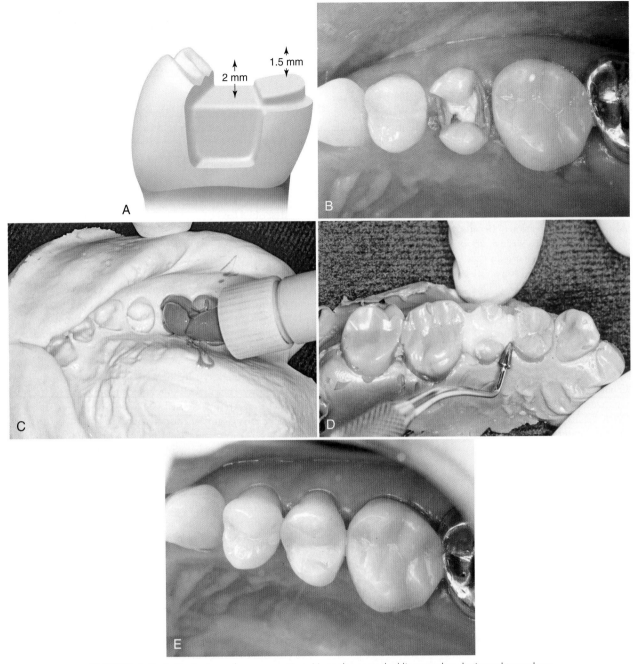

FIGURE 6-3 A, Posterior onlay preparation. Note the rounded line angles designed to reduce internal stress. **B,** Tooth prepared for indirect composite resin veneer. **C,** Vinyl polysiloxane is injected into an irreversible hydrocolloid impression. **D,** Fabrication of the composite resin inlay. **E,** Composite resin inlay bonded into place.

+ Anterior scaler (U-15 Towner/, Hu-Friedy, Inc.)
+ 12- and 30-fluted carbide finishing burs (e.g., ET Esthetic Trimming—Brasseler USA)
+ Fine finishing diamond burs (e.g., ET Esthetic Trimming—Brasseler USA)
+ Intraoral light-curing unit (e.g., Demi Plus LED Dental Curing Light, Kerr Inc.)
   Clinical Technique—ALL-BOND 3—Total Etch Method.
1. Thoroughly clean the preparation with pumice slurry or Cavity Cleanser (Bisco), which should dwell for 30 seconds and excess blotted.

2. Etch the dentin for 5 to 10 seconds using UNI-ETCH with benzalkonium chloride and rinse thoroughly. Remove excess water using a foam pellet or with a high volume suction, leaving the preparation visibly moist.

CLINICAL TIP

Use of an air syringe may desiccate the dentin. A high volume suction or foam pellet to remove excess water followed (if needed) with a dry cotton pellet in a blotting motion will leave the dentin slightly moist.

3. Dispense an equal number of drops of ALL-BOND 3 Parts A & B (1:1) into a mixing well. Immediately replace the caps.

> ### CLINICAL TIP
>
> The caps should be replaced immediately to prevent evaporation of the solvent. Evaporation would change the consistency and the chemical composition of the components.

4. Using a brush, mix ALL-BOND 3 Parts A & B in the well for 5 seconds.
5. Immediately apply 1 to 2 coats to the moist preparation.
6. Gently but thoroughly air dry until there is no visible movement of the material.
7. The surface should appear shiny; otherwise apply additional coats and air dry.
   a. Polymerize for 10 seconds at 500mW/cm².
8. Apply 1 thin coat of ALL-BOND 3 RESIN. Air thin if necessary and polymerize for 10 seconds at 500mW/cm².
9. Block out existing undercuts with a flowable composite resin, according to the manufacturer's instructions.
10. Redefine the preparation, including the enamel margins.
11. Remove the oxygen inhibited layer of the freshly bonded surfaces with an alcohol moistened cotton pellet or gauze.

> ### CLINICAL TIP
>
> The surface with an oxygen inhibited layer will leach more monomer, has inferior properties, and should be removed.

12. Make an impression.
13. Dispense 1 to 2 drops of PRO-V COAT into a mixing well. Immediately replace the cap on the bottle.

> ### CLINICAL TIP
>
> The caps should be replaced immediately to prevent evaporation of the solvent. Evaporation would change the consistency and the chemical composition of the components.

14. Using a brush, apply 1 to 2 coats of PRO-V COAT to the entire preparation.
15. Gently air dry (from 8-10cm from the prep) for 10 to 15 seconds to evaporate the solvent.
16. Proceed with provisionalization. (See section on PROVISIONAL INLAYS AND ONLAYS.

Using ALL-BOND SE—Self Etch Method

Armamentarium.
- Standard prefabricated composite resin laminate veneer setup
- Unfluoridated pumice paste
- Intraoral air abrasion unit (e.g., Microetcher ERC Sand Blaster Danville Engineering) (optional)
- Aluminum Oxide—50 Micron (Danville Materials Abrasive and Polishing Material) (optional)
- Cavity Cleaner (e.g., Cavity Cleanser, Bisco Inc.)
- Bonding Agent (e.g., ALL-BOND SE, Bisco Inc.)

- Flowable composite resin (e.g., Renamel Flowable, Cosmedent Inc.)
- Impression material (e.g., Reprosile, Dentsply)
- Separating agent (e.g., PRO-V COAT, Bisco, Inc.)
  Clinical Technique.
  1. Thoroughly clean the preparation with unfluoridated pumice paste, or a microetcher with 25 micron aluminum oxide or Cavity Cleaner (Bisco), which should dwell for 30 seconds and excess blotted.
  2. Gently dry to remove excess moisture from the tooth preparation and then dispense an equal number of drops of ALL-BOND SE Parts I & II (1:1) into a mixing well. Immediately replace the caps.

> ### CLINICAL TIP
>
> The caps should be replaced immediately to prevent evaporation of the solvent. Evaporation would change the consistency and the chemical composition of the components.

3. Using a brush, mix ALL-BOND SE Parts I & II until uniformly pink. Apply 1 to 2 coats of ALL-BOND SE to the dry preparation and then agitate for at least 10 seconds.
4. Gently but thoroughly air dry until there is no visible movement of the material. The surface should appear shiny; otherwise, apply additional coats of ALL-BOND SE and air dry.
5. Polymerize for 10 seconds at 500mW/cm².
6. Apply one thin coat of ALL-BOND SE LINER. Air thin if necessary and polymerize for 10 seconds at 500mW/cm².
7. Block out existing undercuts with a flowable composite, according to manufacturer's instructions.
8. Redefine the preparation, including the enamel margins.
9. Remove the oxygen inhibited layer of the freshly bonded surfaces with an alcohol moistened cotton pellet or gauze.
10. Make an impression
11. Dispense 1 to 2 drops of PRO-V COAT into a mixing well. Immediately replace the cap on the bottle.

> ### CLINICAL TIP
>
> The caps should be replaced immediately to prevent evaporation of the solvent. Evaporation would change the consistency and the chemical composition of the components.

12. Using a brush, apply 1 to 2 coats of PRO-V COAT to the entire preparation. Gently air dry (from 8-10 cm from the prep) for 10 to 15 seconds to evaporate the solvent.
13. Proceed with provisionalization.

PROVISIONAL INLAYS AND ONLAYS

Provisional restorations are an important and necessary part of any reconstruction. Besides temporarily restoring the tooth/teeth, they serve other important functions including:
- Covering exposed dentin to prevent tooth sensitivity, plaque buildup, cavities, and pulp problems
- Preventing unwanted tooth movement
- Enabling patients to eat and speak normally
- Serving as a diagnostic tool
- Maintaining the health and contours of the periodontal tissue

Provisional inlays and onlay systems are designed with specific properties that are optimized for quick and easy removal. Ideally they should:

+ Be light curable
+ Cure to a semi-hard state
+ Maintain enough flexibility for easy removal
+ Have the ability to be placed without a matrix
+ Be easy to carve and clean up
+ Be eugenol free to allow for the use of resin cements for final cementation.
+ Have excellent retention without cementation
+ Encourage healing of gingival tissue

Fabrication of a Provisional Restoration

Armamentarium.
+ Bis-Acryl materials such as
  + Telio CS Inlay and Telio CS Onlay (Ivoclar Vivadent)
  + Luxatemp Ultra (DMG)
  + Integrity Multi-Cure (Dentsply/Caulk)
  + Venus Temp 2 (Heraeus)
  + Protemp Plus (3M ESPE)
  + Tuff-Temp (Pulpdent)
  + Structur 2 SC (Voco America)
  + PRO-V FILL and PRO-V Flow (Bisco, Inc.)
+ Silicone finishing burs (e.g., Astropol F) or tungsten carbide finishing burs for grinding and excess removal
+ Scalpel (may also be used to remove excess material)

Clinical Technique.
1. Place PRO-V Flow initially to adapt to the internal aspect of the preparation.
2. Place PRO-V FILL in 2- to 3-mm increments. Polymerize each increment for 10 seconds at $500mW/cm^2$.
3. Place the last incremental layer of PRO-V FILL and adjust the occlusion with instruments.
4. After the final adjustment, polymerize for 20 seconds at $500mW/cm^2$.
5. If desired, apply a liquid polish such as BisCover LV. Dispense 1 or 2 drops of BisCover LV into a mixing well. Dip the brush into the BisCover LV. Wipe excess from the brush onto the side of the mixing well. The brush does not need to be saturated; it should be only wet enough to apply one thin coat.
6. Apply one thin coat of BisCover LV in one direction with a smooth stroke. Do not agitate the brush during application.

CLINICAL TIP

It is very important to allow 15 seconds dwelling time for evaporation of solvent after application. Do not air thin because this will disperse the material unevenly causing ripples on the surface.

7. BisCover LV uses the following curing lights and curing times to initiate polymerization:
   a. LED Lights: Using an LED curing light with a minimum output of $500mW/cm^2$, polymerize for 30 seconds at close range (0-2 mm)
   b. Halogen Lights: Using a halogen curing unit, such as VIP junior, with a minimum output of $500mW/cm^2$, polymerize for 30 seconds at close range (0-2 mm)

CLINICAL TIP

If the light intensity is lower and/or curing occurs at a distance (10 mm), polymerize for greater than 30 seconds.

   c. PAC (Plasma Arc) Lights: Using a PAC light, polymerize for 10 seconds at close range (0-2 mm).

CLINICAL TIP

Insufficient curing will leave an air-inhibited layer on the surface of BisCover LV. Upon curing, BisCover LV may produce a brief exothermic reaction, which is minimized by applying in a thin layer. Do not cure on soft tissue.

8. If a second coat is desired, repeat steps 1 to 6.

Removal of the Provisional Restoration

Armamentarium.
+ Standard prefabricated composite resin laminate veneer setup

Clinical Technique.
1. Insert a suitable sharp instrument (probe/scaler) into the material and remove in the line of draw.
2. Proceed with the definitive bonding protocol.

Placement of the Definitive Inlay or Onlay

The placement of inlays or onlays is identical whether they are fabricated in the office or at the dental laboratory using the commercial processes described.

Armamentarium. The armamentarium is the same as that listed for anterior laminate veneers.

Clinical Technique.
1. Remove the provisional restorations (Fig. 6-4*A*).
2. Place the definitive restorations on a clean, dry surface (Fig. 6-4*B*).
3. Place a rubber dam.
4. Thoroughly clean the prepared tooth with pumice.
5. Use 37% phosphoric acid to etch the enamel margins (Fig. 6-4*C*) and to remove the smear layer from the prepared dentin surfaces. Rinse thoroughly and leave the tooth surfaces moist to allow wet bonding.
6. Liberally coat the etched surfaces with a hydrophilic primer from a fourth generation dentin and enamel bonding agent (Fig. 6-4*D*) and dry the primer with oil-free and water-free air until the surface appears glossy without being wet. This indicates that the "hybrid" layer has been established in the dentin and the enamel has been thoroughly coated with the resin in the primer.
7. Apply a dual-curing bonding resin to the dentin and enamel surfaces and the internal surface of the onlay (Fig. 6-4*E*).
8. Mix a dual-cured luting composite resin and apply it to the inner surface of the restoration or to the surface of the prepared tooth (Fig. 6-4*F*).
9. Place the restoration and remove excess luting composite resin with a brush dipped in bonding agent (Fig. 6-4*G*).
10. While the onlay is held in place with an instrument, run dental floss through the proximal areas, pulling in the facial or lingual direction to remove excess resin.

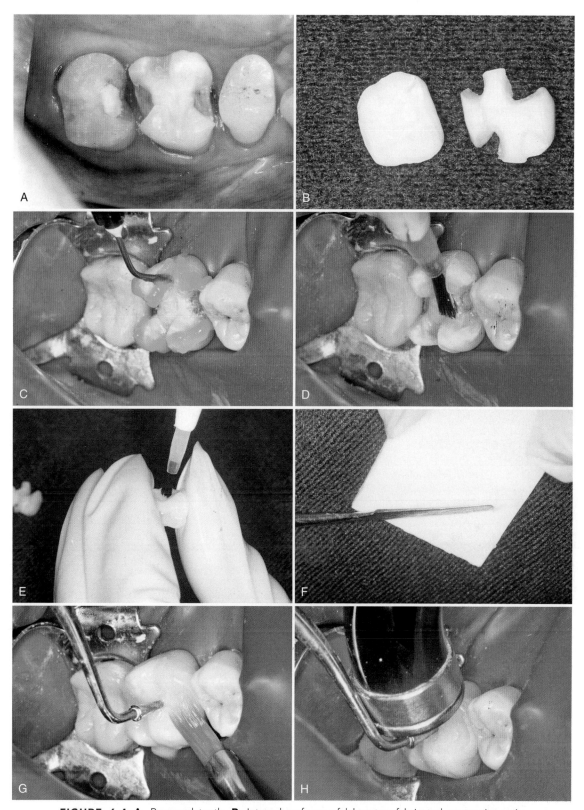

FIGURE 6-4 A, Prepared teeth. **B,** Internal surfaces of laboratory-fabricated composite resin onlays. **C,** Enamel margins are etched with 37% phosphoric acid gel. **D,** Dentin primer is applied. **E,** Bonding resin is applied to the internal surface of the onlay. **F,** Mixing of the dual-cured luting composite resin. **G,** Excess luting composite resin is removed with a brush dipped in bonding agent. **H,** Luting composite resin is polymerized with a visible light source.   *Continued*

FIGURE 6-4, cont'd **I,** Final posterior restoration with various layers displayed. **J,** Excess polymerized luting composite resin is removed with a #12 surgical blade. **K,** Occlusion is adjusted with a carbide finishing bur. **L,** Composite resin onlays are polished with composite resin polishing paste. **M,** Completed onlays. **N,** Preparation of the mandibular arch for two inlays and one onlay. **O,** Finished restorations.

11. Polymerize the restoration for 40 seconds on the occlusal, facial, and lingual surfaces (Figs. 6-4*H* and 6-4*I*).
12. Excess polymerized luting composite resin can be removed with a surgical blade (Fig. 6-4*J*), a scaler, or carbide finishing burs.

CLINICAL TIP

The dual-cured luting composite resin will continue to cure, but finishing can begin 4 minutes after light curing.

---

13. Adjust the occlusion with carbide finishing burs (Fig. 6-4*K*).
14. Polish the finished and adjusted surfaces with normal composite resin polishing techniques, including the use of final polishing paste (Fig. 6-4*L-O*).

THE FUTURE

Composite resins have a promising future in dentistry. The technology has progressed over the years, and bonding agents will ensure strong, long-lasting adhesion to tooth structure. However, ceramic materials such as E Max and monolithic Zirconia provide viable alternatives. Newer materials such as Lava Ultimate CAD/CAM Restorative a resin nano ceramic material combine resin and ceramic materials.

BIBLIOGRAPHY

Berge M: Properties of prosthetic resin-veneer materials processed in commercial laboratories, *Dent Mat* 5:77, 1989.

Bonner P, Kanca J: Dentist reveals methods for fabricating the direct resin inlay, *Cosmet Dent Gen Pract* 5:1, 1989.

Christensen GJ: Tooth-colored inlays and onlays, *J Am Dent Assoc* 4:12E, 1988.

Dimberio RD: A new crown and bridge veneering material, *Quintessence Dent Tech* 4:27, 1979.

First International Symposium on the Clinical Applications of Laboratory Light Cured Composites, December 13, 1984, Valley Forge, PA.

Gallegos LI, Nicholls JI: In vitro two-body wear of three veneering resins, *Quintessence Int* 20:259, 1989.

Gallegos LI, Nicholls JI. In vitro two-body wear of three veneering resins, *J Prosthet Dent* Aug; 60(2):172-8,1988.

Gross J, Malacmacher L: Posterior composite resins: the technique, *Dentique* 1:1, 1985.

James DF: An esthetic inlay technique for posterior teeth, *Quintessence* 14:725, 1983.

Jones RM, Moore BK: A comparison of the physical properties of four prosthetic veneering materials, *Prosthet Dent* 61:38, 1989.

Kanca J: The single visit heat processed indirect composite resin inlay, *J Esthet Dent* 1:13, 1988.

Lappalainen R, Yli-Urpo A, Seppa L: Wear of dental restorative and prosthetic materials in vitro, *Dent Mat* 5:35, 1989.

Michl RJ: Isosit, a new dental material, *Quintessence Int* 9:1, 1978.

Miller M et al: Indirect resin systems, *Reality* 4:52, 1989.

Nash R: Hybrid composites: excellent for veneers, *Lab Man Today* 4:34, 1988.

Nash R: Restorative options for good aesthetics, *Dent Today* 3:1, 1987.

REFERENCES

1. Wendt SL: Time as a factor in the heat curing of composite resins, *Quintessence Int* 20:259, 1989.
2. Watts DC: Coltene seminar, *The Coltene direct inlay system: a report on the properties of the inlay composite material resulting from different curing conditions*, September 1-13, 1988.
3. Duke ES, Norling BK: *Vacuum curing of light activated composite resin veneering resin*, USAF Medical Center and University of Texas HSC published report, San Antonio, Texas.
4. Wendt SF: The effect of heat used as a secondary cure upon the physical properties of three composite resins, *Quintessence Int* 18:351, 1987.
5. Ibsen RL, Neville K: *Adhesive restorative dentistry*, Philadelphia, 1974, Saunders.
6. Albers HF: *Tooth colored restoratives*, ed 7, Cotati, CA, 1985, Alto Books.
7. Simonsen R, Barouch E, Geib M: Cusp fracture resistance from composite resin in Class II restorations, *J Dent Res* 62:761, 1983.
8. Geurtsen W, García-Godoy F. Bonded restorations for the prevention and treatment of the cracked-tooth syndrome, *Am J Dent* 12(6):266-270, 1999.
9. Simonsen R, Barouch E, Geib M: Cusp fracture resistance from composite resin in Class II restorations, *J Dent Res* 62:761, 1983.

7

Porcelain Laminate Veneers Restorations

Kenneth W. Aschheim

In the nineteenth century, porcelain inlays were introduced as an esthetic alternative to metallic restorations. These inlays were formed either by grinding a solid porcelain block[1] or more commonly by fusing porcelain chips to a platinum-gold foil matrix.[2] Extremely brittle restorations, they were contraindicated in high-stress areas. Their imprecise fit resulted in a visible cement line and caries susceptibility because of cement washout. In addition, the absence of an adhesive cement limited these restorations to preparations that provided sufficient frictional retention.

Porcelain use decreased following the introduction of silicate cements in 1908. Although silicates, a combination of silica alumina and calcium fluoride, showed significant solubility in salivary fluids, the fluoride component provided anticariogenicity. Acrylic resins, introduced in 1946, immediately replaced silicate resins as the esthetic material of choice. Although they exhibited better long-term retention, they did not contain fluoride, which resulted in an increased incidence of recurrent decay. Advances in acrylic resin systems, compared with earlier restorations, controlled some of the polymerization shrinkage, but they still exhibited poor overall dimensional stability. In addition, like silicates, acrylic resins required mechanical retention. The introduction of the acid-etch technique and filled composite resins further diminished the use of porcelain as an internal restorative material. Porcelain, in the form of all-porcelain and porcelain-fused-to-metal restorations, was relegated to full coverage restorations.

In the late 1970s, direct and indirect laminate veneers were introduced. Direct veneers, which used light-cured composite resin to overlay the entire facial surface, allowed great flexibility in both shaping and shading teeth. However, they were time consuming and required substantial artistic skill. In addition, they exhibited poor color stability and wear resistance.

Indirect or preformed veneers attempted to overcome some of these limitations.[3] Composed of acrylic, they were treated with ethyl acetate, methylene chloride, or methyl methacrylate and then luted to the etched tooth with a composite resin. Although they exhibited greater color stability and stain resistance than early direct composite resin veneers, the composite resin-to-laminate veneer bond proved to be a fatal weak link.[4] The acrylic veneer also exhibited a dull and monochromatic appearance, poor abrasion resistance,[5] and resulted in unsatisfactory gingival inflammation.

PORCELAIN-BONDED RESTORATIONS

Early research[6] indicated that it was possible to chemically bond silica to acrylic or bis-GMA using a silane coupling agent. Most research[7-9] focused on the direct chemical bonding of porcelain teeth to acrylic denture bases. Early silane bonds prevented seepage of oral fluids between the porcelain-acrylic interface.[10] However, differences in the coefficient of thermal expansion between porcelain and acrylic caused bond deterioration during bench cooling of the heat-cured acrylic.

The need for a technique to repair ceramometal restorations with debonded porcelain prompted interest in the composite resin to porcelain bond. It was discovered that no bond formed between the glazed porcelain and composite resin, even with silane,[10,11,12] unless the surface was roughened.[13]

In 1983, the porcelain-laminate veneer was introduced.[14] It combined the esthetic and positive tissue response of porcelain with the adhesive strength of acid-etch retained restorations and the convenience of a laboratory-fabricated restoration.

BASIC CHEMISTRY

The porcelain-bonded restoration consists of four components
1. An internally etched porcelain veneer
2. A suitable tooth surface
3. A silane-coupling agent
4. A composite resin luting cement

Porcelain

Dental porcelains are composed of natural feldspar (both potassium and sodium aluminosilicate glasses).[15] Early porcelain-laminate veneers used the same porcelains used in all-porcelain restorations. Later, high-strength porcelains specifically designed for bonded restorations were introduced. These materials are stronger than conventional porcelains and composite resin.

Acid Etching

Retention of the acid-etch retained porcelain restoration is accomplished by the creation of microporosities in both the porcelain and enamel. Porcelain porosities are derived from treating the internal surface of the restoration with a 10% acid solution, such as hydrofluoric acid. Studies show that etching with or without the use of a silane coupling agent greatly increases bond shear strength, which can even surpass resin-enamel bond strength (Table 7-1).[16,17]

Salivary contamination of the etched porcelain can significantly reduce bond strength. Application of 37% phosphoric acid for 15 seconds has been shown to restore the etched surface.[18]

Silane Coupling Agents

The function of a coupling agent is to alter the surface of a solid to facilitate either a chemical or physical process.[10] Numerous silane coupling agents exist and are used in dentistry to increase the shear strength of the porcelain-to-composite resin bond.

These agents are believed to be capable of chemically bonding to silica in both the porcelain laminate veneer and the composite resin matrix. Scanning electron micrographs reveal that silane and etching eliminate the polymerization contraction gap, which forms in both etched, nonsilanated and unetched, silanated restorations by allowing the resin to better wet the surface.[17] An in vitro study using two different types of feldspathic porcelain concluded that silane combined with the action of hydrofluoric acid gel is the most effective surface treatment for ceramics.[19]

Composite Resin Luting Cements

Initially, laminate veneers were retained with auto-curing composite resins. Light-activated composite resin luting cements provided increased working time. Numerous viscosities are available. Different shades and opacities allow for color modification of the restoration.

Light-activated resins are ideally suited for most laminate veneers. However, they require sufficient light from a curing light to initiate curing. Therefore they should not be used when the light must travel through a thickness of porcelain that exceeds the manufacturer's recommendations. Factors affecting this maximum depth include the specific light source, the age of the bulb, the shade and opacity of the laminate, and the shade and opacity of the composite resin cement.

BASIC LABORATORY TECHNIQUE

Porcelain-laminate veneers can be fabricated by the laboratory in one of four ways: platinum foil backing, refractory casts, direct castings, or CAD-CAM machining.

Platinum Foil Backing. This method can also be used to construct the all-porcelain crown. A very thin layer of platinum foil is placed on the die. The porcelain is layered on the foil. Then the porcelain-foil combination is removed from the die and fired in an oven. Before try-in, the foil is removed and the porcelain is etched.[20]

The use of platinum foil permits the porcelain to be repeatedly removed from and replaced onto the die during restoration fabrication. This permits easier access to the proximal margins. In addition, the thickness of foil creates a space for opaques and tinting agents.

Refractory Casts. The use of refractory casts is the most commonly used method of porcelain laminate veneer fabrication.[21]

The restoration is fired directly on a refractory die. This eliminates the platinum layer but makes repeated firings difficult once the laminate veneer has been removed from the die unless a duplicate refractory die is fabricated.

The advantages of the refractory cast include tighter contacts and the absence of the gap created by the use of platinum foil. The disadvantages are less room for coloring agents and more difficulty in adjusting proximal areas by the technician.

Direct Castings. Cast ceramic restorations are fabricated using the "lost wax" technique. This eliminates the need for multiple firings but requires extrinsic staining for coloration (see Chapter XX).

> ### CLINICAL TIP
>
> Use a platinum layer to make repeated firings easier after the laminate veneer has been removed from the die.

CAD/CAM Machining. Ceramic restorations can be manufactured either in the dental office or in the laboratory. A cast or video image of the preparation is required, and the restoration always requires modification of the surface porcelain to obtain proper color esthetics. (For a complete discussion, see the section on CAD/CAM systems in Chapter 23.)

ADVANTAGES OF BONDED PORCELAIN RESTORATIONS

The main advantages of bonded porcelain restorations are the following:
1. *Excellent esthetics.* Porcelain offers unsurpassed esthetics. Unlike direct laminate veneers, the porcelain laminate veneers depend less on the esthetic skill of the clinician.

Table 7-1 Effects of Etching and Silane on Bond Shear Strength

Group	Etch	Silane	Bond Shear Strength
A	Yes	No	2907 ± SD 165
B	Yes	Yes	3485 ± SD 340
C	No	No	564 ± SD140
D	No	Yes	978 ± SD390

Data from Hsu CS, Stangel I, Nathanson D. Shear bond strength of resin to etched porcelain [abstract 1095]. In Abstracts of papers: 63rd general session, International Association for Dental Research/Annual session, American Association for Dental Research, Las Vegas (1985) J Dent Res 64: 162-379, 1985.

2. *Excellent long-term durability.* Porcelain is both abrasion resistant and color stable. In addition, porcelain has excellent resistance to fluid absorption.
3. *Inherent porcelain strength.* Porcelain exhibits excellent compressive, tensile, and shear strengths when properly bonded to tooth structure.
4. *Marginal integrity.* Porcelain restorations bonded to enamel exhibit exceptional marginal integrity.
5. *Soft tissue compatibility.* Properly polished porcelain is highly biocompatible with gingival tissue.
6. *Minimal tooth reduction.* Anterior porcelain laminate veneers are considerably more conserving of tooth structure than porcelain-fused-to-metal and all-porcelain full coverage restorations.

DISADVANTAGES OF BONDED PORCELAIN RESTORATIONS

The primary disadvantages of bonded porcelain restorations are the following:
1. *Time.* Multiple visits are required.
2. *Cost.* Laboratory involvement and additional chair time are required when compared with direct restorations, resulting in higher costs to the patient and clinician.
3. *Fragility.* Although strong when bonded to the tooth, bonded porcelain restorations are extremely fragile during the try-in and cementation stages.
4. *Lack of repairability.* Porcelain restorations are difficult, if not impossible, to repair.
5. *Difficulty in color matching.* Although porcelain restorations are color-stable, precise matching of a desired shade tab or an adjacent tooth can be difficult. In addition, shade alteration is impossible after cementation.
6. *Irreversibility.* Tooth reduction, although often minimal, is required.
7. *Inability to trial cement the restoration.* Unlike traditional indirect restorations, bonded porcelain restorations cannot be temporarily retained with a provisional cement for evaluation purposes.

Indications

Porcelain laminate veneers may be indicated in areas traditionally restored with single crowns or composite resin veneers for the following:
1. Correcting diastemata
2. Masking discolored or stained teeth
3. Masking enamel defects
4. Correcting malaligned or malformed teeth

Contraindications

Porcelain laminate veneers may be contraindicated for the following:
1. Patients who exhibit tooth wear as a result of bruxism
2. Short teeth
3. Teeth with insufficient or inadequate enamel for sufficient retention (e.g., severe abrasion)
4. Existing large restorations or endodontically treated teeth with little remaining tooth structure
5. Patients with oral habits causing excessive stress on the restoration (e.g., nail biting, pencil biting)

DIAGNOSTIC AND TREATMENT PLANNING AIDS

Porcelain laminate veneers can be used to change any or all of the following characteristics of a single tooth or multiple teeth:
1. Color (including characterizations and degree of polychromaticity)
2. Size
3. Shape
4. Position within the arch

Wax and Paint Simulation

White orthodontic wax and acrylic paint provide an extremely effective diagnostic and patient education aid. This is especially helpful when evaluating the treatment of single or multiple diastemas, and fractured, misshaped, or malpositioned teeth. The wax can be used to quickly and inexpensively simulate (and thereby "preview") the effects of porcelain laminate veneer placement.

> **CLINICAL TIP**
>
> Prediction of the anticipated outcome of porcelain laminate veneer placement without the use of a preliminary wax simulation is deceptively difficult even for the experienced dentist. A wax "preview," often reveals a favorable prognosis for a clinical situation that initially appears unmanageable with porcelain laminate veneers.

Armamentarium
- White orthodontic tray wax (Hygienic Corp.)
- Mars Black artist's acrylic paint (Liquidtex Artist Materials)
- Plastic instrument (Plastic Instrument PF4, Henry Schein, Inc.)
- One-piece lip retractor (e.g., Self-Span, Ellman International, Inc. or Expandex, Parkell, Inc.)
- Cotton-tipped applicator

Clinical Technique
1. Isolate the teeth with a one-piece lip retractor (Fig. 7-1A).
2. Dry thoroughly with an air syringe.

> **CLINICAL TIP**
>
> Squeeze a ⅛-inch strip of orthodontic wax between the thumb and index fingers. This will quickly form a thin "veneer-shaped" piece of wax.

3. Apply the wax to the teeth and grossly mold to shape with the index finger.
4. Refine the wax with the plastic instrument (Fig. 7-1B,C).

> **CLINICAL TIP**
>
> Simulate shortening of the teeth by applying an appropriate amount of black artist's acrylic paint to the dried tooth surface, using the wooden end of a cotton-tipped applicator (Fig. 7-1D). Turn off the examination light and have the patient separate the teeth until they do not exhibit vertical overlap (Fig. 7-1E). Squinting augments the illusion.

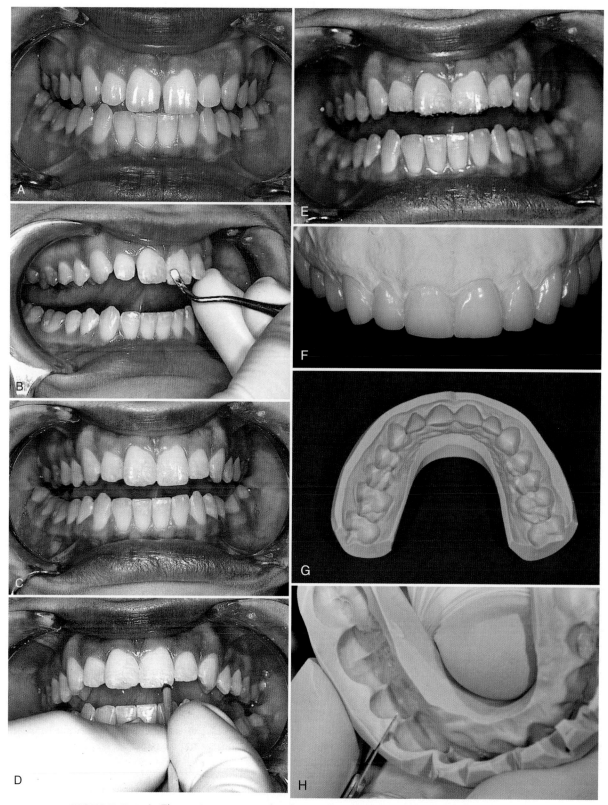

FIGURE 7-1 A, The patient presented with a midline diastema. She also thought her teeth were too long. **B,** The wax is refined with a plastic instrument. **C,** The diastema is closed with white orthodontic tray wax. **D,** Mars black acrylic paint is applied to the teeth with the wooden end of a cotton-tipped applicator. **E,** The black acrylic paint helps the patient envision the esthetic effect of shortening the teeth. **F,** A diagnostic wax-up simulating the proposed final porcelain laminate veneer restorations. **G,** A trayless polyvinylsiloxane (PVS) laboratory putty impression of the diagnostic wax-up to be used as a matrix when fabricating a polyurethane intraoral mock-up of the proposed restoration. **H,** The buccal areas of the matrix are trimmed with the Bard-Parker knife.

Continued

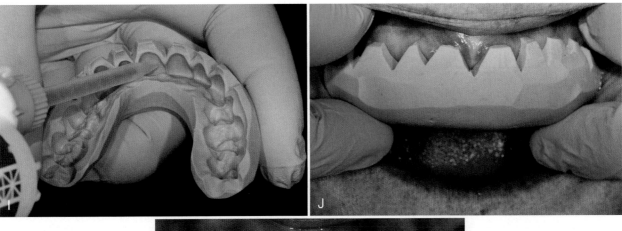

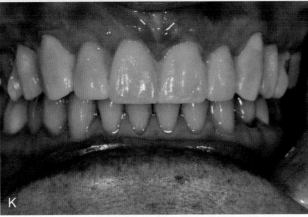

FIGURE 7-1, cont'd I, The appropriate amount of material is placed into matrix. **J,** The matrix filled with the polyurethane acrylic is seated intraorally. **K,** The intraoral mock-up of the proposed definitive restorations. Note how some areas of tooth structure remain uncovered by the polyurethane indicating that the definitive restorations will reproduce the shape of the original tooth structure in those specific areas.

Computer Imaging

Computer imaging provides a two-dimensional prediction similar to the three-dimensional preview provided by wax simulation and acrylic paint. This system has the added advantage of previewing the effects of color and characterization changes and providing a more lifelike prognostication. Computer imaging systems can also provide instant printouts of the predicted changes (see Chapter 22).

Diagnostic Wax-Up / Polyurethane Clinical Mock-Up

CLINICAL TIP

The additional cost of diagnostic wax-ups can often be offset by the time saved when fabricating provisional restorations.

CLINICAL TIP

To simulate shortening of the teeth apply an appropriate amount of black artist's acrylic paint to the dried tooth surface (see Clinical Tip in the section on Wax and Paint Simulation).

Armamentarium
- Diagnostic wax-up
- Polyvinylsiloxane (PVS) laboratory putty (Lab-Putty Hard Silicone Putty, Coltène Whaledent, Inc.)
- Bard Parker Knife with # 15 Scalpel Blade
- Polyurethane provisional restoration material (e.g., Luxatemp Ultra, DMG America)

Clinical Technique
1. The dental laboratory technician fabricates a diagnostic wax-up to simulating the proposed final porcelain laminate veneer restorations (Fig. 7-1F).
2. Adjust the diagnostic wax-up if necessary until it is acceptable to the clinician and the patient.
3. Make a trayless PVS impression of the diagnostic wax-up using laboratory putty (Fig. 7-1G). This will be used as a matrix when fabricating a polyurethane intraoral mock-up of the proposed restoration.

CLINICAL TIP

Care should be taken to produce an impression with a consistent 2 to 3 mm thickness. Finger pressure will be used when the matrix is placed intraorally. If the matrix is too thin, this finger pressure could result in an undesired indentation of an area of the polyurethane mock-up. A matrix that is excessively thick could be overly rigid and difficult to manipulate.

4. Scallop the buccal areas of the matrix with the Bard-Parker knife (Fig. 7-1*H*).

CLINICAL TIP

The buccal "notches" will serve as escape vents for excess polyurethane provisional material. Care should be taken to place the periphery of the matrix as close to the predicted interproximal finishing line as possible (see Figure 7-1*J* for placement).

5. Select the appropriate shade of polyurethane provisional restoration material and place an appropriate amount into the matrix (Fig. 7-1*I*).

CLINICAL TIP

Care should be taken to put the appropriate amount of polyurethane provisional material in the area of the prepared teeth. The amount will vary depending upon whether the contour of the final restoration is to be thicker or thinner than the original tooth. The latter requires far less material than the former.

6. Seat the matrix intraorally and allow the polyurethane material to polymerize (Fig. 7-1*J*). Remove the matrix.
7. Finish and polish the mock-up until it is acceptable to the clinician and the patient (Fig. 7-1*K*).

CLINICAL TIP

Removal of excess material from the interproximal areas at this time will reduce the amount of excess material in the mock-up. A high-speed suction can be used to evacuate excess material; however, an appropriate trap should be installed within the suction head to prevent the accumulation of cured material.

CLINICAL TIP

To simulate shortening of the teeth, apply an appropriate amount of black artist's acrylic paint to the dried tooth surface (see Clinical Tip in the section on Wax and Paint Simulation).

Patient Education

Photography. One of the most effective patient education tools is a book or photograph album containing before and after images of representative cases. These educational materials can be purchased commercially or be produced by the dentist (see also Chapter 22).

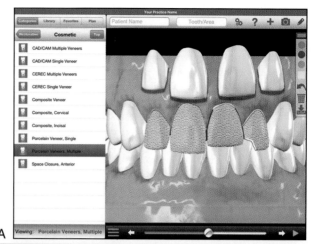

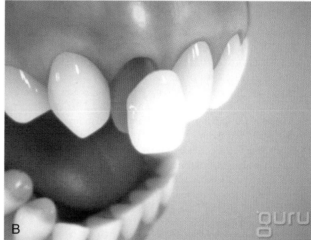

FIGURE 7-2 A, Screen shot from the DDS GP for the IPad. **B,** Screen shot from an animation from the Patient Communication Suite for the PC. (**A,** Courtesy Kick Your Apps, Inc., Poway, CA. **B,** Courtesy Reality Engineering, LLC, Reno, NV.)

Demonstration Porcelain Laminate Veneers. Sample porcelain laminate veneers fabricated to fit on prepared denture teeth or stone casts are valuable patient education aids. They effectively demonstrate the conservative nature of this technique and the lifelike appearance of the definitive restorations.

Tablet Software. Computer tablet demonstration software or computer demonstration software is another patient education modality (for example, DDS GP for the iPad, Kick Your Apps, [Fig. 7- 2*A*] and Guru Patient Communication Suite for the PC, Reality Engineering LLC, Reno [Fig. 7-2*B*]).

TOOTH PREPARATION

The outline form of the porcelain laminate veneer tooth preparation depends largely on the degree of desired color alteration. This consideration particularly influences the location of the interproximal and gingival finish lines.

Static Area of Visibility Versus Dynamic Area of Visibility

The entire facial tooth surface, including the gingival area and the area immediately facial to the contact area with the adjacent tooth (the facial embrasure), is visible if the available light and the perspective of the viewer are optimal. This static area of visibility occurs when the patient is seated in the dental chair under adequate lighting and with the lips fully retracted. The static area of visibility significantly differs from the actual dynamic area of visibility exhibited during normal function.

The dynamic area of visibility of the facial embrasure is partially a function of viewing perspective. It is particularly influenced, however, by shadows cast from surrounding structures. The lip, adjacent tooth contour and position, and gingival architecture, as well as the contour, shade, and position of the tooth under observation are all important factors (Fig. 7-3).

The dynamic area of visibility of the gingival area is governed by the position of the lip during maximal smiling (the high smile line).

Minimal or No Color Change

Proximal Finishing Lines. A proximal chamfer finishing line is preferred except when diastemata are present. Proximal areas adjacent to diastemata should receive a feather-edged finishing line (Fig. 7-4).

Proximal Contact Area. When the shade difference between the tooth (after preparation) and the desired definitive restoration is minimal, proximal chamfer finish lines are placed slightly facial (approximately 0.2 mm) to the contact areas of the adjacent tooth. This provides for the following:

1. Ease in evaluating marginal fit during the try-in stage
2. Access for performing and evaluating finishing procedures
3. Access for home care (margins in "self-cleansing" area)
4. Ease in evaluating marginal integrity during follow-up maintenance visits

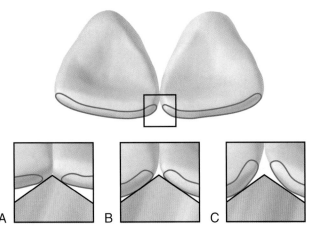

FIGURE 7-3 The dynamic area of visibility (the triangular area) of the facial embrasure is influenced by the depth of the embrasure space and by the shadow cast by surrounding structures including the tooth itself. **A,** The entire embrasure space is visible. The margins of the laminate veneers illustrated in the figure will be visible. To hide this margin, the finishing line must be placed into the contact area. **B,** The embrasure space is only partially visible. The margins of the porcelain laminate veneers illustrated in the figure are just within the nonvisible area. **C,** The majority of the embrasure space is not visible. The margins of the porcelain laminate veneer illustrated in need not have been placed as deeply into the interproximal area.

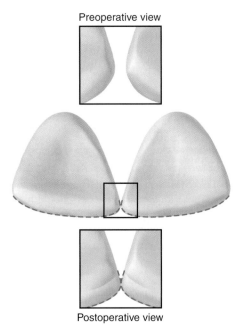

Preoperative view

Postoperative view

FIGURE 7-4 Feather-edged proximal finishing lines are used in proximal areas adjacent to diastemata.

The major disadvantage of this design is the possibility of eventual staining at the tooth-restoration interface. However, the factors influencing the dynamic area of visibility often negate this disadvantage. (See the section on static versus dynamic area of visibility in this chapter.)

Proximal Subcontact Area. The proximal subcontact area (PSCA) consists of the interproximal tooth structure, which is immediately gingival to the contact area with the adjacent tooth. This area is usually not visible from a direct frontal view of the tooth (Fig. 7-5A) and is therefore often left underprepared or totally unprepared. It is visible, however, from an oblique view. Therefore preparation of the PSCA is essential[22] and is particularly crucial when the definitive restoration significantly differs in shade from that of the unprepared tooth structure and to avoid esthetic display of the restoration margins, which may eventually stain (see Fig. 7-5).

CLINICAL TIP

View the preparation of the PSCA from all oblique angles to ensure adequate extension into this often-overlooked area.

Diastemata. The proximal area adjacent to a diastema should receive a feather-edged finishing line (see Fig. 7-4). This finishing line extends from the incisal edge to a point adjacent to the height of the gingival papilla.

Gingival Finishing Lines. A chamfer is preferred for all gingival finishing lines. Supragingival finishing lines provide the same advantages as proximal finishing lines, which terminate facial to the contact areas. In addition, impressions are easier to make with supragingival preparations as compared with subgingival preparations. Supragingival finishing lines also increase the likelihood that restoration margins will end on enamel. The major disadvantage, however, is that any subsequent staining or color changes at the restoration margin will be

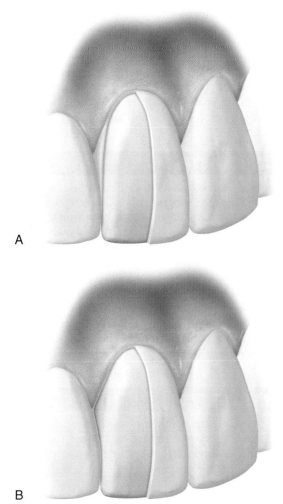

A

B

FIGURE 7-5 A, The proximal subcontact area is visible only from an oblique perspective and is often left unprepared or underprepared. **B,** Proper extension of the preparation into the proximal subcontact area. The proximal subcontact area is often overlooked during tooth preparation.

visible. Therefore supragingival margins are limited to clinical situations in which this area remains concealed by the lip during maximum smiling (high smile line).

When the entire clinical crown is included in the facial display, the gingival margin should be placed 0.1 mm below the free gingival margin. If gingival recession is anticipated, the gingival finishing line can be extended deeper subgingivally as long as the biologic width is not violated.

CLINICAL TIP

Evaluate critically the true position of the lip during maximum smiling (the high smile line) before planning supragingival finishing lines. The true lip position may be deceptive. Patients with unattractive smiles often habitually adapt a high smile line position, which is significantly less revealing of tooth structure than is anatomically possible. After porcelain laminate veneers are placed, the high smile line may significantly elevate, because the patient's psychologic barriers to full smiling have dissipated.

Incisal Preparation. Incisal reduction should ideally provide for 1 mm of porcelain thickness. Therefore if the incisogingival height of the definitive restoration is to be 0.5 mm longer than the existing tooth, only 0.5 mm of incisal reduction is required. If the preoperative teeth are to be lengthened by 1 mm, only a rounding of the incisal edge and placement of a finishing line are required.

A butt joint finishing line provides for the proper thickness of porcelain at the margin to prevent restoration fracture. The finishing line should slope slightly gingivally (approximately 75 degrees from the facial). This augments resistance to facial displacement of the definitive restoration (Fig. 7-6).

After ideal preparation, the incisal outline of the tooth, when viewed from the facial aspect, should be identical to the incisal outline of the proposed definitive restoration, except for a 1-mm incisal reduction. This allows for an even thickness of porcelain. Incisal line angles must be rounded to reduce internal restoration stresses.

Facial Depth Reduction. A facial reduction of approximately 0.5 to 0.7 mm is sufficient for most maxillary teeth and 0.3 mm for smaller teeth, such as mandibular incisors, if adequate thickness of enamel is present. Inadequate thickness of enamel, such as in the gingival one third of the tooth, may require a more conservative tooth reduction. Teeth or portions of rotated tooth surfaces that are in lingual version require proportionately less reduction. Preparation into dentin is sometimes necessary; however, this should involve less than 50% retention of the prepared surface.[16]

The entire finishing line should ideally remain in enamel.

Major Color Change

In addition to considerations of preparation design for minimal color changes, major color differences between the prepared tooth and the desired definitive restoration may also require other adjustments. Visibility of the contact area may necessitate extension of the interproximal finishing line into the contact area to a depth of approximately one-half the labiolingual dimension of the contact area. (See the sections on minimal or no color change and static versus dynamic area

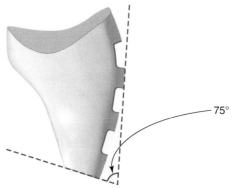

75°

FIGURE 7-6 A butt incisal finishing line should slope approximately 75 degrees gingivally from the facial to provide resistance to restoration displacement and to provide for adequate thickness of porcelain at the margin to prevent restoration fracture.

of visibility in this chapter.) The gingival finishing line can be extended 1 mm subgingivally, assuming the biologic width is not violated. Supragingival margins are indicated, however, if this area remains concealed by the lip during maximal smiling (high smile line). (See Clinical Tip in the section on gingival finishing lines.) The preparation depth may be increased if sufficient thickness of enamel is present. This will allow for an increased thickness of porcelain.

CLINICAL TIP

Tetracycline discoloration occurs in the dentin. The prepared tooth may be darker than the original tooth shade, because the deep tooth preparation that is often necessary in these situations removes a significant amount of the "masking" enamel.

Armamentarium
- Basic dental setup
  Explorer
  High-speed handpiece
  Low-speed handpiece
  Mouth mirror
  Periodontal probe
  Suitable anesthesia (if necessary)
- Lip retractor (e.g., One-piece Self-Span, Ellman International, Inc. Manufacturing Co.; Expandex, Parkell, Inc. or Lip Expanders, Denmat, Inc.)
- High-speed (friction grip) diamond three-tiered depth cutting burs (e.g., LVS-1 [0.3 mm depth cut] and LVS-2 [0.5 mm depth cut], Brasseler USA)
- High-speed (friction grip) two-grit burs (LVS-3, LVS-4, Brasseler USA)
- High-speed (friction grip) diamond wheel bur (e.g., 5909, Brasseler USA
- Unwaxed regular dental floss
- Sharp pencil
- Retraction cord packer (e.g., Fischer's Ultrapak Packer, Ultradent Products, Inc.)
- Nonimpregnated gingival retraction cord (e.g., Ultrapak No. 0 or No. 1, Ultradent Products, Inc.; Gingibraid No. 0 or No. 1, Van R Dental Products, Inc.)
- Gingival retraction instrument (e.g., Zekrya Gingival Protector, DMG America, Inc.) (optional)
- Abrasive polishing disk (ex. Esthetic Polishing Kit (Blue Disk) Brasseler USA)
  Clinical Technique
1. Evaluate patient correct and gingival esthetic issues (Fig. 7-7) (also see Chapter 2 and Chapter 14)

CLINICAL TIP

The true lip position may be deceptive. Patients with unattractive smiles often habitually adapt a high smile line position, which is significantly less revealing of tooth structure than is anatomically possible. After an esthetic rehabilitation, the high smile line may significantly elevate, because the patient's psychologic barriers to full smiling have dissipated (see Fig. 7-18A).

---

2. Administer suitable anesthesia (if necessary).
3. Prepare three horizontal surface depth cuts in the facial surface with a friction grip three-tiered LVS-1 or LVS-2 depth cutting diamond (Figs. 7-8A,B). Depth cuts should be 0.5 to 0.7 mm deep for "ideal" teeth, and 0.3 mm deep for mandibular incisors. Lingually positioned teeth and those with thin enamel require less reduction. See the section on facial depth reduction in this chapter.

CLINICAL TIP

When the three-tiered depth cutting bur is held tangentially to the surface of the tooth, only the middle section of the bur penetrates to its entire depth. This is because of the tooth's convex facial surface (Figs. 7-8C,D). To avoid underpreparation, position the bur two additional times to ensure complete penetration of each section of the bur (Figs. 7-8E-H).

---

4. Prepare three incisal depth cuts with an LVS-3 or LVS-4 diamond bur (Figs. 7-8I-K). The incisal reduction should create a preparation that is 1 mm shorter than the desired definitive restoration.

CLINICAL TIP

To prevent overreduction, draw pencil lines into the prepared enamel guide cuts (Fig. 7-8L) Facial reduction is complete immediately after the pencil lines are removed by the action of the reduction bur.

---

5. Using the depth cuts as a guide, prepare the facial surface with an LVS-3 or LVS-4 diamond bur (Figs. 7-8M,N).
6. Prepare the proximal chamfer finishing lines.
   A. For *diastema*: Prepare a feather-edged finishing line with an LVS-3 or LVS-4 diamond bur. The finishing line should terminate as far to the lingual aspect as possible without creating an undercut area, and it should extend from the incisal edge to the point adjacent to the height of the gingival papilla (see Fig. 7-4).
   B. For *minimal or no color change and no diastema*, see the section on minimal or no color change in this chapter.
      i. Prepare the proximal chamfer finishing line with an LVS-3 or LVS-4 diamond bur to approximately 0.2 mm facial to contact area (Figs. 7-9A,B).
      ii. Prepare the proximal subcontact area with an LVS-3 or LVS-4 diamond bur Fig. 7-9C).
   C. For *major color change and no diastema*, see the section on major color change in this chapter.
      i. Prepare the proximal chamfer finishing line with an LVS-3 or LVS-4 diamond bur to a depth of one half the labiolingual dimension of the interproximal contact area (Figs. 7-9D,E).
      ii. Prepare the proximal subcontact area with an LVS-3 or LVS-4 diamond bur (Fig. 7-9F)
7. Using the depth cut as a guide, prepare the incisolingual finishing line to a modified butt joint with the diamond wheel bur (Fig. 7-9G). The labioincisolingual angle should be approximately 75 degrees (see Fig. 7-6).

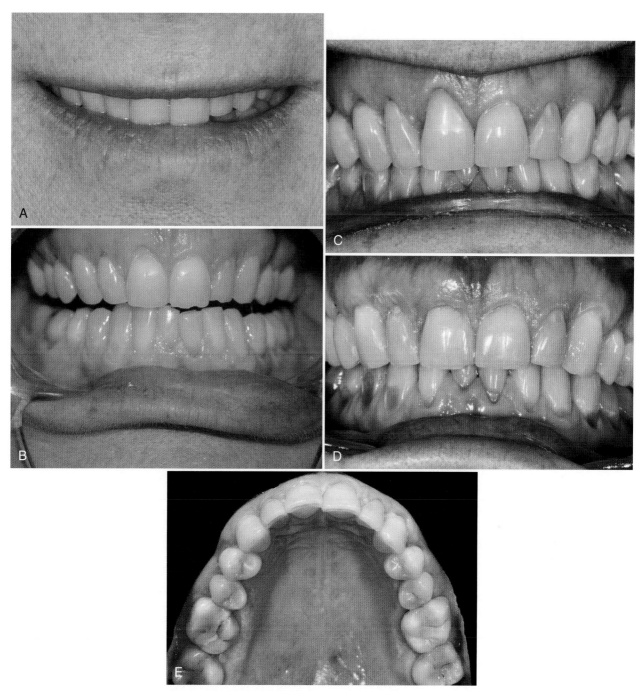

FIGURE 7-7 A, The smile line is evaluated. **B,** Preoperative view of a patient with multiple worn and chipped teeth. **C,** Conservative attempts at restoring worn and facially chipped teeth with composite resin restorations failed to adequately restore esthetics. **D,** Following complete esthetic evaluation and diagnostic wax-up (see Figure 7-1F) gingival grafting was performed. (Surgery courtesy of Scott Kissel, DMD) **E,** Incisal view of the patient.

CLINICAL TIP

A PVS incisal/facial reduction guide can be fabricated from the diagnostic wax up to verify proper reduction (Fig. 7-10*A*) The reduction guide is constructed in the same manner as the matrix used for the polyurethane clinical mock-up described previously (see the section on Diagnostic Wax-Up / Polyurethane Clinical Mock-Up earlier in the chapter). Make a horizontal slice on the labial surface of the reduction guide using a Bard Parker Knife with # 15 Scalpel Blade.

CLINICAL TIP

Be certain that unprepared tooth structure in the proximal subcontact area is not visible from all oblique viewing perspectives. See the Clinical Tip in the section on proximal subcontact area and Figure 7-5)

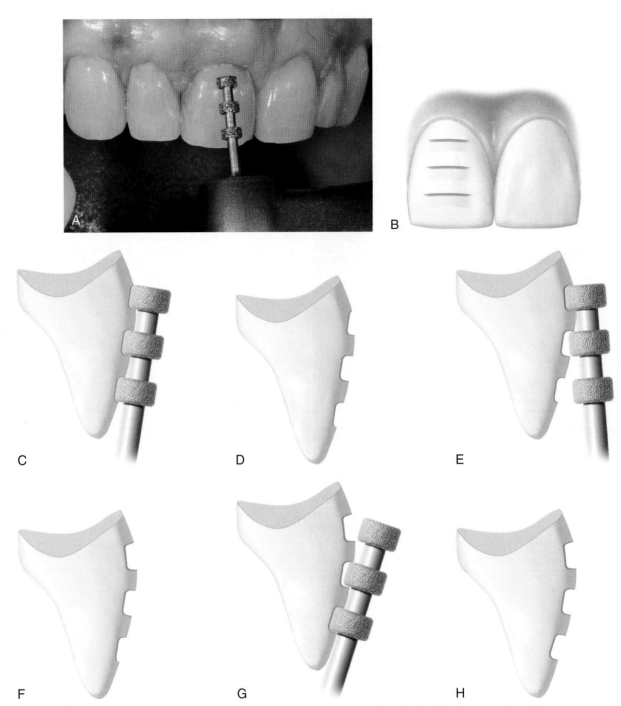

FIGURE 7-8 A, B, Three horizontal depth cuts are prepared in the facial surface. **C,** When the three-tiered depth cutting bur is held tangentially to the surface of the tooth, only the middle section of the bur penetrates to its entire depth. **D,** Only the middle section of the tooth is prepared to the full depth because of the convex facial surface. The incisal and gingival portions of the tooth are underprepared. **E,** The bur is angled a second time to complete the gingival depth cut. **F,** The tooth after two depth cuts. The incisal portion of the tooth remains underprepared. **G,** The bur is angled for the third time to complete the incisal depth cut. **H,** The three depth cuts are equally deep.

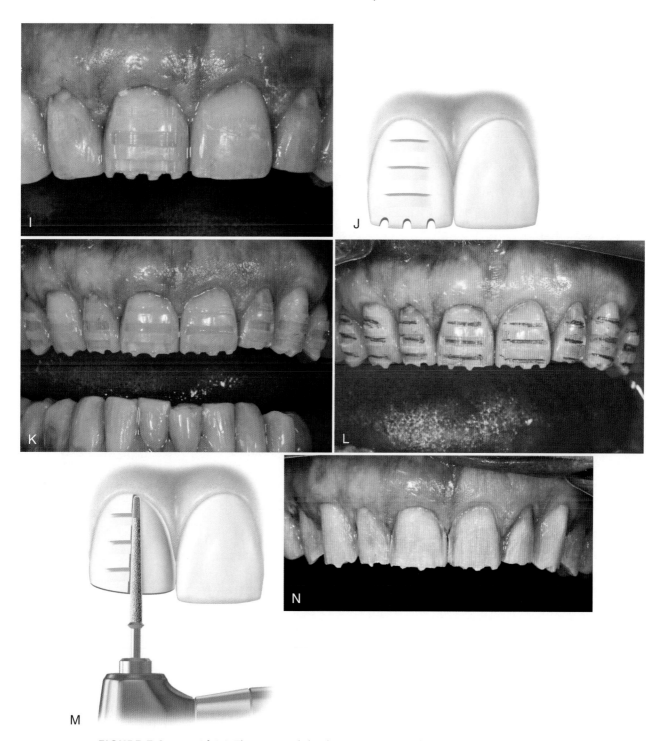

FIGURE 7-8, cont'd I,J, Three vertical depth cuts are prepared in the incisal edge. **K,** Depth cuts are placed on the remaining teeth that will receive laminates. **L,** Facial reduction is complete immediately after the pencil lines are removed by the action of the reduction bur. **M,** The facial surface is prepared using the horizontal depth cuts as a guide. **N,** Facial reduction has been accomplished.

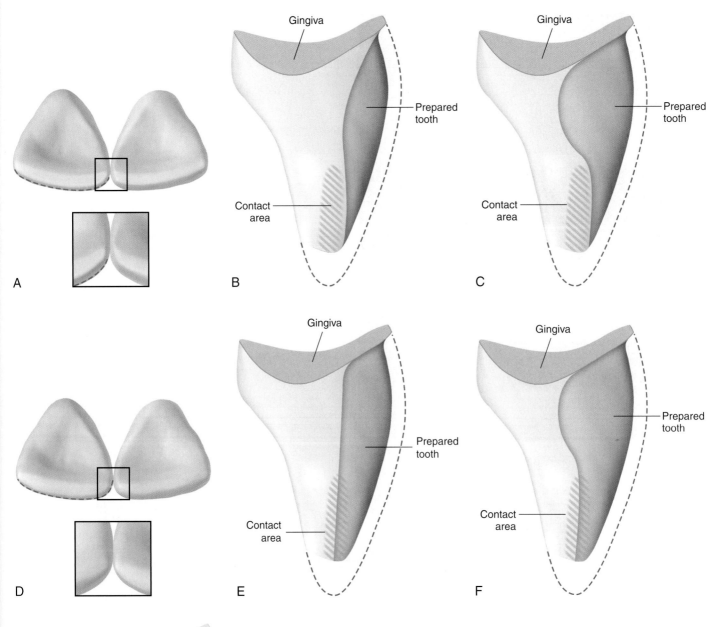

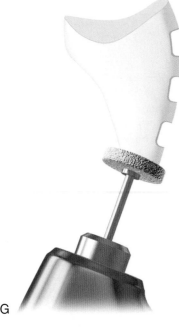

FIGURE 7-9 A, If the final porcelain laminate veneer will be similar in color to that of the prepared tooth, the proximal finishing line terminates 0.2 mm facial to the contact area. **B,** Proximal representation of porcelain laminate veneer preparation before reduction of the proximal subcontact area. The proximal finishing line terminates 0.2 mm facial to the contact area because the final porcelain laminate veneer will be similar in color to that of the prepared tooth. The contact area is indicated with diagonal lines. **C,** Proximal representation of porcelain laminate veneer preparation after proper reduction of the proximal subcontact area. **D,** If the final porcelain laminate veneer will significantly differ in color from that of the prepared tooth, the proximal finishing line terminates within the interproximal contact area at a depth of one half the labiolingual dimension of the contact area. **E,** Proximal representation of porcelain laminate veneer preparation before reduction of the proximal subcontact area. The proximal finishing line terminates within the interproximal contact area at a depth of one-half the labiolingual dimension of the contact area because the final porcelain laminate veneer will be significantly different in color from that of the prepared tooth. **F,** Proximal representation of porcelain laminate veneer preparation after proper reduction of the proximal subcontact area. **G,** An incisal butt joint angled approximately 75 degrees from the facial provides for adequate thickness of porcelain at the margin and resistance to displacement of the restoration.

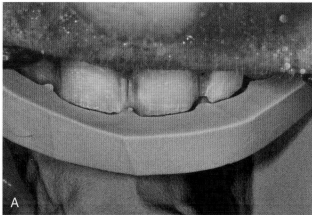

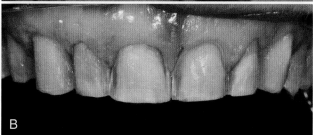

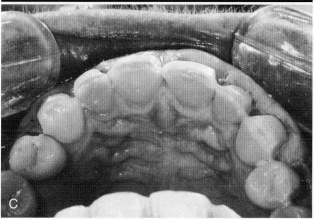

FIGURE 7-10 A, Prepared teeth with PVS reduction guide in place. **B,** Frontal view and (**C**) incisal view of the final preparations prior to cord placement.

8. Prepare the gingival finishing line.
   A. *For supragingival preparations:* Prepare the gingival finishing line to the desired location.
   B. *For subgingival margins:* Gently place gingival retraction cord (see Fig. 7-11C). The cord should extend into the sulcus of the interproximal papillae beyond the proximal finishing line.

CLINICAL TIP

The gingiva can be gently retracted with the gingival retraction instrument (Figs. 7-11A,B).

CLINICAL TIP

For subgingival preparations draw a line with a sharpened pencil at the present location of the gingival margin (currently at the level of the free gingival margin), which will serve as a guide for gingival reduction.

CLINICAL TIP

When the retraction cord is placed, the gingiva will be retracted not only facially but usually also gingivally (Fig. 7-11D).

9. Extend the gingival finishing line (for subgingival preparations only) approximately 0.1 mm subgingivally with an LVS-3 or LVS-4 Diamond bur. Use the pencil line as a guide. Severely discolored teeth may require a 1mm subgingival extension of the finishing line.

CLINICAL TIP

A gingival retraction instrument can be used to retract the gingiva (see Figs. 7-11A,B)

10. Round the incisal line angles with an LVS-3 or LVS-4 diamond bur or an abrasive disk. The thinner LVS-5 or LVS-6 diamond bur may be necessary to access line angles that are close to adjacent teeth (Figs. 7-11E-H).

CLINICAL TIP

Rounding the incisal line angles reduces the internal stress and therefore the fracture potential of the final restoration.[23]

IMPRESSIONING

Armamentarium
+ Retraction cord packer (e.g., Fischer's Ultrapak Packer, Ultradent Products, Inc.)
+ Nonimpregnated gingival retraction cord (e.g., Ultrapak No. 0 or No. 1, Ultradent Products, Inc.; Gingibraid No. 0 or No. 1, Van R Dental Products, Inc.)
+ Scissors
+ Elastomeric impression material (ex. Impregum, 3M ESPE)
Clinical Technique
1. Gently place a retraction cord in the sulcus unless previously placed during preparation.

CLINICAL TIP

Position the cord just beneath the finishing line to avoid interfering with capturing the entire gingival margin in the impression (see Fig. 7-11C).

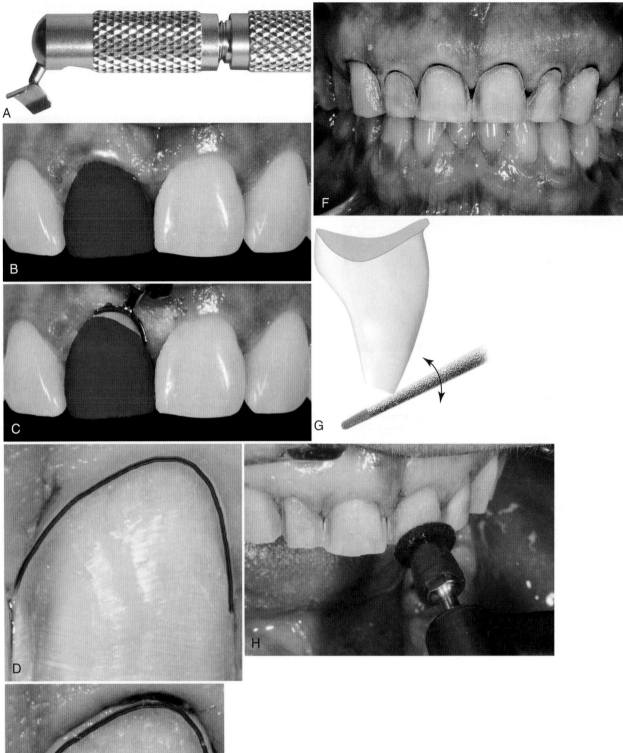

FIGURE 7-11 A, The gingiva can be gently retracted with a gingival retraction instrument (pictured: the Zekrya retraction instrument). **B,** All clinically visible facial tooth structure is painted red. **C,** The Zekrya retraction instrument is used to retract of the marginal gingiva. **D,E,** Simulated pencil marks demonstrate that when retraction cord is placed the gingiva will not only be retracted facially, but usually also gingivally. **F,** The cord should extend into the sulcus of the interproximal papillae beyond the proximal finishing line. The preparation margins are at the level of the free gingival margin and were prepared before placement of the retraction cord. The incisal line angle is rounded with an LVS-3 or LVS-4 diamond bur (**G**) or an abrasive disc (**H**) to prevent internal stresses within the porcelain laminate veneer. (**A,** Courtesy ZenithDental, Distributed by DMG America LLC., Englewood, NJ.)

2. Make the impression with any accurate elastomeric impression material.

> ### CLINICAL TIP
> Leave the retraction cord in place during impressioning. It is usually removed in the impression. However, be certain that all remaining cord is removed before proceeding to the next step.

> ### CLINICAL TIP
> A splinted multi-tooth provisional restoration can often be effectively retained with mechanical retention alone.

Single-Tooth Provisionalization

Armamentarium
- Basic dental setup; see section on major color change
- Plastic matrix or celluloid crown forms (see Chapter 11)
- Sable brush (No. 0)
- Bonding agent
- Hybrid composite resin (e.g., Herculite, Kerr, Corp.)
- Fine diamond finishing burs (e.g., ET Burs, Brasseler USA; Micron Finishing System, Premier Dental Products, Inc.)

Clinical Technique
1. Fit the plastic matrix over the prepared teeth (Fig. 7-12A).

> ### CLINICAL TIP
> The matrix margins should allow for easy removal of excess composite resin.

2. Remove the matrix and place the appropriate shade of composite resin into the matrix.

> ### CLINICAL TIP
> It is often not necessary to etch the enamel, prime the dentin surfaces, or place bonding agent on the teeth before placing the composite resin. Retention of the provisional restoration is solely mechanical.

3. Place the matrix and resin onto the prepared teeth. (If multiple celluloid crown forms are used, all should be placed before curing; after curing, the restoration will be a single splinted unit.)
4. Remove excess composite resin from the *entire* buccal, lingual, and proximal surfaces (Fig. 7-12B).

> ### CLINICAL TIP
> Dip a sable brush or cotton pellet in bonding agent and wipe off all excess composite resin before curing. In addition, featheredge the composite resin on the palatal surfaces with the wetted brush. Precise, smooth marginal adaptation ensures minimal adjustment after curing and prevents gingival inflammation.

5. Light polymerize all surfaces for a minimum of 60 seconds each.

> ### CLINICAL TIP
> Light-cured resin cannot be damaged by excessive light exposure. It is therefore preferable to err on the side of longer exposure times.

6. Verify and correct the occlusion with high-speed diamond finishing burs.

> ### CLINICAL TIP
> Adjustments of the provisional restoration must not alter the previously prepared tooth. If this would not be possible, remove the entire restoration and place a new restoration, making certain that all excess composite resin is removed before curing.

7. Recontour with high-speed diamond finishing burs (if necessary).
8. Instruct the patient that the provisional restoration is for esthetic purposes only and that careful limited function is required (Figs. 7-12C, D).

> ### CLINICAL TIP
> If the provisional restoration dislodges, recement it with a noneugenol provisional cement. Alternatively, etch a 1-mm diameter area of midfacial surface enamel and lute the provisional restoration into place with low-viscosity resin cement.

Multi-Tooth Provisionalization

Armamentarium
- Basic dental setup; see section on major color change
- Study cast or diagnostic wax-up
- Polyvinylsiloxane laboratory putty (Lab-Putty hard Silicone Putty, Coltène/Whaledent, Inc.)
- Polyurethane provisional material (Luxatemp Ultra, DMG America)
- Flowable Polyurethane provisional material (Luxaflow Ultra, DMG America)
- Bard Parker Knife with # 15 Scalpel Blade
- Phosphoric acid etching gel (Ultraetch, Ultradent Products, Inc.)
- Sable brush (No. 0)
- Bonding agent (see Chapter 3)
- Fine diamond finishing burs (e.g., ET Burs, Brasseler USA; Micron Finishing System, Premier Dental Products Inc.)

Clinical Technique
1. Fabricate a PVS matrix from the study cast or diagnostic work-up (see the section on Diagnostic Wax-Up / Polyurethane Clinical Mock-Up in this chapter) for use over the prepared teeth (Fig. 7-13A).
2. Place the appropriate shade and amount of polyurethane provisional material into the matrix (Fig. 7-13B).

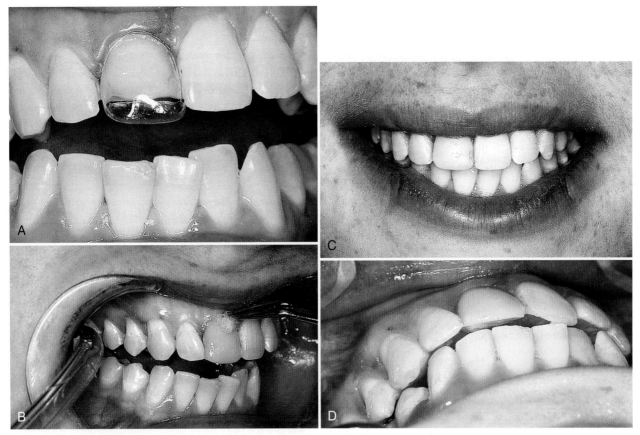

FIGURE 7-12 A, A patient with a single prepared maxillary incisor who required a provisional restoration. A trimmed celluloid crown form is positioned over the prepared tooth. **B,** Excess composite resin is removed with a cotton pellet moistened with bonding agent. Facial (**C**) and incise (**D**) views of the provisional restoration.

3. If the esthetics, retention and marginal fit do not require refinement, skip to step 6. Otherwise, gently remove the provisional restoration (Fig. 7-13D).

4. Following trimming of the provisional restoration (if necessary) the teeth are acid etched with a small pinpoint of etch for the appropriate amount of time (Fig. 7-13F) (see Chapter 3).
5. Place bonding resin on the tooth and "lute "the provisional restorations using the matching flowable polyurethane material. Carefully remove the excess material and polymerize according to the manufacturer's instructions.
6. Verify the occlusion and remove any prematurities.

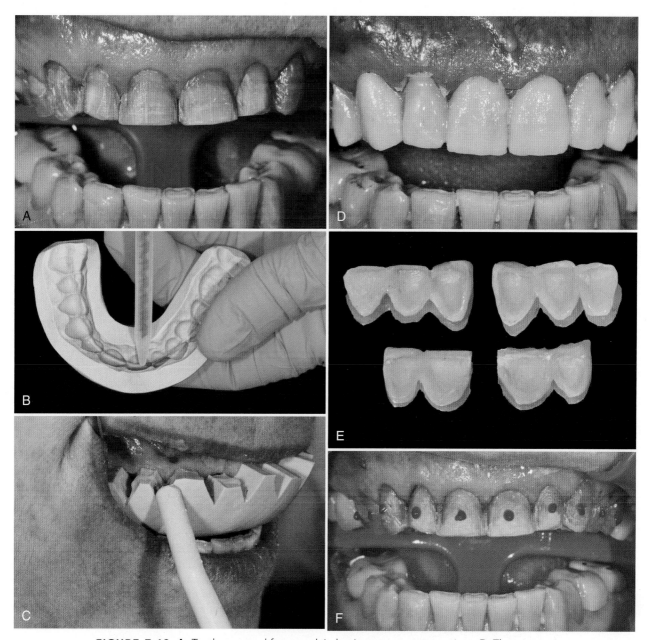

FIGURE 7-13 A, Teeth prepared for porcelain laminate veneer restorations. **B,** The appropriate amount and shade of polyurethane provisional material is placed into the matrix. **C,** The excess material is removed from between the interproximal slits, which serve as vents (see Clinical Tip concerning suction line protection). **D,** The provisional restoration immediately following matrix removal. Although some excess material remains, the pre-removal of excess material with the high speed suction minimizes trimming. **E,** The provisional restoration can be removed in sections, especially if trimming is required. **F,** A small amount of phosphoric acid etchant is placed in the center of the prepared teeth.   *Continued*

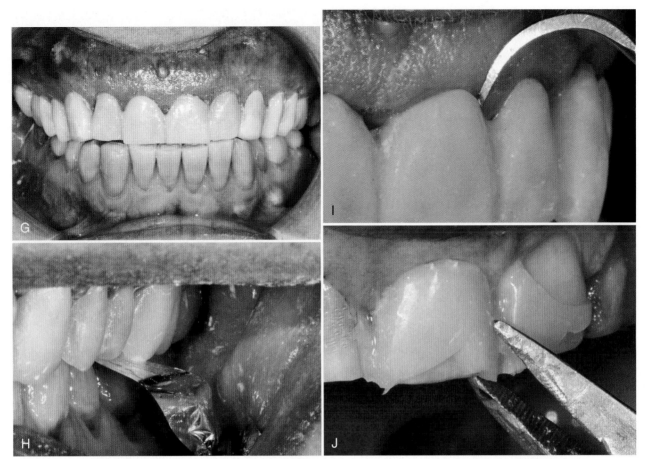

FIGURE 7-13, cont'd G, The provisional restorations. **H,** Ideally, the patient should occlude on natural tooth structure and not on the provisional material. **I,** The provisional restoration is removed with a currette. **J,** The provisional restoration is removed with a hemostat.

7. Provisional restorations can be carefully removed with a curette (Fig. 7-13 *I*) or hemostat (Fig. 7-13 *J*).

> ### CLINICAL TIP
> If a hemostat is use to remove the provisional restorations it is critical that it contacts the provisional material and not the tooth in order to minimize forces on the prepared tooth. These forces could lead to tooth fracture.

> ### CLINICAL TIP
> The failure to remove excess material remaining on the tooth in the area of the "acid etch dots" may prevent proper seating of the final porcelain laminate veneers. Should excess material remain it must be carefully remove using a bur without removing any tooth structure.

LABORATORY COMMUNICATIONS

Natural Versus Idealized Artificial Appearance

Natural teeth are polychromatic and characterized. Canines are usually slightly lower in value or higher in chroma than incisors and premolars. These can be disturbing insights for patients who often desire an idealized artificial appearance (monochromatic, opaque, "coffee cup" white). Both of these alternatives, and the myriad options in between, should be discussed before a final shade selection is made. It may be helpful to elicit the opinion of the patient's friend or family member.

Shade

> ### CLINICAL TIP
> Include in the laboratory prescription both the shade of the tooth after tooth reduction ("stump" shade) and the desired definitive restoration shade. This allows the laboratory technician to attempt to compensate for the underlying discoloration. The Ivoclar Vivodent Natural Die Material guide is ideally suited for this purpose (Fig. 7-14).

To achieve the desired shade change, the percentage of opaquing porcelain can be appropriately adjusted by the dental laboratory technician. The specific ratios vary depending on the type and brand of materials used. Close communication with the dental laboratory technician is essential in this regard.

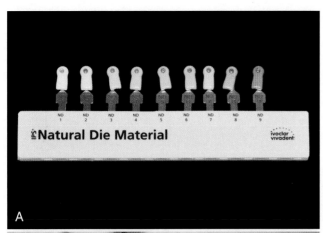

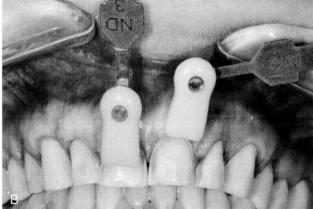

FIGURE 7-14 A, The Ivoclar Vivodent Natural Die Material guide. **B,** Vivodent Natural Die Material shade tab is used to determing the "stump" shade of tooth # 9. Additional tabs can be used to determine the shade of any additional differently shaded areas. The "stump" shade of the cervical third of tooth #8 (which is obscured by the tab) and the entire shade of tooth #10 differed-significantly from the stump shade of tooth #9 and the remaining prepared teeth.

> ### CLINICAL TIP
>
> It is easier to "darken" (lower the value and increase the chroma) than to "lighten" a porcelain laminate veneer by use of internal modification with luting resin. Therefore select the "lighter" alternative when in doubt about a final shade (see Chapter XX).

Shape

Indicate the desired shape and size of each individual porcelain laminate veneer. As a general rule, feminine teeth are more rounded, less textured, and smaller than masculine teeth; however, this is not always appropriate nor is it always desired by the patient (see Chapter XX). Therefore specific characterizations should be specified with images, diagrammatically, or in writing, in the laboratory prescription.

Texture

Texturing scatters reflected light and produces a more natural appearance. If not all of the teeth in the facial display are to be restored, the laboratory personnel should be instructed to match the texture of the adjacent teeth.

> ### CLINICAL TIP
>
> Lack of texturing can produce an artificial appearance, because scattering of light is diminished or absent.

Characterization of Porcelain Laminate Veneers

Characterization and polychromaticity of porcelain laminate veneers can be accomplished by the laboratory technician through the use of different shades of porcelain or by surface staining. The relative thinness of the veneer, however, may limit the extent of polychromaticity attainable in the porcelain. Internal resin shading ideally should be limited to the minor changes that can be accomplished through the use of a single homogeneous shade of luting cement.

TRY-IN CONSIDERATIONS

The porcelain laminate veneers should be tried in and evaluated either with water-soluble, noncuring try-in paste (if available) or with the actual luting agent.

The water-soluble, noncuring try-in paste has the advantage of allowing unlimited time to evaluate the effect of the differing shades. If desired, a number of porcelain laminate veneers, each with a different shade of try-in paste, may be simultaneously evaluated. The pastes will approximate the color of the corresponding luting cement.

The actual luting cement can be used to evaluate the effects of different shades. However, the evaluation must be performed quickly so that the material does not begin to polymerize.

Whether water-soluble, noncuring try-in paste, or the actual luting agent is used, the final result may vary from that which is visualized during this evaluation procedure. This occurs for the following reasons:

1. The shade of the try-in paste may not precisely match that of the corresponding luting resin.
2. The shade of the luting resin may change immediately following curing.
3. The shade of the polymerized resin may change over time.

To partially compensate for these phenomena, a sample of each shade of luting resin should be bench-cured and placed in water and any relative changes noted. These changes can be recorded and considered at the time of try-in to help predict the eventual appearance of the definitive restoration. For example, if the chosen shade of unpolymerized luting agent or try-in paste is higher in value than the corresponding polymerized sample, the definitive restoration will probably be similarly affected and appropriate compensation should be considered. However, other factors, such as the metameric influence (see Chapter XX) of the porcelain and dentin, the thickness of the luting agent layer, and the degree of opacity of the porcelain will further complicate this assessment. These considerations are generally more significant when attempting to match unprepared or previously restored adjacent teeth than when an entire facial display is being restored.

Armamentarium

+ Oil-free pumice

- Water-soluble try-in paste or composite resin luting cement (Insure, Cosmedent, Inc.)
- Extra-fine diamond bur for adjusting porcelain laminate veneers during try-in (Laminate Veneer Kit, Brasseler USA; Micron Finishing System Diamond Burs MF1, MF2, MF3, Premier Dental Products Co.)
- Cotton-tipped applicators

- Acetone or alcohol
- Glycerin (Liquid Strip Syringe Ivoclar Vivadent N.A.) *Clinical Technique*
1. Inspect the porcelain laminate veneers for cracks and imperfections. Place the veneers on the cast and verify appropriate fit individually and collectively (Figs. 7-15A-C).

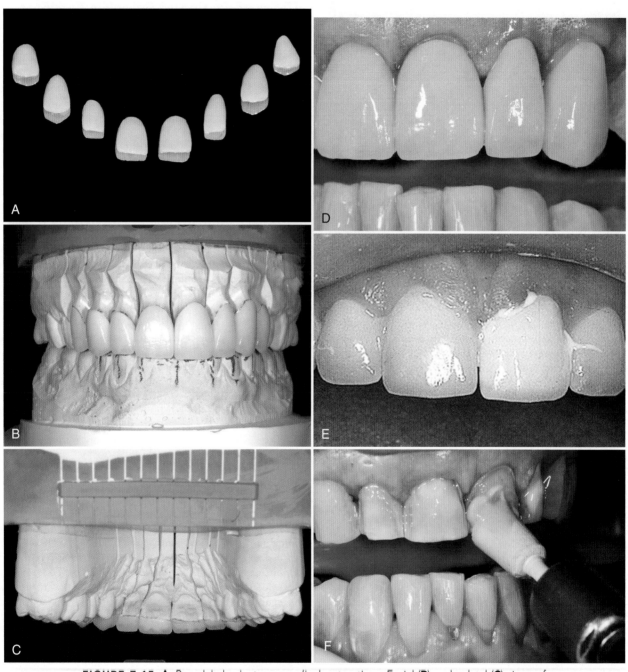

FIGURE 7-15 A, Porcelain laminate veneer final restorations. Facial (**B**) and palatal (**C**) views of the porcelain laminate veneers positioned on the laboratory cast. **D,** The porcelain laminate veneers are placed on the prepared teeth and evaluated for proper fit and appearance. Note the excess try-in paste at the gingival margin. (Part of the retraction device [blue] is visible). **E,** If different cement shades are evaluated simultaneously in adjacent porcelain laminate veneers, comparisons can be easily visualized. **F,** The teeth are cleaned with flour of pumice on a prophylaxis cup using a low speed handpieceto remove all traces of the try-in paste or luting agent.

CLINICAL TIP

Although the porcelain laminate veneers will be cemented with an appropriately shaded luting cement, precise restoration margins are necessary to minimize the exposure of the composite resin cement, which may discolor over time.

2. Thoroughly wet the internal surface of the laminate veneers with water and leave wet.
3. Remove the provisional restoration with a curette (see Fig. 7-13 I) or hemostat (see Fig. 7-13 J). Break the brittle composite resin into smaller fragments if it cannot be removed in one piece.

CLINICAL TIP

If a hemostat is use to remove the provisional restorations it is critical that it contacts the provisional material and not the tooth in order to minimize forces on the prepared tooth. These forces could lead to tooth fracture.

4. Clean all areas of the prepared teeth with flour of pumice on a prophylaxis cup using a low speed handpiece
5. Rinse thoroughly with water and leave wet.

CLINICAL TIP

Prophylaxis pastes contain oil that may contaminate the tooth surface. Therefore do not substitute prophylaxis pastes for oil-free pumice.[24]

6. Moisten the teeth and the internal surfaces of the porcelain laminate veneers with water. Glycerin, a more viscous liquid, may be used if greater retention of the porcelain laminate veneer is desired during this stage.
7. Place the porcelain laminate veneers on the teeth and evaluate for proper fit and color (Fig. 7-15D) Adjustments to the fit can be made with a fine diamond bur.

CLINICAL TIP

Whenever possible, delay adjustments until after the porcelain laminate veneers are bonded into place because of the fragile nature of these restorations before bonding. Therefore perform only those adjustments that are necessary for proper seating of the restorations at this time. Porcelain laminate veneers are much less susceptible to fracture after bonding.

8. Verify shade.
A. *If the shade is correct:* Verify that untinted luting resin will be acceptable by placing untinted water-soluble try-in paste or the actual resin luting cement into the internal surface of the porcelain laminate veneers and placing the veneers on the teeth (Fig. 7-15E).

CLINICAL TIP

If the resin luting cement is used to preview the final result, take care to work quickly so that the material does not begin to polymerize.

CLINICAL TIP

Because the shade of the resin luting cement can change immediately upon polymerization and after time, correlate the final choice of resin cement with bench-cured shade samples. See the section on try-in considerations in this chapter.

B. *If the shade must be altered:* Place the appropriate shade of water-soluble try-in paste or the actual resin luting cement into the internal surface of the porcelain laminate veneers and place the veneers on the teeth.

CLINICAL TIP

If the resin luting cement is used to preview the final result, take care to work quickly so that the material does not begin to polymerize.

CLINICAL TIP

Evaluate different cement shades simultaneously in adjacent porcelain laminate veneers, in order to easily visualize comparisons. This is best accomplished with try-in pastes that allow unlimited working time.

CLINICAL TIP

Because the shade of the resin luting cement can change immediately upon polymerization and after time, correlate the final choice of resin cement with bench-cured shade samples. See the section on try-in considerations in this chapter.

CLINICAL TIP

If you cannot attain an acceptable shade, the laminate veneer can be custom stained in the office or by the laboratory.

9. Clean the internal surfaces with a cotton-tipped applicator followed by a water spray, and finally in an ultrasonic cleaner with acetone or alcohol. Apply 37% phosphoric acid for 15 seconds to remove any salivary contamination from the etched surface.

CLINICAL TIP

The "etching" of the etched porcelain surface of a porcelain laminate veneer is much more durable than the "etching" of etched enamel. Cleaning (as described in step #9) will not damage the etched surface.

10. Clean the teeth again with oil-free pumice (Fig. 7-15F) wash and dry with oil-free air.
11. Clean proximal surfaces with a finishing strip.

CUSTOM LABORATORY STAINING

A large discrepancy in hue or chroma requires custom staining either at chairside or by the laboratory technician. Most laminate veneers are fabricated on a refractory cast, which is destroyed when the veneer is removed, so a new cast must be fabricated unless a duplicate refractory model was fabricated.[25]

Armamentarium
+ Basic dental setup; see the section on major color change
+ Low-speed green stone
+ Basic custom shading setup (see Appendix A)
+ Porcelain laminate investment material
+ Air abrader (e.g., Microetcher, Danville Materials)
+ Porcelain etch (10% hydrofluoric acid)

Clinical Technique
1. Mix investment material and carefully place a small amount of investment on the lingual aspect of the porcelain laminate veneer.
2. Shape the remaining investment into a block and place the porcelain laminate veneer on this block with the facial side of the restoration facing out.
3. Trim excess investment to completely expose the facial surface. This is best done before the investment sets.
4. Carefully remove the glaze on the buccal surface with a low-speed green stone.
5. Modify the porcelain laminate veneer as necessary and fire (see Appendix A).
6. After "bench cooling," carefully remove the porcelain laminate veneer from the investment.
7. Carefully air abrade the internal aspect of the porcelain laminate veneer to remove any remaining investment material.
8. Try-in the porcelain laminate veneer. If the shade is still not acceptable, repeat steps 1 through 7.
9. Verify with the porcelain manufacturer whether re-etching of the internal aspect of the porcelain laminate veneer with hydrofluoric acid is necessary. Do not allow the etchant to contact the external surfaces.

CEMENTATION

Armamentarium
+ Basic dental setup; see the section on major color changes
+ Oil-free pumice
+ Interproximal abrasive strips (Sof-flex Strips, 3M ESPE)
+ Dead soft matrix strips (e.g., dead soft metal matrix strip, DenMat) or clear plastic matrix strips (e.g., Clear Mylar Strips, Patterson, Inc.) or Polytetrafluoroethylene (PTFE) tape[26-28]
+ Silane coupling agent (ex Silane, Ultradent Products, Inc.)
+ 37% Phosphoric acid etching gel (ex. Ultraetch, Ultradent Products, Inc.)
+ Dentin/enamel bonding agent (e.g., One-Step, Bisco, Inc.)
+ Set of shaded resin luting cement (e.g., Insure, Cosmedent, Inc.)
+ Interproximal abrasive separating strip (e.g., QwikStrip Serrated White, Axis Dental, Inc.)
+ Diamond-tipped laboratory Tweezers (e.g., Tweezers (554069) Ivoclar/Vivadent)
+ Curette (Paradise Dental Technology, Montana Jack R138)

Clinical Technique

1. Apply Phosphoric acid to the internal surface of all the porcelain laminate veneers (if required) according to the manufacturer's instructions (Fig. 7-16B).
2. Rinse the porcelain laminate veneer to remove all excess acid gel.

3. Apply silane coupling agent to the internal surface of all the porcelain laminate veneers according to the manufacturer's instructions (see Fig. 7-16E; Fig. 7-16F).

4. If the tooth surface has been contaminated, clean the facial and lingual tooth surfaces again with flour of pumice on a prophylaxis cup using a low speed handpiece.
5. Place matrix strips (dead soft metal matrix, clear plastic matrix or polytetrafluoroethylene [PTFE] tape) between the first teeth to restored and the adjacent teeth (Fig. 7-16G).

6. Etch the enamel and dentin (if exposed) for 15 seconds (Fig. 7-16H) (see Chapter 3).
7. Wash with water and or water/air spray for a minimum of 10 seconds for gel or liquid etchants (Fig. 7-16I) (see Chapter 3).
8. Air dry (Fig. 7-16J).

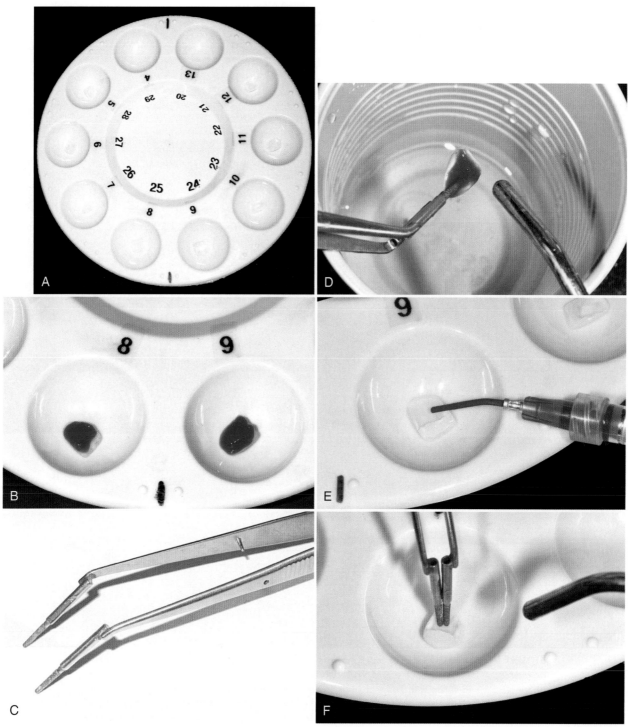

FIGURE 7-16 A, Placement of a porcelain laminate veneer on an incorrect tooth can easily occur after the luting cement is applied. To avoid this problem, use an artist palette (above) or draw and label circles on the bracket table cover. **B,** 37% phosphoric acid etch applied to the internal surfaces of the porcelain laminate veneer. Some silane coupling agents require acid etch activation of the porcelain surface. **C,** Diamond tipped laboratory tweezers (e.g., Tweezers 554069, Ivoclar/Vivadent). **D,** The high coefficient of the tweezers' friction tips provide excellent gripping capabilities that can withstand a strong water-spray without the need for excessive compression forces. **E,** Silane coupling agent is applied to the internal surface of the porcelain laminate veneer according to the manufacturer's instructions. **F,** The porcelain laminate veneer can be stabilized when using an air syringe to evaporate the silane solvent silane by holding the restoration in place with a gentle downward force. *Continued*

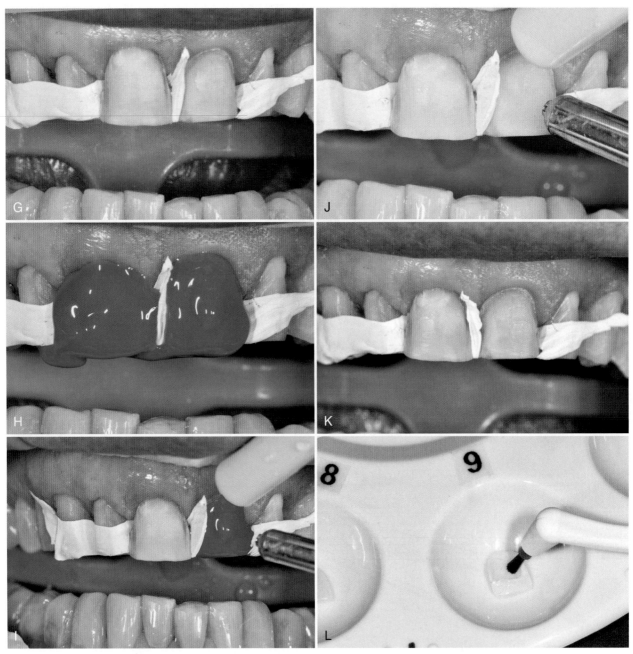

FIGURE 7-16, cont'd G, PTFE tape (shown) or matrix strips are placed between the first teeth to be restored and the adjacent teeth. **H,** The enamel and dentin (if exposed) is etched with 37% phosphoric acid for 15 seconds. **I,** The etchant is removed with water. **J,** The preparation is dried with oil-free air. **K,** Fresh matrix strips are placed into all interproximal areas. **L,** Bonding agent is applied to the internal surface of the porcelain laminate veneers according to the manufacturer's instructions.

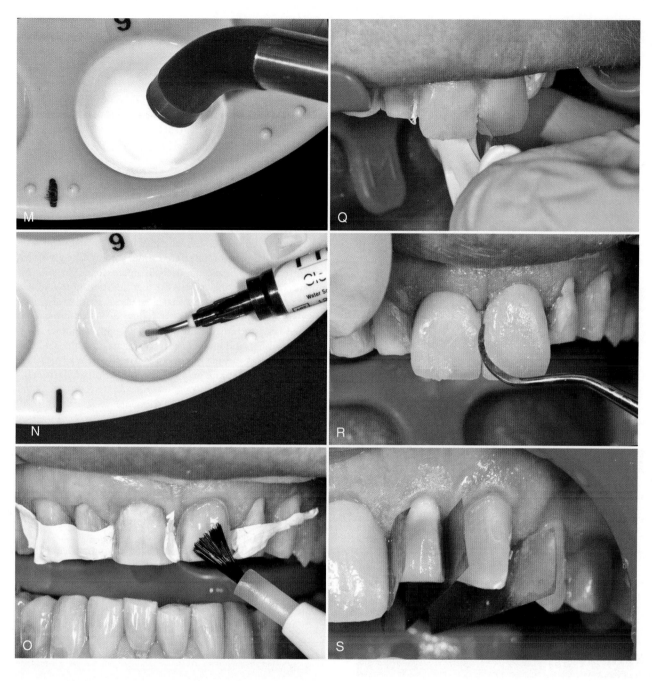

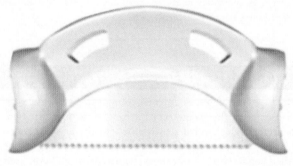

FIGURE 7-16, cont'd **M,** Light polymerize the resin per manufacturer's instructions. **N,** The preselected shade of luting cement is applied to the internal surface of the porcelain laminate veneer. **O,** Bonding agent is applied to the tooth structure according to the manufacturer's instructions. **P,** An interproximal abrasive separating strip (e.g., QwikStrip Serrated White, Axis Dental, Inc) is used to separate the laminates. **Q,** Excess cement is removed using an interproximal abrasive separating strip (e.g., QwikStrip Serrated White). **R,** Excess polymerized composite resin is initially removed from the marginal areas with a curette. **S,** Alternatively, dead soft metal matrix strips can be used between adjacent teeth.

Controlled positioning of the 37% phosphoric acid is facilitated by the use of a gel.

9. Repeat the etching process and rewash the enamel if it is not "frosty" white.
10. Place new matrix strips between all interproximal areas (Fig. 7-16K).
11. Selectively rewet the dentin with a cotton pellet as per manufactures instructions.
12. Apply bonding agent to the internal surface of the porcelain laminate veneers and light polymerize according to the manufacturer's instructions (Figs. 7-16L and M).
13. Apply the preselected shade of luting cement to the internal surface of the porcelain laminate veneer (Fig. 7-16N).

Place the porcelain laminate veneers underneath an opaque cup to prevent premature curing of the resin.

14. Place dentin/enamel bonding agent onto the tooth according to the manufacturer's instructions (Fig. 7-16O).
15. Carefully place the porcelain laminate veneers onto the teeth and fully seat to place.

To ensure proper seating of the porcelain laminate veneer, first use finger pressure with a pulsing motion on the incisal edge in an incisogingival direction. Then press with a pulsing motion on the facial surface in a labiolingual direction. Repeat these steps as necessary.

16. Hold the porcelain laminate veneer in place and polymerize the incisal tip from a facial direction for 10 seconds.
17. Remove excess luting cement with a sable brush moistened with bonding agent.

Dipping the brush into bonding agent before removing excess cement prevents "pulling" of the cement, which could create marginal voids.

18. Polymerize the remaining luting cement from the buccal, lingual, and incisal directions according to the manufacturer's instructions.

Light-cured resin cannot be damaged by excessive light exposure. It is therefore preferable to err on the side of longer exposure times.

19. Remove the matrix strips.

20. Remove excess flash with a curette. (Fig. 7-16R).
21. Repeat steps 2 through 17 for the remaining porcelain laminate veneers. Two adjacent teeth can be placed simultaneously (Fig. 7-16S).

Try-in the restorations that will be luted next. Even minimal amounts of excess luting agent from the previously luted porcelain laminate veneers can prevent the proper seating of subsequent veneers.

FINISHING AND POLISHING

Postcementation intraoral finishing of both porcelain and resin at the tooth-restoration interface can be accomplished with rotary instruments. Scanning electron microscope and spectrographic reflectance analyses reveal that adjusted porcelain can attain a surface smoothness that is superior to that of glazed porcelain if a specific protocol is followed.[29] This protocol is outlined later and involves the use of progressively finer abrasives. Finishing and polishing instruments include diamond burs, a 30-fluted carbide bur and a 2-μm to 5-μm particle size diamond polishing paste on a webbed rubber prophylaxis cup.

Armamentarium
+ Composite resin carving instruments (e.g., TCA, TCB, TCD, American Dental Manufacturing)
+ Diamond finishing burs (Micron Finishing System Diamond Burs MF1, MF2, MF3, Premier Dental Products Co.)
+ 30-fluted carbide bur (e.g., ETUF6 and 379UF, Brasseler USA)
+ Interproximal abrasive strips (Sof-Flex Strips, 3M ESPE)
+ Unwaxed regular dental floss
+ Porcelain polishing paste (e.g., Truluster, Brasseler USA; Instaglaze, George Taub Products)
+ Webbed rubber prophylaxis cup (e.g., Young Dental Mfg. Co.)

Clinical Technique
1. Carefully finish the facial margins with the MF1 finishing diamond in a high-speed handpiece at low speed (regulated by applying appropriate pressure on the rheostat) with water coolant.
2. Finish the lingual areas with a fine "football-shaped" diamond.
3. Dry the marginal areas to evaluate for smoothness and repeat steps 1 and 2 if necessary.

Hold the finishing instruments (composite resin carving instruments or the handpiece) in the dominant hand (right hand for right-handed dentists, left hand for left-handed dentists) and the evaluation instrument (explorer) in the other hand. This allows for efficient repetitive alternations between the evaluation instrument and the finishing instrument. If all instruments are held with only the dominant hand, repeated instrument transfers can become tedious, resulting in inadvertent overlooking of restorative material overhangs (Figs. 7-17A,B).

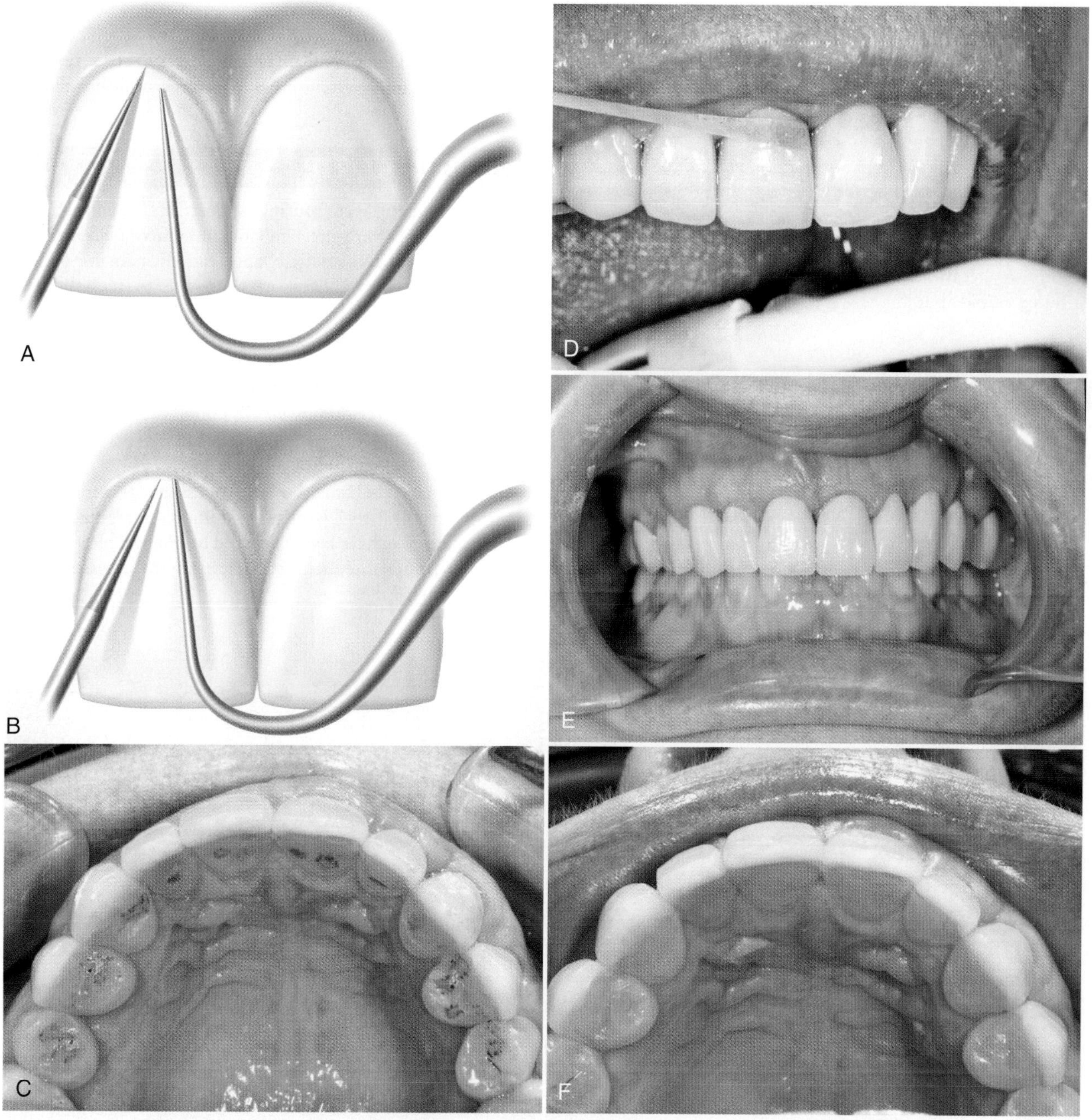

FIGURE 7-17 A, The finishing/polishing instrument is held in the dominant hand while the explorer is held in the other hand. Two-handed instrumentation allows for efficient repetitive alternation between the evaluation instrument and the finishing/polishing instrument. This expedites the tedious, repetitive "margin polishing/margin evaluation" process. **B,** The finishing/polishing instrument is held in the dominant hand while the explorer is held in the other hand. Two-handed instrumentation expedites the tedious, repetitive "margin polishing/margin evaluation" process. **C,** Whenever possible, maximal intercuspation and excursive movements should be on natural tooth surfaces. **D,** The proximal areas are finished and polished with interproximal abrasive strips. **E,** The completed maxillary porcelain laminate veneers in maximum intercuspation. (Also see Figure 7-18A and the completed maxillary and mandibular restorations shown in Figures 7-18M and N.) **F,** Maxillary Incisal view of the completed restorations.

4. Evaluate the occlusion with articulating paper in both centric occlusion and in all eccentric excursions. Adjust porcelain, if necessary, with an extra-fine "football-shaped" diamond bur.
5. Repeat steps 1 through 4, substituting first an M2 finishing diamond, then an M3 finishing diamond, and lastly, a 30-fluted carbide bur.

> ### CLINICAL TIP
>
> Do not substitute a 7- or 12-fluted carbide bur, which tends to chip or cleave the porcelain, for the recommended 30-fluted carbide bur.[29]

> ### CLINICAL TIP
>
> Whenever possible, maximal intercuspation (Fig. 7-17C) and excursive movements should be on natural tooth surfaces. This may not be possible with certain occlusal schema, such as canine-protected occlusion.

6. Finish and polish the proximal areas with interproximal abrasive strips (Fig. 7-17D).

7. Evaluate the interproximal contact areas with unwaxed dental floss and repolish if necessary.
8. Polish with a diamond polishing paste on a prophylaxis cup using intermittent pressure to prevent heat buildup.

> ### CLINICAL TIP
>
> Defer cosmetic recontouring, if possible, for approximately 1 to 2 weeks after porcelain laminate veneer placement. The initial dramatic cosmetic change can elicit in the patient a psychologic ambivalence and a desire to reestablish the previous appearance. Allowing the patient time to adjust to the new appearance usually eliminates this initial reaction. (This familiar response is commonly seen after the creation of a drastically new hairstyle.) Recontouring at this time therefore may result in overcorrection.

9. Reevaluate the finishing and polishing procedures in approximately 1 to 2 weeks for additional marginal discrepancies that may have been obscured by gingival bleeding or may result from subsequent water sorption by excess luting resin (Figs. 7-17E,F).

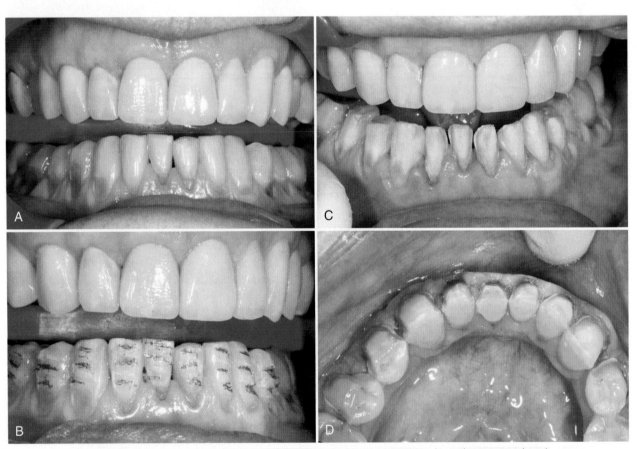

FIGURE 7-18 A, Maxillary porcelain laminate veneers restorations have been completed. Mandibular porcelain laminated veneers restorations are planned. **B,** Depth cuts are prepared and marked with pencil lines. **C,** The mandibular anterior and premolar teeth are prepared. **D,** Incisal view of the preparations.

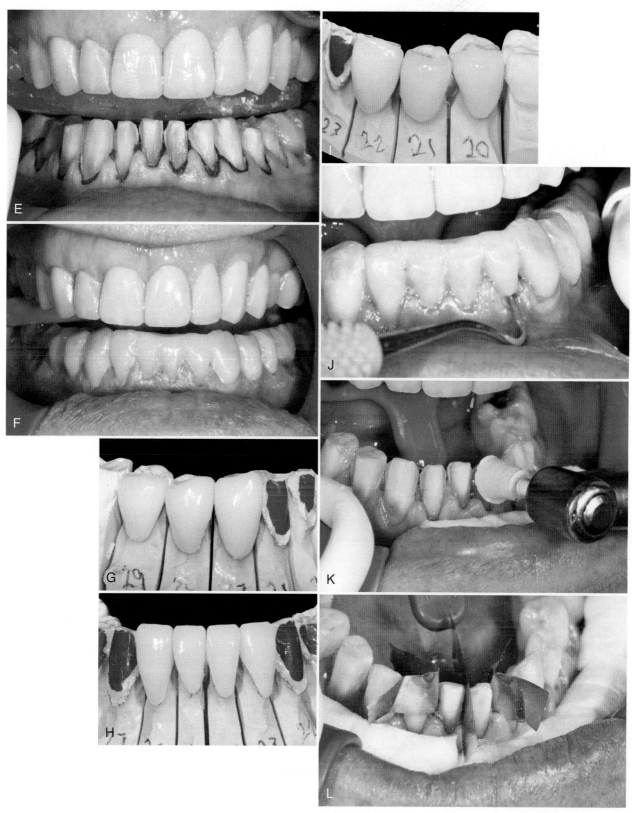

FIGURE 7-18, cont'd E, Retraction cord has been placed. **F,** Provisional restorations have been placed. **G-I,** The definitive restorations on the laboratory dies. **J,** The provisional restorations are removed. **K,** The prepared teeth are cleaned with flour of pumice on a prophylaxis cup using a low speed handpiece. **L,** Dead soft matrix strips (or other separating materials) are placed between the prepared teeth.   *Continued*

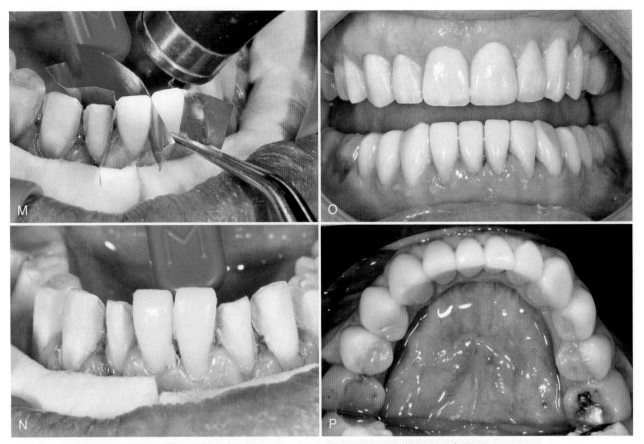

FIGURE 7-18, cont'd M, The porcelain laminate veneers are cemented. **N,** Excess cement around the restoration margins will be removed. **O,** Frontal view of the completed maxillary and mandibular porcelain laminate veneers. **P,** Incisal view of the completed mandibular porcelain laminate veneers.

CLINICAL TIP

Evaluate critically the true position of the lip during maximum smiling (the high smile line) before planning supragingival finishing lines. The true lip position may be deceptive. Patients with unattractive smiles often habitually adapt a high smile line position, which is significantly less revealing of tooth structure than is anatomically possible. After porcelain laminate veneers are placed, the high smile line may significantly elevate, because the patient's psychologic barriers to full smiling have dissipated.

MANDIBULAR PORCLAIN LAMINATE VEENERS

The steps for producing mandibular porcelain laminate veneers are identical to those in the maxillary arch except for differences in the amount of tooth structure reduction (see section on Tooth Preparation earlier).

Armamentarium
♦ Identical Armamentarium as in previous sections on Tooth Preparation, Impressioning, Provisional Restorations, Laboratory Communications, Try-In Considerations, Cementation, Finishing And Polishing

Clinical Technique
1. Administer suitable anesthesia (if necessary) (see Fig. 7-18*A*).

2. Prepare the teeth (Figs. 7-18*B-D*). Also see the sections on Tooth Preparation earlier in this chapter.

3. Place retraction cord (Fig. 7-18*E*) and make impressions. (See the section on Impressioning earlier in this chapter.)

4. Fabricate a suitable provisional restoration (if necessary). (See the section on Provisional Restorations earlier in this chapter; Fig. 7-18*F*.)

5. Send the impressions or casts to the dental laboratory where restorations will be fabricated and returned for evaluation, try-in, and cementation. (See the sections on Laboratory Communications, Try-In Considerations, Cementation, Finishing and Polishing earlier in this chapter; Fig. 7-18*G*.)

6. Remove the provisional restoration are removed. (See the section on Try-In Considerations earlier in this chapter; Fig. 7-18*H*.)

7. Verify the fit of the restorations.

8. Clean the teeth with flour pumice flour of pumice on a prophylaxis cup using a low-speed handpiece. (See the section on Try-In Considerations earlier in this chapter; Fig. 7-18*I*.)

9. Place the appropriate separating strips (Fig. 7-18*J*).

10. Seat, verify, and cement the porcelain laminate veneers and (see the section on Cementation earlier in this chapter; Fig. 7-18*K*).

11. Remove excess cement (Fig. 7-18*L*).

12. Finish and polish the restorations (see the section on Finishing and Polishing earlier in this chapter; Figs. 7-18*M,N*).

CLINICAL CASE STUDY

A 54-year old woman presented with malpositioned maxillary anterior teeth. Her medical history was noncontributory. She refused any type of orthodontic treatment. Maxillary porcelain laminate veneers were treatment planned, fabricated, and placed (Fig. 7-19).

CONCLUSION

Significant advances in porcelain technology have permitted increased versatility in its use as a restorative material. When combined with acid-etch bonding techniques, porcelain laminate veneers are a more conservative and highly esthetic alternative to full coverage restoration in appropriate clinical situations.

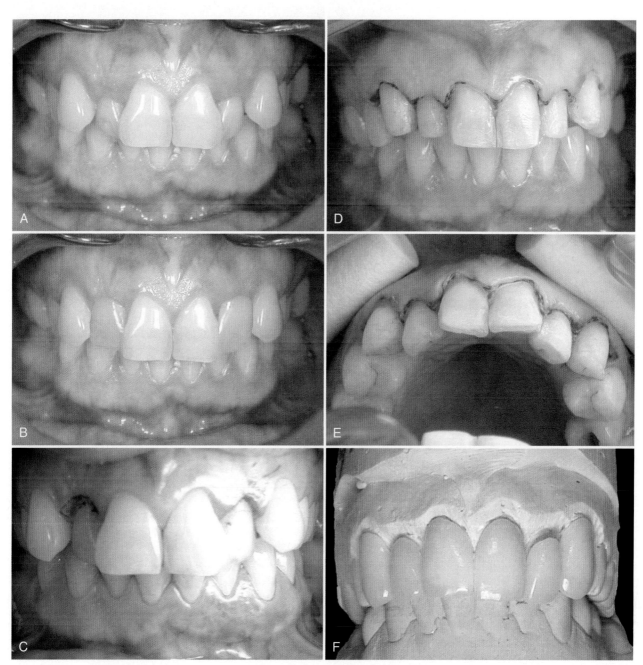

FIGURE 7-19 A, Preoperative view of the patient's teeth. **B,** A computer simulation demonstrates a potential treatment result (see Chapter 22). **C,** Electrosurgical gingivectomies were performed prior to tooth preparation. Frontal (**D**) and incisal (**E**) views of the porcelain laminate veneer tooth preparations. **F,** The porcelain laminate veneers on the laboratory casts.
Continued

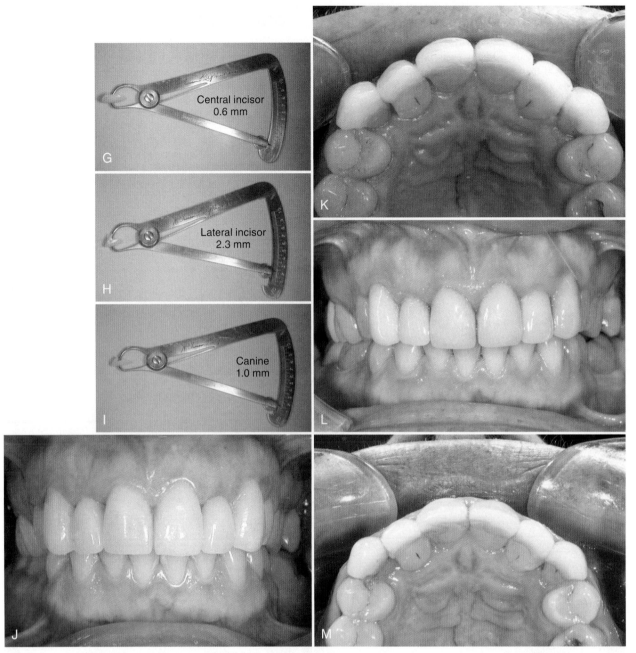

FIGURE 7-19, cont'd G-I, The veneers have different thicknesses to compensate for their relative positions. Frontal (**J**) and incisal (**K**) views obtained one week after placement of the porcelain laminate veneers. Frontal (**L**) and incisal (**M**) views obtained 13 years after placement of the porcelain laminate veneers.

REFERENCES

1. McGehee WH, True HA, Inskipp EF: *A textbook of operative dentistry*, ed 3, New York, 1950, The Blakiston Co.
2. Faunce FR: Tooth restoration with preformed laminate veneers, *Dent Surv* 53(1):30, 1977.
3. Boyer DB, Chakley Y: Bonding between acrylic laminates and composite resins, *J Dent Res* 61:489, 1982.
4. Cannon, ML, Marshall GW Jr, Marshall SJ, Cooley RO: Surface resistance to abrasion of preformed laminate resin veneers, *J Prosthet Dent* 52:323, 1984.
5. Bowen RL: *Report 6333. Development of silica resin direct filling material*, Washington, DC, 1958, National Bureau of Standards.
6. Paffenberger GC, Sweeney WT, Bowen RL: Bonding porcelain teeth to acrylic denture bases, *J Am Dent Assoc* 74:1018, 1967.
7. Meyerson RL: Effects of silane bonding of acrylic resins to porcelain on porcelain structure, *J Am Dent Assoc* 78:113, 1969.
8. Quinn F, McConnell RJ, Byrne D: Porcelain laminates: a review, *Br Dent J* 161:61, 1986.
9. Newbury R, Pameijer CH: Composite resins bonded to porcelain with silane solution, *J Am Dent Assoc* 96:288, 1978.
10. Highton RM, Caputo AA, Matyas J: Effectivness of porcelain repair systems, *J Prosthet Dent* 42:292, 1979.
11. Barreto MT, Bottaro BF: A practical approach to porcelain repair, *J Prosthet Dent* 48:349, 1982.
12. Jochen DG, Caputo AA: Composite resin repair of porcelain teeth, *J Prosthet Dent* 38:673, 1977.
13. Simonsen RJ, Calamia JR: Tensile bond strength of etch porcelain, *J Dent Res* 62:297, 1983.
14. Jordan RE, Suzuki M, Senda A: Clinical evaluation of porcelain laminate veneers: a four year recall report, *J Esthet Dent* 1:126, 1989.
15. Stangel I, Nathanson D, Hsu CS: Shear strength of the composite bond to etched porcelain, *J Dent Res* 66:1460, 1987.

16. Nichols JI: Tensile bond of resin cements to porcelain veneers, *J Prosthet Dent* 60:443, 1988.

17. Garber DA, Goldstein RE, Feinman RA: *Porcelain-laminate veneers*, Chicago, 1988, Quintessence.

18. Horn HR: Porcelain-laminate veneers bonded to etched enamel, *Dent Clin North Am* 27:671, 1983.

19. Jardel V, Degrange M, Picard B, Derrien G: Correlation of topography to bond strength of etched ceramic, *Int J Prosthodont* 12:59, 1999.

20. Phillips RW: *Skinner's science of dental materials*, ed 7, Philadelphia, 1973, Saunders.

21. Wildgoose DG, Winstanley RB, van Noort R: The laboratory construction and teaching of ceramic veneers: a survey, *J Dent* 25:119, 1997.

22. Nixon RL: Tooth preparation for porcelain veneers, *Forum Esthet Dent* 4:5, 1986.

23. Highton R, Caputo AA, Matayas J: A photoelastic study of the stresses on porcelain laminate preparations, *J Prosthet Dent* 58:157, 1987.

24. Calamia JR: Materials and techniques for etch porcelain facial veneers, *Alpha Omegan* 4:81, 1988.

25. Scharf J: In-office custom staining of porcelain laminate veneers, *Dent Today* 9:28, 1990.

26. Dunn, WJ, Davis JT, Casey JA: Polytetrafluoroethylene (PTFE) tape as a matrix in operative dentistry, *Oper Dent* 29:470, 2004.

27. Brown, Dennis E: Using plumber's teflon tape to enhance bonding procedures, *Dent Today* 21:76, 2002.

28. Stean, H: PTFE tape: a versatile material in restorative dentistry, *Dent Update* 20:146, 1993.

29. Haywood VB, et al: Polishing porcelain veneers: an SEM and specular reflectance analysis, *Dent Mater* 4:116, 1988.

Porcelain-Full Coverage and Partial Coverage Restorations

Vincent Celenza and Howard N. Livers

ALL-CERAMIC RESTORATIONS

Fueled by the esthetic revolution and intense media pressure for beautiful teeth, smile makeovers and elective procedures such as porcelain veneers (see Chapter 7) and tooth-whitening methods (see Chapter 13) have never been more commonplace. In randomized clinical studies, subjective assessments by patients demonstrate a clear preference for all-ceramic crowns when compared with porcelain fused to metal restorations.[1] All-ceramic systems are the primary choice for anterior tooth restoration or enhancement but now are increasingly considered for posterior teeth as well. Additionally, dentists now have expanded uses for multiple unit all-ceramic applications in selected situations. There are a number of all-ceramic systems available to restorative dentists. The primary difference among all-ceramic systems is in their method of manufacture and whether they exist in a monolithic (single layer of material) or multiphase system (layered porcelain on a high strength ceramic core).

Superior esthetics over traditional porcelain fused to metal (PFM) is routinely achieved with all-ceramic restorations.[2] Certain all-ceramic crown materials, especially ($Li_2Si_2O_3$), possess superior translucency throughout the material, not only limited to the incisal edges as in the situation of porcelain fused to metal restorations. Light transmission and translucency enable dentists to achieve superior esthetics and shade matching with adjacent natural teeth (Fig. 8-1).

High strength ceramic cores require less tooth reduction than PFMs, which require a minimum of 1.5 to 2.0 mm of axial reduction. This reduction is necessary to create space for layers of opaque and veneering porcelains over an opaque metal core. Lithium disilicate and leucite-reinforced ceramic cores possess superior strength.[3-6] Alumina and zirconia cores possess superior strength as well but do not have the translucent characteristics of lithium disilicate.

The cost of high noble metals such as gold has increased dramatically in recent years. Without the costs associated with precious metal, the all-ceramic crown can be less costly.

IPS e.Max

IPS e.Max (Ivoclar Vivadent) is an all-ceramic system consisting of five different components:
+ e.Max Press (lithium disilicate glass-ceramic ingot for the "press" technique)
+ e.Max Zirpress (fluorapatite glass-ceramic ingot for the press technique)
+ e.Max CAD (lithium disilicate glass-ceramic block for the CAD/CAM technique)
+ e.Max Zir CAD (zirconium oxide block for the CAD/CAM technique)
+ e.Max CERAM (fluorapatite veneering ceramic)

IPS e.Max CAD is a lithium disilicate glass-ceramic for CAD-CAM applications. The ingots are produced using sophisticated glass technology, which prevents the formation of defects in the ingots. Because the ingots are only partially crystallized, the blocks are easily machined. The ingots at this point are in their blue, translucent state. The partial crystallization process leads to the formation of lithium metasilicate crystals, which are responsible for the material's relatively high strength and marginal integrity.

Following milling, the restorations are tempered and thus reach a fully crystallized state. At this point the lithium disilicate crystals are formed. Although improvements have been made in all categories, the most notable is in the material strength wherein 360 MPa has been achieved, allowing a number of restorative possibilities. Achievable fit is excellent when properly fabricated.[7] If the core is cut back after pressing or waxed and pressed to less than full contour, porcelains may be baked in layers to achieve depth of color in the definitive restoration

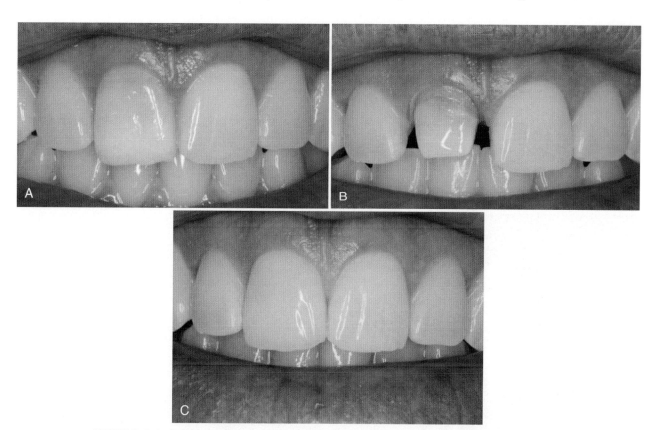

FIGURE 8-1 A, This endodontically treated central incisor had darkened over time and was unsightly to the patient. **B,** A full coverage restoration was deemed necessary to block the darkened cervical region. **C,** The final result is acceptable in lithium disilicate using ingot A-1 LT and minor incisal feldspathic additions. LT, Low translucency.

("layering technique"). In addition to full coverage restorations, e.Max is particularly well suited for posterior inlays, onlays, and anteriorly for porcelain veneers.[5] A simple acid etching (using 5% hydrofluoric acid) of all the internal aspects of the restoration during bonding or "luting" procedures enhances retention (Fig. 8-2A).

Following the complete removal of all preexisting alloy and excavation of any caries present, the teeth are isolated and the internal surfaces are etched with 10% phosphoric acid for 15 to 30 seconds, rinsed well, and lightly air dried. This is followed by application of *Gluma* desensitizing liquid (Heraeus Kulzer Inc.) using a microbrush or equivalent, to all exposed dentin surfaces.

Next, radiopaque light-polymerized reinforced glass ionomer (Fuji II LC, GC America, Inc.) is mixed, powder/liquid, then syringed using a needle syringe (AccuDose, Centrix, Inc.) into the cavity preparation to create a base and fill any undercuts. It

is immediately light polymerized and prepared to create ideal preparation designs (Fig. 8-2B). The impression is made and poured in stone or scanned intra-orally and reproduced digitally to reproduce the clinical situation (Fig. 8-2C). Alternatively, the stone cast may be scanned and the digital information used to manufacture the restorations using CAD-CAM technology, milling from a block.

Waxing, spruing, pressing, divesting, fitting, and margin refinement are all done utilizing the sectioned stone cast where dies are removable and may be inspected and handled individually (see Fig. 8-2C). The second, solid, uncut cast is used to verify interproximal contacts in the laboratory (Fig. 8-2D).

At the restoration delivery appointment, provisional restitutions are removed and the cavity preparations are thoroughly cleaned with Tubulicid (Dental Therapeutics AB) using a microbrush or equivalent. This chemical removes the superficial smear layer without opening tubules, while cleaning and distributing fluoride simultaneously. Next, the restorations are tried in individually and adjusted where necessary for complete seating (see the section on Crown Try-in and Placement later in this chapter). Once all the restorations have been tried in together and are ready to be placed permanently, they are internally acid etched with IPS ceramic etching gel (5% Hydrofluoric acid) for 20 seconds, rinsed, and air dried. As a recommendation, these internal surfaces should be "conditioned" using Monobond Plus (silanization) for 60 seconds then air dried. Next, the internal surfaces of the teeth including enamel are etched with 10% phosphoric

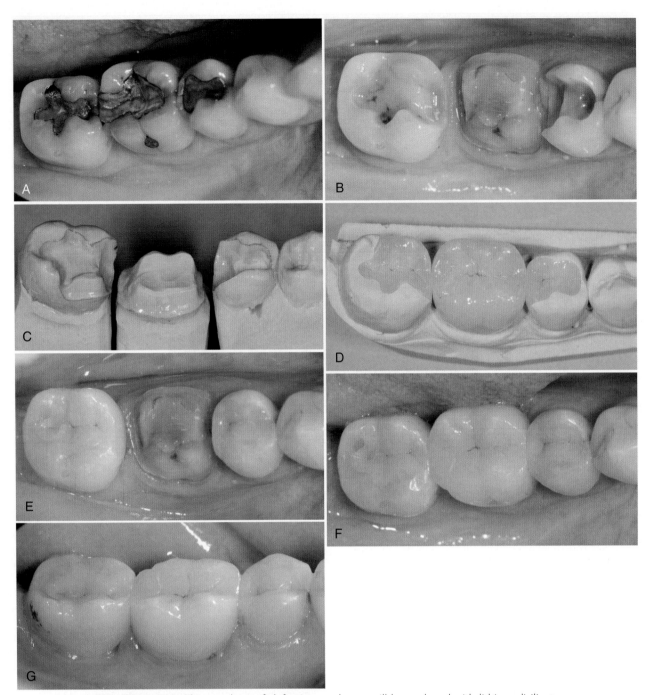

FIGURE 8-2 A, This quadrant of defective amalgams will be replaced with lithium disilicate e.Max restorations. **B,** The second premolar is prepared for a two-surface inlay; the first molar will be a full crown and the second molar will be an MO with mesiolingual cuspal coverage, making it an "onlay." **C,** The sectioned stone die cast on which the patterns will be waxed and sprued for pressing. **D,** Restorations are placed and checked on the solid uncut stone cast to verify interproximal contacts in the laboratory. **E,** The first premolar is seated first. **F,** Finished restorations, occlusal view. **G,** Finished restorations, lingual view.

acid for 15 to 30 seconds, rinsed well, and lightly air dried. Immediately apply Gluma desensitizing liquid on dentin surfaces using a microbrush. Studies have shown that Gluma that touches enamel surfaces will have no effect on the bond strength of the restorations to the tooth.[7] One-Step universal light-polymerized dental adhesive (Bisco, Inc.) is then applied with a microbrush to all internal surfaces to be bonded (enamel, dentin, and base) and is light-polymerized for 60 seconds.

> **CLINICAL TIP**
>
> Brush a tiny amount of lubricant (Vaseline) on proximal surfaces of the restoration to facilitate easy cement removal, taking care not to allow any lubricant to get inside the restoration. An easy way to ensure this does not happen is to lubricate the proximal surface while the restoration is firmly seated on the working die.

Dual luting composite resin cement or Variolink (Ivoclar Vivadent) are well-suited luting agents for these types of restorations. The luting cement is best filled into a needle syringe (ex., AccuDose) and delivered into the isolated cavity preparation. The restoration is then placed and fully seated using a metal-pointed instrument pressing into the central fossa to ensure complete seating. A plastic disposable bristle brush (Bendabrush, Centrix, Inc.) may be used to wipe away excess cement and while still applying seating pressure, floss should be passed between teeth to clear the interproximal excess before light curing.

CLINICAL TIP

In a multi-restoration quadrant like this where interproximal contacts are involved, placing the inlay and onlay first (Fig. 8-2E) is recommended before placing the full crown between them for several reasons: First, full seating may be visually ensured more easily. Second, finishing of the interproximal margin intraorally may be facilitated as well. Last, it is easier to place, check, and add contacts, if necessary, for a full crown than it is for an inlay. Furthermore, the technician would not be constrained by the contours of a full crown restoration the way he or she would be for a narrow two- or three-surface inlay.

CLINICAL TIP

When interproximal contacts are involved in a multi-restoration quadrant, place the inlay and onlay first before placing the full crown between them. Full seating may be visually ensured more easily, finishing of the interproximal margin intraorally is facilitated and it is easier to place, check, and add contacts, if necessary, on a full crown than it is for an inlay. The laboratory technician has fewer constraints when contouring a full crown restoration than with a narrow two or three surface inlay or onlay.

Once all the restorations have been luted into place and excess cement has been cleared, final occlusal refinements need to be made. For this, use two-color, double-sided articulating paper Accufilm II (Parkell, Inc.) and 7-micron–thick metal foil (Almore International Inc.), football-shaped diamond burs, (e.g., Fine 8369DF-31-025, and Extrafine 369DEF-31-025 [Brassler USA]) and rubber wheels (Dialite LD adjustment, finishing, and polishing kit [Brassler USA]) all designed specifically for use with lithium disilicate. See the section on Occlusal Adjustments later in this chapter (Figs. 8-2F and G).

Porcelain Laminate Veneers

In addition to inlays and onlays, e.Max can be used for porcelain laminate veneers (Fig. 8-3). e.Max is available in a variety of ingot choices ranging from translucent to opaque (HT, LT, MO, and HO). Due to the material's somewhat low-value quality, depth of color and translucency can be achieved giving lifelike results. The more opaque ingots can block unwanted substrate color, for example, gold posts or dark, discolored dentin, typically seen in endodontically treated teeth. The degree to which these dark substrate colors may be blocked may be a function of the skill of the dental ceramist when compared with what might be achieved with more conventional metal-ceramic systems.

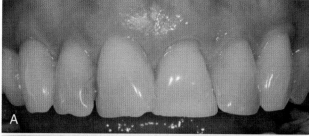
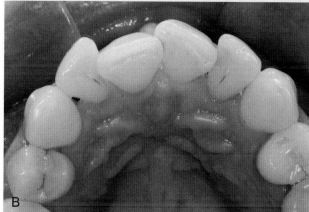
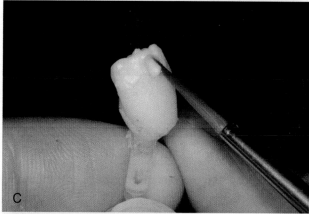
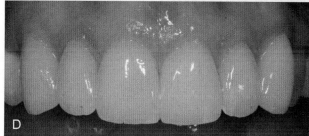

FIGURE 8-3 A, The six anterior incisors will be esthetically enhanced using porcelain laminate veneers compensating for tooth misalignment through tooth preparation. **B,** Rotations and overlap are apparent in this occlusal view. **C,** The core was cut back and translucent porcelains were added to create incisal translucency. **D,** Final e.Max restorations waxed and pressed with minimal additions for incisal effects.
Continued

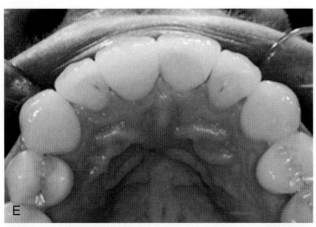

FIGURE 8-3, cont'd E, Incisal view showing lingual extension and degree of tooth preparation "wrapping" in order to effect changes in alignment and proportion.

Besides e.Max there are a number of other restorative material options, which possess a high-strength ceramic core and are available as either a monolithic or a layered technique. These include LAVA (3M ESPE), Cercon (Dentsply Ceramco) and Procera (Nobel Biocare).

Zirconia

An all-ceramic system known as Procera AllCeram (Nobel Biocare) has been available since 1993.[8-15] Unique to this method is the use of computer-assisted design and computer-assisted manufacturing (CAD/CAM) to fabricate a densely sintered, high-purity aluminum oxide coping, which is later veneered with porcelain. A scanner "reads" the stone die into a specialized unit that processes the data and creates either a two-dimensional cross-section or a three-dimensional view on a computer monitor. The shape of the crown (e.g., an emergence profile angle) may be selected and modified before actual coping fabrication (CAD). The production unit (originally in Sweden but now milling centers are available throughout the world), receives this information via modem and the coping is fabricated and mailed to the dentist without the need for any stonework leaving the dentist's office (see Chapter 23).

 The primary advantage in this methodology is the ability to ensure quality control in the coping manufacturing process using industrial standards, which eliminates the many operator variables possible in coping fabrication. The marginal preparation design may be more chamfer-like than a true shoulder because of the increased strength of this sintered understructure. Sharp internal line angles and stress points are undesirable because they create internal stress in the coping. The zirconia coping or understructure has proved to be very strong but the feldspathic porcelains layered on the coping have been less than fully reliable.[16] Delamination or chipping is common (Figure 8- 4A)

Originally, coping design was implicated as the primary reason for delamination. Greater attention given to porcelain support improved but did not eliminate the problem. More recently, use of zirconia in monolithic designs has been gaining popularity. The milling of blocks produces a full contour restoration, which is colored by new techniques developed for this purpose.[16] New techniques in copy milling have enabled technicians to reproduce patterns for multiple unit frameworks and implant frameworks

or complete monolithic designs (Figs. 8-4B-K).[17] It is expected that this monolithic restoration simply will not chip or break in any way.

Continued research and study in the use of zirconia has led to new technology and techniques, bringing us closer and closer to esthetics we have come to expect with more conventional feldspathic materials. A major advantage with this material is its virtually indestructible strength.

Light Absorption and Refraction

The metal component of PFM restorations prevents the transmission of light. Even diffusion of light through the porcelain is diminished when metal is present beneath the veneering porcelain.[18,19] The marginal soft tissues adjacent to subgingivally placed metal collars often appear dark, especially if the gingival tissues are thin. This effect may occur in PFM restorations with facial butt joint designs, because the small amount of porcelain covering the metal is opaque and creates a shadow of the root surface by blocking the normal transmission of light through the facial gingival tissues (Fig. 8-5A and B).

All-ceramic crowns and natural teeth allow the transmission of light to occur because of the absence of a metal coping. The ability to allow light to pass through itself varies with different materials. For example, feldspathic porcelains characteristically refract light differently than cast glass or pressed ceramics and natural enamel. The unorganized, random crystalline form of porcelain refracts approximately 25% of the available light and opacifying porcelain refracts even less. e.Max refracts as much as 75% of entering light, because its organized crystalline form has a refractive index similar to that of enamel.[20] Zirconia restorations do not possess the same optical qualities as lithium disilicate. Researchers have concluded that light transmission is significantly diminished in zirconia restorations.[21,22] LAVA restorations (3M ESPE) are the most translucent of the zirconia restorations at 0.3-mm and 0.5-mm core thicknesses. Studies [23] have also demonstrated that the thickness of the zirconia core directly affects translucency. Therefore monolithic zirconia restorations are opaque and, as such, are usually less desirable for use in the esthetic zone.

Biocompatibility

Rough, uneven, porous surfaces tend to encourage bacterial colonization. Poor margin adaptation or design, improperly glazed porcelains, and rough acrylics contribute to gingival inflammation.[24] Clinically, superb gingival response and esthetics routinely occurs when margins are placed well above attachment levels and, as such, do not invade or infringe upon the biologic width. Biofilm formation differs significantly among restorative materials.[25,26] Polished zirconia exhibits sharply reduced plaque accumulation compared with metal-ceramics, making it ideal for subgingival margin placement.[27]

Control of Margin Placement

The gingival extent of the interproximal shoulder of a full crown restoration may be deeper than ideal because of caries or a preexisting deep restoration. Deep subgingival margins complicate retraction, impression techniques, and margin evaluation. Biologic width violation and compromised oral hygiene access can result in gingival inflammation, pocket formation, and other

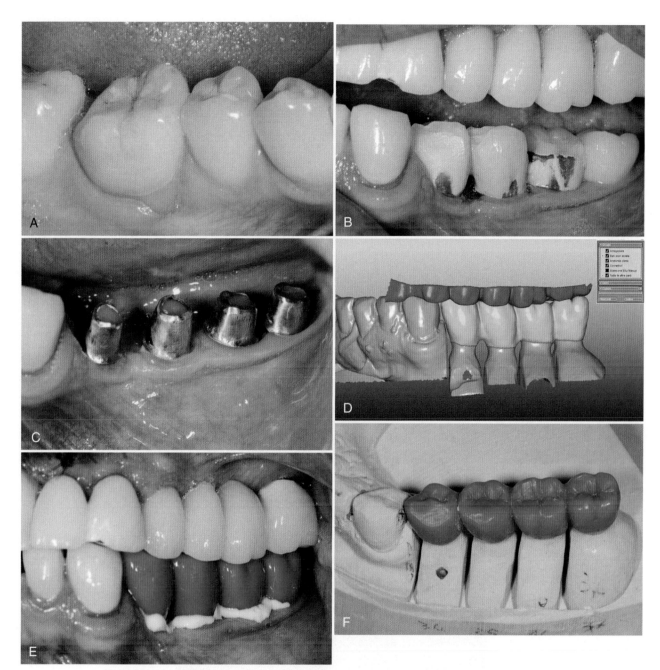

FIGURE 8-4 A, Chipping or fracturing of feldspathic porcelains fired over zirconia cores is a common occurrence. **B,** This patient exhibited porcelain fractures and shearing from the poorly designed metal framework, but more so from his relentless bruxing habits. **C,** Four custom waxed and cast gold abutments were fabricated and placed over the four implants. **D,** Articulated casts were scanned and using CAD-CAM technology a "prototype" of reinforced acrylic was milled from a block. **E,** The milled acrylic prototype fits precisely on the stone dies. **F,** Fit Checker (a silicone paste used to indicate film thicknesses, frictional rubs, or binding) was utilized to verify the fit of the prototype intraorally. If an improper fit was detected such as a rock (fulcruming around one of the abutments), the prototype can be sectioned and reattached in vivo using virtually any acrylic to make the correction. Additionally, any desired modifications to the occlusal surfaces may be made by additions or subtractions.

Continued

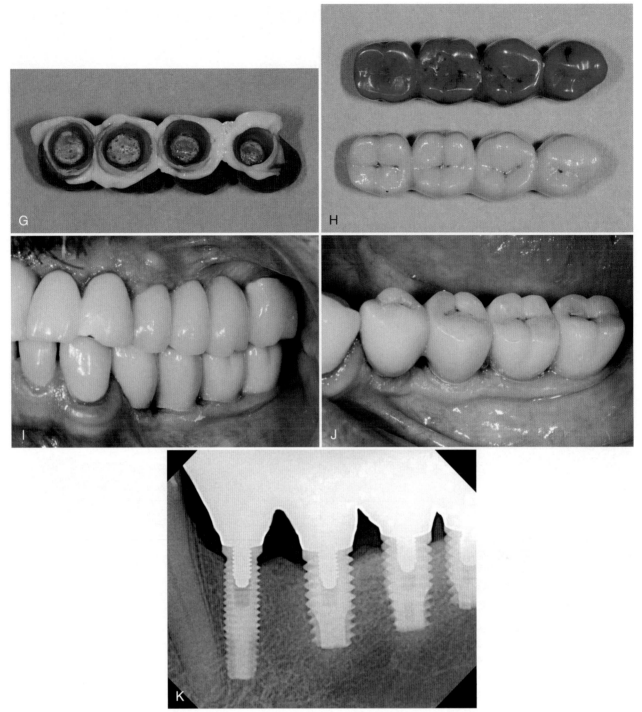

FIGURE 8-4, cont'd G, Fit appears acceptable, as the film thickness of the "fit-check" is minimal and all four units appear fully seated. **H,** The green prototype was then "copy-milled" to produce a monolithic result. External shading and stains were fired to produce acceptable esthetics. **I,** When the prototype has been properly designed, carefully checked, and modified as necessary intraorally, an exact copy can be milled from a zirconia block and once finished can be placed in the mouth. **J,** Occlusal view of the restoration in Figure 8-4 J. **K,** Radiograph demonstrating the excellent fit of the zirconia fixed partial denture to the gold abutments.

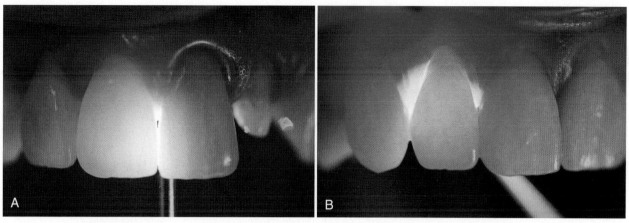

FIGURE 8-5 A, Transillumination of a metal-ceramic crown on the maxillary left central incisor at the try in stage. Lack of light transmission is apparent. **B,** Transillumination of a lithium disilicate crown on the maxillary right lateral incisor. Note the obvious passage of light through the restoration.

periodontal problems.[28-31] If the preparation has ideal substrate color, it is usually not necessary to place the preparation into the gingival sulcus. An exception to this occurs when a restoration is used to correct a diastema. A subgingival margin allows for a more gradual increase in restoration interproximal emergence contour by avoiding an abrupt transition of tooth to restorative material. In addition, especially when using lithium disilicate or another translucent core, and assuming ideal tooth substrate color, the margin placement can be supragingival, thus avoiding any physical challenge to biologic width.[32,33]

Ideal Preparation Requirements

Preparations for single tooth restorations have evolved primarily with the goal of creating excellent natural esthetics. Retention is aided by parallel axial wall design, dentin bonding techniques, and acid etching the internal portion of the restoration if possible[34] Restorations made of zirconia, are currently not internally etchable. The finishing line can be 90 degrees to the external unprepared axial root surface, with rounded internal line angles. Thin margins or beveled preparations are contraindicated because they would create an unacceptably weak ceramic margin.

Perhaps the most difficult aspect of the butt joint preparation design is the shoulder or actual butt joint. When viewed from the occlusal, adequate reduction is important to guard against breakage during function, because classically, thin areas tend to chip as the tooth flexes. A 360-degree chamfer with a minimum depth of 1 mm is recommended; however, 1.5 mm is ideal, because the restoration will be thicker and therefore stronger. More research is needed to determine the ideal preparation depth, because the increased strength of the materials suggest that less tooth reduction and thinner restoration wall thickness may be acceptable. In addition, greater thickness always provides the ceramist with a better opportunity to achieve more lifelike esthetics and affords greater ability to block underlying unfavorable substrate color. However, greater material thickness achieved by more reduction than recommended (over preparation) may lead to pulpal involvement and can weaken the tooth.

TECHNIQUE

Armamentarium
- Standard dental setup
  - Explorer
  - Mouth mirror
  - Periodontal probe
  - Suitable anesthesia
  - High-speed handpiece
  - Low-speed handpiece
  - "Great White" #2 carbide for prior crown removal (S.S. White Technologies Inc.)
  - Diamond burs:
  - Chamfer, round end taper, 5856L-31-018 (Brasseler USA)
  - Modified chamfer, 5878K-31-018 (Brasseler USA)
  - Cingulum reduction bur, football, 6379-31-023 (Brasseler USA)
  - Incisal reduction bur, #35010-31-5 and 30006-106 (Brasseler USA)
  - Occlusal reduction bur, 30010-018424U0 or 36006-011817U0 (Brasseler USA)
  - White polishing points, 649-31-420 (Brasseler USA)
  - Protection/visualization cord, No. 000 Ultrapak, black, nonimpregnated (Ultradent Products, Inc.)
  - Deflection/retraction cord, No. 1 Ultrapak, blue, nonimpregnated, (Ultradent Products, Inc.)
  - Carver (American Eagle Instruments, Inc.).
  - Scissors
  - Cotton pliers

Clinical Technique
Anterior Preparation (Fig. 8-6)
1. Place protection cord; see the section on Impressioning in this chapter. This may need to follow interproximal axial reduction first in order to break the interproximal contact and allow easy cord placement.
2. Reduce the tooth a minimum of 1.0 mm facially and axially. (Note: Reduction of more than 2.0 mm is considered overreduction and can substantially weaken the integrity of the remaining tooth structure, possibly leading to fracture of the

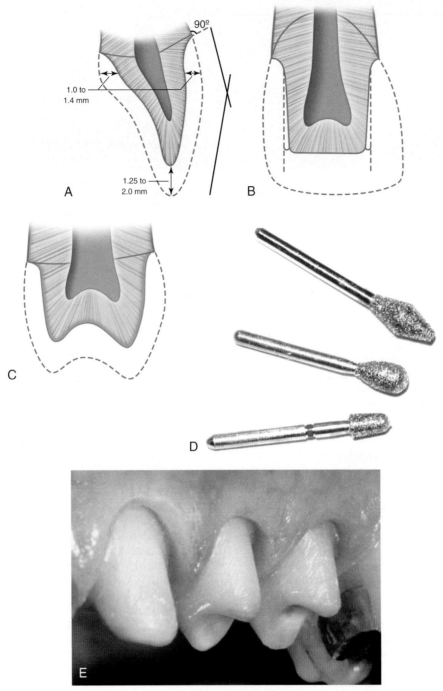

FIGURE 8-6 A, Lateral view of an anterior tooth preparation. **B,** Facial view of an anterior tooth preparation. **C,** Lateral view of a posterior tooth preparation. **D,** The bottom two burs are round-ended (Brasseler USA: 30010-018424U0 or 36006-011817U0) and are well suited for posterior reduction. A conventional occlusal-reduction diamond shaped bur (Brasseler USA 811-017278U0) is not. **E,** Posterior occlusal reduction should be "scooped out" buccolingually as is evident in these premolar preparations. This ensures adequate occlusal thickness without sacrificing axial wall height or restricting the ceramist's ability to include anatomically correct groove carving in the restoration.

abutment. Additionally, pulpal involvement and sensitivity become potential problems.)

3. Reduce the tooth 1.5 to 2.0 mm incisally if sufficient tooth structure exits.

> **CLINICAL TIP**
>
> Overreduction is contraindicated because it could lead to excess unsupported restorative material, which could fracture during function and, additionally, will reduce retention by shortening the axial wall height of the tooth.

4. Reduce the tooth at least 1.0 mm palatally to create sufficient space for material thickness to resist tensile (lateral) forces.
   Note: Axial reduction on the facial surface follows two planes (see Fig. 8-6B).

> **CLINICAL TIP**
>
> Ensure all prepared surfaces are smooth, rounded, and flowing. Avoid creating sharp corners where stress concentrations can occur.

> **CLINICAL TIP**
>
> Pay particular attention to the facial-to-lingual transition at the prepared incisal edge. Avoid thin edges or sharp points in this area; these can easily lead to crown seating problems because often these areas are not precisely replicated in the stone die. If the die is an exact reproduction of the clinical tooth, you can appreciate how easily thin or pointed stone areas may inadvertently be abraded. This in turn will lead to inaccurate internal aspects of crowns with excess material at the incisal edge. This excess material will prevent full crown seating. Stress concentrations may also occur at these points[35,36] (see Figs. 8-6B, 8-10B, and 8-11).

Posterior Preparation

1. Place protection cord; see the section on Impressioning in this chapter. This may need to follow interproximal axial reduction first in order to break the interproximal contact and allow easy cord placement, and eliminate the worry of inadvertent gouging of an adjacent tooth.
2. Reduce the tooth a minimum of
   a. 1.0 to 1.5 mm axially using a 5856L-31-018 (Brasseler USA)
   b. 1.5 to 2.0 mm occlusally using a 30010-018424U0 (Brasseler USA) to allow sufficient bulk (thickness) in the restoration to resist tensile (lateral) forces
   c. Axial reduction on the buccal surface of a mandibular tooth follows two planes. (see Fig. 8-6C) unless the tooth is in cross-bite in which case the lingual reduction should follow two planes. The situation is reversed for a maxillary tooth.

> **CLINICAL TIP**
>
> "Scoop out" posterior occlusal reduction buccolingually. This ensures adequate occlusal thickness of the restoration while avoiding sacrificing axial wall height or restricting the ceramist from creating anatomic groove carving (see Fig. 8-6E).

> **CLINICAL TIP**
>
> Terminate the finishing line of the preparation entirely on sound tooth structure. Ending on cements, bases, or metallic substructures does not ensure a positive seal against microleakage. Crown lengthening procedures alone or in combination with forced eruption procedures can help enhance marginal integrity while avoiding violations of biologic attachment dimensions.[37-39]

Impressioning: The Double Cord Technique

The butt joint or rounded shoulder preparation design allows little or no room for error in reading the final preparation in die material. Therefore, the entire extent of the prepared tooth must be clearly visible in the impression. Additionally, to create accurate marginal fit and to control emergence profile, impressioning a small amount of unprepared tooth structure beyond the finishing line is of equal importance. When compared with preparation designs incorporating bevels, full and partial shoulder preparations, sloping shoulders, or chamfer design preparations require a greater level of technical expertise to achieve accurate fits, because less room for error exists. Excellent impressioning requires superior performance in tooth preparation and soft tissue control.

Circumferential placement of a thin retraction cord (the "visualization" or "protection" cord), followed by a second thicker cord (the "displacement" cord) allows visualization of the finishing lines and creates adequate gingival retraction with sufficient space for impression material. Immediately before impressioning, only the larger cord is removed.

Armamentarium
- Standard dental setup (see the section on Ideal Preparation Requirements earlier in this chapter)
- Suitable hemostatic agent (Hemodent, Premier)
- Scissors
- Plastic metal instrument to be used for soft tissue deflection
- Suitable impression material (e.g., Impregum with Permadyne (3M ESPE)

Clinical Technique
1. Gently place the thin No. 000, contrasting color (black) cord, which was previously dipped into a hemostatic liquid solution (Hemodent, Premier Dental Products, Inc.).

> **CLINICAL TIP**
>
> To further guard against soft tissue trauma, use a plastic instrument held in the hand not holding the handpiece to *deflect* the gingival cuff away from the rotating bur (Fig. 8-7A). This can allow bloodless tooth preparation even in sub-gingival areas.
>
> This static positioning of the plastic instrument (see Fig. 8-7A) is an excellent way to begin learning the skill of protecting soft tissues while preparing teeth. Once this begins to feel more comfortable, moving the plastic instrument in tandem with the moving handpiece will be the next step toward developing good soft tissue control skills.

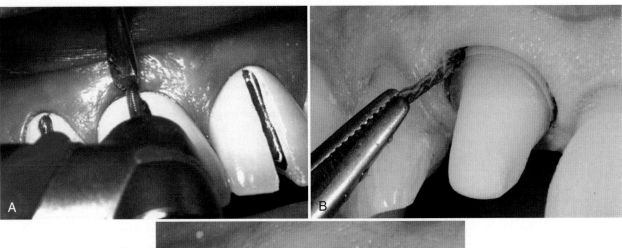

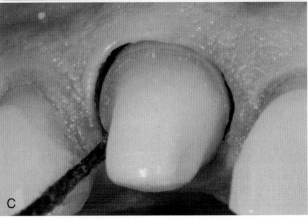

FIGURE 8-7 A, A plastic instrument (metal) positioned in this way with one hand, "deflects" and protects the marginal soft tissues, while the bur in the handpiece in the other hand cuts through the metal-ceramic crown subgingivally to remove it without causing any bleeding. **B,** Removal of the larger "displacement" cord exposes the thin "visualization cord" beneath it, which remains in place during the impression making. **C,** With the removal of the second larger "retraction" or "displacement" cord nearly complete, unprepared tooth structure beyond the finishing line is clearly visible and ready for impressioning.

> ### CLINICAL TIP
>
> Place the cord *before* the initiation of any subgingival tooth preparation. This will visually locate and protect the subjacent junctional epithelium because this thin cord sits on, and is apically limited by it.

2. After tooth preparation has been completed, true retraction needs to be accomplished to create room for the impression material lateral to the tooth and beyond the finishing line. Lateral displacement of the gingival cuff is accomplished by the placement of the second, wider cord. Because the true purpose of this cord is to displace tissue, this cord is referred to as the "retraction" or "displacement" cord (Figs. 8-7B and C).
3. Place the second displacement/retraction cord. This is nonimpregnated and dry but is moistened with air/water spray after placement.
4. Remove the retraction cord (second, top cord) after at least 4 minutes, while leaving the protection cord in place (see Figs. 8-7B and C). Make the impression with any standard impression material (Fig. 8-8). This is known as the "single cord technique."

5. Carefully inspect the impression with magnification for completeness, absence of voids, or obvious distortions.

> ### CLINICAL TIP
>
> Supragingival preparation designs simplify impression procedures and whenever possible are the preferred designs from both restorative and periodontal standpoints. Consider supragingival preparations when axial wall height is sufficient and esthetic demands permit.

PROVISIONAL RESTORATIONS

Properly contoured and well-fitting provisional restorations may be regarded as templates for final restorations.[40-42] These provisional restorations should protect prepared tooth structure and maintain the tooth's position in the arch. Fit is particularly critical when margins are placed subgingivally, because slight openings or short margins allow gingival tissues to proliferate and invaginate. Undercontouring of the provisional restoration allows soft tissue overgrowth circumferentially, which will invariably result in trapping of soft tissue tags during restoration try-in. Soft tissue that interferes with full seating at the delivery

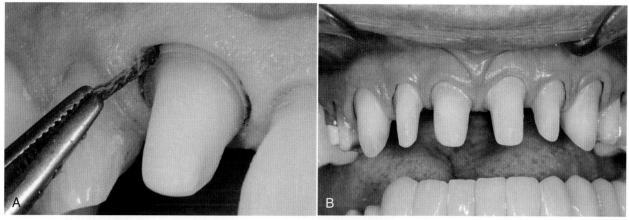

FIGURE 8-8 A, The full extent of the prepared teeth have been captured in this impression, which was made using only one cord. **B,** This is the clinical situation just after the impression was removed and black cords are still in place. If tooth preparations are thoroughly and carefully performed, followed by accurate provisionalization with well-fitted margins, complete and accurate impressions are readily readable and all tooth preparation details are easily captured in the material even though only one cord was placed.

visit should be retracted and/or removed prior to cementation procedures. Failure to remove these tags, which prevent full seating of the crown and create an area of potential marginal leakage, can result in restoration failure.

> ### CLINICAL TIP
>
> Study casts of provisional restorations; record tooth length, width, emergence profile, contour, esthetic arrangement, occlusion, and incisal guidance (disclusion). This information may be very helpful to laboratory technicians in the fabrication of definitive restorations especially in the anterior region.

Die Preparation

All aspects of the prepared tooth must be captured in the impression and faithfully reproduced in die stone. Tooth preparation design determines die preparation design. Ditching beneath the finishing lines is contraindicated in butt joint, shoulder, or chamfer preparation designs because this process would result in weak, friable, and thin die stone at the finish line (Fig. 8-9A). Furthermore, unprepared tooth structure captured apical to the finish line may provide valuable information pertaining to the emergence profile of the tooth (Fig. 8-9B).

> ### CLINICAL TIP
>
> "Clear" excess stone from the finish line of dies with rounded shoulder or chamfer preparation designs with a large rubber wheel (Brasseler USA porcelain polisher white 0301-220). Leave the unprepared tooth structure near the finish line untouched where possible so that it is clearly discernible (Figs. 8-9C and D).

> ### CLINICAL TIP
>
> Lead pencil outlining at the margin is contraindicated because lead that joins the wax pattern at the margin, once invested, will not burn out in the oven and can lead to short castings because lead is an antiflux.

Crown Try-in and Placement
Contact Areas
Armamentarium

+ Standard dental setup (see the section on Ideal Preparation Requirements earlier in this chapter)
+ Colored spray powder (e.g., Occlude, Pascal Co., Inc.)
+ Unwaxed dental ribbon
+ Polishing wheels (e.g., Brasseler USA porcelain polisher white 0301-220, pink 0306-220, or DiaLite R17D, Axis Dental)

Clinical Technique
1. Try in the final crown with gentle finger pressure.
2. Check margins with a fine tip explorer to confirm full seating.
3. Check contact areas with floss while holding the crown in place. (The dental assistant should hold the crown in place with finger pressure while the operator passes floss through the contact area.)
4. Locate areas of tight contact by applying a light powder mist of Occlude indicator powder to the interproximal surfaces of the crown.
5. Reseat the crown, remove it, and observe the interrupted powder area created by the tight contact (Figs. 8-10A and B).
6. Adjust the "mark" with polishing wheels. (Dialite HP Knife-Edge Ceramic Polishers [Axis Dental], Brasseler USA Extra-coarse L26XCHP, Coarse L26CHP, Medium L26MHP, Fine L26FHP).
7. Reseat the crown and check the contact area with floss.
8. Recheck the margin with an explorer.
9. The occlude powder can easily be removed by simply wiping the contact area with dry gauze.
10. If the contact is light, make corrections by firing add-on porcelains.

Internal Fit

The color of conventional silicones or indicator pastes closely approximates the internal color of all-ceramic crowns, making

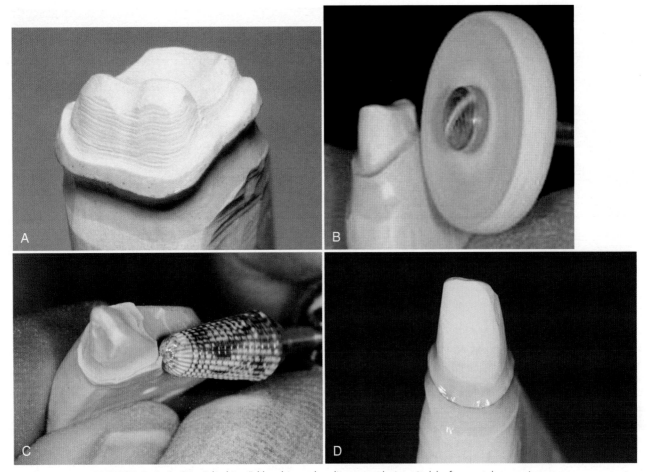

FIGURE 8-9 A, Die "ditching" like this molar die example is suitable for metal-ceramic restorations and associated tooth preparation designs that feature bevels, but is unsuitable for preparations that move closer toward shoulder designs such as those preparations designs recommended for full-ceramic restorations. **B,** Use a large rubber wheel (Brasseler USA porcelain polisher white 0301-220) to clear excess stone away from the finish line for dies with rounded shoulder or chamfer preparation designs. In this way, the finishing line will not be vulnerable to chipping because there will be supporting stone beneath it. **C,** This large straight handpiece carbide bur from Brasseler USA (H79GSQ-021892U0) is also very nice for clearing away stone from the finishing line when preparation is a light chamfer and something closer to "ditching" is desired. **D,** Preparation of the stone die margin clearly delineated, outlined with a red pencil, then a thin coat of stone sealer (Clear Coat Model Hardener, American Dental Supply, Inc.) is painted around the margin and chamfer area to protect and prevent the marked finishing line from rubbing off.

them ineffective in detecting areas in which the restoration binds. (Note: A new dark gray colored silicone gel has been introduced to the market that will allow high spots or places of friction to be visually discerned. This would be fine if the correction were to be made inside the crown, but for reasons about to be discussed the adjustment should be made to the tooth preparation itself, and for that reason a medium used to show the offending area, which "transfers a mark" from the crown to the tooth, is preferable). However, because the occlusal surface and all axial surfaces have been die spaced, theoretically the only areas of the crown that may interfere with full seating are the unspaced areas of the die or where the stone die does not accurately represent the true clinical situation. Sharp edges in the tooth preparation can lead to inaccuracies because stone can be easily rubbed away or merely dissolved away from the running water used in the cast trimming process (Fig. 8-11*A-E*).

> ### CLINICAL TIP
>
> It is preferable to adjust the tooth rather than the restoration because adjustment of the internal area in the restoration may lead to future fracture of the restoration due to potential initiation of crack propagation.[35,36]

> ### CLINICAL TIP
>
> The binding area or rub mark internally at the incisal edge is indicative of a discrepancy between the tooth and the die. The best and easiest way to compensate for this is to modify the tooth intraorally rather than try to grind out the incisalmost portion of the crown. The rub mark noted in the crown will correlate with a colored mark left at the exact offending area of the tooth.

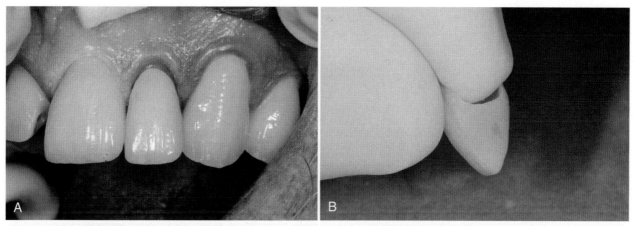

FIGURE 8-10 A, This lateral incisor crown has been lightly dusted with Occlude on the interproximal surfaces and the crown is being tried-in. Clearly, the contacts are preventing the complete seating of the crown. **B,** The rub mark is easily discernable in this photo and may be adjusted chairside using rubber wheels.

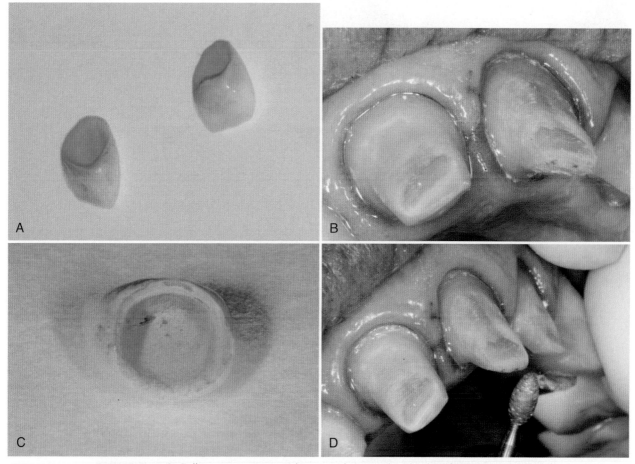

FIGURE 8-11 A, Full crowns, veneers, inlays or onlays, can be checked for full seating after interproximal contacts have been adjusted, by spraying all internal surfaces with a colored powder spray such as Occlude to disclose high spot interferences or rubs, which through frictional binding prevent full seating of the restoration. **B,** A discrepancy at the incisal edge of the tooth preparation in the stone die led to a "teetering" of the crown at try-in. The causative areas at the incisal edges are clearly visible. **C,** The internal surface of the crown after try-in with green powder clearly shows an offending area, which is preventing the full seating of the restoration, at the deepest portion of the crown at the incisal edge. The "rub" mark has a corresponding "transfer" mark, which can be seen on the tooth itself. The operator has a choice to either adjust the crown internally or adjust the tooth directly. **D,** The choice to adjust the tooth directly intraorally is easily accomplished dry at low speed and rarely requires anesthesia.

Continued

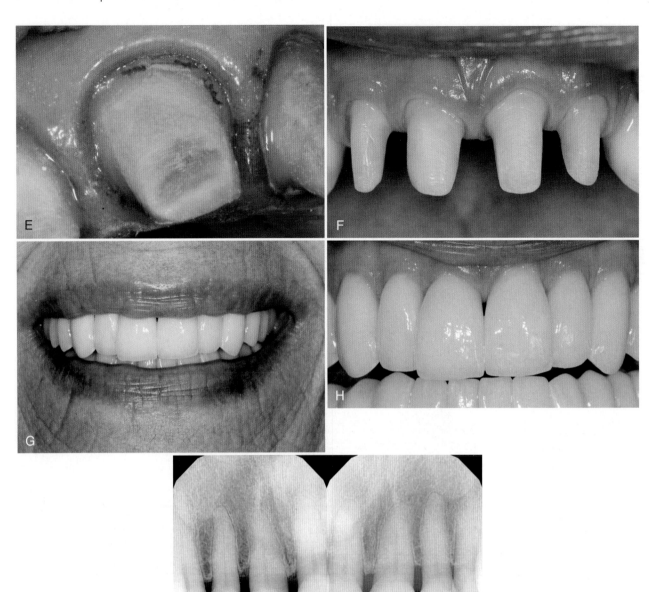

FIGURE 8-11, cont'd E, After the offending area of the tooth was adjusted, the crown was reseated to check for improved fit. Green powder at the shoulder area is only possible if the crown seats fully. **F,** Prepared teeth using #5878K-31-021 bur followed in the chamfer area only with 8878K-31-021 (Brasseler USA). **G,** Smile view showing a "natural" appearance of incisors achieved by incorporating subtle irregularities. One central incisor is slightly longer; the distal areas of the central incisors slightly overlap the laterals. **H,** The health of the marginal soft tissue is a reflection of the accuracy of the fit of our restorations. Maintained with excellent patient home care, these soft tissues appear healthy and free of any inflammation. **I,** Note the precise fit of the e.Max crowns on these anterior teeth after final cementation (see Chapter 12).

Armamentarium
+ Standard dental setup (see the section on tooth preparation earlier in this chapter)
+ Football shaped diamond bur to be used at slow speed for adjustment (e.g., Brassler USA 379-31-023 or 368-31-023).
+ Colored indicator spray (e.g., Occlude)
+ Alcohol
+ Cotton pledget
+ JSP Steam Cleaner (optional) (JSP)

CLINICAL TIP

If the crown is to be permanently placed by etching and bonding techniques, it is best to complete all fitting steps in which spraying internally with powders is planned, before internally etching the crown for luting purposes. It can be difficult to remove colored powders when the crown has already been etched. Additionally, the cleanest etched surface will be achieved when done last just prior to luting, because saliva picked up from multiple try-ins contaminates the surface and prevents the best bond achievable.

Clinical Technique
1. Spray the internal aspect of the crown with a thin mist of a colored spray especially on the shoulder and incisal edge area (see Fig. 8-10*B*).
2. Seat the crown with gentle finger pressure.
3. Remove the crown and carefully inspect all areas for rub marks (see Fig. 8-10*C*).
4. Gently adjust the binding areas where the powder marks have been transferred to the tooth (see Fig. 8-11*A*) with a football diamond or similar bur using slow speed (see Figure 8-11*C*).
5. Anesthesia is usually unnecessary.
6. Repeat, if necessary.
7. Check the margins with an explorer tip to confirm full seating and note the transfer of powder to the shoulder or chamfer area (see Fig. 8-11*F*).

CLINICAL TIP

The transfer of green powder from the crown to the shoulder area of the prep visually indicates full seating (see Fig. 8-11*C*).

CLINICAL TIP

The Occlude may be easily removed from inside the crown using a steam machine. If this is not available, a cotton pledget dipped in alcohol and rubbed inside the crown will also suffice.

8. Verify radiographically.

Clean, careful preparations with accurate, complete impressioning (see Fig. 8-8*A*) coupled with careful and faithful die replication, margin delineation (see Fig. 8-9*A*), and precise laboratory steps, can yield impressive results both esthetically and radiographically (Figs. 8-11*G-I*).

The importance of careful and thorough fitting of the crowns as well as contact and occlusal adjustment is crucial. The dentist-technician working relationship must be cultivated, nourished, and developed for high quality restorative results to become routine.

Occlusal Adjustments

Once interproximal contacts and internal fit are satisfactory, make occlusal corrections.

Armamentarium
+ Standard dental setup (see the section on Tooth Preparation earlier in this chapter)
+ Two-color, double-sided articulating paper (Accufilm II, Parkell, Inc.)
+ Football-shaped diamond burs—e.g., Brasseler USA Fine 8369DF-31-025, and Extra-fine 369DEF-31-025 (Fig. 8-12).
+ Rubber wheels (e.g., Brasseler USA Dialite Lithium Disilicate (LD) Adjustment, Finishing and Polishing Kit) which includes:
  + LD11MLD.RA a medium grit grinder to adjust LD that creates much less heat than other instruments
  + W16MLD.RA Medium Point
  + W16FLD.RA Fine Point
  + W17MLD.RA Medium Cup
  + W17FLD.RA Fine Cup
+ 7-micron–thick *shimstock* metal foil (Almore Co.)
+ Hemostat

Clinical Technique. In the situation of simple restorative dentistry or "conformative dentistry" in which the position of maximum intercuspation irrespective of joint position is intended, the patient is asked to "close their teeth together," without guidance of the jaw closure or influencing the closure in any way. The inclines of opposing teeth guide the jaws to their most fully closed tooth-relation position.
1. With two-color, double-sided articulating paper held in place with a hemostat, have the patient gently "tap" the teeth into occlusion. (Note: If the restorations to be evaluated are in the maxillary arch, place the red side of the paper up and the black or darker color down to mark the opposing teeth in the mandible (Fig. 8-13*A*).
2. Remove the paper and note red marks on maxillary teeth (Fig. 8-13*B*) and black marks on mandibular teeth (Figure 8-13*C*).

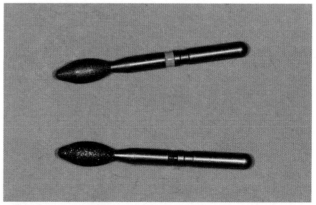

FIGURE 8-12 These fine and extra fine diamonds were developed by Brasseler USA specifically for occlusal adjustment of lithium disilicate restorations.

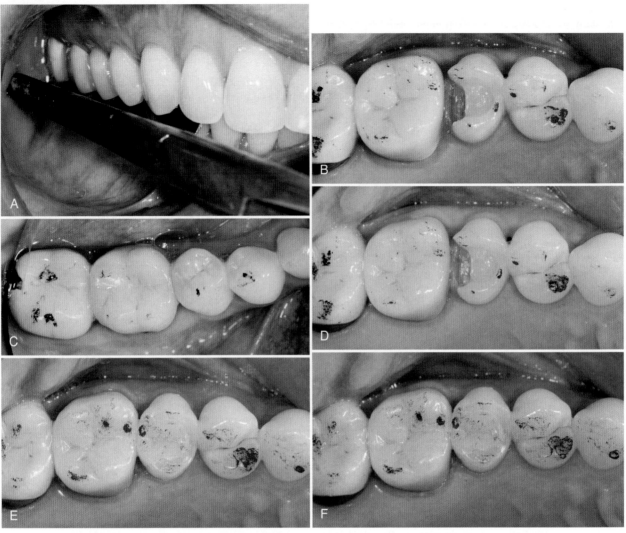

FIGURE 8-13 A, The patient in maximal intercuspal position. The red/black articulating ribbon is interposed between the closed teeth and held firmly with a hemostat. **B,** Red markings on the maxillary teeth of patient in Figure 8-55. **C,** Black marks on the mandibular teeth were made simultaneously and correspond to the red marks on the maxillary teeth in Figure 8-56. **D,** After again occluding, markings of the opposing teeth superimpose. After seating the restoration, the markings should be the same after the patient occludes again (Figure 8-57). **E,** After placement of the restoration, the procedure in Figure 8-54 is performed again marking the maxillary teeth in red and simultaneously marking the mandibular teeth in black. **F,** These black-on-red marks were made when the patient closed without the articulating paper in place allowing the black marks on the mandibular teeth to superimpose over the red marks of the maxillary teeth. Note that the new restoration makes contact on the distal marginal ridge at the same time as the other clearly demonstrated contacts in the arch (*black-on-red*) are made.

3. Again have the patient simply close his or her teeth together, this time without the articulating paper in place. This causes a superimposition of the opposing occlusal markings, black marks over red where true contact is made (Fig. 8-13D). It is very important to note that several marks will not superimpose. This is because these areas of the opposing teeth do not actually make contact, are therefore not interferences, and should not be adjusted. Only "true" contacting surfaces superimpose "black on red" and should be adjusted if they are interfering with the patient's ability to achieve maximum intercuspation.

> ### CLINICAL TIP
>
> Do not adjust non-superimposed marks (i.e., red only); these are erroneously caused by the thickness of the paper and do not represent true contacting surfaces.

> ### CLINICAL TIP
>
> Dry teeth surfaces with 2×2 gauze and apply a thin film of Vaseline to both sides of the articulating paper. This facilitates the transfer of the colorant to the dry tooth surface.

> ### CLINICAL TIP
>
> Make sure the red side of the articulating paper marks the arch where the restoration is being placed, with black facing the opposing teeth. Upon superimposition of the colors, "black-on-red" is easy to read. It is more difficult to read if done in reverse.

4. Adjust the restoration with fine diamonds and rubber wheels where necessary.
5. Confirm occlusal contact by having the patient close into the position of maximal intercuspation with a strip of *shimstock* foil held in place by a hemostat. With the patient's teeth held closed, the inability to remove the foil should prove contact is present. Check the teeth adjacent to the crown being placed in the same manner to verify that those teeth are not prevented from making full contact by a restoration nearby that may not yet be fully adjusted (see Fig. 8-13).
6. Once the position of maximum intercuspation has been achieved and confirmed, check for interferences in lateral excursions. Canine protected occlusion is usually most desirable when possible, because canines, through their anterior guidance, create "lift-off" in lateral excursions (freedom from contacts in excursive movements) avoiding the possibility of potentially harmful, off-axis deflective posterior tooth contacts. In the absence of anterior guidance, such as with an anterior open bite situation or Class III maxillomandibular relation, group function may be created by adjusting inclines of posterior teeth in excursions to create an even distribution of contacts and therefore forces, in lateral excursions.

Close visual inspection will reveal "true" contacts wherever black superimposes on the previously marked red areas. Where black did not superimpose over red marks indicate areas of false marking and are brought about by the thickness of the articulating paper. These marks should not be adjusted. Only the points of "black on red" are true contacts and may be adjusted if deemed necessary, or used as a visual confirmation that all the teeth in the quadrant are in occlusion, as in the example in Figure 8-13F. If a restoration is in hyperocclusion, or "too high," the only black-on-red mark in the quadrant would be on the restoration. No other black-on-red marks would be created upon closure with the articulating paper removed because true contacts would not be possible with an offending "high" point of contact present.

Physical confirmation may also be verified by holding a piece of *shimstock* (Almore, International, Inc.) in a hemostat and placing it between the teeth when the patient occludes. If there is resistance to removal of the foil, then there is certainty that tooth contact exists. In this way each tooth and its associated contact may be tested one at a time around the arch.

Color

The luting agent may have an effect on the final color and translucency of the restoration and this must be considered prior to permanent placement. Water-soluble try-in pastes are useful in this regard.

> ### CLINICAL TIP
>
> Place a drop of water into the fully fitted and adjusted e-Max crown or veneer to directly visualize its relative translucency. Water will act to "pull" the underlying substrate color through the restoration to simulate what a translucent luting agent (e.g., Variolink, Ivoclar Vivadent) might produce as a final outcome. More opacious cements like *glass ionomer* (GC Fuji Plus, GC America) can be previewed similarly before actual final cementation, to better predict the esthetic result and help avoid potentially irreversible decisions about final color.

However, restorations made of reinforced aluminous-oxide core designs tend to be less translucent. They often are "milky" and are relatively unaffected by the color of the luting agent selected.

The qualities that differentiate these materials may be used to advantage. For example, when using full coverage to restore a tooth for which the adjacent teeth to be "matched" have low value characteristics, e.Max (Ivoclar Vivadent) would probably produce the best results because of its inherent translucency, especially in the cervical third of the tooth. This is technically a difficult effect to create with materials that are inherently high value or bright. Similarly, zirconia-based crowns would probably best match teeth that are high in value, brighter, creamier, or more opacious, especially in the cervical third. Additionally, these materials can better mask unwanted underlying tooth influences, such as dark dentin or cast cores, than can the more translucent materials.

If color modifications beyond that which may be achieved through luting agents alone are necessary, these restorations may be stained, tinted, or characterized and refired in the ceramic oven to produce the best results. If acceptable "matches" cannot be achieved, a different choice of ingot may be indicated (e.g., one that is more translucent or one that is more opacious).

> ### CLINICAL TIP
>
> Compare the degree of brightness or translucency of the cervical third of the tooth to be restored with the adjacent teeth. This determination will help decide which restorative material will likely be the most esthetic choice. Low value, high translucency—consider lithium disilicate; high value, more opaque—consider zirconia.

LUTING

Low viscosity luting agents are the preferred materials to secure any of the aforementioned restorations. High-viscosity cements such as polycarboxylates are generally considered too thick and may create hydrostatic pressures, which could interfere with or prevent full seating of the restoration. Composite resin luting agents, such as Variolink (Ivoclar Vivadent), or resin-modified glass ionomer cements such as GC Fuji Plus (GC America) or RelyX (3M ESPE), may be used for permanent restoration placement. E.Max restorations permit light curing through the restoration; thus light-activated cements may be considered. These restorations may also be internally acid etched, which when combined with a total tooth-etching procedure and composite resin luting agent, is probably the most retentive system currently available. Resin-modified glass-ionomer cements may provide sufficient retention with less incidence of postoperative sensitivity.

"Previewing" the final restoration by inserting it with a retrievable temporary cement (i.e., Tempbond, Tempbond NE, Kerr Corp.), has many benefits including checking of interproximal contacts, checking comfort and precision of the occlusal scheme, evaluating restoration fit and tooth sensitivity, and verifying color and tooth arrangement. Nonetheless, modifications are still possible if deemed necessary before committing to permanent cement. Many times by going through this "trial" period of a few days to several weeks depending on the patient and the situation, costly remakes can be avoided. Furthermore, this additional care demonstrates to our patients that we are committed to their well-being and are interested in doing all that we can to deliver the best work that we are capable of.

> ### CLINICAL TIP
>
> Yellow pliers by GC America are well suited for provisionally cemented crown removal. Rinsing with warm water prior to removal helps soften the provisional cement, which makes removal much easier (Fig. 8-14).

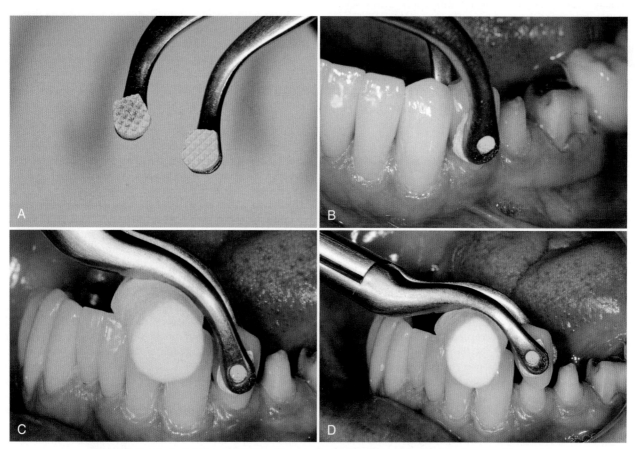

FIGURE 8-14 A, Friction is increased by coating the rubber replaceable grippers with emery powder. **B,** Placement of the grippers at or below the height of contour of the dry, provisionally cemented crown to be removed is the second step after warming the crown and its cement by having the patient rinse with hot water. **C,** Placing a cotton roll on the tooth anterior to the crown to be removed will protect the teeth and act as a fulcrum to facilitate a vertical path of removal. **D,** Keeping a firm grip with the pliers, pressing downward with a slight rotation, the softened provisional cement inside the crown will detach and permit the relatively easy removal of the crown.

It is important to emphasize that this procedure is made possible by the incredible crown strength of these restorations. In the past, a technique like the one described may have led to creation of cracks in the porcelain or worse, catastrophic crushing of the crown. It is also worth noting that eugenol-containing cements are contraindicated as a temporary cement if those restorations are planned for etching and bonding procedures, because that combination has been shown to decrease bond strengths.[43,44]

Zirconia crowns are not internally etchable. Additionally, sandblasting, which microscopically roughens the internal surface, is not recommended to maximize mechanical retention of these crowns because it has been shown that crack propagation begins at the internal surfaces of crowns that are sandblasted.[45] The decision whether or not to etch enamel and/or dentin for any of these crown systems is left to the practitioner.

CONCLUSION

As alternatives to conventional porcelain-fused-to-metal crowns, strong, well-fitting and lifelike all-ceramic materials continue to gain popularity. Dentists are increasingly confident choosing lithium disilicate (e.Max) for many of their anterior and posterior single unit needs, and monolithic zirconia for multiple unit posterior applications is gaining traction as well.

Presently there is no one restorative material choice suitable for all applications. A thorough working knowledge of these materials will allow the practitioner to fully benefit from current dental technology and ultimately achieve the finest results for our patients.

REFERENCES

1. Kregelstein, C, et al: Subjective Assessment of All-Ceramic Restorations, Presented at International Association for Dental Research Meeting, 2009.
2. McGehee WH, True HA, Inskipp EF: *A textbook of operative dentistry*, ed 3, New York, 1950, The Blakiston Divison, McGraw Hill.
3. IPS e.max System: Ivoclar Vivadent. http://www.ivoclarvivadent.us/emaxchanges everything. Accessed December 13, 2013.
4. Silva NR, Bonfante E, Rafferty BT, et al: Conventional and modified veneered zirconia vs. metal ceramic: fatigue and finite element analysis, *J Prosthodont* 21(6):433-439, 2012.
5. Culp L, McLaren EA: Lithium disilicate: the restorative material of multiple options, *Compend Contin Educ Dent* 31(9):716-725, 2010.
6. Silva NR, Thompson VP, Valverde GB, et al: Comparative reliability analyses of zirconium oxide and lithium disilicate restorations in vitro and in vivo, *J Amer Dent Assoc* 142(4 Suppl):4S-9S, 2011.
7. Kobler A, Schaller HG, Gernhardt CR: Effects of the desensitizing agents Gluma and Hyposen on the tensile bond strength of dentin adhesives, *Amer J Dent* 21(60):388-392, 2008.
8. Andersson M, Oden A: A new all-ceramic crown: a dense-sintered, high-purity alumina coping with porcelain, *Acta Odontol Scand* 51(1):59-64, 1993.
9. Zeng K, Oden A, Rowcliffe D: Flexural tests on dental ceramic, 434-439, 1996.
10. May KB, Russell MM, Razzoog ME, Lang BR: Precision of fit: the Procera AllCeram crown, *J Prosthet Dent* 80(4):394-404, 1998.
11. White S, Caputo A, Chun Li Z, Yu Zhao X: Modulus of rupture of the Procera All-ceramic system, *J Esthet Dent* 8(3):120-126, 1996.
12. Wagner WC, Chu TM: Biaxial flexural strength and indentation fracture toughness of three new dental core ceramics, *J Prosthet Dent* 76(2):140-144, 1996.
13. May KB, Razzoog M, Lang BR, Wang R: Marginal fit: the Procera all-ceramic crown, abstract 2379, *Inter Assoc Dent Res ADR* 1997.
14. Prestipino V, Ingber A, Kravitz J: Clinical and laboratory considerations in the use of a new all-ceramic restorative system, *Pract Periodontics Aesthet Dent* 10:567, 1998.
15. Sadan A, Hegenbarth EA: A simplified and practical method for optimizing aesthetic results utilizing a new high strength all-ceramic system, *Pract Periodontics Aesthet Dent* 10(suppl):4, 1998.
16. Guess PC, Kulis A, Witkowski S, Wolkewitz M, Zhang Y, Strub JR: Shear bond strengths between different zirconia cores and veneering ceramics and their susceptibility to thermocycling, *Dent Materials* 24(11):1556-1557, 2008.
17. Moving to monolithic: New price-competitive materials and techniques give laboratories affordable and automated CAM solutions, *Inside Dent technology* 2(1):70-71, 2011.
18. McLean JW: *The science and art of dental ceramics*, vol 2, Chicago, 1980, Quintessence Publishing.
19. Geller W, Kwiatkowski S: The Willi's glas crown: a new solution in the dark and shadowed zones of esthetic porcelain restorations, *Quintessence Dent Technol* 11:233, 1987.
20. Spyropoulou PE, Giroux EC, Razzoog ME, Duff RE: Translucency of shaded zirconia core material, *J Prosthet Dent* 105(5):304-307, 2011.
21. Dogen S et al: Translucency measurement of zirconia and lithium-disilicate using densitometry and spectrophotometry, *IADR abstract*, 2011.
22. Baldissara P, Llukacej A, Ciocca L, Valandro FL, Scotti R: Translucency of zirconia copings made with different CAD/CAM systems, *J Prosthet Dent* 104(1):6-12, 2010.
23. Moeller M, Razzoog ME, Duff RE: Translucency of Procera zirconia and alumina core materials, *IADR abstract*, April 1-4, 2009.
24. Flores-de Jacoby L, Zafiropoulos GG, Ciancio S: Effect of crown margin location on plaque and periodontal health, *Int J Periodontics Restorative Dent* 9:197, 1989.
25. Bremer F, Grade S, Kohorst P, Stiesch M: In vivo biofilm formation on different dental ceramics, *Quintessence Int* 42(7):565-574, 2011.
26. Busscher HJ, Rinastiti M, Siswomihardjo W, van der Mei HC: Biofilm formation on dental restorative and implant materials, *J Dent Res* 89(7):657-665, 2010.
27. Kosyfaki P, del Pilar Pinilla Mart√≠n M, Strub JR: Relationship between crowns and the periodontium: a literature update, *Quintessence Int* 41(2):109-126, 2010.
28. Nevins M: Interproximal periodontal disease—the embrasure as an etiological factor, *Int J Periodontics Restorative Dent* 2:9, 1982.
29. Ingber JS, Rose LF, Coslet JG: The "biologic width"—a concept in periodontics and restorative dentistry, *Alpha Omegan* 70(3):62-65, 1977.
30. Kramer GM: A consideration of root proximity, *Int J Periodontics Restorative Dent* 6:9, 1987.
31. Kramer GM: Rationale of periodontal therapy. In Goldman HM, Cohen DW, editors: *Periodontal therapy*, ed 6, St Louis, 1980, Mosby.
32. Gargiulo AW, Wentz FM, Orban B: Dimensions and relations of the dentogingival junction in humans, *J Periodont* 32:261, 1961.
33. Nevins M, Skurow HM: The intracrevicular restorative margin, the biologic width, and the maintenance of the gingival margin, *Int J Periodont Restor Dent* 4:30, 1984.
34. Malament KA, Socransky SS: Survival of Dicor glass-ceramic dental restorations over 14 years, Part I. Survival of Dicor full coverage restorations and effect of internal acid-etching, tooth position, gender, and age, *J Pros Dent* 81(1):23-32, 1999.
35. Rekow ED, Silva NR, Coelho PG, et al: Performance of dental ceramics, *J Dent Res* 90(8):937-952, 2011.
36. Guess PC, Zavanelli RA, Silva NR, et al: Monolithic CAD/CAM lithium disilicate versus veneer Y-TZP crowns: comparison of failure modes and reliability after fatigue, *Int J Prosthodont* 23:434-442, 2010.
37. Ingber JS: Forced eruption: Part II. A method of treating non-restorable teeth—periodontal and restorative implications, *J Periodontal* 47(4):203-216, 1976.
38. Pontoriero R, Celenza F Jr, Ricci G, Carnevale G: Rapid extrusion with fiber resection: a combined orthodontic-periodontic treatment modality, *Int J Periodontics Restorative Dent* 7:30–43, 1987.
39. Wagenburg BD, Eskow RN, Langer B: Exposing adequate tooth structure for restorative dentistry, *Int J Periodontics Restorative Dent* 9:323, 1989.
40. Skurow HM, Nevins M: The rationale of the periodontal provisional biologic trial restoration, *Int J Periodontics Restorative Dent* 8:1, 1988.
41. Reider CE: Use of provisional restorations to develop and achieve esthetic expectations, *Int J Perio Rest Dent* 9:2, 1989.
42. Shavell HM: Mastering the art of tissue management during provisionalization and biologic final impressions, *Int J Periodontics Restorative Dent* 3:25, 1988.
43. Peutzfeldt A, Asmussen E: Influence of eugenol-containing temporary cement on bonding of self-etching adhesives to dentin, *J Adhesive Dent* 8(1):31-34, 2006.
44. Meyerowitz JM, Rosen M, Cohen J, Becker PJ: The effect of eugenol containing and non-eugenol temporary cements on the resin-enamel bond, *J Dent Assoc S Africa* 49(8):389-392, 1994.
45. Chintapalli RK, Marro FG, Jimenez-Pique E, Anglada M: Phase transformation and subsurface damage in 3Y-TZP after sandblasting, *Dent Mater* 29(5):566-572, 2013.

9

Ceramometal Full Coverage Restorations

Ira D. Zinner, Richard D. Miller, Stanley Markovits, Mitchell S. Pines, Yale E. Schnader, Patrick E. Reid, Paul Federico, William Baum

To the patient, cosmetic considerations in anterior fixed prosthodontics are as important, if not more important, than the functional aspects. The finest fitting restoration with exquisite porcelain carvings can meet with total patient dissatisfaction if it does not conform to the expected esthetic results. The esthetic goals of both doctor and patient have never been greater than they are today. This has fueled a search for new materials and methods to fulfill the desires of the dental team. The veneering materials with the highest esthetic value are the weakest components of restorations and require support from the core material. Core materials, be they metal, zirconia, or lithium disilicate, are the least esthetic components of the restoration. This chapter only deals with metal as the core material. Minimizing the amount of core material used would seem to minimize the problem. A thin 1.5 mm to 2 mm layer of veneering ceramic over a well-designed core is sufficient to create a life-like restoration. The use of a silhouette coping, one mimicking the profile of the prepared tooth, does not provide optimum support for the veneering ceramics. A coping should be designed to create an even layer of ceramics over a convex surface that is well rounded and void of any sharp angles. This core design presents the ceramist with many challenges. The core material must allow no more than 2 mm of porcelain on the occlusal surface: therefore the articulation must be precise. The core must be veneered to allow optimal light transmission while concurrently blocking visualization of the core.

BASIC CHEMISTRY

The basic chemical components of ceramometal porcelains are potassium-sodium aluminosilicate glasses (Table 9-1). Combinations of metallic and nonmetallic oxides are added as opacifiers (Table 9-2).

The conventional all-ceramic and acrylic resin full and partial coverage restorations, although esthetically pleasing, may fail under heavy occlusal stress because of low tensile and shear strengths.[1] Newer porcelain materials are stronger but still cannot be used to create multiple-unit fixed prostheses.[2] Full cast restorations offer sufficient strength but lack the esthetic appearance required in today's society. Ceramometal dental restorations, however, offer both strength and acceptable appearance.[3]

The strength of the porcelain-to-metal bond is close to the tensile strength of the opaquing porcelain. Fracture usually occurs within the body of the porcelain. If this is not the case, an error in fabrication technique usually is to blame.[1,4,5] Ceramic and metal alloys must have properties that allow for both physical and chemical compatibility. The fusion temperature of the ceramic (usually lower than 100° C)[1] is lower than the metal casting temperature, which prevents the cast metal substructure from melting during porcelain application.[3] Ceramometal porcelains contain more soda and potash than typical all-ceramic blends; this increases thermal expansion to a level compatible with the metal alloy (the coefficient levels of thermal expansion for several porcelains are presented in Table 9-3). The coefficient of thermal expansion of the ceramic is 13 to 14 $\times$ 10^{-6}/°C. This should be approximately 0.5 to 1 $\times$ 10^{-6}/°C less than the coefficient of thermal expansion of the casting alloy, which places the brittle ceramic into slight compression at the ceramometal interface when it cools. Ceramic is much stronger under compression than under tension.[3] In addition, because it is brittle and tends to form minor stress-concentrating defects, the ceramic is much stronger when applied to a rigid metal framework. This framework, upon wetting with porcelain, reduces the internal ceramic defects and supports the brittle porcelain, thus adding strength to the restoration.[1] Conversely, the metal of a knife-edged finishing line or a bevel contains insufficient bulk to resist small

Table 9-1 **Ingredients Of Dental Porcelains**

Ingredient	Dental Porcelain (Weight %)	Decorative Porcelain (Weight %)
Feldspar	81	15
T body 1Quartz	15	14
Kaolin	4	70
Metallic Pigment	<1	1

Data from Craig RG, editor: Restorative dental materials, ed 9, St Louis, 1985, Mosby.

deflections during seating. Porcelain should not be applied to these thin margins because if resistance to seating is encountered, flexing of the metal can cause the porcelain to flake off.[4]

Opaque porcelains, which mask the metal coping, contain metallic oxide opacifiers. New opaque porcelains can be used effectively in layers as thin as 100 μm. However, this opaque porcelain must be covered by at least 1 mm of body porcelain to mask its reflectiveness.

Vitrification in ceramic restorations refers to a liquid phase caused by reaction or melting which, on cooling, forms a glassy phase. If this formation is disturbed by the addition of too much modifying oxide, devitrification (crystallization) can occur.[4] The ceramic porcelains are sensitive to devitrification because of their alkali content, which can cause clouding with additional porcelain firings. Repeated firing of high-expansion ceramometal

porcelains at maturing temperature increases the likelihood of devitrification.[4]

Traditional dental ceramometal porcelains were formulated as a compromise between optimum properties and metal compatibility. The coefficient of thermal expansion of the porcelain had to be raised to approximate that of the ceramometal alloy. The ceramic metal had to be alloyed to cast at a higher temperature than conventional gold-copper alloys so that it could withstand the higher porcelain firing temperatures and reduced thermal expansion to meet that of the porcelain. Current ceramometal alloys have had their coefficient of thermal expansion adjusted to be compatible with conventional ceramometal porcelains (see Table 9-3).

CERAMOMETAL ALLOYS

Ceramometal alloys must have a high modulus of elasticity to prevent deflection (are rigid) which could result in loss of portions of the porcelain veneer. Although the modulus of elasticity of commercial ceramometal alloys vary, they are clinically acceptable at a minimum thickness of one-half millimeter. Use of copings thinner than one-half millimeter risks perforation when fitting the restoration.

Ceramometal alloys should not melt during porcelain application or exhibit creep at high temperatures. (Creep is a strain that results in deformation or flow of the material over time when subjected to a constant stress). The most important aspect of the alloy chosen is that it must not distort, melt or exhibit creep with the high temperatures needed for its fusion with porcelain. That is, it must fit the tooth accurately after the porcelain is added.

Table 9-2 **Composition of Dental Ceramics for Fusing to High-Temperature Alloys**

Compound	Biodent Opaque BG 2 (%)	Ceramco Opaque 60 (%)	V.M.K. Opaque 121 (%)	Biodent Dentin BD 27 (%)	Ceramco Dentin T 69 (%)
SiO_2	52.00	55.00	52.40	56.90	62.20
Al_2O_3	13.55	11.65	15.15	11.80	13.40
CaO	–	–	–	00.61	00.98
K_2O	11.05	09.60	09.90	10.00	11.30
Na_2O	05.28	04.75	06.58	05.42	05.37
TiO_2	03.01	03.01	02.59	00.61	
$7rO_2$	03.22	00.16	05.16	01.46	00.34
SnO_2	06.40	06.40	15.00	04.90	00.50
Rb_2O	00.09	00.04	00.08	00.10	00.06
BaO	01.09	01.09	–	03.52	–
ZnO	–	00.26	–	–	–
UO_3	–	–	–	–	–
B_2O_3, CO_2, and H_2O	04.31	03.54	03.24	09.58	05.85

Data from Nally JN, Meyer JM: Recherche Experimentale sur la Nature de la Liaison Ceramo-Metallique, Schweiz Monatsschr Zahnheilkd 80:250-277, 1970.

Table 9-3 Porcelain Coefficient of Thermal Expansion

Low Coefficient
Ceramco
Denpac
Vita
Excelco
Medium Coefficient
Pencraft
Duceram
Synspak
High Coefficient
Biobond
Williams
Crystar

CLINICAL TIP

A thin marginal apron may distort during porcelain application and result in an inaccurate fit. To avoid this, copings should be waxed with thick margins, and then thinned (after porcelain application) during final finishing. The metal apron on an 80-degree bevel should not be covered with porcelain since it may fracture. Only a 45-degree facial bevel may be covered with opaque and porcelain and will not fracture.

When a ceramometal alloy is heated during porcelain firing, its modulus of elasticity must be high (rigid) enough to resist metal deformation. However, as the restoration cools, the alloy should be able to deform a small amount to relieve the stress produced by the thermal contraction of the porcelain. If the modulus of elasticity of the alloy is too high, it will be ungiving and be unable to relieve this stress. Thus, the stress remains in the porcelain and may lead to crazing.[3]

Creep is seen in metals at temperatures close to their melting point. It can be controlled by avoiding extremely long firing cycles. Creep is a time-dependent strain that occurs under stress and results in deformation or flow of the material.[6] It is shown by a material that continues to deform even though the stress on it remains the same. High-temperature creep is flow that occurs at elevated temperatures. For gold alloys, high-temperature creep occurs at about 1800° F. It can be reduced by varying alloy composition so that a dispersion strengthening effect occurs at the high temperature.[1,7,8]

All intraoral restorative metals, including ceramometal alloys should be resistant to tarnish and corrosion in the mouth.[3]

Classification of Ceramometal Alloys

The two basic types of ceramometal alloys are the precious alloys and the base metal alloys.

Precious Alloys. Because original ceramometal restorations contained high proportions of noble metal, their clinical characteristics are well documented; they show good resistance to oxidation, tarnish, and corrosion.[4] The noble metals are gold, platinum, palladium, iridium, rhodium, osmium, and ruthenium. Their physical properties are all similar, although the nongold noble alloys require a modified investment to withstand the higher casting temperatures. Ceramic alloys are very hard and strong compared with ADA Type I, Type II, and Type III gold; they are similar to Type IV gold. The coefficient of thermal expansion of ceramic alloys is less than that of any of the four types of gold. The noble metals and silver are often referred to as precious metals. Typical ceramometal alloy characteristics are presented in Table 9-3.[2]

Base Metal Alloys. Base metal alloys consist of nickel, chromium, molybdenum, cobalt, and beryllium. They can be used to obtain satisfactory fit, but laboratory procedures for base metals are much more technique sensitive than those for the noble alloys. High casting shrinkage of the base metal alloys necessitates special investments and casting methods. When nickel-based alloys are subjected to heat treatment during the porcelain firing cycles, the strength and hardness of the alloy diminishes. The base metal alloys' oxide thickness is more difficult to control, which creates problems with additional porcelain firings.[4]

Dental ceramometal restorative alloys may be further classified by their major constituents and the chronology of their development (Tables 9-4 and 9-5).[2]

Group 1: Gold Noble

Composition
1. 96% to 98% noble metal
   a. 84% to 86% gold
   b. 4% to 10% platinum
   c. 5% to 7% palladium
2. 2% to 3% base metal

Properties. Gold noble alloys, which were developed in the 1950s, are weaker and have less sag resistance (the property of a ceramometal alloy to resist flow under its own weight during soldering and porcelain application)[3] than the more recently developed ceramometal alloys. Gold noble alloys are the easiest to cast and solder and have a yellow color that aids in obtaining the lighter tooth color shades. These alloys are the most costly because of their high noble metal content. The Group 1 alloys were developed by both J.F. Jelenko and Co. and J. Aderer, Inc.[2]

Group 2: White Noble

Composition
1. 80% noble metal
   a. 51% to 54% gold
   b. 0% platinum
   c. 26% to 31% palladium
2. 14% to 16% silver

Properties. Platinum, the most costly metal, was eliminated in the Group 2 alloys. The gold content was reduced and the palladium portion increased. The overall noble metal proportion was reduced by adding silver. These alloys have improved mechanical properties with higher strength and greater sag resistance. They are easy to fabricate and are less costly than Group 1 alloys. However, the silver may cause some porcelain greening, and the gray color of the alloy makes it harder to obtain

Table 9-4 **Ceramometal Alloys**

Group	% Noble Metal	Contains Silver (Greening)	Technique Sensitivity	Porcelain Type (Coefficient of Thermal Expansion)	Color	Minimum Thickness (mm)
1	96-98	No	Low	Conventional	Yellow	.5
2	80	Yes	Low	Conventional	White	.5
3	53-60	Yes	Medium	High	White	.5
4	90	No	Low	Low or Conventional	White	.5
5	0	No	High	Conventional	White	.4
6	0	No	Medium to High	Conventional	White	.5
7	78-88	Some contain Ag	Medium	Conventional	White	.5
8	0	No	High	Very Low?	White	?
9	84-92	Some contain Ag	Low	Very High, Low Fusing	Yellow	.5

lighter tooth color shades.[2] The Group 2 alloys were developed by Joseph Tuccillo in 1976 at J.F. Jelenko and Co.[9]

Group 3: Palladium-Silver Alloys

Composition

1. 53% to 60% noble metal
   a. 0% gold
   b. 0% platinum
   c. 53% to 60% palladium
2. 30% to 37% silver
3. 10% base metals

Properties. These alloys contain palladium, silver, and a small amount of base metals. They are easy to cast and solder, have acceptable mechanical properties, and are the least expensive of the noble alloys. Previously, the coefficient of thermal expansion of palladium-silver alloys was higher than that of gold alloys, necessitating the use of porcelains with a correspondingly higher coefficient of shrinkage. Current alloys have a lower coefficient which is compatible with conventional ceramometal porcelains. The silver content may cause greening of the porcelain, requiring judicious use of metal conditioners.[2] Metal conditioner is an opaque porcelain with a high concentration of pink pigment that is used to negate the green discoloration of the porcelain caused by the silver content. These alloys can absorb gases in their liquid state and then release the gases during solidification, which may cause bubbles to form in the porcelain during its application.[10] Palladium alloys are prone to carbon contamination, which affects the porcelain-to-metal bond; therefore carbon blocks and graphite crucibles must not be used with these materials. Absorbed gases can also be minimized by not overheating the alloy and not holding the molten metal for long periods before casting. The Group 3 alloys were developed by Clyde Ingersoll of Williams Gold Inc., in 1975.[11]

Group 4: Gold-Palladium Alloys

Composition

1. 90% noble metals
   a. 45% to 52% gold
   b. 38% to 45% palladium

2. 0% silver
3. 10% base metals

Properties. Both silver and platinum were eliminated from Group 4 alloys. The mechanical properties (e.g., modulus of elasticity, yield strength), the ease of fabrication, and the dimensional accuracy make these the most promising of all the noble alloys. They originally had a lower coefficient of thermal expansion than Group 1, 2, or 3 alloys, making them compatible only with lower shrinkage porcelains. The Group 4 gold-palladium alloys were developed by Paul Cascone at J.F. Jelenko and Co. in 1978.[12] In 1985, the alloy was improved[12] by increasing the coefficient of thermal expansion, making it more compatible with conventional porcelains. These alloys are white gold in color.

Group 5: Nickel-Chromium Alloys

Composition

1. 0% noble metal
2. 100% base metal
   a. 60% to 82% nickel
   b. 11% to 20% chromium
   c. 2% to 9% molybdenum
   d. 0% to 2% beryllium

Properties. The use of nickel-based alloys was explored in the 1950s, but lack of a suitable investment and technique delayed their successful development. Advancements in casting investments and the soaring gold prices of the 1970s spurred the acceptance of nickel alloys. These alloys are comprised of nickel, chromium, molybdenum, and beryllium. The beryllium-containing alloys, in general, cast better and have a greater porcelain-to-metal bond strength than the non–beryllium-containing alloys. This accounts for the great degree of difference in mechanical properties in this group. These alloys are the hardest alloy group, have a very high modulus of elasticity, and have a higher melting temperature than the other alloy groups. The presence of nickel introduces the possibility of nickel hypersensitivity in allergic patients, and the small amount of beryllium adds the hazard of beryllium toxicity in the dental laboratory if proper ventilation is not established. Laboratory procedures are

Table 9-5 Properties of Ceramometal Alloys(F)

Group	Type	Example	Au (%)	Pt (%)	Pd (%)	Ag (%)	Cr (%)	Ni (%)	Co (%)	Be (%)	Ti (%)	Proprietary Metals
1	Gold noble	Jelenko *	88	5	6							0
		Degudent †	78	10	9							2
		Rx CG *	87	7	5							
		Bio 86 ‡	86	11								0
												3
2	White noble	Cameo *	53		27	16						4
		Ceramco White	51		31	15						3
		RxWCG ‡	52		30	14						
												4
3	Palladium silver	JeIstar *			60	28						12
		Degustar			52	38						10
		Rx Palladent B*			60	28						
												12
4	Gold palladium	Olympia *	52		39							9
		Deva M †	47		45							8
		RxSF 45	45		45							
												10
5	Nickel chromium	Rexillium ‡						75	14	2		9
6	Cobalt	Genesis					27		53			20
		Nouarex ‡					25		55			20
7	High palladium	Legacy *	2		85							12
		Deguplus 2	1		80							18
		Aspen ‡	6		75	7						
												11
8	Titanium	R/1 ‡									100	Slight
		R/2 ‡									90	10
9	Ceramic Type IV Gold	Bio 75G ‡	75	9								16
		Degunorrn †	73.8	9		9.2						
												8

(S) = Soft, (H) = Hard, (F) = Hardness after firing. Values are rounded to nearest whole number. Data supplied by manufacturers.
*Manufactured by J.F. Jelenko and Co.
†Manufactured by Degussa Dental, Inc.
‡Manufactured by Jeneric/Penton, Inc.

Melting Range (EF)	Casting Temperature (EF)	Vickers Hardness	Yield Strength (psi)	Elongation (%)	Coefficient of Thermal Expansion	Density (gm/cm*)
2100-2150	2300	182	65,300	5	14.7	19.2
2100-2300	2550	200	68,150(5)	7(S)		18
			84,100(H)	3(H)		
2100-2150	2300	165	40,000	5		18.5
1870-2030		190(S)	74800(S)	9(S)	14.5	18.9
		215(H)	84500(H)	7.5(H)		
2200-2300	2400	220	80,000	10	14.7	16.7
2300-2345	2550	130(0)	30,450(0)	35(S)		14.5
		220(H)	61,630(H)	10(H)		
		220(F)				
2200-2300	2400	220	80,000	10		13.8
2250-2380	2500	189	67,000	20	14.8	10.7
2100-2250	2550	200(S)	56,550(S)	25(S)		11.2
		250(H)	81,200(H)	10(H)		
		220(F)				
2200-2275	2500	165	0	10		10.5
2320.2380	2450	220	83,000	20	14.1	13.5
2230-2390	2550	185(S)	53,650(S)	31(S)		14.4
		275(H)	94,250(H)	10(H)		
		260(F)				
2200-2300	2550	250	80,000	10	14.6	13.5
2250-2350	2500	240	74,000	9-12		7.8
2415-2550	2600	350	61,000	9	14.6	8.8
2425-2475	2675	260	90,000	7		8.8
2020-2360	2450	270	95,500	20	14.2	11
2110-2355		260(F)	83.380(S)	30(S)		11.5
		260(F)	83,350(H)	30(H)		
		260(F)				
2115-2275		250	80,000	21		11
3035		175	50025	15	9.85	4.51
2800-3000		330	129920	9	10.22	4.51
1841-1967	2192-2237	125(S)	40029(S)	22(S)	16.6	16.7
		200(H)	63089(H)	14(H)		
1650-1815	2010	230(C)	49300(S)	14(S)	16.4	16.7
		150(S)	72500(H)	6(H)		
		200(H)				

extremely technique sensitive.[2] These alloys produce suitable restorations when nickel hypersensitivity is not a problem and when a low-cost alloy is desired. The dental laboratory should be knowledgeable about the proper handling of these alloys.

Group 6: Cobalt-Based Alloys

Composition
1. 0% noble metal
2. 100% base metal
   a. 55% to 64% cobalt
   b. 25% to 34% chromium
   c. 2% to 9% molybdenum

Properties. In general, the castability, solderability, and porcelain-to-metal bond strength of the cobalt-based alloys are not as good as those of the nickel-based, beryllium containing alloys. Cobalt-based alloys are harder and more technique sensitive than Group 5 alloys.[2]

Group 7: High-Palladium Alloys

Composition
1. 78% to 88% noble metal
   a. 76% to 88% palladium
   b. 0% to 2% gold
2. 0% to 1 % silver
3. 12% to 22% base metal

Properties. The high-palladium alloys are extremely hard and have very high yield strength. They do not cast as well as the gold alloys and are more technique sensitive in laboratory fabrication. These alloys are compatible with most conventional porcelain systems.

BASIC CONSIDERATION IN FULL COVERAGE PREPARATIONS

Diagnostic Phase

Prior to initiating any tooth preparation, the restorative dentist should thoroughly discuss and understand the patient's expectations and cosmetic desires. A thorough history, as well as the patient's attitude toward prior treating clinicians, should be recorded. In addition, a full series radiographic examination should be obtained, using appropriate instrumentation. Ideally, two sets of diagnostic casts should be made: One set should be mounted on a semiadjustable articulator using verified intraoral records and the second set should be used for a diagnostic wax-up to demonstrate to the patient the desired esthetic results. If the patient's expectations are unrealistic or if the patient's opinion differs from that of the dentist, the dentist should be able to advise the patient and explain the limitations in terms of the cosmetic result. If the patient cannot accept the result set forth by the dentist, then no further dentistry should be pursued with this patient (see Chapters 27 and 28)

Photography. Close-up extraoral and intraoral photographs (see Chapter 22) should be taken prior to any dental treatment as part of the patient's record. These photos are first employed during case presentation between the patient and the clinician. They may be used to aid communication between the dentist and laboratory technician. Photographs should also be taken following completion of treatment and maintained as part of the patient's record (see Chapter 27).

Diagnostic Casts. Prior to tooth preparations, an irreversible hydrocolloid impression should be made of both dental arches and mounted on a semiadjustable articulator. If changes are required for cosmetic purposes, an additional diagnostic cast is altered with white carving wax to create the desired effect. If soft tissue modifications are anticipated, these changes should be included on the cast using pink base plate wax. The completed diagnostic wax-up of the desired soft and hard tissue changes may then be used by the treating clinician as a guide for treatment planning and case presentation.

Periodontal Considerations

The presence of unesthetic, pathologic, periodontal structures precludes a cosmetic result. Thus, prior to performing any fixed prosthodontic procedures, all periodontal tissues should be in a state of optimum health and be able to be maintained in that condition by the patient.

Inflammation may be caused by temporary cement or impression material that remains in the gingival sulcus area or by placement of less than optimal provisional restorations.

Provisional Restorations

Provisional restorations are a critical part of restorative dental procedures (see Chapter 10). They must be carefully fit to the prepared tooth or teeth, accurately occlude the opposing arch, properly contact the adjacent teeth, and have finished marginal areas that will not irritate gingival tissue. Unfortunately, many clinicians feel that these "temporaries" are unimportant and need not be precisely fabricated. This will ultimately result in an unnecessary expenditure of time correcting subsequent failures associated with these restorations. These often include recementation appointments and cosmetic remakes due to tissue migration. Corrections should be made prior to proceeding with construction of the definitive prostheses. There should be stability after placement of the provisional prostheses in terms of tooth shade, contour, occlusion, and esthetics. Ideally, especially in more complex multiunit restorations, prior to any tooth preparation, a set of diagnostic casts should be mounted on an articulator. The clinician should determine a shade and then fabricate a silicone index of the unprepared teeth. The designated teeth are prepared on the cast and the dental laboratory technician processes a heat-polymerized acrylic resin provisional prosthesis. Following intraoral tooth preparation or preparations, the processed provisional prosthesis is fitted and then relined intraorally with an appropriate auto-polymerizing acrylic resin. It is removed, carved, polished and checked intraorally. The provisional prosthesis should be cemented with non-eugenol temporary cement.

> ### CLINICAL TIP
>
> Eugenol-based cement will soften the resin and make it more difficult for the practitioner to add additional resin.

Long-term provisional prostheses should be metal supported to prevent the necessity of repeated repairs.

The carved provisional prosthesis should simulate the desired definitive prosthesis, both in shade and in contours. Any alterations needed should be made on the provisional prosthesis prior to fabrication of the definitive restoration.

More than one set of provisional prostheses may be needed due to subsequent alterations for creation of the desired cosmetic effect. Once this is achieved, then the provisional prosthesis is a template, or a guide, for the shade, contours, occlusion, and incisal guidance of the definitive prosthesis.

Tooth reduction, especially the area of the anterior teeth influencing incisal guidance, is verified with the provisional prosthesis. If, when wearing and functioning with this prosthesis, the area incisal to the cingulum becomes thin or perforated, then this area of the tooth must be re-prepared prior to impression taking. If the tooth preparation is altered, the provisional prosthesis is relined with the appropriate autopolymerizing acrylic resin of the selected shade.

The marginal termination of the provisional fixed prosthesis ends at the apical extent of the preparation. Underextension may results in tooth sensitivity, possible pulpal damage, and the growth of the gingival tissues over the shoulder of the preparation. Overextension may cause periodontal problems, gingival recession, and a compromised esthetic result.

Tooth Reduction

The laboratory technician must be provided sufficient room for both metal and porcelain, even if intentional prophylactic endodontic treatment is necessary. Opaquing porcelain need only be 100 microns thick, but unless it is covered by an optimum thickness of surface porcelain, the definitive restoration will appear flat and unlifelike[13] or artificial. Insufficient tooth reduction forces the laboratory technician to create either an overcontoured, periodontally unacceptable restoration or a properly contoured, unesthetically opaque restoration.[14] In either case, under-reduction in the gingival third precludes creation of a straight emergence profile that is necessary to ensure gingival health.[15,16]

Overreduction is also undesirable because it can lead to insufficient retention and resistance form as well as an increased risk of pulpal involvement. In addition, if porcelain is thicker than 1.5 mm because of inadequate tooth structure or insufficient metal buildup, the risk of porcelain fracture is increased.

Laboratory Considerations. A team approach should be employed both in conventional as well as implant-supported rehabilitations. The restorative dentist must be able to communicate and work with the dental technician as a team member. The team approach begins at the diagnostic and treatment planning phase and continues through the completion of treatment. In order to achieve maximum results, both functionally and cosmetically, the technician and the clinician should understand what the desired end result should be. The team should also understand what the patient's desires and goals are. It should be determined prior to any dental treatment

if the patient's goals are achievable and reasonable. Is the patient compliant and rational or is there an antagonistic attitude toward dentists and dentistry or unrealistic expectations? In addition, if alterations of the prosthesis or postinsertion repairs or corrections are needed, the technician who created the prosthesis should be the person to perform the technical work. The clinician should know the quality, exact brand, and manufacturer of all the materials used in the fabrication of the prosthesis. Precise communication between the laboratory and clinician is mandatory. The dentist should record the technical aspects of prosthesis in the patient's treatment record. If a dentist other than the one involved with fabrication of the prosthesis assumes the dental care of a patient, it is particularly advantageous if the original dentist can provide complete information about the prosthesis. Any necessary repairs can then be accomplished with a greater degree of success if this information is available.

Impression Procedures

Two types of impression materials are recommended for fixed prosthodontics: reversible hydrocolloid and elastomeric materials such as polyether and the polyvinyl siloxane.

These materials require the clinician to work in a clean, periodontally healthy field. Periodontal problems should be treated prior to any tooth preparations. If full coverage restorations are fabricated and inserted in the presence of soft tissue pathology, facial gingival recession may occur after treatment of the inflammation. Complete healing of the gingival treatment area must occur before finalizing tooth preparation. This will lessen the chance of soft tissue shrinkage and an obvious exposed margin. Preparations should terminate at or about 0.5 mm below the gingival margin. All preparations should be cut as an ideal full shoulder preparation with a one millimeter bevel. Any deviation from the ideal is created after the dentist cuts an ideal preparation. The bevel is the only part of the preparation that may extend subgingivally. When a restoration margin will be visible during function, a 45-degree facial bevel is employed rather than a facial butt joint, because there is a common termination of metal, opaque, and porcelain. This bevel also permits the clinician to secure a closing angle at the margin to reduce recurrent caries. Thus no metal color will show facially. Bevels are created with a 12 fluted blunted plug finishing bur, not with diamond rotary instrumentation, Retraction cord is not used to retract soft tissues, but to maintain the sulcus created with the beveling instrument. Only number 1 or number 2 cord is necessary to maintain the sulcular space for impression materials (Fig. 9-1).

All impressions should be full arch impressions and the opposing cast made from an irreversible hydrocolloid impression. All dies should be trimmed by the dentist, not the technician. If the technician trims the dies, errors in margin termination may occur.

After the die cast is poured and prior to separating and trimming dies, the cast should be mounted in an "indexed" mounting system such as Accu-Trac or Pindex systems (Coltene/Whaledent, Inc.) or EZ Di-Lok system (Di-Equi Dental Products).

Preparations

There are four types of finishing lines used for full coverage porcelain fused to metal restorations
1. Knife-edged finishing line (Fig. 9-2A)
2. Chamfer preparation (Fig. 9-2B)

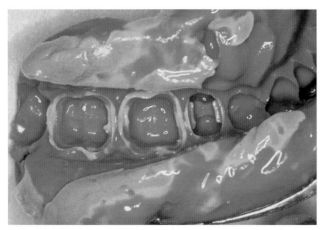

FIGURE 9-1 To obtain adequate impressions of the gingival margin, a No. 1 or No. 2 retraction cord is necessary to maintain the sulcular space.

3. Full shoulder preparation (Fig. 9-2C)
4. Full shoulder with a bevel preparation (Fig. 9-2D)
5. Full shoulder with a three quarter bevel modified with a facial butt joint preparation for esthetics

Knife-Edged Finishing Line.   The knife-edged preparation is a tapered preparation that has maximum tooth reduction at the occlusal or incisal portion and tapers to zero cutting at the gingival termination. This type of preparation is usually used after periodontal surgery. In this situation the gingival margin is usually on root surface. First an ideal full shoulder preparation is made at the cervical area of the tooth to ensure that sufficient tooth structure is removed. Then additional tooth structure is removed with a flame shaped finishing bur to create a long bevel. The gingival termination of the preparation is where the previous

shoulder ender, which is now ending in a knife-edged taper. There is no additional bevel. The problem with this preparation is that because of the taper, there is more tooth structure removed at the occlusal aspect; there is greater risk of pulpal involvement. Failure to remove enough tooth structure may result in an overcontoured restoration.

Chamfer Preparation.   The chamfer preparation reduces more tooth structure in the gingival third than the knife-edged preparation. It does not allow as much room as a full shoulder preparation for the buttressing of metal in the gingival one third that is needed to produce the rigid metal framework for porcelain. If a chamfer stone is used to create a deep chamfer yielding a low-stress concentration preparation, a reverse lip may be cut. A low-stress concentration preparation is one in which the walls are more parallel than in a high-stress concentration preparation, and the shoulder is between 90 and 110 degrees, with an internal rounded line angle. Removing the lip may result in a preparation that is more subgingival than desired. A more tapered chamfer preparation results in a high-stress concentration preparation. A high-stress concentration preparation is overly tapered and the shoulder to axial wall line angle is less than 90 degrees. The shoulder slopes incisally. This type of preparation as well as the knife-edged finishing line may result in marginal metal distortion during firing, depending upon the depth of the gingival portion of the preparation. The finishing area (gingival area) of the preparation requires a buttress or thickness of metal to avoid distortion when baking porcelain.

Full Shoulder Preparation.   The full shoulder preparation has the most of the same attributes as the full beveled shoulder preparation (with the exception of the bevel), without the disadvantages of the anterior bevel. It is used for a butt joint ceramic type of restoration.

Full Shoulder with a Bevel Preparation.   The ideal preparation for porcelain fused to metal restoration is a full shoulder with a bevel. The main difference between a shoulder

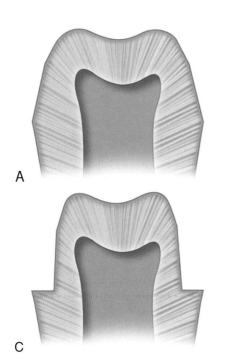

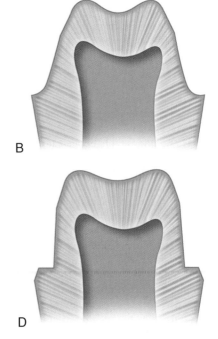

FIGURE 9-2 A, Tapered knife-edged preparation. **B,** Chamfer preparation. **C,** Full shoulder preparation. **D,** Full shoulder with bevel preparation.

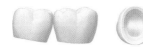

FIGURE 9-3 Optimal interproximal form for biologic contours of definitive full coverage restorations. The contact area allows for an occlusal embrasure and a gingival embrasure, which allows room for a healthy interproximal papilla. An internal view of the castings shows a beveled shoulder with the same thickness throughout the preparation. The gingival embrasure has a wide contact area to aid cleansability and enhance the health of the surrounding interproximal papilla. The buccolingual embrasure enhances food deflection and periodontal health.

preparation and a chamfer preparation is in the gingival third and is the additional tooth reduction necessary to create a shoulder between the horizontal and vertical line angles formed by the shoulder and the axial wall. The additional reduction provides room for additional metal, which buttresses the shoulder and supports the porcelain. The shoulder preparation may have a shoulder of 90 to 120 degrees (Fig. 9-3) The advantages of a full shoulder with a bevel preparation are:

1. The creation of adequate room in the gingival third for proper contouring of the restoration to maintain periodontal health with a straight emergence profile
2. The creation of room in the gingival third for proper porcelain application and esthetics
3. The creation of a buttress of metal in the gingival area to avoid distortion of the metallic framework during the baking of porcelain and the seating of castings
4. The creation of a more parallel, less tapered preparation enhancing retention of the restoration.[19]

Bevel Types (Table 9-6)

Forty-Five Degree Facial Bevel. To avoid displaying a facial metal collar, a full shoulder preparation combined with a facial 45-degree bevel and an 80-degree proximal and lingual or palatal bevel (Fig. 9-4A) is cut. Facially, the porcelain, opaque, and metal are brought to a common termination with predictable fit, contour, and color. Because the vertical amount of marginal metal is so narrow, the opaque is barely visible in the finished restoration. The facial 45-degree bevel is like a sloped shoulder and allows creation of the desired esthetic result. Also, from a laboratory viewpoint it is less technique sensitive than a butt joint.[17]

A porcelain margin accumulates less plaque, results in less margin exposure caused by gingival recession that occurs over a period of time, and is less objectionable cosmetically. Porcelain stacking and firing does not distort the facial margin of the 45-degree bevel. The 45-degree bevel with porcelain over the metal collar has greater esthetic potential, as well as the same marginal adaptation, as the 80-degree bevel with an all-metal collar.[17] The use of the 45-degree facial bevel provides a closing angle facially similar to the creation of a closing angle around the remainder of the preparation, but it has opaque and porcelain baked on it for cosmetics. The advantage of this bevel facially over the facial butt joint is the incorporation of a facial closing angle.

Eighty-Degree Facial Bevel with Porcelain Covering the Metal Collar. The complete bevel prepared with a plug finishing bur has an 80-degree or greater convergence angle (Fig. 9-4B). Porcelain baked onto this facial apron will fracture off due to the flexure of the metal in the apron area.

Table 9-6 **Finishing Line Variations for Shoulder and Shoulder with Bevel Preparations**

Type	Indications
Butt joint	Anterior splints up to six units
45-Degree facial bevel	Esthetics is paramount; this is a preferred substitute for a butt joint. It also is less technique sensitive.
80-Degree facial bevel with porcelain	Not recommended because of possibility porcelain will fracture
80-Degree facial bevel with metal	For short preparations to increase retention, endodontic teeth with posts, better closing angles, and postperiodontally treated teeth with long clinical crowns.

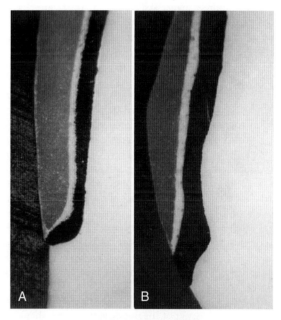

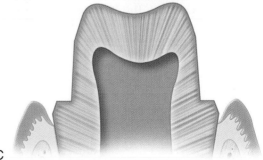

FIGURE 9-4 Specimen sectioned for light microscopic examination shows a full shoulder preparation with a facial 45-degree bevel and a proximal and lingual 80-degree bevel. Black is metal; white is opaquer; gray is porcelain. **A,** Magnified view of a prepared tooth showing a lingual margin with an 80-degree bevel and a metal collar (original magnification × 25). **B,** 80-degree facial bevel with metal collar. **C,** Proper placement of the finishing line. The bevel should extend only about 0.5 mm into the facial sulcus area.

Eighty-Degree Facial Bevel with Metal Collar. For small and large splints or fixed prostheses, a full shoulder with 360-degree encirclement by a bevel is required for closure at the termination of the preparation. The bevel should extend only about 0.5mm into the facial sulcus area (Fig. 9-4C). The metal collar is not a limiting factor in the fabrication of a fixed prosthesis. It can be used in a single full coverage restoration or for fixed partial prostheses.

Full Shoulder with a Bevel and a Facial Butt Joint Preparation. The bevel is prepared on the proximal and palatal or lingual surfaces of the preparation, but not on the facial surface. The facial surface terminates in a butt joint shoulder finishing line to avoid showing a facial metal collar. In addition, for porcelain to be esthetically acceptable, 1.5mm of thickness must be obtained for the opaque layer and body porcelain. This space does not exist at the margin of a bevel or knife-edged finishing line preparation if optimum crown contours are created. This type of finishing line is satisfactory for single or multiple unit splints of up to six units especially when the facial gingival tissue is thin or almost transparent. For larger splints over six units, a butt joint is not recommended because of the contraction of the metal during baking of porcelain and the concomitant lack of marginal integrity.

Pontic Design

Ridge Lap Pontic. Ante stated "A pontic must restore the dentition to proper form and function while preserving the esthetic quality of the tooth it replaces, ensure its sanitation, and be biologically acceptable to the tissue.[18] Ideally, a pontic would exactly duplicate the tooth it replaces. However, the residual ridge (Fig. 9-5) over which the pontic will be placed is usually convex.[19] Consequently, that surface of the pontic contacting the mucosa would be concave if the pontic were to recreate the natural tooth shape at the gingival area. This maximum tissue contact pontic design, known as the ridge lap or saddle pontic, is undesirable because a concave surface is difficult to clean, resulting in soft tissue irritation with concomitant periodontal problems.[20]

Modified Ridge Lap Pontic. In the modified ridge lap design[21] the facial aspect of the pontic assumes the shape of the replaced tooth and contacts. This allows for maximum esthetics. The tissue contact is minimal and the underside of the pontic only follows the convex anatomy of the residual ridge on the buccal half of the residual ridge. The remainder of the lingual portion of the pontic (the area of the pontic above and lingual to the height of the ridge) is convex. This lingual portion of the pontic is easily cleansed, however, some problems surface soon after insertion of the prosthesis.

1. Despite hygienic procedures, the concave tissue surfaces of the pontics invariably become coated with plaque and debris. The corresponding ridge surfaces usually become red and inflamed.[22]
2. The triangular area of the linguopalatal surface traps food particles and also annoys the patient's tongue.
3. The pontic may not provide adequate air seal for desired or correct phonation during speech.
4. The space that exists between pontic and ridge or pontic and abutment may permit droplets of saliva to be forced through during speech sounds, causing annoyance and embarrassment.[23]

Stein Pontic. The Stein pontic is a variation of the modified ridge lap pontic. It is designed for sharp edentulous ridges, exhibits minimal tissue contact, and offers acceptable esthetics. It is contraindicated in edentulous ridges with broad buccolingual dimensions.

Sanitary Pontic. The sanitary pontic has no tissue contact. It possesses the occlusal form and function of the tooth it replaces, but has a rounded gingival surface that does not extend to the residual ridge. This pontic is used when an esthetic replacement is not required. Thus it may be used in mandibular molar areas when desired. Maintenance of a hygienic condition of the ridge is usually satisfactory when the pontic, with rounded contours, is kept 2 to 3 mm above the ridge. When the pontic tissue clearance is less than 2 mm, it contributes to food entrapment.

Ovate Pontic. The most functional and esthetic pontic is the ovate pontic. It requires plastic reconstructive surgery of the ridge to create a concavity. In the preparation of an ovate pontic, an egg-shaped form is produced on the tissue surface that blends into the cervical third of the pontic and the tissue surface of the pontic is glazed and polished to a smooth finish. When properly placed, the pontic appears to emerge from the surgically created corpus of the ridge, affording a more natural and pleasing effect. Cleansing of soft tissue and the pontic is expedited and effective. A properly contoured ovate pontic automatically creates interdental papillae which fill the embrasures, thereby eliminating the dark space triangles between teeth, reducing the escape of saliva during speech, and reducing occasional lisping sounds. The ovate pontic is a necessity in patients with a high smile line. It is contraindicated in or against a knife-edged ridge. It is important that the residual ridge is capable of being augmented in buccolingual thickness to contain the ovate pontic within the body of the ridge (see Chapter 17).

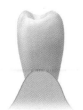 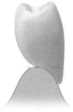 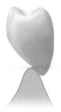 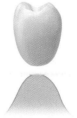 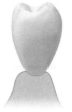

A. Ridge lap pontic   B. Modified ridge lap pontic   C. Stein pontic   D. Sanitary pontic   E. Ovate pontic

FIGURE 9-5 Relationship of pontic design to residual ridge.

Framework Considerations

One of the very important steps in the construction of a ceramometal restoration is the design of the metal frame-work. The metal frame must resemble the completed restoration except for the labial, lingual, and occlusal surfaces of abutments and pontics, which are 1.5 mm smaller, and the incisal surface, which is 2 mm smaller, to allow for the support of porcelain and creation of a uniform shade. The connection areas are placed toward the lingual surface with adequate room for opaque, porcelain, and a deep facial embrasure in order to create individuality and the illusion of depth in the definitive porcelain-fused-to-metal restoration. If the dentist is concerned about porcelain fracture, the connection areas can be waxed, cast up to the occlusal surface posteriorly for support, and to occlusally contact the opposing teeth (Figs. 7-11 to 7-13). If the metal is gold plated, it can mimic the interproximal occlusal embrasure space. Anteriorly, the connection areas should not interfere with the gingival embrasures or incisally with translucency or the incisal embrasure.

The work authorization should specify the placement and height of interproximal struts, the presence of metal occlusal contacts (when fabricating a posterior ceramometal restoration), and the type of metal desired. For anterior restorations the work authorization should also include the need for metal lingual contact, depending on the individual anterior guidance factors. Posteriorly, the contact areas between adjacent teeth or restorations should be in metal, not porcelain. If the contact point is porcelain instead of metal and the porcelain marginal ridge area fractures, a food impaction area will result, and the crown must be replaced. For this reason, the interproximal metal struts on individual crowns should extend to within 1 mm of the occlusal surface of the porcelain and should contain the contact area or point that *is* required. When the technician returns the ceramometal casting to the dentist, it should be tried in the mouth for gingival fit, contour, occlusion, and contact with adjacent teeth. The adaptation of the internal surface of the casting should be checked using Cavitec cement (Kerr Corp.), Multiform paste, or a polysiloxane paste (i.e., Pressure Indicating Material, Coltene/Whaledent, Inc.), as indicating materials. Next, using a small bur, the dentist should scribe the termination of porcelain on the labial surface of the casting at the facial gingival margin. This mark is a guide for the technician for terminating facial porcelain because no porcelain should be baked, onto the apron of the crown casting; this area is thin and flexible, and porcelain baked on it *will* fracture. By scribing the termination of the veneering material intraorally, allowance is made for a small gold collar or finishing line that is hidden in the sulcus area.

CLINICAL TIP

To compensate for high light reflection, caused by thin layers of translucent porcelain covering an opaque mask, select shades that are slightly lower in value than the surrounding teeth.[13] This should not result in reduced brightness of the restoration.

CLINICAL TIP

Intraoral scribing eliminates the laboratory guesswork about subgingival termination of the porcelain and results in maximal esthetics.

CLINICAL TIP

After the porcelain' veneer has' been baked and glazed, a gold-plating solution maybe used to impart a yellow color to gray ceramometal casting. The gray color of the metal adds darkness to the gingiva. The plated yellow gold color gives a softer, "self-masking" appearance that is more acceptable to the patient.

BASIC CONSIDERATIONS IN TOOTH FORM

Patient Personality and Gender

The oral examination, history, and ascertaining the patient's esthetic requirements and expectations are essential when attempting to provide the most esthetic and functional prosthesis possible.

Endless combinations and variations of physical attributes exist in men and women, but a complete analysis also accounts for personality factors. In general, masculinity is associated with vigorous, strong, and robust qualities, whereas femininity is translated in terms of softness, delicacy, and curvature of anatomic form (see Chapter 2).

By selecting and modifying a tooth form, the dentist is creating an image for the patient. By placing the two maxillary central incisors boldly in a dominating position, usually facing forward, around which the lateral incisors are rotated and elevated slightly above the plane of occlusion, the sense of vigorous domination is established in the position of the maxillary central incisors. A small maxillary lateral incisor confers the appearance of femininity, whereas lateral incisors that are almost as broad as central incisors confer ruggedness and masculinity. A patient with a "delicate" appearance often has lighter skin and, consequently, lighter teeth.

The maxillary canines are important because they are easily visible from a frontal or lateral view, and serve as a gateway to the posterior teeth. By turning the tip of the canine inward, one may prevent a toothy and possibly anthropoidal[24] appearance; however, the mesial aspect of the canine should not be hidden when viewed from directly in front of the patient.

An important factor to consider in all situations is the age of the patient. The dentist is seeking to create, when necessary and approved by the patient, the desired illusion of a natural tooth in the oral environment. Age and concomitant changes bring challenges to the creative dentist attempting to fabricate an artistically acceptable prosthesis. Studying changes wrought by time, and their visibility in relation to the planned porcelain restoration, may suggest appropriate modifications such as cuspal reductions caused by wear, reduction of translucent incisal edges of anterior teeth, color change, possible change in the shape of papillae, and, of course, changes in chroma and value.

A study of the position of natural teeth reveals:[24]

1. Roundness of the arch form denotes femininity; squareness denotes masculinity.
2. Incisal edges of maxillary teeth of females follow the curve of the lower lip.
3. When females speak, smile, or laugh, they expose more maxillary teeth than males do. The maxillary first premolars should be contoured to conform with the canines.
4. In males, a square incisal silhouette with prominence of the maxillary central incisors and canines may indicate a bolder and more vigorous personality.

Up until recent times, it was an inspiring challenge to the dentist to duplicate as closely as possible the qualities of the natural teeth, resulting in unobtrusive functional and harmonious restorations (see Chapter 2). Currently there is an increasing desire by many patients to obtain large, B1, B2, B3, B4 (New Porcelain Bleach Shades/Shade Guide, Ivoclar Vivadent) restorations.

Alignment of Gingival Margins. Alignment of the gingival margins usually enhances the cosmetic result. When discrepancies are visible, refer the patient for periodontal correction prior to beginning tooth preparation (see Chapters 14 and 21).

HUE, CHROMA, AND VALUE

Preston and Bergen[25] have provided the following definitions (see Chapter 2):

1. Hue. "That dimension of color used to distinguish one family of color from another." The physical hue order is, by the common names, violet, blue, green, yellow, orange, and red. It is usually defined by the color family name.
2. Chroma. "That quality by which one distinguishes a weak hue from a stronger more intense hue. It is the amount of a basic hue added to gray. If more colorant is added, a stronger, more intense hue (higher chroma) results." It is also referred to as "saturation." Chroma denotes the concentration or strength of the basic hue. Intense color indicates a higher chroma or saturation.
3. Value. "That quality by which one distinguishes a light color from a dark color; a gray scale that extends from black to white. It has nothing to do with the amount of gray in a color—only the relative level of brightness, lightness or brilliance. It is not a quantitative, but rather a qualitative description. Value is found by comparing the chosen color to a color of similar brightness." Colors of low value are more like black; colors of high value are more like white. Value, a quality of grayness, is an important factor of color, both to the dentist and the technician, who should be able to separate value from other dimensions and detect and control differences that could prove disastrous to shade matching.

One of the simplest modifications is to raise the chroma of the dominant hue. The modification of the chroma that is too high is more difficult. If a lower chroma is needed, the color must be neutralized by its complement. The most obvious color one might use to raise value is white. The technician should be fully versed in the many ways of managing dentists' requests for modifications and characterizations and communication should be thoroughly clear (see Chapter 2 and Appendix A).

Poor esthetics is exacerbated when too light a shade has been selected and modified by staining and coloring; this combination creates artificiality. However, the current trend towards fulfilling patients' desires for pure white shade B1, B2, B3, B4 (New Porcelain Bleach Shades/Shade Guide, Ivoclar Vivadent) with no staining or characterizations can substitute for traditional realism. The dentist should differentiate the hue, value, and chroma of the patient's natural teeth and then apply these factors to the porcelain restoration.[26] Concentrating on these aspects for 5-second intervals helps to prevent retinal fatigue (retinal adaptation), thus permitting shade differences to be more readily detected. One of the most important factors to communicate to the technician is the type of tooth enamel being matched (i.e., opaque, translucent, dull, or highly reflective).

No matter how beautifully the color has been incorporated in the porcelain restoration or how skillfully the tooth has been contoured, a high glossy glaze is incompatible with the appearance of the enamel of the surrounding teeth if the latter are comparatively dull. With the use of the bleach shades, the only method the clinician has to differentiate between adjacent porcelain veneered crowns is by creation of facial, gingival, and incisal embrasures of varying depths.

Ceramometal procedures require the thinnest layer of porcelain opaquing materials that block out the metal casting surface. Covering this opaque masking with a thin layer of translucent body and incisal porcelain permits the restoration to become highly reflective. As such, the tooth cannot be compatible with its adjacent natural teeth.

CLINICAL TIP

To compensate for high light reflection, caused by thin layers of translucent porcelain covering an opaque mask, select shades that are slightly lower in value than the surrounding teeth.[13] This should not result in reduced brightness of the restoration.

Positioning the restoration more lingually and increasing the incisal curvature directs the light in various directions away from the viewer. The contour and texture of the outer porcelain surface defines the character of the restoration and contributes vitality to its appearance. Each tooth is individualized and characterized by a distinct outline form. The incisal form and tooth position influence esthetics more than any other aspect, because the tooth is silhouetted against the dark shadow of the oral cavity.

Creation of Dental Illusions

The apparent size of teeth (length and width) may be influenced by contours of the teeth and the effects of light reflections. For example, the maxillary central incisors reflect light anteriorly, superiorly, inferiorly, and laterally. By contouring the facial aspects to deflect the light in directions other than forward (e.g., curving the lateral aspects into embrasures), the tooth may be made to appear narrower and longer. Using contouring to reflect light superiorly in the gingival third and inferiorly in the incisal curve, should give the illusion of a shorter and broader maxillary tooth. In the situation of malpositioned teeth, it may be necessary to create the illusion of a wider tooth in a small space. This can be effected by bringing the contact points as far facially as possible and flattening the surfaces to reflect all the light facially. A diastema can often be eliminated by porcelain crowns that make contact in the lingually positioned embrasure, and that have narrow facial aspects to reflect a smaller tooth. The curves moved laterally into the embrasures permit the light to be deflected away from the viewer.[13] The facial forms of the adjacent crowns should curve into one another in the areas of the proximal contact rather than be separated by a thin straight disk. However, this may not improve esthetics when managing small square central incisors with a diastema between them. In these situations, closure, may create an unesthetic result.

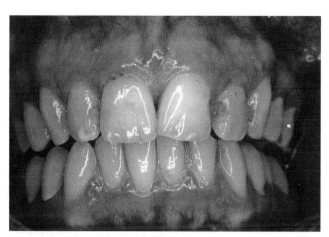

FIGURE 9-6 Preoperative facial view of a patient requiring porcelain fused to gold crowns.

Surface texturing that is similar to adjacent natural teeth is an important feature of the restored tooth. It produces interplay of light and creates pleasant color matching experiences.

Horizontal and vertical lines affect the apparent width or length of the tooth being fabricated.

In addition to the variables of color and contour, the technician should be informed of all aspects involving the compatibility of the porcelain with various aspects of the remaining natural teeth (Fig. 9-6).

CLINICAL TIP

Surface texturing should be slightly more emphasized on the restorations than that which is present on the adjacent tooth being matched because light is reflected differently from tooth enamel and glazed porcelain (enamel).

A removable prosthesis affords the advantage of trial seatng in determining the size and form of the restorative teeth. Corrections can be made in wax in the process of repositioning, reshaping, or replacing the denture teeth. In fixed prosthodontics, provisional acrylic resin coverage serves a similar diagnostic step. By adjusting the plastic, the dentist may satisfy the patient's esthetic expectations. An impression and a poured stone cast may serve as further instructional guidance for the laboratory technician.

A valuable aid in creating esthetic restorations is to place a degree of importance on the personality of the patient. Esthetic factors usually correlate with the patient's facial form and the degree of facial symmetry. Rounded, blunt, or sharp distoincisal line angles of the anterior teeth will greatly vary the visual perception of facial esthetics. Incisal embrasures should vary from one side of the tooth and arch to the other. The degree of space from the mesiofacial incisal line angle must contain both horizontal and vertical variations of this space.

Extrinsic staining and shading will highlight or illuminate the cosmetic result only when all the aforementioned factors have been satisfied. Incisal translucency, enamel hypocalcifications, enamel crazing lines, and areas of wear can be accurately created in an esthetic restoration. Overcharacterization can mar the result and produce an unwanted, unsightly effect.

Poor esthetics occurs when the teeth lack individuality. Poor esthetics is exacerbated when shade is too light or too dark and by a lack of proper embrasures, surface texture, and contours. When all the above occur, the restoration appears flat, unindividualized, and of uniform color, giving the appearance of a single mass of porcelain, or what is known as "Chiclets." An acceptable cosmetic result is obtained in the following ways.

1. Avoid flatness by optimum fabrication of the curvature of the facial surfaces, which reflect light differently.
2. Use deep orange-brown stain interproximally to enhance the individuality of the prosthesis.
3. Create deep incisal embrasures for individuality; the length and curvature of the incisal surfaces should follow the smile line of the lower lip.
4. Avoid gingival inflammation by providing adequate interproximal space for the papillae and gingival embrasures. The gingival terminations must not be overextended or shy of the margin, or too bulky, which results in gingival problems. The facial gingival heights must be the same. The porcelain-fused-to-metal restorations should aid in maintenance of an optimal periodontal environment.[27] This requires use of a straight emergence profile, optimum gingival embrasure contour to maintain the interdental papilla, and not over contouring the facial gingival contour.

Management of Misaligned Teeth

Diastemata. Several methodologies may be used to create a favorable cosmetic result when diastemata are present or when teeth are rotated. The optimum method of treatment is to employ adult orthodontics, whether minor tooth movement or full banded complete therapy (see Chapter 15).

After tooth movement is complete, the teeth are held in place for at least 6 months by a fixed retainer. If the teeth are to be covered eventually, metal and acrylic resin fixed provisional restorations may be used as the fixed retainer. The major problem with adult orthodontics for closure of diastemata or correction of rotated or overlapped anterior teeth is the common need for splinting the teeth to maintain their positions after tooth movement, because they have a tendency to revert to their original positions.

Cosmetically, if the diastema between two short, square shaped central incisors is to be closed, the end result is usually not as esthetic as the patient and clinician desire. If it is necessary to close this type of diastema, crown lengthening should be done prior to any tooth preparation. For a pleasing result, it behooves the dentist to create longer teeth.

Protruded Teeth. When a tooth is facially protruded, the surrounding facial soft tissue is thin. This is especially common with maxillary canines. Orthodontic therapy is the treatment of choice (see Chapter 15). If this tooth is to be covered with a restoration for realignment and cosmetics without orthodontic treatment, sufficient tooth structure must be removed to allow not only for metal and porcelain, but also for the realignment. Prophylactic endodontic therapy is often necessary. Also, the facial margin of the restoration cannot be carried subgingivally without the risk of gingival recession due to the thinness of this facial soft tissue. In addition, a pronounced facial bulge at the gingival margin of the definitive restoration cannot be avoided because of the facial angulation of the underlying root.

Tooth Reduction

Armamentarium

* Standard dental setup
  * Explorer
  * Mouth mirror
  * Periodontal probe
  * Appropriate anesthesia
  * High-speed handpiece
  * Low-speed handpiece
* Suitable size impression trays
* Diamond burs
  * A football-shaped diamond stone, coarse or medium (e.g., 63-68-023 large or 63-68-016 small, Brasseler USA).
  * A shoulder diamond or a cylinder stone (e.g., 835-010, Brasseler USA).
  * A 1-mm diameter shoulder diamond with a 3-degree taper (e.g., 6849-016, Brasseler USA) for molars or the smaller 811-033 (Brasseler USA) for premolars. The 45-degree bevel is formed with either the Premier Dental Products two striper DCB.5 or the Brasseler USA 30005 48.

Clinical Technique

1. Administer the appropriate anesthesia.
2. Create two 1-mm 3-degree taper facial guide cuts with the shoulder diamond bur. The first cut follows the facial angle from the height of contour to the incisal edge. The second cut parallels the long axis of the tooth from the gingival margin to the height of contour. This ensures sufficient removal of tooth structure and a 3-degree taper.
3. For anterior teeth, prepare a third depth guide cut on the lingual surface from the gingival margin to the height of the cingulum, using the same shoulder diamond stone as for the facial surface. Prepare a fourth depth guide cut from the height of the cingulum to the incisal edge with a 1.2-mm shoulder stone.

   For posterior teeth, prepare two depth guide cuts on the lingual surface as described for the facial surface. Create an additional depth cut at least 1.5 mm deep on the occlusal surface to ensure adequate occlusal reduction.

4. Finish the preparation, except for the area incisal to the cingulum of the anterior teeth, by following the depth guiding cuts.

5. For anterior teeth, reduce the height of the incisal edge by at least 2 mm.
6. For anterior teeth, prepare the area from the incisal edge to the cingulum with a football-shaped stone. The depth of preparation in this area must accommodate for the incisal guidance created in the diagnostic wax-up, as well as provide room for the metal, opaque, and porcelain of the restoration. If the pulp is large, a metal lingual surface may have to be used to avoid pulp exposure. If the mandibular anterior teeth will not be covered with porcelain, the centric occlusal contacting area on the palatal aspect of the maxillary crowns should be metal so reduce the incisal of the mandibular anterior teeth.
7. For anterior teeth, verify tooth reduction, especially that area influencing the incisal guidance, with the transitional prosthesis. If the section incisal to the cingulum becomes thin or perforated, re-prepare this area or alter the treatment plan (e.g., metal lingual, intentional endodontics, or selective grinding of opposing teeth) prior to impressioning the preparation.
8. Contour and polish the provisional restorations, and cement them with sedative non-eugenol temporary cement (see Chapter 10).
9. Dismiss the patient and evaluate the esthetics, tooth contours, gingival health, and occlusion at the next office visit.

Bevel Placement

Once the esthetics of the provisional restorations is acceptable to both the dentist and the patient, create a finishing line.

Armamentarium

* Standard dental setup (see the preceding section on Tooth Reduction)
* Blunted 12-fluted steel finishing bur (e.g., Premier Dental Products Two Stripper DCB) which is manufactured with a blunted tip, or a carbide finishing bur (GTB NYU; Brasseler USA).

Clinical Technique

1. Prepare a bevel on the mesial, palatal, and distal margins with a blunted 12-fluted steel plug or fine diamond finishing burs (Fig. 9-7A).
2. Use a clockwise direction for beveling and a counterclockwise rotation for gingival curettage.
3. Hold the bur parallel to the path of insertion (Fig 9-7B). The bevels and subgingival buccal shoulder must not violate the biologic width (see Chapter 14).

Tissue Management and Impressioning

Armamentarium

* Standard dental setup (see the previous section on Tooth Reduction)

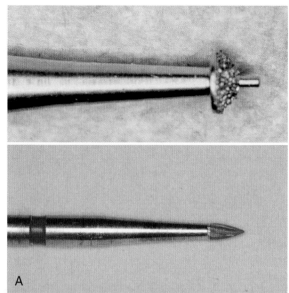

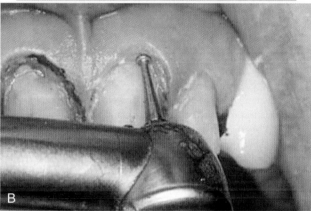

FIGURE 9-7 **A,** Rotary instruments used to create a facial 45-degree bevel. Premier Dental Products Two Stripper DCB .5 (*top*) and Brasseler USA GTB NYU (*bottom*). **B,** Preparing a facial 45-degree bevel on a different patient. The Two Stripper DCB .5 bur is held perpendicular to the shoulder.

+ No.1 gingival retraction cord
+ No. 2 gingival retraction cord
+ Suitable impression material

Clinical Technique

1. Bevel placement creates adequate room in the sulcular area for the impression material.

CLINICAL TIP

Gingival retraction cords are not used for gingival retraction at the time of impressioning, but rather to maintain the space created while beveling.

2. There should be no gingival bleeding at the time of impression making. If the soft tissues are healthy and were managed without extending the margins of the preparation more than 0.5 mm into the gingival sulcus, the gingiva will not bleed.
3. Only a No. 1 or No. 2 cord is necessary to maintain the sulcular space for the impression material.
4. The single strand of cord should be fully visible when in place. It is not used for retraction, but rather to maintain the prepared sulcus.

5. Make a final full arch impression of the preparations.
6. Make an irreversible full arch irreversible hydrocolloid impression of the opposing arch.
7. Prior to sectioning the cast for trimming preparation dies, the casts should be mounted in an "indexed" mounting system (e.g., Accu-Trac or Pindex systems (Coltene/Whaledent, Inc.) or EZ Di-Lok system (Di-Equi Dental Products).

CLINICAL TIP

"Ditching" the dies is important in two respects: It gives the dental technician a finishing point and it insures that the finished restoration does not extend beyond the preparation which risks the creation of periodontal problems.

8. After securing the dies, trim and ditch them below the end of the preparation.

CLINICAL TIP

To ensure proper delineation of the margins, the individual dies should be trimmed by the dentist. Casts can be returned from the laboratory with removable dies ready for trimming or the dentist can send completed casts using an "indexed" mounting system (e.g. Accu-Trac or Pindex systems (Coltene/Whaledent, Inc.) or EZ Di-Lok system (Di-Equi Dental Products). With practice, casts can usually be poured, indexed, and the dies trimmed in one day, with little alteration in the practitioner's schedule.

Die Trimming and Preparation

Armamentarium
+ Denture vulcanite bur
+ No. 6 handpiece round bur
+ Die spacer—0.25 mm thickness (George Taub Products)
+ Cyanoacrylate

Clinical Technique

1. Trim the die first with a vulcanite bur.
2. Ditch below the bevel with a No. 6 round bur.
3. Paint a single layer of die spacer over the entire die, except for auxiliary cuts, at the shoulder and bevel.
4. Paint a thin layer of cyanoacrylate over the termination of the bevel to prevent chipping or scraping away of this area during laboratory procedures.
5. Articulate the full arch casts (with trimmed dies) and send instructions to the laboratory for wax-up and fabrication of the ceramometal castings.

Work Authorization

The work authorization should specify the placement and height and width of interproximal struts, metal occlusal contacts (when fabricating a posterior ceramometal restoration), and the type of metal that the dentist desires. For anterior restorations, the work authorization should also include the need for metal lingual contact, depending on the individual anterior guidance factors. Emphasize to the laboratory that the contact areas between adjacent teeth or restorations should be in metal and not in porcelain, posteriorly.

CLINICAL TIP

If the contact point is in porcelain instead of metal and the porcelain marginal ridge area fractures, a food impaction area results and the crown will have to be remade. Therefore, the interproximal metal struts on individual crowns should extend up to within 1 mm of the occlusal surface of the porcelain and should contain the contact area or point that is required.

Try-In of Castings

Armamentarium
+ Standard dental setup. (see the above section on Tooth Reduction)
+ Indicating paste: Cavitec cement (Kerr Corp.); Fit Checker (GC America)
+ No. 1 round bur

Clinical Technique
1. Check the adaptation of the internal surface of the casting using either Cavitec cement or Fit Checker as indicating materials.
2. Check the castings in the mouth for gingival fit, contour, occlusion, and contact with adjacent teeth.
3. Using a small bur, scribe the desired location of the termination of porcelain on the facial surface of the casting, at the facial gingival margin.

In metal ceramics, the opaque layer reflects light while light passing around it creates a shadow which delineates the core. A florescent powder can be applied over the opaque layer that will reflect more light than the opaque layer alone, lighting up the veneering material and obscuring the coping.

Light reflecting back from the metal core will be visible. Ceramists can decrease the amount of light reflection but cannot increase it. A metal casting core that is high in value can easily be made lower in value. Dentin powders are used for creating the chroma and enamel powders control the value. It requires years of study and experience for a master ceramist to develop the skills necessary to create lifelike restorations.

The core material must be chosen according to the demands of the restoration. After a diagnostic wax-up has been completed, the dimensions of the connection points can be calculated. Metal ceramics requires 2 mm^2, Zirconia 3 mm^2, and lithium disilicate 4 mm^2. The desired shade and the supporting tooth structure (dowel/ core stump) shade must be evaluated by the dental team. All team members must evaluate the merits of the available core materials and choose the most appropriate one. Each core material has limitations and challenges in its fabrication and the ceramist must feel comfortable with the choice. Use of CAD/CAM requires skill and judgment by the dental team. CAD software can automate the labor but should not be allowed to dictate design. The steps for fabrication of the restoration are different for the chosen core materials. A wide verity of metals and zirconia are available. The dental team must be confident in the knowledge of the specific handling requirements of the chosen materials to maximize success.

CLINICAL TIP

A scribed line serves as a guide for the technician for the cervical termination of facial porcelain and allows the thin metal collar or finishing line to be hidden in the sulcus.

Soft Tissue Casts and Shade Selection

CLINICAL TIP

Crown contours are critical for establishing esthetics and maintaining gingival health. A soft tissue cast is helpful in this regard, especially in anterior teeth. Create the soft tissue cast after the castings are tried in and found to be clinically acceptable.

Armamentarium
+ Standard dental setup (see the previous section on Tooth Reduction)
+ Suitable luting agent
+ Autopolymerizing acrylic resin (e.g. Duralay, Reliance Dental Mfg. Co.)
+ Suitable impression material (e.g., irreversible hydrocolloid)
+ Metal retention device (e.g., flat headed screws or bent dowel pins)
+ Soft Denture Reline Acrylic (e.g., Coe Soft, GC America)
+ Self-curing pink acrylic (e.g., Jet Pink Acrylic, Lang Dental Manufacturing Co., Inc.)
+ Yellow stone

Clinical Technique
1. Lute the castings together intraorally with red autopolymerizing acrylic resin.
2. Make an overall irreversible hydrocolloid impression with the castings reseated firmly into the index.
3. Flow a soupy mix of red autopolymerizing acrylic resin into the occlusal two-thirds of the casting and insert a flat headed screw or bent dowel pin into the stone cast for retention.
4. Cover the gingival area surrounding the castings with a mixture of two parts resilient autopolymerizing denture liner and one part hard pink autopolymerizing acrylic resin.[28]

CLINICAL TIP

Apply the mixture with a standard disposable syringe. Then sprinkle acrylic beads onto the surface to facilitate union with the subsequent die stone cast.

5. Make an irreversible hydrocolloid impression of the provisional restoration and send casts to the laboratory.
6. Select a shade and prepare a proper laboratory prescription, including required characterization.

CLINICAL TIP

With a small No. 1 round bur, scribe the porcelain termination line on the facial surface of the casting at the facial gingival margin. This line will serve as a guide for the technician for the cervical termination of the facial porcelain and allow the thin metal collar or finishing line to be hidden within the sulcus.

Porcelain Try-In

Armamentarium
+ Standard dental setup. (See the previous section on Tooth Reduction.)

Clinical Technique

1. The laboratory should only use low-speed handpiece fine green stones or fine diamond stones to recarve the bisque bake porcelain.
2. Correct the points or areas of contact until unwaxed extra fine dental floss just snaps through.
3. Refine the crown contours intraorally with appropriate high-speed diamond stones and copious amounts of water to avoid overheating and fracturing the veneering material.
4. Refine the occlusion. If the cast is inaccurate, make another impression. If the articulation is incorrect, remount the cast prior to returning it to the laboratory.

CLINICAL TIP

Perform extensive additions directly on the cast, using ivory wax. Make an irreversible hydrocolloid impression of these altered restorations and make a cast. This creates a guide for the technician to make the required alterations.

CLINICAL TIP

Perform extensive additions directly on the cast, using ivory wax. Make an irreversible hydrocolloid impression of these altered restorations and pour a cast. This creates a guide for the technician to make the required alterations.

5. When splinting a posterior quadrant, the metal interproximal struts can be maintained up to and including the occlusal surface for maintenance of occlusal stability in patients with a high risk of porcelain fracture (see the section on Framework Considerations earlier in the chapter). Correct centric occlusal discrepancies on the articulator, on which the casts had been previously mounted according to verified maxillomandibular recordings.
6. Correct small discrepancies in eccentric movements intraorally.
7. Return the bisque bake restoration to the laboratory with the proper work authorization, including the required alterations and a shade guide tab and/or a drawing of the selected color indicating placement of gingival, body, and incisal shades, and character variations.

CLINICAL TIP

To maintain a natural appearance and surface texture, use the natural glaze of the porcelain, rather than painting on a low-temperature glaze after applying surface stains.

CLINICAL TIP

If the original bisque bake does not match the selected color, return the chosen shade guide tab to the laboratory. Alternatively, an acrylic shade guide tab can be modified to the correct shade of the provisional restoration using an acrylic resin stain kit (e.g., Minute Stain, George Taub Products).

Box 9-1 "Average" Casting Spaces	
Smallest Shear Space	10 Microns
Inlays Detectable Occlusally	21 Microns
Interproximal Gingival	26 Microns
Average Human Hair	35 Microns
Visible Space	50 Microns
Crown Space Detectable Gingivally	76 Microns
Excellent Crown Casting	100 Microns
Average Crown Casting Before Burnishing The Margins	200 Microns

Trial Cementation and Final Cementation

The use of magnification, sharp explorers and bite-wing radiographs are necessary to verify the restorations acceptability. It has been determined that the "average" casting

Solubility and shrinkage at cement lined margins is critical. One might consider scarfing margins with immaculate bevels, interior shimming, venting, and retention cuts.

Use a trial cementation on multiple unit restorations for the final evaluation of esthetics, occlusion, and other potential processing errors. Dental cementation involves luting metals, porcelains as well as bonding for veneers and plastics. The manipulation of the materials, working and setting times, rheologic (flow) and wetting properties, breakdown and mechanical resistance, and dissolution in foods and oral fluids must be considered by the dentist. High strength in tension, shear, compression and biologic acceptability is desirable.

The Smear Layer. Prime components of the smear layer are residual temporary cement, eugenol, bacterial, cutting debris, saliva, blood, plaque, etc. These should be removed with flour of pumice (no fluorides) and 3% hydrogen peroxide and finally flushed clean with copious water. The dentinal tubules, clogged with debris, if cleaned with polyacrylic acid or methyl ethyl ketone (Cavidry, Parkell, Inc.) may cause future pulpal sensitivities. It is best to use 3% hydrogen peroxide and cotton to dry the preparation, as opposed to drying with compressed air, in order to for the dentin to remain hydrated (see Chapter 3).

The Prosthetic Casting. After the fit has been evaluated and adjusted, the casting may be prepared for cementation. A sand or aluminum oxide blaster should be used to clean out the interior surface of the casting thereby eliminating any residual chlorides and casting debris. The surface should appear "frosted" to enhance adherence of the cement. If there are multiple connections, dental floss contact wrappings may be used to afford easy post-cementation cleanup. Precision attachments are best filled very carefully with red Duralay lubricant to avoid cement intrusion. Be careful that finger manipulation does not smear this grease into the cementable crowns.

After the patient approves the completed restorations, a variety of cements can be used for final cementation (Fig. 9-8). For a complete discussion and a step by step technique of cementation see Chapter 12.

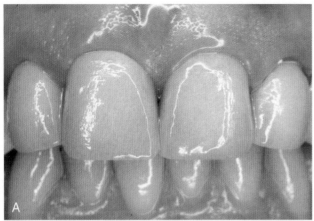

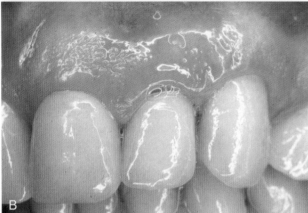

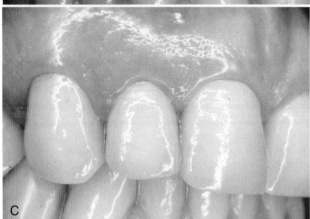

FIGURE 9-8 A, Frontal view of completed restoration. **B,** Left lateral view of completed restoration. **C,** Right lateral view of completed restoration.

CONCLUSION

It is possible to create strong, well-fitting, and lifelike restorations using any of a number of presently available alternatives to conventional porcelain fused to metal restoration materials. However, the available materials have different characteristics. A thorough working knowledge of the use of these materials will allow the practitioner to fully benefit from current dental technology to ultimately achieve the best results and deliver the finest care for patients.

REFERENCES

1. Sakaguchi RL, Powers JM: *Craig's restorative dental materials*, ed 13, St Louis, 2012, Mosby, pp 255, 263-264, 466.
2. Asgar K: *Casting materials*. International State of the Art Conference on Restorative Dental Materials, Bethesda, Md, Sept 8-10, 1986, National Institutes of Health, pp. 105-123.
3. Phillips RW: *Skinner's science of dental materials*, ed 8, Philadelphia, 1982, Saunders.
4. McLean JW: *The science and art of dental ceramics. Vol 2: Bridge design and laboratory proceedings in dental ceramics*, Chicago, 1980, Quintessence.
5. Cascone PJ: The theory of bonding for porcelain to metal systems. In Yamaha H, Grenoble, P, editors: *Dental porcelain: the state of the art*. University of Southern California Conference Proceedings, a compendium of the Colloquium held at the University of Southern California School of Dentistry on Feb. 24-26, 1977, Los Angeles, Calif.
6. Avner SH: *Introduction to physical metallurgy*, New York, 1974, McGraw Hill.
7. Williams DY: *Materials in clinical dentistry*, New York, 1979, Oxford University Press.
8. Vickery RC, Badinelli LA: Nature of attachment forces in porcelain-gold systems, *J Dent Res* 47:683, 1968.
9. Tuccillo JJ: *Dental restorations combining dental porcelain and improved white gold alloy*, US Patents No 3,961,420 and No 3,981,723 (1976).
10. Tuccillo JJ: Comments at the International State of the Art Conference on Restorative Dental Materials, National Institutes of Health, Sept. 8-10, 1986, Bethesda, Md, pp. 151-155.
11. Ingersoll CJ: *Tarnish-resistant palladium base dental casting alloy*, US Patent No 113,929,474 (1975).
12. Cascone PJ: *Low dental alloy*, US Patents No 4,523,262, and No 4,539,176, (1978, 1985.
13. Eissman HS, Rudd KD, Marrow RM: *Dental laboratory procedures in fixed partial dentures*, vol 2, St Louis, 1980, Mosby.
14. Perel ML: Periodontal considerations of crown contours, *J Prosthet Dent* 26:627, 1971.
15. Wheeler RC: Complete crown form and the periodontium, *J Prosthet Dent* 11:722, 1961.
16. Yuodelis RA, Weaver JD, Sapkos S: Facial and lingual contours of artificial complete crown restorations and their effects on the periodontium, *J Prosthet Dent* 29:61, 1973.
17. Panno FV, Vahidi F, Gulker I, et al: Evaluation of the 45-degree labial bevel with a shoulder preparation, *J Prosthet Dent* 56:655, 1986.
18. Ante IH: The fundamental principles, design, and construction of crown and bridge prostheses, *Dent Items Interest* 1:215, 1928.
19. Atirams H, Kopezyk R, Kaplan A: Incidence of anterior ridge deformities in partially edentulous patients, *J Prosthet Dent* 57:191, 1987.
20. Stein RS: Pontic-residual ridge relationship: a research report, *J Prosthet Dent* 16:251, 1966.
21. Langer B, Calagna L: The subepithelial connective tissue graft, *J Prosthet Dent* 44:363, 1980.
22. Hirshberg SM: The relationship of oral hygiene to embrasure and pontic design: a preliminary study, *J Prosthet Dent* 27:26, 1972.
23. Seibert IS, Cohen DW: Periodontal considerations in preparation for fixed and removable prosthodontics, *Dent Clin North Am* 31:529, 1987.
24. Heartwell CM, Rahn AO: *Syllabus of complete dentures*, ed 4, Philadelphia, 1986, Lea & Febiger.
25. Preston JD, Bergen SF: *Color science and dental art*, St Louis, 1980, Mosby.
26. Pincus CL: *Achieving the ultimate esthetic smile*, Proceedings of the Second International Congress of Prosthodontics, Las Vegas, Nev, Oct. 19-21, 1979.
27. Seide LJ, editor: *A dynamic approach to restorative dentistry*, Philadelphia, 1980, Saunders.
28. Pameijer JHN: *Periodontal and occlusal factors in crown and bridge procedures*, Amsterdam, 1985, Dental Centre for Postgraduate Courses.

Acrylic and Other Resins: Provisional Restorations

Paul R. Chalifoux

Achievement of esthetic and functional excellence in fixed prosthodontics is the reward for meticulous attention to detail at each stage of treatment. A high-quality provisional restoration is crucial to this success. The interim crown or fixed partial denture must be a mirror image of the definitive restoration, with the only variable being the material (Fig. 10-1A,B,C).

Failure to do so may result in periodontal damage, pulpal irritation, occlusal aberrations, and patient dissatisfaction.

BASIC CONCEPTS

The provisional (treatment) restoration provides for the following:

1. **Pulp protection and sedation of the prepared abutments while the definitive restorations are being fabricated.** An adequate thickness of provisional material and good marginal integrity affords protection against thermal insult and bacterial and salivary invasion of the dentinal tubules.
2. **Evaluation of the tooth preparation and parallelism of abutments.** Designing the treatment restoration to be similar to the definitive restoration gives the operator an immediate opportunity to assess (and correct if necessary) the tooth preparation for undercuts, adequate enamel/dentin reduction, and mutual paths of insertion.
3. **Immediate replacement of missing or extracted teeth.** The inclusion of pontics in the provisional restoration provides immediate replacements in edentulous spaces, which

aids in stabilizing and preventing drifting of abutments and opposing teeth and maintaining gingival architecture (Fig. 10-2).

4. **Improvement of esthetics in interrupted and debilitated dentitions.** The provisional restoration provides immediate coverage with an esthetic resin crown for maligned, eroded, discolored, poorly restored, and damaged abutments.
5. **A healthy environment for the periodontium.** Crowded and maligned abutments, overhanging margins of existing restorations, and areas of erosion or abrasion are replaced with properly contoured resin crowns compatible with periodontal health.
   - Provisional restorations maintain gingival position and health. Gingiva collapses onto subgingival tooth structure if it is not supported by a provisional restoration. Gingiva collapsed onto prepared tooth structure interferes with the insertion of a definitive restoration.
   - Proper contours and full extension to cover preparation margins maintains gingival health. Food impaction occurs when restorations are under contoured. Plaque accumulation and a lack of gingival stimulation creates inflammation when surfaces are over contoured. Open, short, porous, and rough margins also create gingival inflammation.
   - Proper interproximal contact is critical to papillae health. Contacts must be within 5mm of the crestal interproximal bone to maintain gingival papillae shape. Proper provisional restoration fit, shape, and polish further reduces chances of papillae inflammation.
6. **A means of evaluation and reinforcement of the patient's oral home care in maintaining an interim fixed restoration as a prerequisite to the permanent restoration.** The patient's dexterity and motivation may be inadequate to provide the meticulous daily preventive maintenance necessary

---

This chapter is partially based on the chapter, Acrylic and Other Resins: Provisional Restorations by David Federick, which appeared in the second edition of *Esthetic Dentistry: A Clinical Approach to Techniques and Materials.*

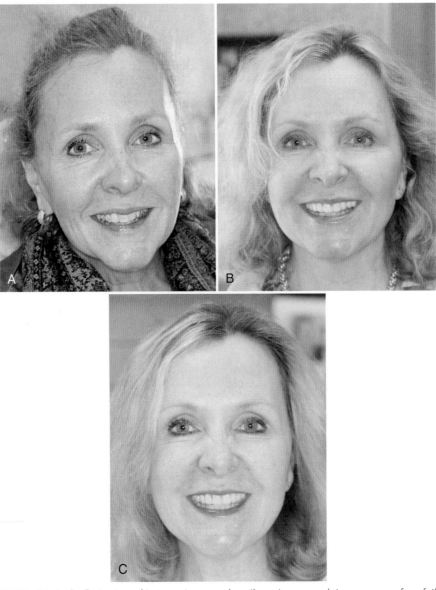

FIGURE 10-1 A, Patient seeking an improved smile using porcelain veneers after failed attempts at Invisalign. **B,** Provisional restorations provided a guide for definitive treatment. **C,** Patient's smile was improved with 10 porcelain veneers.

to care for a fixed partial denture. In these situations, placing a removable prosthesis may be prudent.

7. **Facilitation of periodontal therapy by providing access to and total visibility of surgical sites.** Removal of the provisional restoration gives the periodontist an unobstructed surgical field in which to perform soft and hard tissue corrective procedures.

8. **Stabilization of mobile teeth during and after periodontal therapy.** The splinting action of joining two or more teeth increases resistance to an applied force and offers a stabilizing effect and reorientation of stress vectors.[1] This action is important when fibers of the periodontal ligaments are in the process of reattaching to the cementum of a periodontally treated abutment. A tooth made stable by a splinting procedure may undergo a reinsertion of periodontal fibers, whereas a mobile abutment has little chance of reattachment.[2]

9. **Facilitation of development and evaluation of an occlusal scheme.** Various occlusal schemes and excursive guides can be evaluated by adding provisional materials to or removing provisional materials from the occlusion and contours of the provisional restoration.

10. **Evaluation of vertical dimension, phonetics, interocclusal distance, and esthetics.** The information gleaned during the alteration and finalization of the provisional restorations can be used to develop the subsequent definitive restorations.

11. **Aid in determining the prognosis of questionable teeth.** Changes in mobility patterns, osseous graft "takes," redefined lamina dura, periodontal ligament thickness, success of endodontic therapy, success of hemisection and bicuspidization procedures, pocket depth decreases, and alleviation of signs and symptoms of periodontal disease may be

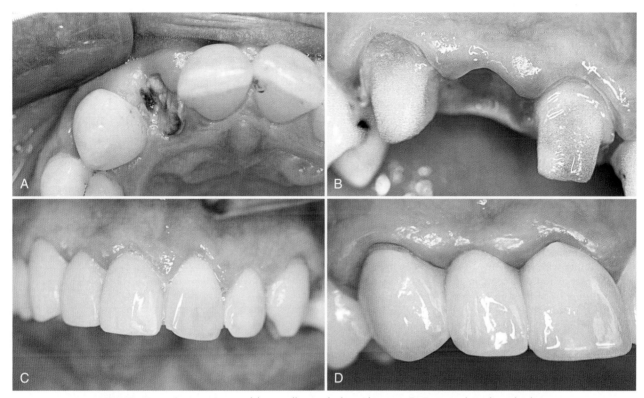

FIGURE 10-2 A, A nonrestorable maxillary right lateral incisor. **B,** Prepared teeth and edentulous area formed by a provisional restoration with an ovate pontic eight weeks post extraction. **C,** Three-unit heat processed provisional restoration controlling gingival contours. **D,** Definitive all-porcelain bridge.

determined during the provisional restorative phase of therapy. These factors aid the clinician in making decisions about retaining questionable abutments.

12. **Allow proper mastication.** Mastication is limited by provisional restoration strength and retention. Restorative materials must resist fracture and dislodgment during function. Forces on a provisional restoration are reduced by avoidance, chewing habits, protection from parafunctional forces, and food selection.

13. **Maintain adjacent, opposing, and abutment teeth position.** Proper provisional restoration occlusion, fit, and interproximal contacts prevent abutment, adjacent, and opposing teeth from shifting and supererupting.

REQUIREMENTS FOR A PROVISIONAL RESTORATION

The interim restoration must maintain gingival health. The basic requirements of a morphologically correct and physiologically acceptable provisional restoration are as follows:

1. **Marginal adaptation.** Marginal adaptation is achieved by careful attention to the details of the margins and reline/remargination procedures when applicable.

2. **Retention.** A provisional cement must always be used to ensure a barrier to intrusion of saliva and bacteria. Thick layers of cement do not correct a poorly made, ill-fitting provisional restoration.

   a. **Material strength and flexibility.** Retention is directly proportional to material strength and indirectly proportional to material flexibility. If applied force results in restoration flexing and breaking of the cement seal, it will dislodge.[3]

   b. **Preparation design.** Retention of a provisional restoration is indirectly proportional to degree of convergence of the walls of the preparation (i.e., less convergence creates greater retention) and directly proportional to the surface area. Cuts and boxes increase retention.

   c. **Cement strength.** Cement strength and cement to tooth and cement to provisional material interfaces strength affects retention. Provisional cements are designed to have weak mechanical strength, which when combined with the flexibility of provisional restorative materials allows for easy removal. However, the cement must be strong enough to resist displacement during reasonable function.

   d. **Displacement forces are affected by their duration, frequency, intensity, and direction.** A provisional restoration must withstand the test of time if an extended period of service becomes necessary. Clinical judgment is required to determine which cement is appropriate for a given clinical situation.

3. **Nonporous and dimensional stability.** A good grade of provisional material that is properly polymerized provides a superior restoration capable of extended service. Analysis of forces is critical to success. Forces of bruxism, which are 10 times normal forces, must be avoided. Construction of an interim night guard is required.

4. **Esthetics.** Attention to anatomic details encourages a patient's cooperation and acceptance of the provisional restoration.

5. **Physiologic contours and embrasures.** Adequate sluiceways and deflecting contours (that are not overcontoured) enhance the health of the periodontium.
6. **Ease of refinement.** Ease of refinement is especially important for a patient with a periodontal prosthesis whose provisional splint is fabricated and delivered before periodontal surgery. The healing periodontium usually exhibits controlled gingival recession for pocket elimination. The abutments must then be altered by apically extending the finishing lines and relining the original provisional splint to cover the newly exposed tooth surfaces.
7. **Biologic occlusion.** The occlusal scheme developed in the provisional restoration must include a stable centric occlusion, an acceptable vertical occlusion dimension, unobstructed excursive movements, and proper cusp-fossae development for efficient mastication.
8. **Compatibility with supporting tissues.** Rough, unpolished margins, overcontoured crowns, impinged embrasures, and a poor fit must be avoided in the provisional restoration to promote periodontal health.
9. **Ease of cleaning by the patient.** The patient must be able to maintain a plaque-free environment using routine preventive home care devices and techniques. Advise patients that extended use of chlorhexidine oral rinses stains provisional restorations.

CLINICAL TIP

A final layer (glaze) of the light-cured, unfilled methyl methacrylate resin (TempSpan Glaze) produces the best resistance to staining.

BASIC CHEMISTRY

Polymers used to produce provisional restorations are categorized by chemistry or method of cure. Method of cure includes chemical, heat, light or dual cure activated. Chemical categories of these polymers includes acrylic, composite resin, and polycarbonate. Polymer chemistry includes methacrylate resin (methylmethacrylate, ethylmethacrylate, vinyl methacrylate, butylmethacrylate) and composite resin (bis-GMA, bis-acryl, urethane dimethacrylate) (Table 10-1).

Auto-Cured Resin in Provisional Restorations

Acrylic polymers were introduced to dentistry in 1931. Polymethyl methacrylates are supplied in powder and liquid components. The powder (polymer) is polymethylmethacrylate plus benzoyl peroxide (initiator). The liquid (monomer) is methylmethacrylate plus hydroquinone (inhibitor). Other temporization materials are supplied in powder/liquid or paste/paste form.

Acrylics were difficult to use because the conversion of acrylic monomer to polymer resulted in 24.8% shrinkage. Shrinkage in plastics, in particular acrylics, occurs as a result of the difference between single molecule intermolecular van der Wall's distances of 4 angstroms and long chain molecules with intermolecular distances of 1.9 angstroms. Larger molecules and fillers such as prepolymerized particles reduced

Table 10-1 Provisional Crown and Bridge Resins: Selective Samples

Type	Brand	Manufacturer
Methyl methacrylate	Duralay	Reliance Dental Mfg. Co.
	Jet	Lang Dental Mfg. Co., Inc.
	Tab	Kerr Corp.
	Alike (radiopaque)	GC America
	Coldpac Trim Plus Temp Art Unifast, Unifast LC	Yates-Motloid Bosworth Co. Sultan Healthcare GC America
Ethyl methacrylate	Provisional Bridge Resin	Dentsply Caulk
	Splintline Lang	Lang Dental Mfg. Co.
Vinyl ethyl methacrylate	Snap	Parkell Inc
	Trim, Trim II	Bosworth Co.
	Dura-Seal	Reliance Dental Mfg. Co.
Bis-GMA (auto-cured)	Pro-Temp	Premier Dental Products
	Temphase	Kerr Corp.
	Luxatemp	DMG America
	Super-T	American Consolidated Mfg.
Bis-GMA (light polymerized)	Triad (light polymerized)	Dentsply Trubyte
	Isotemp (DC)	3M ESPE
	Astron LC (dual polymerized)	Astron Dental Corp.
Iso-butyl Bisacryl	Temp Plus Protemp Luxatemp Integrity Access Crown Protemp 3 Garant Ultra Trim Perfectemp Cool Temp Natural Fill-In, Temphase SmarTemp TempSpan Structure Systemp. C&B	Ellman International Inc. 3M ESPE DMG America Dentsply Caulk Centrix, Inc. 3M ESPE Bosworth Co. Discus Dental Coltène/Whaledent Kerr Corp. Parkell Inc. Pentron Clinical Voco GmbH Ivoclar Vivadent

shrinkage, thereby enhancing ease of use. Acrylic currently is packaged with a liquid (methyl methacrylate), which is mixed with a powder (polymethylmethacrylate) composed of prepolymerized particles. Acrylics are not used as fillings because they lead to pulpitis and periodontitis caused by their generation of heat during cure and acidic and porous properties.[4,5] Originally, non-bisGMA acrylic material was used for sealants, adhering orthodontic brackets to teeth and in denture prosthesis.

There are several variations of acrylics include polymethyl methacrylate, polyethyl methacrylate, polyvinyl methacrylate and isobutyl methacrylate.

The selection of an acrylic resin for crown and bridge temporization is based on many factors. Shade availability, handling ease, polymerization time, exothermic heat production, and anticipated length of service of the provisional restoration are major considerations. The operator may choose an extended putty stage resin to facilitate manipulations and may prefer a rapid-set resin for repairs. The properties of the various classes of acrylic resins available for crown and bridge temporization should be evaluated and compared before selection Table 10-2.[6]

Setting Stages of Auto-Cured Resin (Powder/Liquid)

1. **Doughy, or putty, stage.** In the doughy, or putty, stage a mixture of acrylic resin can be manipulated by hand, sticks to nonlubricated fingers, and has lost all surface gloss.
2. **Rubbery stage.** In the rubbery stage the resin is 60% to 70% set and can be removed from the mouth. The excess is easily trimmed with sharp scissors and immediately repositioned over the abutments for complete polymerization.

Light-Cured Composite Resin/Auto-Cured Composite Resin in Provisional Restorations

Dr. Rafael L. Bowen combined acrylic resins with epoxy and glass beads to produce an esthetic composite resin with good physical properties. BIS-GMA resin, a mixture of bisphenol A and glycidyl methacrylate diluted with glycol methacrylate was combined with glass beads to reduce shrinkage. The resulting composite resin proved to be hydrolytically unstable. Subsequently, combinations of resins and fillers, including several that cross-linked polymer chains such as triethylene glycol dimethacrylate and ethylene glycol dimethacrylate produced a successful dental composite resin.

Bis-GMA type restorative materials have definite applications in short-term crown and bridge temporization. Unlimited working time and favorable manipulative properties may make light-cured composite resins an alternative to conventional auto-cured crown and bridge resins. Bis-GMA provisional resins may also be used in the following situations:

1. For intraoral repair of fractured provisional fixed partial dentures
2. For reestablishing proximal and contact areas
3. For remargination procedures
4. For veneering conventional provisional crowns and bridges to provide an exceptionally esthetic and durable restoration

CLINICAL TIP

When auto-cured or light-cured composite resins or both are used in the previously mentioned applications, a primer layer of bonding primer should be placed on the polymethyl methacrylate to be repaired or veneered.

Bisacryl. Bisacryls are resin composites and are the new generation of composite provisional materials. There are several versions of dual activated, light activated or chemically activated. They are filled with glass fillers, which improve physical characteristics, are easier to work with, strong, odorless, dimensionally stable, esthetically pleasing, exhibit minimal shrinkage and heat generation and can be fiber reinforced. Bisacryls are packaged in a paste-paste formulation, which is mixed in a double barrel gun with a mixing tip. It undergoes a 3-stage polymerization reaction. The first phase is a free-flowing paste that becomes elastic within 60 to 75 seconds. The second phase is a cross-linking polymerization reaction allowing the polymer to reach a high compressive strength. A final phase of polymerization allows the resin to reach its final hardness within 5 minutes after initial mixing so the restoration can be adjusted and polished before cementation.

Bisacryl materials are highly oxygen inhibited. Outer layers should be removed prior to finishing and polishing by wiping with an alcohol gauze.

Polycarbonate. Polycarbonate is a plastic used to construct orthodontic brackets, denture bases, and prefabricated provisional crowns (Table 10-3). It is synthesized from Bisphenol A and is a very strong and highly esthetic material, ideal for anterior use. Polycarbonate anterior and premolar crowns of various sizes are relined and can be added to or reduced.

CLINICAL TIP

A polycarbonate preformed crown is selected when maximum strength is required, the tooth resembles the shape of the polycarbonate crown and approximates a Vita A2 shade (VITA classical Shade Guide, Vident).

Aluminum and Stainless Steel. Aluminum and stainless steel crowns (see Table 10-3) are most often used for long-term temporization of severely structurally compromised primary teeth. They are not esthetic, which limits use for teeth that are not visible in the facial display. Stainless steel crowns are used for long-term temporization but they are difficult to adapt and fit. Aluminum is soft and therefore easy to fit and adjust but wears quickly.

Heat Processed Resin. Heat processed resin provisional restorations are fabricated in the dental laboratory. They are constructed on models of prepared teeth or on study models of pre-preparation teeth, which are subsequently prepared by the laboratory technician. They are then directly relined by the clinician. The laboratory procedure requires creating teeth in wax, investing into a mold, melting out the wax, placing resin into the mold and heating, usually by boiling overnight. The resin is divested, trimmed, shaped, and polished. In advanced techniques, preformed facial shells or facings are placed onto facial surfaces.

Combinations of Materials. Materials can be combined. Composite resin is veneered over provisional restorations to improve appearance. Material is added to cover margins, alter tooth dimension, create proper occlusion, or clinically reline provisionals for proper fit.

Table 10-2 Properties of Acrylic Resins for Provisional Restorations

Material	Curing Shrinkage	Strength	Exothermic Heat	Stiffness	Reline and Repair Strength	Color Stability	Stain Resistance	Polishability	Abrasion Resistance	Cost
Polymethyl methacrylate	Medium	High	High	High	Excellent	High	High	High	Medium-high	Low
Polyethyl methacrylate										
Polyvinyl methacrylate	Medium	Medium-high	Medium-high	Medium	Excellent	Medium-high	Medium-high	Medium-high	Medium	Low
Isobutyl methacrylate	Medium	Medium	Medium	Medium	Excellent	Medium	Medium	Medium	Medium	Low
Bis-GMA composite resins (auto-cured)	Low	Medium	Low	Medium (brittle)	Poor	Medium	Low-medium	Medium-high	Medium	High
Bis-GMA (dual cured or light cured)	Low	Medium	Low	Medium (brittle)	Poor	Medium-high	Low-medium	Medium-high	Medium	High

Table 10-3 **Preformed Crowns and Crown Forms**

Type	Brand	Manufacturer
Polycarbonate	ION Crown (anterior and premolar)	3M ESPE
	Polycarbonate Crowns	Directa AB
	B-Crowns (anterior)	Bosworth Co.
	Molar-B-Crowns (posterior)	Bosworth Co.
	Alu-Plast (tooth color, posterior) Polycarbonate Crowns Polycarbonate Crowns Polycarbonate Crowns	Hahnenkratt GmbH JS Dental Manufacturing, Inc. Solodent Scott's Dental Supply
Plastic/acetate	Caulk Crown Forms	Dentsply Caulk
	Strip Crowns	Henry Schein, Inc.
	Directa Coform	JS Dental Manufacturing, Inc.
	Odus Pella 3M Strip Crown Kit	E.C. Moore Co., Inc. 3M ESPE
Metal	Aluminum Crowns	Parkell Inc.
	ISOFORM (posterior)	3M ESPE
	Unitek Crowns	3M ESPE
	Gold Anodized	3M ESPE
	Temgold-Gold Anodized Aluminum Crowns	DSC Dental Supply Co.
	Stainless Steel and Aluminum Aluminum Shell Crowns Stainless steel crowns	Denovo Dental, Inc. Integra Miltex Acero XT Store

GENERAL TECHNIQUES

Provisional restorations can be fabricated directly intraorally without a matrix (direct technique), using a preformed matrix made on study models and then formed intraorally (indirect direct technique), or completely fabricated on prepared models and/or then relined intraorally (indirect technique).

1. **Direct placement.** Acrylics, polycarbonate, celluloid forms, composite resins (chemical, light, or dual cure)—Preferred material: chemical cure acrylic

   Direct placement fabricates provisional restorations directly on teeth. Direct techniques include the block technique, veneering using a preformed shell such as polycarbonate crowns, metal preformed crowns, and celluloid forms.

   A block technique usually uses acrylic, which is mixed to a doughy consistency, squeezed over the teeth, and repeatedly placed and removed during setting to disengage uncorrected undercuts. A dentist must be able to manually manipulate the material, apply it to a tooth, produce a general shape and remove it, which limits materials

such as bisacryl and many composite resins. Bisacryl and composite materials remain in a fluid state, which makes manipulation impossible without a matrix. There are occasions for which composite can be hand built and shaped. The resulting restoration is trimmed, shaped, and polished. (See Acrylic Block technique later in this chapter.)

2. **Direct matrix.** All polymers—Preferred: Bisacryl

   Direct matrix involves fabrication a provisional restoration intraorally using a preformed matrix. A plaster model is not required to form the matrix. Missing tooth structure is restored on a temporary basis with a restorative material such as an acrylic or bisGMA composite resin. (Fig. 10-3A)

   A matrix is formed by placing impression material in a full, quadrant, or triple tray. Irreversible hydrocolloid is the most common impression material used but other materials such as vinyl polysiloxane can be used. It provides adequate accuracy and is inexpensive compared to other impression materials. Irreversible hydrocolloid impressions are wrapped in a wet paper towel or placed in a humid environment to avoid moisture loss and distortion. Vinyl polysiloxane (silicone), polyether, or rubber base impression materials provide ease of use and a quick technique (Fig. 10-3B,C). After tooth preparation, provisional restorative material such as bisacryl (or acrylic) is placed into an impression and the impression is reseated intraorally. Upon initial set of the provisional restorative material, usually about 60 seconds for bisacryl, the impression is removed and the material is allowed to harden. When using acrylic, an impression is moved up and down every 15 seconds to minimize engagement of undercuts and removed after 2 minutes.

   The provisional restoration is trimmed, shaped, and polished (see Fig. 10-3C).

> ### CLINICAL TIP
>
> When making the impression, note the location of the tooth, which is closest to but not included in, the impression. Use this tooth as a reference when subsequently reseating the impression loaded with the provisional material.

   Acrylic is difficult to use in an impression matrix as undercuts on adjacent teeth lock the material into position if it is not removed before setting. Setting time of acrylic varies depending on the mixture and temperatures of surrounding areas.

   As an alternative technique, a putty impression is made as a sectional impression with no tray and then relined with a syringable vinyl polysiloxane (silicone) impression (e.g., Aquasil, Dentsply International) material to form a matrix. The matrix is formed with a patient in an open or occluding position.

3. **Indirect Direct Matrix.** All Polymers—Preferred: Acrylic, Bisacryl

   Indirect direct matrix procedures are completed in a dental office or in a dental laboratory. (Fig. 10-4A). A missing maxillary first molar will be replaced with a three unit

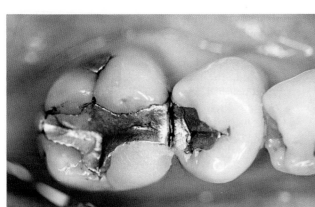
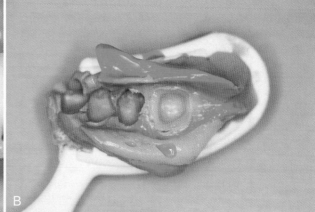
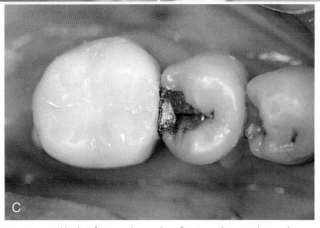

FIGURE 10-3 A, A mandibular first molar with a fractured mesiolingual cusp is provisionally restored with composite resin before fabricating a silicone matrix in a Triple Tray (Premier Dental Products). **B,** Triple Tray impression with 60 second cured bisacryl provisional restoration immediately after removal from the mouth. **C,** The final bisacryl provisional restoration.

fixed partial denture. A study model is prepared, a tooth added in the edentulous space and the teeth restored to ideal contours for construction of a matrix.

A matrix is formed indirectly on a study model. A provisional restorative material is placed in the matrix, which is then placed directly over prepared teeth.

An impression is made and used at the time of, or prior to, a patient appointment. For situations in which teeth are structurally deficient or teeth are missing, a prosthetic tooth, wax, composite resin, clay, or similar material is added to the model to restore teeth. A matrix is fabricated on the model and then used to form the provisional restoration intraorally.

When diagnostic wax ups are completed on mounted models, an impression is made of the model and a duplicate model produced (forming a matrix on a model with diagnostic wax ups may damage the wax up). A duplicate model is used for fabrication of the matrix. (Fig. 10-4B).

It is difficult to replicate detail with a vinyl vacuum thermoplastic matrix. It is easy to reproduce detail with a high quality impression material. Attention to detail in producing a model and detailed matrix results in a provisional restoration, which requires little to no adjustment.

Dental laboratory heat processed resin provisional restorations are strong and very esthetic. They are constructed as a shell on study models prepared by a laboratory technician leaving space for intra-oral relining.

4. **Indirect.** All Polymers—Preferred Acrylic, Heat processed resin, Bisacryl

Indirect provisional restorations are fabricated on models and can be completed in a dental laboratory or a dental office (Figs. 10-4C,D).

When a provisional restoration is fabricated in a dental office during a patient appointment, a regular or fast set plaster is used to pour a model of the prepared teeth. A matrix is formed on a pre-preparation study model or diagnostic wax up, filled with provisional restorative material and placed onto a model of prepared teeth. (Figs. 10-5A-D)

The provisional restoration is cured, shaped and finished. (Fig. 10-5E)

It is ready to be tried in intraorally, adjusted and cemented. (Fig. 10-5F)

The provisional restoration is a map to replicate in the definitive restorations. (Fig. 10-5G).

An indirect technique, dental laboratory fabricated provisional restoration, is constructed of heat processed resin to maximize

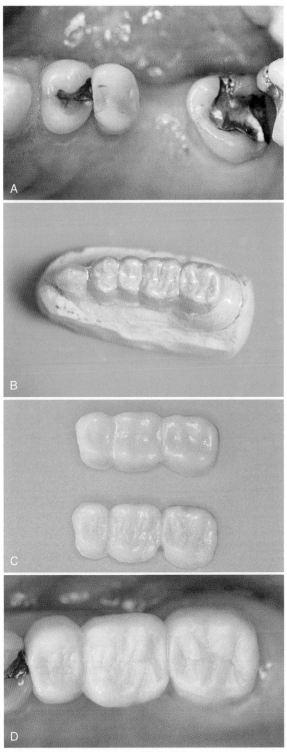

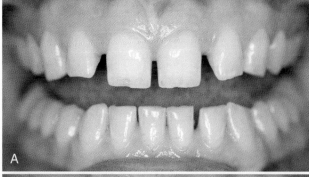

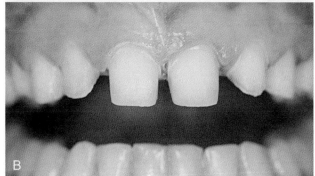

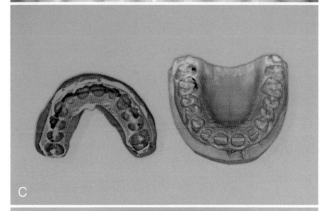

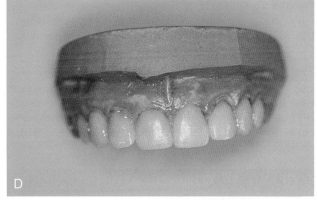

FIGURE 10-4 A, A missing maxillary first molar will be restored with a three unit fixed partial denture. **B,** A vinyl vacuum formed thermoplastic matrix on a plaster cast. The cast was fabricated from an impression of a diagnostic wax tooth replacement on the original study model. **C,** The maxillary provisional restoration with little detail was formed with a vinyl vacuum formed thermoplastic matrix. The detailed mandibular provisional restoration was formed with a silicone matrix. **D,** The final provisional restoration was fabricated using a silicone matrix and required minimal finishing.

FIGURE 10-5 A, Multiple diastemata and small teeth will be restored with bonded porcelain. **B,** Final teeth preparations. **C,** Putty silicone matrix fabricated from a diagnostic wax up and an impression of the prepared teeth. **D,** Provisional restoration on a model of prepared teeth after removal from the matrix.
Continued

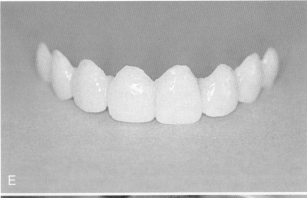

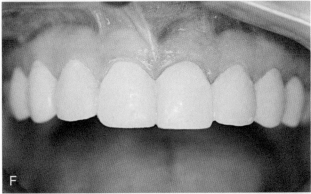

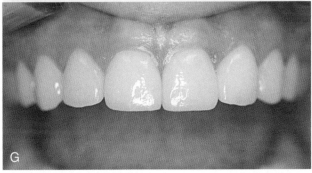

FIGURE 10-5, cont'd E, The provisional restoration after minor finishing, polishing and glazing. **F,** The provisional restoration cemented. **G,** Definitive bonded all-porcelain restorations.

strength and esthetics. It is formed on models of prepared teeth from a definitive impression. These restorations are commonly used during extensive periodontal treatment, evaluation of questionable teeth, or long-term evaluation of opened vertical dimension.

CLINICAL TIP

The matrix must be stable when used intraorally. Extend the matrix one to two teeth beyond the prepared teeth and cover 2 to 3 mm of gingival tissues. Create larger coverage of the gingival tissue if there are no teeth adjacent to the prepared teeth.

CLINICIAL TECHNIQUES

There are many techniques and materials used to construct provisional restorations (Tables 10-4 to 10-7). A restorative

Table 10-4 Miscellaneous Materials and Devices

Brand	Manufacturer
Identic Syringable Impression System	Dux Dental
Burlew Dry Foil	Jelenko
Aquapres	Lang Dental Mfg. Co., Inc.
Triad VLC System	Dentsply Trubyte
Metal/Mesh Reinforcing Bars	Ellman International Inc.
Hand Instruments	3M ESPE
Perfectone Molds	George Taub Products
Novatech Collection	Hu-Friedy Mfg. Co.
Flexible Dappen Dish	George Taub Products
Acrylic Provisional Adjustment & Polishing Kit	Brasseler USA
Titanium Alloy Provisional Posts	Coltene/Whaledent

Table 10-5 Crown Removers

Brand	Manufacturer
Kline Crown Remover	Brasseler USA
Baade Pliers	S.S. White
Wynman Crown Gripper	Premier Dental Products
Morrell Crown Remover	Premier Dental Products
Crown Remover	Ellman International Inc. Mfg.
Automatic Crown Removers	J.S. Dental Manufacturing, Inc.
Richwil Crown and Bridge Remover Metalift Crown and Bridge Removal System CORONAflex	Almore International, Inc. Metalift KaVo Dental V

Table 10-6 Indicating Pastes and Moisturizing Lubricants (Liquid)

Brand	Manufacturer
High Spot (spray)	Dux Dental
Mizzy (spray)	Buffalo Dental Manufacturing Co., Inc.
Crown & Bridge Lube	Dux Dental
Masque	Bosworth Co.

Table 10-7 **Stent Formers**

Type	Brand	Laboratory
Vacuum	Vacuum Forming Unit	Patterson Dental Supply Co.
	StaVac	Buffalo Dental Manufacturing Co., Inc.
	Pro Form Vacuum Form	Keystone Industries
Manual	Press-Form Kit	Ellman International Inc.

situation and dentist preferences dictate which materials and techniques are used. Selection of material and technique is based on the ability to maximize esthetics, strength, ease of construction, longevity, cost, and retention. It is prudent to consider the location and number of teeth, missing teeth, and the forces that will be applied (Box 10-1).

Preformed Crowns and Crown Forms

An acceptable interim restoration can be produced using polycarbonate, a celluloid strip, or metallic crowns. Although this procedure may result in gingival abuse if improperly performed, a cautious clinician who allots adequate time for the procedure can produce a serviceable restoration.

Polycarbonate Crowns (Anterior Teeth and Premolars)

To achieve adequate retention, fit, and physiologic contours, the preformed crown must be altered, relined, trimmed, and polished before cementation.

Armamentarium
- Standard dental setup
  Cotton rolls
  Dappen dish (silicone)
  Explorer
  High-speed handpiece
  Low-speed handpiece
  Mouth mirror

Box 10-1
Preferred Techniques in Various Situations

Single Anterior Tooth
Polycarbonate, Composite resin Veneered, Bisacryl
Multiple Anterior Teeth
Laboratory Constructed, Matrixed Bisacryl, Polycarbonate
Single Posterior Tooth
Matrixed Bisacryl, Acrylic Block Technique
Multiple Posterior Teeth
Matrixed Bisacryl, Acrylic Block, Laboratory
Missing Teeth
Anterior
Laboratory Constructed, Matrixed Bisacryl
Posterior
Laboratory Constructed, Matrixed Bisacryl

Periodontal probe
2″ × 2″ gauze
Crown and bridge scissors (Brasseler USA)
- Petroleum jelly (e.g., Vaseline petroleum jelly, Unilever, Inc.) or silicone gel (e.g., Silicone V Lubricant, V Lubricant, Inc.)
- Acrylic resin of choice (see Table 10-1)
- Polycarbonate crown kit (3M ESPE)
- Polycarbonate crown mold guide
- Boley gauge (optional) (Henry Schein, Inc.)
- No. ½ Hollenback carver
- Acrylic bur setup low-speed straight handpiece
  Low-speed tapered carbide bur—rounded tip, 4-mm base (e.g., H79E-040 carbide "E" cutter, Brasseler USA)
  Low-speed tapered carbide bur—rounded tip, 2.3-mm base (e.g., H261D-023 carbide "D" cutter, Brasseler USA)
  Low-speed diamond bur—pointed tip 3.7-mm base (e.g., 852-037 medium grit diamond, Brasseler USA)
  Low-speed round carbide bur—rounded (No. 10) tip, 2.7-mm head (e.g., H 1-027 carbide cutter, Brasseler USA)
  Low-speed straight carbide bur—flat (No. 557) tip, 1-mm base (e.g., H31-010 carbide cutter, Brasseler USA)
  Low-speed inverted cone carbide bur—flat (No. 34) tip, 0.8-mm base (e.g., H2-008 carbide cutter, Brasseler USA)
- Acrylic finishing setup. See the section on Finishing and Polishing in this chapter.
- Shade correction setup (optional). See the section on Color Correction and Shade Characterization in this chapter.
- Provisional cementation setup. See the section on Cementation in this chapter.

Clinical Technique
1. Select the correct size crown from the kit. A mold guide or Boley gauge facilitates the selection (Figs. 10-6A-C).
2. Adjust the crown gingivally and proximally with a low-speed diamond or carbide bur (e.g., H79E040, H261D023, 852037, Brasseler USA), and remove a thin layer of internal acrylic with a handpiece round bur (02710, Brasseler USA) so that it fits over the prepared tooth and does not bind.
3. Protect the dentin and adjacent soft tissue with a layer of petroleum jelly or silicone liquid.
4. Fill the crown shell with a mixture of acrylic resin. Wait until the surface monomer dissipates (i.e., the surface sheen disappears), and then carefully seat it on the preparation. As a guide to proper seating, note that the incisal edge or occlusal surface relates correctly to the adjacent teeth.

CLINICAL TIP

For easier cleanup, use a rubber or silicone dappen dish instead of glass. (Acrylic does not stick to rubber or silicone.)

5. When the reline acrylic resin achieves the rubbery stage, trim excess away from the margin with a No. ½ Hollenback carver.

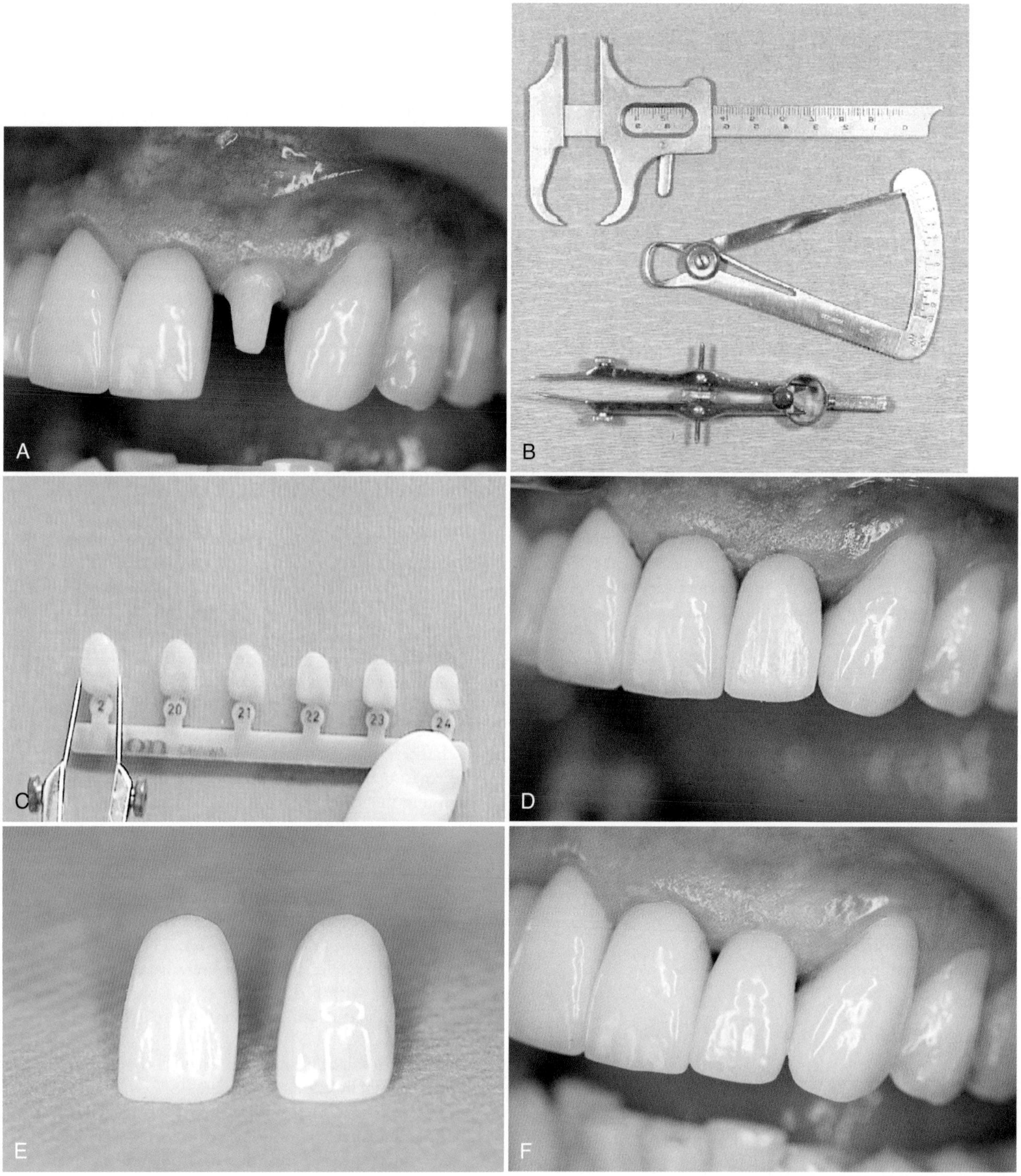

FIGURE 10-6 A, A maxillary left lateral incisor is prepared to accept an all-porcelain crown. **B,** Gauges used to compare the space between the central incisor and the canine and the width of polycarbonate shells. **C,** A gauge set to the width of the lateral incisor space in order to compare the widths of the lateral incisors on a polycarbonate mold guide. **D,** The relined polycarbonate provisional restoration cemented on the prepared tooth. **E,** The polycarbonate provisional restoration (left) and the definitive all-porcelain crown should be virtually indistinguishable. **F,** The all-porcelain crown cemented on the prepared tooth.

While the acrylic is setting, remove and replace the provisional crown. This will accomplish the following:
1. Protect the tooth from the exothermic reaction of the setting resin.
2. Prevent the provisional crown from locking into undercuts of adjacent teeth.
3. Prevent the provisional crown from locking onto resin core material.

6. Remove the unit when the reline material has set.
7. Trim and smooth.
8. Reline or remarginate if necessary. See the section on Remargination in this chapter.
9. Finish and polish the restoration. See the section on finishing in the chapter.
10. Custom stain or characterize if necessary. See the section on Color Correction and Shade Characterization in this chapter.
11. Cement (Fig. 10-6D). See the section on Cementation of provisional restorations in this chapter.
   The provisional restoration should resemble the anticipated definitive restoration (Figs. 10-6E,F).

Celluloid (Clear) Strip Crown (Anterior Teeth and Premolars)

Armamentarium
+ Standard Dental Setup. See the section on Preformed Crowns and Crown Forms in this chapter.
+ Petroleum jelly (e.g., Vaseline petroleum jelly, Unilever, Inc.) or silicone gel (e.g., Silicone V Lubricant, V Lubricant, Inc.)
+ Acrylic resin of choice (see Table 10-1).
+ Celluloid crown kit (3M ESPE)
+ Boley gauge (optional)
+ Crown and bridge scissors (e.g., No. 325, Brasseler USA)
+ No. ½ Hollenback carver
+ Acrylic bur setup. See the section on Preformed Crowns and Crown Forms in this chapter.
+ Acrylic finishing setup. See the section on finishing procedures in this chapter.
+ Shade correction setup (optional). See the section on Color Correction and Shade Characterization in this chapter.
+ Provisional cementation setup. See the section on cementation of provisional restorations in this chapter.
   Clinical Technique. The clinical technique is similar to that described for polycarbonate crowns with the following exceptions:
1. Trim the appropriate strip crown with scissors to achieve the correct length.
2. Perforate the incisal edge with an explorer, and open the proximal surfaces with a #6 round bur so that the acrylic resin establishes proximal contacts.
3. After the acrylic resin has set, remove the restoration, cut away the celluloid shell.

Acrylic Block Technique

The acrylic block technique involves freehand carving of an acrylic block constructed directly on abutments. Acrylic is mixed to a smooth, firm, doughy consistency, pressed over the prepared teeth, relined for an accurate fit, and hand shaped. In a rubbery stage, it is removed and trimmed with scissors. It is repeatedly removed and replaced until polymerization is complete. The acrylic block technique is quick and effective but requires training and experience.

Mix acrylic powder into liquid until all powder is wet. To create a doughy stage, mix powder and liquid to a firm flowing consistency and let it sit for 1 to 2 minutes. It will thicken to a doughy phase without becoming granular (which will occur if excess powder is added).

Armamentarium
+ Standard Dental Setup. See the section on Preformed Crowns and Crown Forms in this chapter.
+ Petroleum jelly (e.g., Vaseline petroleum jelly, Unilever, Inc.) or silicone gel (e.g., Silicone V Lubricant, V Lubricant, Inc.)
+ Acrylic resin of choice (see Table 10-1)
+ Impression material: irreversible hydrocolloid or silicone impression material
+ No. 15 scalpel
+ Acrylic bur setup. See the section on Preformed Crowns and Crown Forms in this chapter.
+ Acrylic finishing setup. See the section on finishing procedures in this chapter.
+ Shade correction setup (optional). See the section on Color Correction and Shade Characterization in this chapter.
+ Provisional cementation setup. See the section on cementation of provisional restorations in this chapter.

Clinical Technique
1. Match tooth color to an acrylic shade guide.

Acrylic may not match a stock shade guide so a custom shade guide is constructed.

2. Mix and place acrylic into a mold of a tooth. A tooth mold is constructed by making an impression of an existing shade tab.
3. Add a stick to hold the new acrylic shade tab. Use a toothpick, shaft from a cotton swab, and so on.

Teeth lighten when dehydrated, so shade matching is completed before tooth preparation.

4. Prepare teeth to accept a definitive restoration.
5. Place gingival retraction cord if a tooth preparation extends subgingivally.
6. Coat prepared teeth and adjacent soft tissues with petroleum jelly or silicone.
7. Mix the acrylic of choice by adding small increments of powder to liquid. Mix until it is a doughy consistency.
8. Roll the acrylic into a ball or shape to approximate the size of the tooth or teeth to be constructed.

9. Press the acrylic onto the prepared teeth.
10. Have the patient close onto the acrylic to establish a proper occlusion dimension.
11. While the acrylic is seated on the tooth, press the facial and lingual surfaces. This avoids lifting of material.
12. Remove the acrylic from the teeth and trim excess material with scissors.
13. Mix and place a thin layer of acrylic into the teeth side of the provisional while in the doughy phase and reseat it over the teeth.
14. Move the acrylic up and down every 10 to 20 seconds to disengage acrylic from any possible undercuts on the prepared and the adjacent teeth.
15. Remove the acrylic when heat is first generated. At this point, it feels warm.

Allow it to completely cure extraorally. Placing it in hot water will decrease the curing time. The acrylic will feel hard when completely cured. Although the heat generated from the curing acrylic of the first mix accelerates cure of reline material, the reline acrylic (step 13 above) placed inside the provisional restoration will remain soft longer than the original acrylic (Figs. 10-7A-C).

CLINICAL TIP

Run water over a ball of acrylic if it is sticky.

CLINICAL TIP

Place a provisional into hot water to accelerate its cure.

CLINICAL TIP

Coating a provisional with petroleum jelly reduces porosity from exposure to air. Place petroleum jelly when initial heat from the curing reaction is felt.

16. When the acrylic has completely cured, trim it with acrylic burs.
    a. Trim excess acrylic on the facial, lingual, mesial, and distal to the margins.
    b. Shape the facial, lingual, and interproximal contours with acrylic trimming burs and sandpaper disks.

CLINICAL TIP

Do not touch the contact areas.

CLINICAL TIP

When trimming various contours of a provisional restoration, look from various directions to observe contours. Depth perception is difficult when observing from one direction.

    c. For posterior teeth, shape the occlusal surfaces beginning with the external surfaces of the cusps and the ridges forming the perimeter of the occlusal table.
    d. Form a central cut in the center of the occlusal surface with a pointed acrylic bur.
    e. Form the facial and lingual cuts with a pointed acrylic bur.
    f. Round between the cuts and form the secondary cuts (Fig. 10-7D).
17. Polish the acrylic provisional restoration with a rag wheel on a lathe using fine pumice to create the definitive contours. The edge of the rag wheel polishes cuts; the flat surface of the rag wheel polishes large surfaces such as the facial and lingual contours (Figs. 10-7E, F).
18. Isolate the teeth with cotton rolls, wash and gently dry leaving the teeth slightly moist.

CLINICAL TIP

Overdrying will incorporate air into dentinal tubules causing sensitivity.

19. Mix the cement and place a layer inside the provisional restoration.
20. Place the restoration onto the prepared teeth and press it into position.
21. Remove excess cured cement with an explorer and floss.
22. Check and adjust the occlusion.

CLINICAL TIP

Acrylic "catches" in diamond burs so carbide burs are preferred for adjusting.

23. Polish the adjusted provisional restoration.

Direct Preparation/Impression Technique

The use of an impression as a matrix is the most popular method of positioning polymerizing polymers over tooth preparations to produce a multiunit provisional splint. Any elastic impression material in a stock impression tray or in putty materials is acceptable. Either the direct or the indirect method may be performed.

Armamentarium
- Standard Dental Setup. See the section on Preformed Crowns and Crown Forms in this chapter.
- Petroleum jelly (e.g., Vaseline petroleum jelly, Unilever, Inc.) or silicone gel (e.g., Silicone V Lubricant, V Lubricant, Inc.)
- Polymer of choice
- Impression material: irreversible hydrocolloid or silicone impression material
- No. 15 scalpel
- Acrylic bur setup. See the section on Preformed Crowns and Crown Forms in this chapter.
- Acrylic finishing setup. See the section on finishing procedures in this chapter.
- Shade correction setup (optional). See the section on Color Correction and Shade Characterization in this chapter.
- Provisional cementation setup. See the section on cementation of provisional restorations in this chapter.

Clinical Technique
1. Make an impression of the unprepared abutments using irreversible hydrocolloid or silicone impression material intraorally the mouth or on a study model (Figs. 10-8A-C).

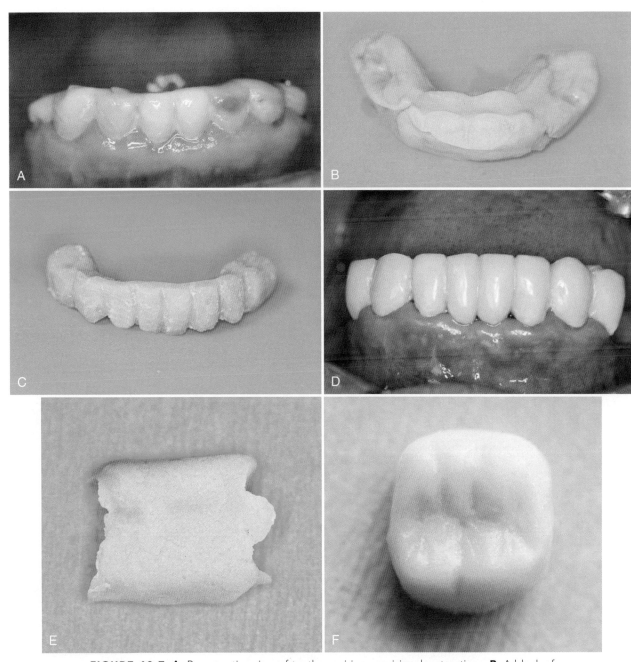

FIGURE 10-7 A, Preoperative view of teeth requiring provisional restorations. **B,** A block of acrylic positioned on the prepared teeth was removed and initially trimmed with scissors while in a rubbery stage. **C,** The acrylic provisional restoration after initial contouring with acrylic burs. **D,** Single tooth acrylic block technique immediately after removal from a prepared mandibular first molar. **E,** The acrylic provisional restoration four weeks after immediate restoration of extracted teeth #21, 24, 25, and 28. **F,** Acrylic block provisional restoration after shaping and polishing.

2. Remove unnecessary elastic material from the impression (e.g., interproximal tags, border extensions) to make reseating easier.
3. Store until tooth preparation is completed.
4. Prepare teeth (Fig. 10-8D).
5. Protect the prepared abutments with petroleum jelly or silicone emulsion if acrylic is used.
6. Pour a mixture of acrylic resin into the impression and when no sheen is present, carefully insert the impression to ensure full and accurate seating over the preparations. If bisacryl is used, mix and place immediately.
7. Remove the splint at the rubbery stage, and trim any excess resin with sharp scissors.
8. Return the splint to the impression and position the tray over the preparations.
9. When fully set, remove the splint and finish in the usual manner (Fig. 10-8E).

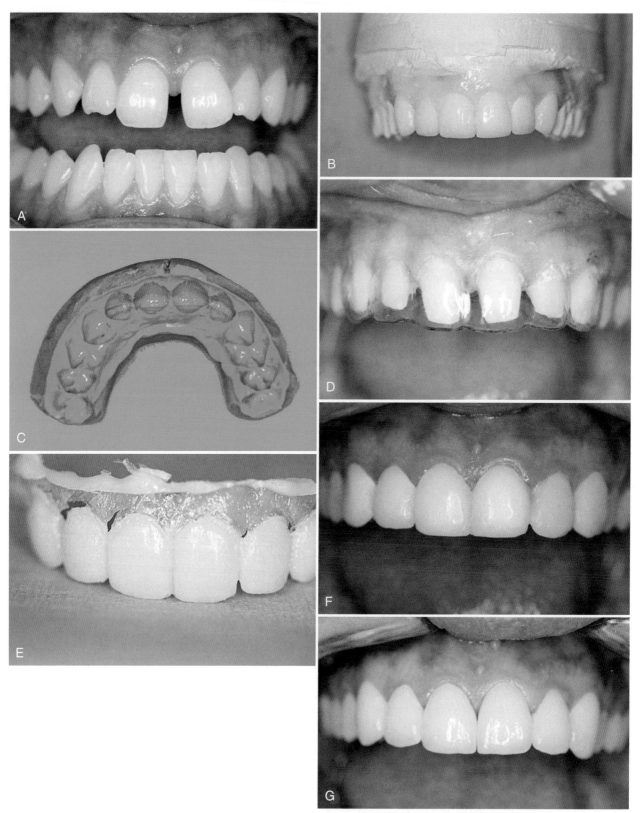

FIGURE 10-8 A, Anterior teeth with large diastemata. Severe wear of the lateral incisors combined with anterior teeth spacing will be restored with bonded porcelain. **B,** A diagnostic wax-up used to confirm treatment. A silicone matrix is formed on a duplicate cast. **C,** The putty silicone matrix. **D,** Vinyl vacuum-formed thermoplastic matrix tried on prepared teeth to evaluate for adequate reduction. **E,** The untrimmed bisacryl provisional restoration removed from the matrix after being formed directly over the prepared teeth. **F,** The provisional restoration cemented on the prepared teeth. **G,** The definitive bonded porcelain restorations on the six anterior teeth.

10. Reline or remarginate if necessary. See the section on Remargination in this chapter.
11. Finish and polish the restoration. See the section on finishing procedures in this chapter.
12. Custom stain or characterize if necessary. See the section on Color Correction and Shade Characterization in this chapter.
13. Cement. See the section on Cementation of provisional restorations in this chapter (Figs. 10-8*F*, *G*).

Composite Resin Veneered Anterior Restorations

Composite resin veneered over the facial surface of a provisional restoration provides maximum esthetics. The technique is preferred over a polycarbonate provisional when a tooth is substantially different in color than a Vita A2 shade or significantly different in shape from a preformed shell.

There are two veneering techniques:
1. A provisional restoration is constructed of a polymer material in the usual manner. The facial surface is reduced using an acrylic bur, sandpaper disk, or diamond bur depending on the material. A correct shade of composite resin is selected, applied over the facial surface, and finished.

2. Composite resin can be placed into a matrix to form the facial surface first (Fig. 10-9*A*).
   A matrix with uncured composite resin on the facial aspect is tried onto prepared teeth to ensure composite resin clearance. The matrix is removed from the mouth and the composite resin is light cured.

CLINICAL TIP

When a matrix is clear vinyl, the composite resin is polymerized from the outside while seated on the prepared teeth. Coat areas of composite resin that are part of a prepared tooth to prevent veneering composite from adhering. When a matrix is not clear, the composite resin is cured for 20 seconds extraorally, aiming the light at the internal surface of the matrix. It is best to have space between the composite resin and prepared teeth surfaces. If composite resin is against the prepared teeth, press it with a composite instrument to create a gap. If there is a large amount of composite resin such that it is extending into interproximal areas, remove some composite, press, and reseat. Do this several times if necessary to create a gap.

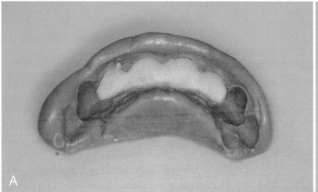
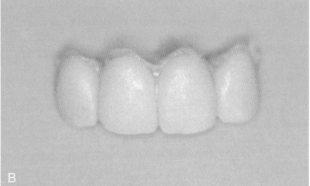
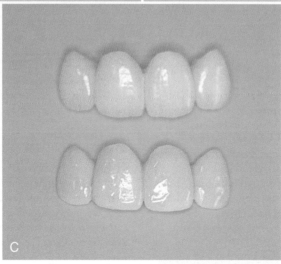

FIGURE 10-9 A, A silicone matrix filled on the facial surfaces with composite resin will be evaluated intraorally to ensure clearance with prepared teeth, removed, and light cured. **B,** The composite resin faced provisional restoration immediately after relining on the abutments. **C,** The composite resin veneered provisional restoration (*bottom*) which served as a guide for the definitive splinted all-porcelain crowns (*top*).

Cured composite resin is not washed or disturbed to maintain an oxygen inhibited layer, which joins to relining materials. It is important to have space between composite resin and a prepared tooth surface so there is room for reline material.

It is important to have space between composite resin and a prepared tooth surface so there is room for reline material.

The matrix containing the cured composite resin is then filled with acrylic or bisacryl and placed over the prepared teeth. The provisional restoration is removed, trimmed, polished and fit (Figs. 10-9B,C).

Armamentarium
+ Standard Dental Setup. See the section on Preformed Crowns and Crown Forms in this chapter.
+ Petroleum jelly (e.g., Vaseline petroleum jelly, Unilever, Inc.) or silicone gel (e.g., Silicone V Lubricant, V Lubricant, Inc.)
+ Polymer of choice
+ Impression material: irreversible hydrocolloid or silicone impression material
+ No. 15 scalpel
+ Acrylic bur setup. See the section on Preformed Crowns and Crown Forms in this chapter.
+ Acrylic finishing setup. See the section on finishing procedures in this chapter.
+ Soft Flex disks (3M ESPE)
+ 7901 Midwest bur
+ Shade correction setup (optional). See the section on Color Correction and Shade Characterization in this chapter.
+ Provisional cementation setup. See the section on cementation of provisional restorations in this chapter.

Clinical Technique: First Technique
1. Select an appropriate shade using a shade guide matching the selected composite resin (Fig. 10-10A).
   a. Materials may not match a stock shade guide so a custom shade guide should be made.
   b. Teeth lighten when dehydrated so a shade is completed prior to tooth preparation.
2. Prepare teeth to accept a definitive restoration (Fig. 10-10B).
3. Place gingival retraction cord if a tooth preparation is subgingival.
4. Construct a provisional restoration of acrylic, bisacryl, polycarbonate, resin, or like materials as described previously.
5. Reduce the facial surface of a provisional restoration with an acrylic bur or sandpaper disks.
6. Select composite resin to match the desired esthetics.
   a. Note that composite resin is translucent and will show through underlying material. A cut back provisional should be a close color match before composite resin is applied.

A ball creates a point contact when applied to a facial surface which spreads out when pressure is applied to minimize entrapment of air.

7. Roll composite resin into a ball.
8. Air inhibition of composite resin cure results in weakness or compromised esthetics.
9. Unfilled resin (bonding agent) applied to the surface of a trimmed provisional restoration

A wet surface minimizes air entrapment and creates a more complete contact of materials.

10. Place the composite resin ball in the middle of the facial surface.
11. Spread composite resin with finger pressure guiding its direction to completely cover the facial surface.
12. Definitive sculpturing is completed with a composite resin instrument (Fig. 10-10C).
13. Light cure all areas of the composite resin for 10 seconds.
14. Try in the provisional restoration intraorally to check composite resin extension and esthetics (Fig. 10-10D).

For difficult restorations, complete composite resin shaping intraorally to maximize esthetics prior to light curing.

15. Shape the composite resin with burs and sandpaper disks. Maximum shaping of uncured composite resins results in minimal shaping after curing.
    a. Diamond burs are used for initial shaping and placement of surface texture.
    b. Smooth interproximal surfaces and line angles with flame-shaped finishing burs (#7901, Midwest Dental).
16. Polish composite resin with cups, points, wheels, brushes, and polishing paste.
17. Isolate teeth with cotton rolls, wash and gently dry.
18. Mix cement and place it inside the provisional restoration.
19. Place the provisional restoration onto the prepared teeth and press it into position.
20. Remove excess cement.
21. Check and adjust the occlusion with articulating paper.
22. Complete final polishing with multi-fluted finishing burs and Burlew wheels.
23. Check the provisional restoration esthetics to ensure it resembles the anticipated definitive restoration (Figs. 10-10E,F).

Indirect/Direct Technique

Secure preoperative diagnostic casts for patients with coronally debilitated teeth or edentulous spaces. The cast can be corrected to the ideal anatomic form using inlay wax, resin, denture teeth, or preformed polycarbonate or metallic crowns. The corrected cast serves as the model, which is impressed. The impression is used to position the polymerizing acrylic resin onto the prepared teeth.

Armamentarium. The armamentarium is the same as that listed for the direct technique.

Clinical Technique. Use the same clinical technique as that described for the direct technique, except use the corrected cast as the source of the impression.

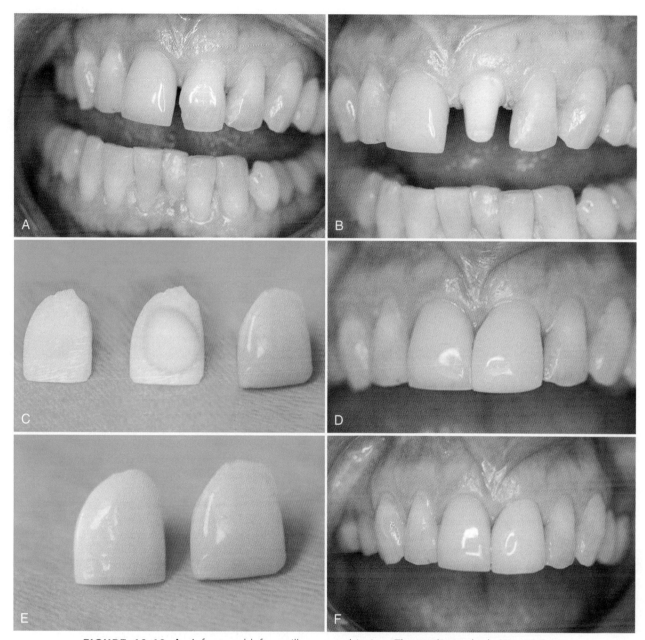

FIGURE 10-10 A, A fractured left maxillary central incisor. The teeth are shade Vita A3.5.
B, The central incisor prepared for an all-porcelain crown. **C,** A provisional restoration that was
fabricated after cutting back on the facial surface and covering with composite resin by placing
a ball of composite resin on the surface, spreading it, curing and finishing. **D,** A composite resin
veneer provisional restoration cemented on the prepared tooth. **E,** The definitive crown (left)
and the provisional restoration (right) should be virtually indistinguishable. **F,** The definitive all-
porcelain crown.

Plastic Matrix Technique

Some clinicians think that elastic materials are inadequate and
inaccurate for carrying acrylic resin during the fabrication of
provisional splints. Disadvantages include the following:
1. Voids and bubbles that are not easily detected until the polymerization of the resin is complete, yielding a porous, unesthetic surface
2. Occlusal discrepancies caused by distortion or incomplete
   reseating of the impression
3. Cumbersome procedures allowing minimal or no visibility or
   access to the polymerizing resin

The use of a clear plastic matrix to carry acrylic resin eliminates these disadvantages and provides the following additional
advantages:
1. The clear matrix serves as a tooth preparation (reduction)
   guide.
2. Acrylic resin polymerizes into a smooth, void-free surface
   against the plastic.

3. The matrix is reusable for fabrication of replacement provisional restorations.
4. Auxiliary personnel can easily make the matrix.
5. The matrix is inexpensive to produce.[7]

Ellman Press-Form System

Armamentarium
+ Standard Dental Setup. See the section on Preformed Crowns and Crown Forms in this chapter.
+ Petroleum jelly (e.g., Vaseline petroleum jelly, Unilever, Inc.) or silicone gel (e.g., Silicone V Lubricant, V Lubricant, Inc.)
+ Acrylic resin of choice (see Table 10-1)
+ Diagnostic cast
+ Press-Form System (Ellman International Inc.)
+ Plastic sheets (in various sheet thicknesses): 0.02 inch for short spans, 0.03 inch for medium spans, 0.04 inch for long spans
+ Blue inlay wax (optional)
+ Bunsen burner
+ Denture or metallic crown forms or polycarbonate crowns (optional)
+ Clay or Mortite
+ Acrylic bur setup. See the section on Preformed Crowns and Crown Forms in this chapter.
+ Acrylic finishing setup. See the section on finishing procedures in this chapter.
+ Shade correction setup (optional). See the section on Color Correction and Shade Characterization in this chapter.
+ Provisional cementation setup. See the section on cementation of provisional restorations in this chapter.

Clinical Technique
1. Prepare a stone or plaster cast.
2. Make any necessary corrections to the tooth structure.

CLINICAL TIP

If the coronal anatomy must be corrected with inlay wax, duplicate the cast in plaster or stone before adapting the heated plastic sheet. However, if resin denture teeth or preformed crowns are used to correct the original cast, it is not necessary to duplicate the cast before adapting the heated plastic.

3. Block out peripheral undercuts with clay or Mortite stripping.
4. Select the appropriate plastic sheet. Use a 0.02-inch plastic sheet for a one- to six-unit splint. For longer spans, use a 0.03- to 0.04-inch thick sheet.
5. Securely insert the plastic sheet into the frame.
6. Use silicone spray to coat the cast and both sides of the plastic sheet.
7. Heat the plastic sheet on one side until opacity begins to disappear (2 to 4 seconds).

CLINICAL TIP

Do not allow the sheet to overheat or sag excessively, which causes it to tear or buckle. This creates a distorted, inaccurate matrix that may also adhere to the cast.

8. Place the plastic sheet on the cast, and aggressively apply putty for 10 seconds to mold the sheet to the cast.
9. Allow the sheet to cool for 20 seconds; peel away the putty and lift the sheet off the cast.
10. Trim the plastic sheet with scissors.

CLINICAL TIP

Trim the borders to within 2 to 3 mm of the gingival margins.

Include one tooth mesial and one tooth distal to the terminal abutments of the fixed partial denture. If no teeth are adjacent to terminal preparations, leave a 5-mm "drape" of plastic covering the distal soft tissue area. Carefully round all sharp corners of the matrix to prevent intraoral soft tissue lacerations.

11. Prepare the teeth.
12. Protect the prepared abutments with petroleum jelly or silicone emulsion.
13. Pour a mixture of acrylic resin into the matrix.

CLINICAL TIP

+ Place wet wads of paper towels into the stent adjacent to the terminal abutments, which confines the resin until it reaches the putty stage.
+ Place the acrylic in the stent.
+ When the surface sheen disappears, remove the paper towels.
+ Carefully seat the stent and acrylic over the preparation in the correct path of insertion.

14. Carefully position the plastic matrix carrying the acrylic resin over the preparations to ensure full and accurate seating.
15. Seat the matrix with finger pressure only on the plastic extensions over the unprepared teeth adjacent to the terminal abutments.
16. Remove and replace to avoid locking into an undercut.
17. Remove the matrix and resin at the rubbery stage so that excess resin can be trimmed with sharp scissors.
18. Return the resin splint to the plastic matrix, and reseat both over the preparation.

CLINICAL TIP

While the acrylic is setting, remove and replace the matrix/resin and direct a stream of water over the matrix containing the polymerizing acrylic resin. See the Clinical Tip in the section on Preformed Crowns and Crown Forms.

19. When fully set, remove the splint and finish in the usual manner.
20. Remarginate if necessary. See the section on Remargination in this chapter.
21. Finish and polish the restoration. See the section on finishing procedures in this chapter.
22. Custom stain or characterize if necessary. See the section on Color Correction and Shade Characterization in this chapter.
23. Cement. See the section on Cementation of provisional restorations in this chapter.

Vacuum Former Unit

The vacuum former unit is particularly suited to producing long-span matrices. The technique involving the vacuum former unit is more time consuming than the hand-molded method and yields a closely adapted sheet.

> **CLINICAL TIP**
>
> The vacuum former unit is ideal when study casts exist and visualization through the clear matrix is used to analyze proper reduction of abutments.

Armamentarium. The armamentarium is the same as that listed for the Ellman Press-Form System with the exception of:
- A vacuum forming unit (i.e., Dental Vacuum Forming Unit, Buffalo Dental B Manufacturing Co., Inc.)
- Optional electronically heated knife (i.e., Therma-knife tray trimmer, Buffalo Dental Manufacturing Co., Inc.)

Clinical Technique
1. Prepare a stone or plaster cast.

> **CLINICAL TIP**
>
> The coronal anatomy can be corrected on the model. See the Clinical Tip in the section on Plastic Matrix Technique.

2. Preheat the unit by activating the calrod element (heating element).
3. Drill a hole 1 inch in diameter in the center of the palate of a maxillary cast. A mandibular cast should be a horseshoe shape.
4. Block out peripheral undercuts with clay or Mortite stripping.
5. Spray the cast with silicone.
6. Select the plastic sheet. Use a 0.02-inch plastic sheet for a one- to six-unit splint. For longer spans use a 0.04- to 0.06-inch thick sheet.
7. Secure the plastic sheet into the frame, and reposition the frame upward to the highest position just below the calrod.
8. Allow the plastic sheet to sag only 0.5 inch before guiding the frame with the sheet down over the cast.

> **CLINICAL TIP**
>
> Do not allow the sheet to overheat or sag excessively, which causes it to tear or buckle. This creates a distorted, inaccurate matrix that may also adhere to the cast.

9. Quickly lower the frame over the cast.
10. Activate the vacuum.

> **CLINICAL TIP**
>
> Leave the calrod element on for an additional 30 seconds, and vacuum for 1 minute. This step allows for proper adaptation and cooling of the plastic.

11. When the sheet has cooled, remove it from the cast. Cut away the excess sheet material to aid in removal.
12. Trim the plastic sheet.

> **CLINICAL TIP**
>
> Trim the borders to within 2 to 3 mm of the gingival margins. See the Clinical Tip in the section on Plastic Matrix Technique. An electronically heated knife provides easier trimming.

13. Prepare the teeth.
14. Protect the prepared abutments with petroleum jelly or silicone emulsion.
15. Pour a mixture of acrylic resin into the impression.

> **CLINICAL TIP**
>
> Place wet wads of paper towels into the stent on the teeth adjacent to terminal abutments. See the Clinical Tip in the section on Plastic Matrix Technique.

16. Carefully position the plastic sheet carrying the preparations to ensure full and accurate seating.
17. Remove the matrix and resin at the rubbery stage so that the excess resin can be trimmed with sharp scissors.
18. Return the splint to the plastic sheet and reseat both over the preparations. Repeatedly remove and reseat it to disengage from any possible undercuts.
19. When fully set, remove the splint and finish in the usual manner.
20. Reline or remarginate if necessary. See the section on Remargination in this chapter.
21. Finish and polish the restoration. See the section on finishing procedures in this chapter.
22. Custom stain or characterize if necessary. See the section on Color Correction and Shade Characterization in this chapter.
23. Cement. See the section on cementation of provisional restorations in this chapter.

Indirect Technique

Employing the indirect technique allows a clinician to avoid direct contact between freshly cut dentin with the acrylic resin monomer or avoid the potentially damaging effect of the exothermic heat of polymerization on pulpal tissue. This method should also be considered when making long-span splints of six or more units (and fresh extraction sites are present) or to decrease chair time for both patient and dentist. The method involves securing an impression of the prepared teeth, preparing a quick-set plaster cast, and making the provisional restoration on the cast.

Advantages
1. The prepared teeth and tissues do not have contact with surface monomer and polymerization heat.
2. Leaving the resin splint on the cast throughout the procedure minimizes polymerization shrinkage; distortion is minimized.
3. Oral contaminants (e.g., blood, saliva) do not contact polymerizing acrylic resin.
4. An auxiliary staff member can perform this extraoral procedure, thereby freeing the dentist for other productive procedures.

Disadvantages
1. The procedure is time consuming.
2. Extra materials and devices and increased cost are involved.

Armamentarium
+ Standard Dental Setup. See the section on preformed crown and crown forms in this chapter.
+ Cord placement instrument
+ No. 0, 00, 000 gauge retraction cord
+ Impression material: irreversible or reversible hydrocolloid or silicone impression material (e.g., Identic Syringable System, Dux Dental)
+ Petroleum jelly (e.g., Vaseline petroleum jelly, Unilever, Inc.) or silicone gel (e.g., Silicone V Lubricant, V Lubricant, Inc.)
+ Tin foil substitute (e.g., Al-Cote, Dentsply Caulk; Coe-Sep, GC Amercia; Liquid Foil, Lang Dental Mfg. Co., Inc.)
+ Acrylic resin or bisacryl of choice (see Table 10-1)
+ Acrylic bur setup. See the section on Preformed Crowns and Crown Forms in this chapter.
+ Acrylic finishing setup. See the section on finishing procedures in this chapter.
+ Shade correction setup (optional). See the section on Color Correction and Shade Characterization in this chapter.
+ Provisional cementation setup. See the section on Cementation of provisional restorations in this chapter.

Clinical Technique
1. Prepare the teeth.
2. Place the retraction cord into the sulcus below the preparation margins (0, 00,000 gauge)
3. Make a full arch impression using an elastomeric impression material.

> ### CLINICAL TIP
>
> To secure a more accurate impression (especially of the marginal detail), use the Identic Syringable Impression System (Dux Dental).

4. Have the assistant mix Identic irreversible hydrocolloid with cold water and fill a stock impression tray. (Water-cooled trays are not required in this technique.)
5. Using a syringe, place tempered Identic syringable hydrocolloid around the prepared tooth, taking care to fill the sulci, and place the tray containing the irreversible hydrocolloid over the teeth.
6. Leave the tray in place for 2 minutes.
7. Pour the impression with a fast set plaster or stone.

> ### CLINICAL TIP
>
> Use slurry water (i.e., water mixed with a small amount of finely ground set plaster, such as waste water from a model trimmer) to accelerate the cast setting.

8. Trim the cast.
9. Apply a tin foil substitute.
10. Using any of the techniques listed previously, construct the provisional restoration on the model as if it was being done intraorally.
11. Reline or remarginate if necessary. See the section on Remargination in this chapter.
12. Finish and polish the restoration. See the section on finishing procedures in this chapter.
13. Custom stain or characterize if necessary. See the section on Color Correction and Shade Characterization in this chapter.
14. Cement. See the section on Cementation of provisional restorations in this chapter.

Laboratory-Produced Shell and Reline Technique

The professional dental laboratory can assist the dentist in achieving excellence with acrylic resin provisional restorations (Table 10-8). The dentist relines a processed acrylic resin shell (provided by the laboratory) with an auto-polymerized resin on the prepared teeth. The shell can be auto-polymerized or heat processed on study casts to the dentist's prescription. Heat processing provides increased strength, durability, and stain resistance and is particularly appropriate for long-term use (Figs. 10-11*A,B*).

Another technique uses hollow plastic denture teeth as "veneers" to which the laboratory adds resin to fill out the shell's proximal and lingual contours. A length of 15-gauge, half-round stainless steel wire can be incorporated into multiple-unit splints to add strength and stiffness (Fig. 10-11*C*).

Kevlar (Dupont) and Polyethylene Fiber (Ribbond, Ribbond, Inc.) reinforcement can also be used. Nylon mesh (Splint Grid) and stainless steel mesh (Splint Mesh) (Ellman International Mfg. Co.) also provide a degree of reinforcement to acrylic resin provisional fixed partial dentures.

Armamentarium
+ Standard Dental Setup. See the section on Preformed Crowns and Crown Forms in this chapter.
+ Diagnostic cast
+ Acrylic resin of choice (see Table 10-1)
+ Acrylic bur setup. See the section on Preformed Crowns and Crown Forms in this chapter.
+ Acrylic finishing setup. See the section on finishing procedures in this chapter.
+ Shade correction setup (optional). See the section on Color Correction and Shade Characterization in this chapter.
+ Provisional cementation setup. See the section on cementation of provisional restorations in this chapter.

Clinical Technique
1. Provide the dental laboratory with preoperative diagnostic casts, centric occlusion and protrusive records, shade and characterization information, and detailed instructions for the production of an acrylic resin shell.
2. The technician corrects anatomic contour on the study casts.
3. The technician underprepares the abutments on the cast (with a 1-mm reduction) to provide space for resin (Fig. 10-12*A*).

Table 10-8 Laboratory-Processed Custom Provisional Shells

Brand	Laboratory
Resista-Temps	Indianapolis: http://resista-temps.com/
Glidewell Laboratories (Bio-Temp)	California: www.glidewelldental.com/

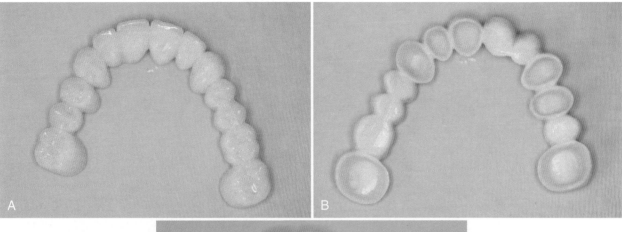

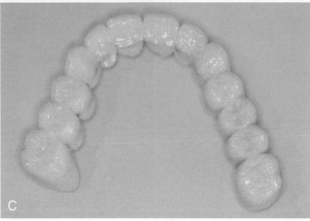

FIGURE 10-11 A, The occlusal view of a laboratory processed provisional restoration. **B,** The internal surface of the laboratory processed provisional restoration in part A before intraoral relining on the prepared teeth. **C,** Wire reinforcement strengthens this laboratory heat processed provisional restoration.

4. The technician fabricates the splint using one of the various previously described methods.
5. Initial finishing can be performed before sending the restoration to the dental office.
6. Reline intraorally on the prepared abutments (Figs. 10-12B,C).
7. Finish and polish the restoration. See the section on finishing procedures in this chapter.
8. Custom stain or characterize if necessary. See the section on Color Correction and Shade Characterization in this chapter.
9. Cement. See the section on cementation of provisional restorations in this chapter (Fig. 10-12D, E).

Other Clinical Situations

Porcelain or Composite Resin Laminate Veneer Provisional Restoration. Porcelain laminate veneer provisional restorations provide no mechanical resistance to displacement forces as opposed to crowns which have a definitive path of insertion and withdrawal. Loss of retention occurs from failure of cement, the cement to tooth interface or the cement to provisional restoration interface.

Spot bonding creates better retention when using resin cements or composite resin provisional restorations. The small bonding area in the center of a tooth limits retention, which allows a provisional veneer to be removed. Composite resin provisionals are rigid, which improves retention.

Armamentarium
+ Standard Dental Setup. See the section on Preformed Crowns and Crown Forms in this chapter.
+ Acrylic or bisacryl of choice
+ Acrylic finishing setup. See the section on finishing procedures in this chapter.
+ Shade correction setup (optional). See the section on Color Correction and Shade Characterization in this chapter.
+ Provisional cementation setup. See the section on cementation of provisional restorations in this chapter.

Clinical Technique
1. Create a direct or indirect matrix as described earlier in this chapter.
2. Create a provisional restoration as described earlier in direct and indirect matrix techniques.
3. Apply 37% phosphoric acid to a 2- to 3-mm circular area in the center of each tooth.
   a. Leave acid on dentin for 10 seconds.
   b. Leave acid on enamel for 30 seconds.
4. Apply a desensitizing agent such as Gluma to dentin.
   a. Apply a bonding agent as directed by a manufacturer.

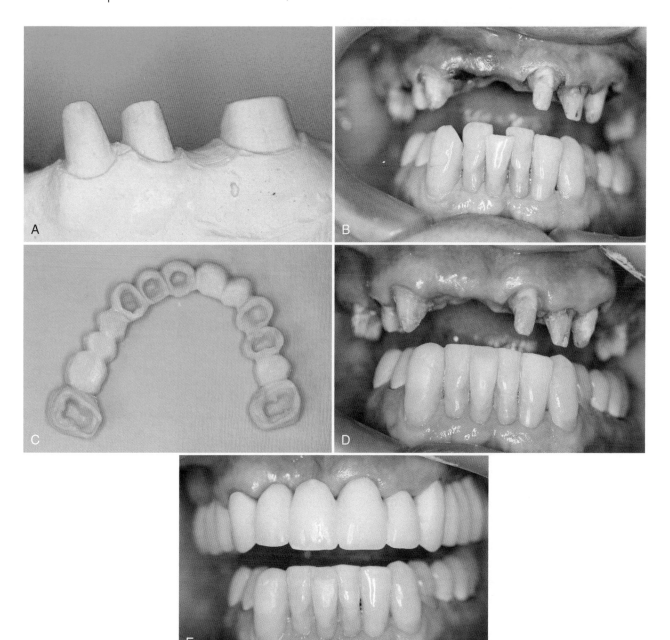

FIGURE 10-12 A, A duplicate of the study model with the teeth prepared by a dental laboratory technician. The teeth have been reduced by a depth of 1 mm and to the height of the gingiva. **B,** Prepared teeth and extraction areas before immediate replacement with a provisional restoration. **C,** The provisional restoration after relining with acrylic, trimming with acrylic burs and polished with sandpaper disks. **D,** The prepared teeth and edentulous areas two months post extraction with the laboratory processed provisional restoration in place. Note that the mandibular anterior teeth have been restored with composite resin and recontoured to improve the occlusion. **E,** Heat processed provisional restoration 2 months after initial placement.

CLINICAL TIP

Do not use a self-etching bonding agent as the whole tooth will be bonded. The bond will be too strong to allow for removal of the provisional restoration.

5. Apply dual cure resin cement to the inner surface of each tooth the provisional restoration. Alternatively, use a flowable composite resin if all surfaces are accessible to light curing.

6. Place the provisional restoration onto the prepared teeth.

7. Light cure the incisal area for five seconds to gel the resin cement and tack the laminate veneer in place.

8. Remove excess cement from the marginal area with a brush followed by an explorer.

9. Light cure all surfaces of the provisional restoration for 10 seconds.

Alternative Method Porcelain or Composite Resin Laminate Veneer Provisional Restoration. The procedure is the same as a composite resin veneer but a weak bond is created to allow removal. Composite resin is applied to a prepared tooth in bulk and shaped with a composite resin instrument. Final shaping is accomplished with sandpaper disks and polishing points, cups and disks. It is spot bonded to allow for removal.

Clinical Techniqueone solu

1. Plan treatment for restoration (Fig. 10-13*A*).
2. Prepare teeth for porcelain laminate veneers (Fig. 10-13*B*).
3. Apply 37% phosphoric acid in a 2- to 3-mm circular area in the center of each tooth (Fig. 10-13*C*).
   a. Leave acid on dentin for 10 seconds.
   b. Leave acid on enamel for 30 seconds.
4. Apply a desensitizing agent such as Gluma to exposed dentin.
5. Apply bonding agent to the complete prepared area as directed by the manufacturer.

CLINICAL TIP

Do not use a self-etching bonding agent, because the complete prepared surface will be bonded. The bond will be too strong to remove a provisional restoration.

CLINICAL TIP

Do not light cure the bonding agent before cementing a provisional. Collagen fibers on exposed dentin collapse when a provisional is placed creating a weaker reversible bond.

---

6. Select an appropriate composite resin.
7. Roll composite resin into a ball.
8. Place the ball onto the center of a tooth.
9. Spread the ball with a finger guiding it completely over the prepared tooth structure.
10. Remove the excess and shape with a composite resin instrument.
11. Light cure the composite resin for 10 seconds.

Shape and polish with sandpaper disks, finishing burs and polishing cups, points and wheels (Fig. 10-13*D*).

Provisional Restorations for Coronally Debilitated Teeth

When minimal coronal dentin is available, the retention of the provisional restoration is compromised. Standard retention techniques must be altered or augmented to compensate for a lack of resistance and retentive form.

Endodontically Treated Teeth. Between the required two appointments, a provisional restoration is mandatory (especially for anterior teeth) for restorations involving a dowel and core. It is not always feasible to immediately provide a final dowel and core for endodontically treated teeth before temporization.

1. If the restorability of a tooth is questionable, an interim post/crown is less expensive than a restoration that may subsequently be lost with tooth removal.
2. During lengthy periodontal treatment periods of questionable teeth, the interim resin post/core is mandatory.

When fabrication or placement of a dowel/core is delayed, a titanium alloy provisional post or fiber reinforced resin post

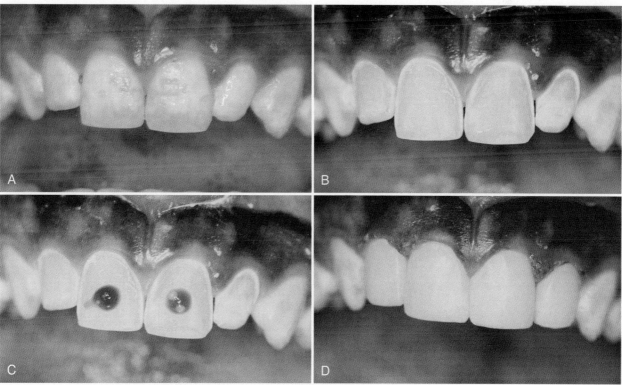

FIGURE 10-13 A, Four maxillary incisors with mottled enamel will be restored with porcelain laminate veneers. **B,** Porcelain laminate veneer preparations. **C,** 37 % Phosphoric acid is placed for spot bonding of the composite resin provisional restorations. **D,** Composite resin provisional restorations.

may be used to add retention to the acrylic resin provisional restoration. Accessory provisional aluminum pins are also available (Para-Post systems, Coltene/Whaledent). These devices are incorporated into provisional restorations during reline technique (Fig. 10-14). The provisional post/crown must be monitored (as any temporarily cemented provisional restoration) regularly for cement washout and caries development.

Nonendodontically Treated Teeth. To provisionally restore teeth that, despite having little coronal structure, do not require endodontic therapy, an interim pin-retained, light-cured composite resin "crown" may be used. This restoration can later be prepared as a pin-retained core on which a definite restoration can be placed.

Mechanical Interlocks

There are times when provisional restorations cannot resist applied forces. Retention is improved with mechanical interlocking. Dimple interlocks are created by drilling holes through a provisional restoration to create dimples in build-up material of prepared teeth and placing composite resin through the hole in the provisional restoration and into the dimples. Dimples are created into composite resin cores or other restorative materials but not into tooth structure. Interproximal interlocks are created by creating an interproximal box in a provisional restoration. The box is filled with composite resin so it will engage undercuts of about 1 mm on an adjacent tooth.

Composite resin is trimmed and shaped after placement to ensure proper occlusion and open gingival embrasures which allows access for floss threading. A provisional restoration is flexible enough that with firm force composite resin interlocks disengage for provisional restoration removal.

Armamentarium
+ Standard Dental Setup. See the section on Preformed Crowns and Crown Forms in this chapter.
+ Acrylic or bisacryl of choice
+ Acrylic finishing setup. See the section on finishing procedures in this chapter.
+ Shade correction setup (optional). See the section on Color Correction and Shade Characterization in this chapter.
+ Provisional cementation setup. See the section on cementation of provisional restorations in this chapter.

Clinical Technique
1. Construct a provisional restoration in the usual manner as described earlier in the chapter.
2. Cut a box into the mesial (and distal if added retention is required). The box should be similar to a class II amalgam preparation and extend gingivally enough so composite resin placed in the box will engage 1 mm of undercut on an adjacent tooth.
3. Cement the provisional crown with provisional cement and remove the polymerized cement.
4. With a composite resin instrument, place enough composite resin into the box to fill it without allowing excess to flow into the gingival areas.
5. Trim the excess composite resin from the facial, lingual and gingival areas and light cure.

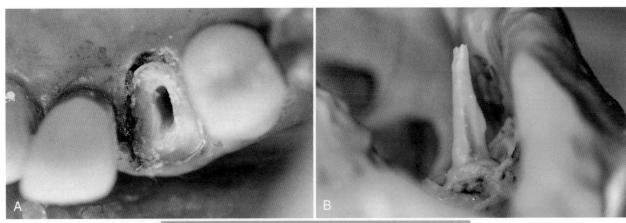

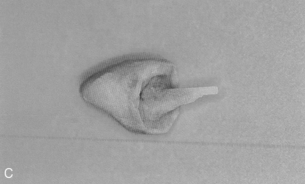

FIGURE 10-14 A, Maxillary left canine prepared to accept a cast post. **B,** A silicone impression of the canal revealing the tapered canal shape. **C,** A completed provisional restoration with a properly shaped, fiber reinforced provisional post.

6. Adjust the occlusion, finish and polish in the usual way as described above.
7. Demonstrate to the patient to the proper use of the floss threaders.

Provisional Restorations for Edentulous Spaces

Pontic Design. Interproximal contact areas are constructed wider buccolingually than the solder joint of the permanent splint to provide strength for the splint. The tissue-contacting surface of a pontic must be flat or convex (never concave) to permit efficient cleansing with floss and other home care devices (Fig. 10-15). See discussion on pontic design in (see Chapter 9).

Temporization of Osseointegrated Implants

After the prescribed healing period required for osseointegration, the reentry surgical procedure is performed, and healing abutments are placed. The patient may be required to wear a modified relined interim removable prosthesis before placement of the definitive restoration. This may be particularly desirable when implants are in the anterior sextant. One solution to this scenario is the placement of an interim acrylic resin fixed prosthesis incorporating transitional cylinders (Table 10-9). These components may be used by the dentist in a direct chairside

fabrication of an acrylic resin prosthesis or when prescribed for laboratory fabrication.[8]

Whether fabricated directly (chairside) or by a dental technician, the provisional prosthesis provides many benefits to the patient. Wearing a modified fixed prosthesis when indicated eliminates the need for healing abutments. The patient can immediately use the osseointegrated implants with a preview of the definitive prosthesis. Function and esthetics can be altered in the interim restoration until the patient and clinicians are satisfied. In addition, this "fixed-type" prosthesis provides an excellent training and evaluation guide for the home care regimen. It may also be retained as a backup prosthesis in case repair or modifications are required for the definitive prosthesis (Fig. 10-16).

Intraoral (Direct) Technique

The intraoral technique is a modification of the plastic matrix technique, which uses either a vacuum former unit or an Ellman Press-Form System. It requires the fabrication of a clear plastic matrix that represents the correct anatomic form desired in the provisional restoration.

Armamentarium. The armamentarium is the same as that listed for the vacuum former unit or Ellman Press-Form System with the following exceptions:
+ Appropriate retention screws
+ Guide pin (BIOMET 3i)
+ Titanium transitional cylinder (BIOMET 3i)

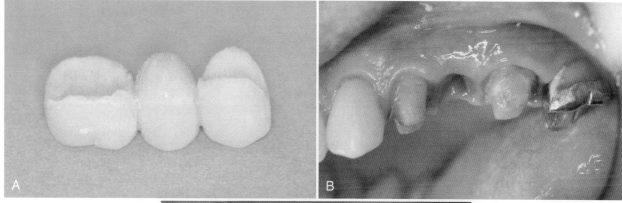

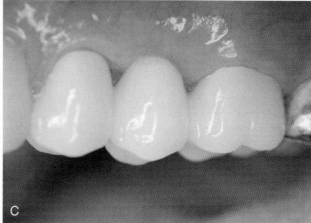

FIGURE 10-15 A, A three unit immediate provisional restoration with an ovate pontic to guide soft tissue healing. **B,** Prepared teeth and edentulous area eight weeks post extractions. **C,** Definitive all-porcelain bridge with ovate pontic conforming to the shape of the healed tissues.

Table 10-9 Components for Implant-Retained Provisional Restorations

BIOMET 3i Provisional Components	Clinical Application
PreFormance Provisional Components	PreFormance Post, PreFormance Cylinder
Low Profile QuickBridge Provisional Components Provide Temporary Cylinders	QuickBridge Cylinder and Cap Provide Abutment Temporary Cylinder

- Cotton pellets and silicone plugs (e.g., Fermit, Ivoclar Vivadent)

Clinical Technique
1. Secure the appropriate transitional cylinders to the abutments. Determine the reduction in height necessary, remove cylinders, and adjust them with a sintered diamond disk.
2. Secure to implant with guide pin.
3. Use the clear plastic matrix to carry acrylic resin intraorally (cut a hole in the matrix to allow it to seat over the cylinder).

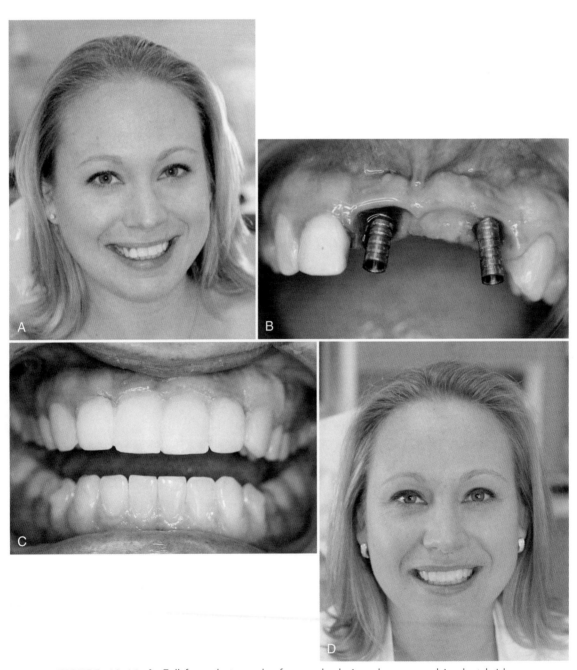

FIGURE 10-16 A, Full face photograph of a poorly designed crown and implant bridge. **B,** Implant provisional fixtures placed and modified to accept a provisional restoration. **C,** Provisional restorations on teeth #4 to 13 fabricated with composite resin faced bisacryl. **D,** Full face photographs of diagnostic provisional restorations.

4. Allow the resin to set to just after the rubbery stage before unscrewing and removing the assembly. Allow complete exothermic polymerization to occur extraorally.

5. When fully set, contour the acrylic resins and refine the occlusion.

6. Finish and polish the restoration. See the section on finishing procedures in this chapter.

7. Custom stain or characterize if necessary. See the section on Color Correction and Shade Characterization in this chapter.

8. Insert and secure the restoration with retention screws. The access opening can be obturated with cotton pellets and silicone plugs, or Fermit (Ivoclar Vivadent).

Indirect Technique

The professional dental laboratory can produce acrylic resin interim restorations that seat directly to the implant head or to abutments secured to implants.

Armamentarium. The armamentarium is the same as that listed for the indirect technique with the following exceptions:

+ Impression material: polyether or vinyl polysiloxane
+ Irreversible hydrocolloid
+ Border wax or injectable silicone
+ Appropriate retention screws
+ Access blocker (optional)

Clinical Technique

1. Fabricate a short-term removable prosthesis. This is usually a modified or relined existing removable partial prosthesis.

2. Make a polyether or vinyl polysiloxane impression of the impression coping.

3. Make an irreversible hydrocolloid impression of the opposing arches; make interocclusal records and select the correct shade.

4. Connect the abutment analogs or implant analogs to the impression copings.

5. Pour impressions; articulate the master and opposing casts.

6. Attach transitional cylinders to analogs and complete a full-contour wax-up.

7. Invest, boil out, flask, pack with resin, and process.

8. Recover and finalize the prosthesis.

9. Deliver the custom prosthesis to the patient.

10. Secure the restorations to the abutments or implants with retention screws.

Remargination. If marginal discrepancies are noted, an intraoral repair procedure (remargination) is required.

Armamentarium

+ Standard Dental Setup. See the section on Preformed Crowns and Crown Forms in this chapter.
+ Dappen dish
+ Universal Polishing Paste (Ivoclar, Inc.)
+ Assorted red sable brushes (No. 00 to No. 2)
+ Acrylic resin of choice (see Table 10-1)
+ Acrylic bur setup. See the section on preformed crowns and crown restorations in this chapter.

Clinical Technique

1. Roughen the resin surrounding the defect with an acrylic cutting bur.

2. Mix a moderately fluid acrylic resin, and paint it onto the dry defect area.

3. Additional mixed resin may be placed in the gingival sulcus adjacent to the defect.

4. Seat the splint so that the fluid resin sets in the defect.

5. Remove when set; trim and finish the restoration to the correct margins.

CLINICAL TIP

Light-cured resins are an excellent, efficient material for repairing marginal defects. If light-cured composite resins are used to remarginate defects (or restore contacts, repair fractures, and adjust occlusal defects) of polymethyl methacrylate provisional restorations, the defect must first be primed with bonding primer before the composite resin is applied.

Repairs. Provisional restorations are easily repaired and modified by adding flowable or regular composite resin (Fig. 10-17A). Composite resin adherence to provisional materials is not strong. The provisional restoration is roughened with a diamond bur to increase surface area in order to improve the retention of the composite resin repair (Fig. 10-17B). In high stress areas, mechanical retention is created with pot holes or lateral retention cuts. It is crucial that the composite resin engages the mechanical locks (10-17C).

Finishing and Polishing Procedures. To ensure biologic compatibility the provisional restoration must be finished so that the contour and marginal excellence approach that of the definitive cast restoration. Various laboratory carbides, diamond stones, and diamond-coated disks are used to establish physiologically acceptable contours (Table 10-10 and Fig. 10-17C; see Table 10-3). Following intraoral occlusal adjustment to establish centric relation and excursive border movement, the occlusal surfaces are refined and defined with burs. See the acrylic bur setup discussion in the section on Preformed Crowns and Crown Forms in this chapter. Correct esthetic coronal anatomic shape is achieved with a series of flat planes rather than rounded surfaces.

Facial textures, supplementary anatomy, and development cuts are sculpted with carbide burs. Smoothing is accomplished with a slurry of medium pumice on a wet chamois wheel with a dental laboratory lathe.

To avoid breaking the acrylic resin splint, all smoothing and polishing must be done on the slow-speed lathe setting. Interproximal surfaces are smoothed and polished with pumice wheels, sand paper disks, and Sof-Lex (3M, Inc.) disks on a straight handpiece. High-luster polishing is accomplished with a dry rag wheel coated with Universal Polishing Paste, a white diamond bar on the dental lathe, or glazing resin (Table 10-11). However, custom staining is always performed after polishing but before glazing.

Color Correction and Shade Characterization. To create an exceptionally esthetic, lifelike acrylic resin provisional restoration that pleases the most demanding patient, the operator can apply surface colorants (Table 10-12). This is readily accomplished with the Taub Minute Stain Kit (George Taub Products) or the Lang Jet Adjuster Kit (Lang Dental Mfg. Co., Inc.).

These quick-setting, colored acrylic liquids are applied with a brush to modify the shades of acrylic provisional restorations. The stains adhere or bond to all dental resins, including ethyl and methyl methacrylate, polycarbonates, vinyl methacrylate copolymers, resin crowns and laminates, denture bases, acrylic

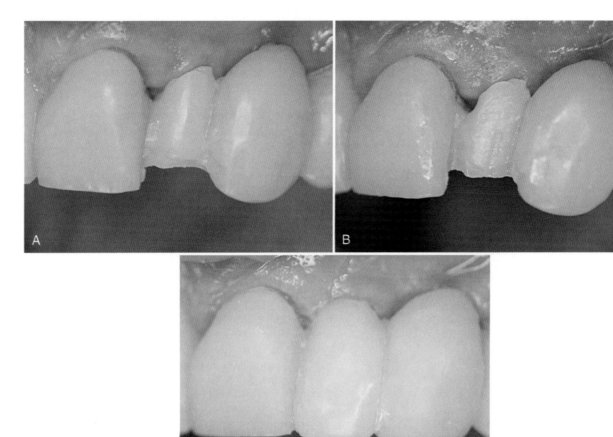

FIGURE 10-17 A, A fractured long term provisional restoration on a 95-year-old patient. **B,** The existing material is roughened with a diamond bur, etched to increase surface energy and bonding agent applied. **C,** Composite resin replacement of the lateral incisor.

Table 10-10 Finishing and Polishing

Brand	Manufacturer
Cutting/Finishing Bur	Ellman International Inc..
Pure Buff Lathe Wheels	Almore International, Inc.
Sof-Lex Discs	3M ESPE
Fine Pumice	Kerr Corp.
White Diamond Bar	Laboratory Products
Sulci Discs	Burlew Co.

Table 10-11 Acrylic Resin Glaze

Brand	Manufacturer
Cyanodent (Fast/Slow)	Ellman International Inc..
Glaze	George Taub Products
Justi Modifying Stain Kit	American Tooth Industries
Tempspan Glaze	Pentron Clinical

Table 10-12 Shade Alteration Kits

Brand	Manufacturer
Minute Stain Kit	George Taub Products
Jet Adjusters	Lang Dental Mfg. Co., Inc.
Prisma)	Dentsply Caulk

denture teeth, and composite resins. These stains can be applied intraorally or extraorally (Fig. 10-18).

Armamentarium
+ Standard Dental Setup. See the section on Preformed Crowns and Crown Forms in this chapter.
+ Assorted red sable brushes (No. 00 to No. 2)
+ Acrylic color correction kit (Taub Minute Stain Kit or Lang Jet Adjusters Kit)

Clinical Technique
1. Finish and polish the restoration. See the section on finishing in this chapter.
2. Make certain the surface is clean.

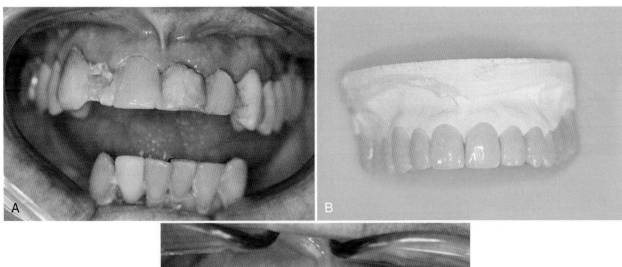

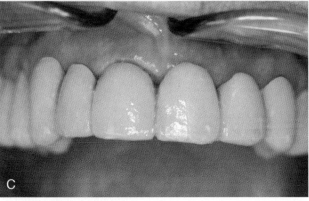

FIGURE 10-18 A, Defective composite resin bonding with extensive caries. **B,** Wire reinforced laboratory processed provisional restoration of the clinical situation in Fig. 10-11C. **C,** Custom stained provisional restoration on prepared teeth.

> **CLINICAL TIP**
>
> Gently shake bottles of stain to disperse pigments. Only shake bottles vigorously when intense, concentrated colors are desired.

3. Dip the brush into the bottle, wipe off excess pigment at the bottle neck, and bleed additional excess from the brush onto the ceramic or glass mixing slab. Pigments should be evenly dispersed with a very light, quick brush stroke. Additional layers can be applied following 10-second drying periods.

   Cementation. Cements with or without eugenol can be used for cementation of provisional restorations (Table 10-13). Cements containing eugenol are indicated for relief of pulpal sensitivity. However, the eugenol may inhibit the setting of the acrylic during subsequent reline and remargination procedures. Non-eugenol formulations are easier to remove from the acrylic resin.

Armamentarium
+ Standard Dental Setup. See the section on Preformed Crowns and Crown Forms in this chapter.
+ Cord placement instrument (optional)
+ No. 0 gauge retraction cord (optional)
+ Provisional cement: non-eugenol or eugenol type

+ Petroleum jelly (e.g., Vaseline petroleum jelly, Unilever, Inc.) or silicone gel (e.g., Silicone V Lubricant, V Lubricant, Inc.)
+ Dental floss
+ Dental floss threader
+ Cement removal instrument
+ Small cement spatula
+ No. ½ Hollenback or red sable brushes
+ #7 wax spatula

Clinical Technique
1. Isolate the teeth with cotton rolls, and dry them with the air syringe.

> **CLINICAL TIP**
>
> Lubricate the provisional splint externally with mineral oil or petroleum jelly to facilitate the removal of excess cement after setting.

> **CLINICAL TIP**
>
> Place lengths of dental floss between the prepared teeth before cementation of the splint to facilitate dislodging interproximal excess cement.

Table 10-13 Provisional Cements

Type	Brand	Manufacturer
Eugenol	Temrex ZOE Plus	Temrex Corp.
	Embonte	Dux Dental
	Flow-Temp	Premier Dental Products
	TempBond	Kerr Corp.
	Trial Cement	Opotow Corp.
	TempoCem, Tempocem soft Embonte, Embonte 2 Rely X Temp E	DMG America Dux Dental 3M ESPE
	Temrex Rely X Temp	Temrex Corp. 3M ESPE
Non-eugenol	Zone	Dux Dental .
	Nogenol	GC America
	Freegenol	GC America.
	Flex-Span CMT	Pentron Clinical
	TempBond Clear	Kerr Corp.
	Neo-Temp	Water Pik, Inc.
	Provicol TempoCem NE Freegenol, Temp, Avantage, Nogenol Integrity TempGrip RelyX Temp NE TempoSIL 2 Systemp.cem, System. link TempSpan	VOCO GmbH DMG America GC America Dentsply Caulk 3M ESPE Coltene/Whaledent Ivoclar Vivadent Pentron Clinical

---

CLINICAL TIP

Place a section of nonimpregnated retraction cord into the sulcus before cementation of the provisional restoration. Retrieving this cord during excess cement removal ensures that no cement remains; however, failure to remove the cord can have adverse periodontal consequences.

---

2. Prepare a eugenol or non-eugenol provisional cement according to the manufacturer's instructions.
3. Deliver a thin film of cement to the restoration with a #7 wax spatula or plastic instrument (Brasseler USA).
4. Seat the restoration on the preparations and direct the patient to gently close into the centric occlusal position.
5. After the cement has set, gently remove the excess with an explorer or No. ½ Hollenback carver. Floss threaders and unwaxed dental floss effectively cleanse cement from interproximal spaces.
6. Make certain no excess subgingival cement remains because it may contribute to gingival irritation and recession.

Laboratory Prescription and Communication. Properly fabricated provisional restorations can be used as a three-dimensional laboratory prescription. A stone cast duplicate of the cemented provisional restorations aids the dental technician in developing crown contour, emergence profile, transitional line angles, proportion, lip and smile lines, disclusion guides, and esthetics in the definitive restoration (Fig. 10-19). This serves to minimize chairside adjustments and remakes. An acrylic tab accurately conveys the desired shade to the laboratory.

Proper communication with the laboratory is accomplished with a laboratory prescription, study models of a provisional restoration, photographs and verbal communications if necessary (see Fig. 10-19B). The laboratory prescription includes shade selection, a description of color variation, occlusal patterns, and notes of changes in tooth position and shape. Photographs of the provisional restoration, adjacent teeth and shade guides held next to teeth enhance communication. Study models of the provisional restorations are mounted on an articulator and a silicone index is fabricated to guide length and position of the permanent restoration the dental laboratory (see Figs. 10-19C,D). It is important that the laboratory technician have a complete understanding of normal tooth position, color and shape. A laboratory prescription discusses differences.

Modular Provisional Implants

Patients seeking implant-retained prostheses are often hesitant to initiate treatment because of the lengthy osseointegration period requiring the use of a removable interim prosthesis. This factor may cause patients to seek alternative care. It is now possible to offer patients the option of never being without an implant-supported provisional prosthesis between the time of the initial implant placement and stage 2 surgical exposure. There are several brands of mini implants available. The Modular Provisional Implant and Prosthetic System (MTI-MP) from Dentatus USA provides a system for the implantologist and restorative dentist to deliver the following benefits:

1. The MTI-MP provides immediate interim stable restorations immediately after implant placement (Fig. 10-20).
2. The MTI-MP eliminates the need to wear a tissue-supported prosthesis that may transmucosally "load and stress" the submerged implants.
3. The MTI-MP implant prosthesis presents a preview of the definitive prosthesis and can be altered to analyze the form desired in the definitive restoration.
4. The pure titanium MTI-MP implants serve as stabilizers for bone and membranes in guided tissue regeneration procedures.

The MTI-MP system is not currently accepted by the American Dental Association (ADA), but it is FDA 510K approved. The system contains components that permit implantologists and restorative dentists to fabricate fixed and removable immediate interim implant-retained restorations.

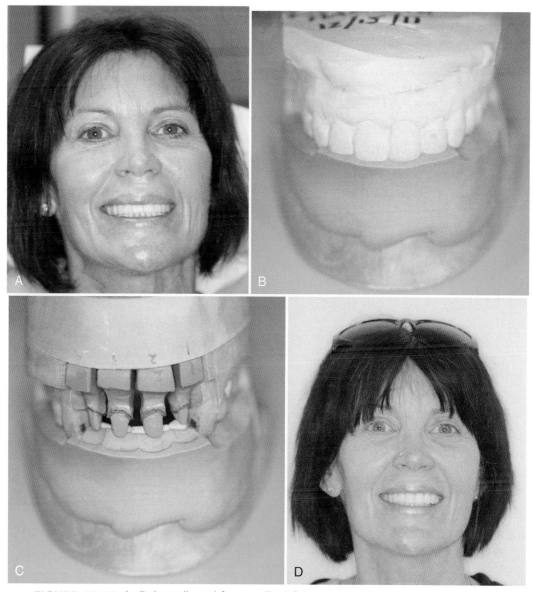

FIGURE 10-19 A, Esthetically and functionally deficient anterior crowns. **B,** Study model of accepted provisional restoration indexed with silicone for reproduction in the definitive restorations (see Fig. 10-9). **C,** Model of the definitive crown preparations mounted to a silicone index on the opposing model to act as a guide for the definitive restorations. **D,** Improved smile with splinted all porcelain crowns as guided by composite resin veneered provisional restorations.

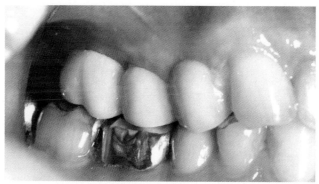

FIGURE 10-20 One-week postoperative view of three-unit (teeth #3, #4, and #5) polymethyl methacrylate provisional splint retained by three Modular Transitional Implant and Prosthetic System (MTI-MP) titanium transitional implants.

CONCLUSION

An esthetic, biologically compatible, physiologically sound interim restoration satisfies the patient, ensures tissue health, and favorably enhances the definitive restoration delivery and cementation times. Experience gained during this critical phase of therapy aids the clinician in accepting perioprosthetic challenges confidently.

The restorative dentist must never rationalize that the provisional restoration is "only temporary," a mindset than can easily lead to failure of treatment goals. The acrylic resin provisional restoration should be considered a "permanent restoration made of temporary material."[9]

REFERENCES

1. Federick DR, Caputo AA: Stress distribution to the supporting tissues of abutment stabilized with fixed splints, *J Calif Dent Assoc* 8:33, 1980.
2. Amsterdam M, Fox L: Provisional splinting: principles and techniques, *Dent Clin North Am* 4:73, 1959.
3. Chalifoux PR: Maximum esthetics, strength and interlock retention, *Inside Dentistry* 6(4):52-55, 2010. http://www.dentalaegis.com/id/2010/04/maximum-esthetics-strength-and-interlock-retention. Accessed October 10, 2013.
4. Altinas SH, Yondem I, Tak O, et al: Temperature rise during polymerization of three different provisional materials, *Clinical Oral Investig* 12(3):283-286, 2008.
5. Stanley HR, Serdlow H, Bounocore MG: Pulp reactions to anterior restorative materials, *J Am Dent Assoc* 75(1):132-141, 1967.
6. Burgess JO: Provisional materials, *The Dental Advisor* 12(1), 1995.
7. Federick, DR: Temporization, *The Dental Advisor* 9(1), 1992.
8. Federick DR: Provisional/transitional implant retained fixed restorations, *J Calif Dent Assoc* 23:19-22, 1995.
9. Schneider DN: Full-coverage temporization—an outline of goals, methods, and uses (Part 1), *Quint Int* 11:27, 1980.

11

Acrylic and Other Resins: Removable Prosthetics

Frank Lauciello

The art and science of esthetic dental principles are identical, whether discussing natural teeth or fixed or removable restorations. Removable prosthodontics can serve as a valuable tool for illustrating the principles of esthetics. The simplicity of repositioning denture teeth allows the various esthetic effects of different tooth positions to be easily interpreted. Many early contributors to the literature have emphasized the importance of setting denture teeth so that they appear natural.[1-6] Many of the universal concepts of dental esthetics have evolved from these efforts to naturalize dentures. Figure 11-1 gives a general outline of the various options for tooth positions of the maxillary anterior teeth.

The individual tooth positions and inclinations will be described in relationship to a horizontal reference plane. This reference plane is recorded from the patient and transferred to an articulator. Many different techniques and articulator components exist, and are beyond the scope of this chapter. However, a very practical technique that can be applied to most articulation systems will be presented.

ESTHETIC REFERENCE PLANE

The occlusal plane by definition is the average plane established by the incisal and occlusal surfaces of the teeth or in the case of the edentulous patient, the surface of wax occlusion rims contoured to guide in the arrangement of denture teeth.[7] The occlusal plane can be viewed in both the frontal and sagittal planes. The incisal surfaces, when viewed in the frontal plane, should have a pleasing parallelism to the patient's facial features (interpupillary line, eyebrows, hairline, etc.) (Fig. 11-2).

The posterior occlusal surfaces when viewed in the sagittal plane should, on average, correspond to an imaginary plane established by the inferior border of the ala of the nose (or the average between the two) and the superior border of the tragus of each ear (Camper's plane).[7] Although the accuracy of Camper's plane as representative of the occlusal plane is arguable, it is adequate

for this proposed technique. This ideal plane will be referred to as the *esthetic reference plane* (ERP) (see Fig. 11-2). Fabricating a restoration that is parallel with the patient's ERP (especially when viewed in the frontal plane) is critical to the esthetic success of the restoration. Restorations that deviate from this horizontal plane are typically the result of improper or inadequate communication with the dental laboratory technician. Therefore it is imperative that the patient's ERP be recorded by the clinician and then communicated to the technician. The simplest and least expensive tool that facilitates this evaluation is the Biteplane (Ivoclar Vivadent) or Fox Plane (Dentsply International).

The Biteplane rests on the surfaces of the maxillary teeth or in the case of complete dentures, the maxillary wax rim. The external wings of the Biteplane help to amplify the visual relationship of the patient's maxillary incisal/occlusal plane to their ERP (Fig. 11-3*A,B*).

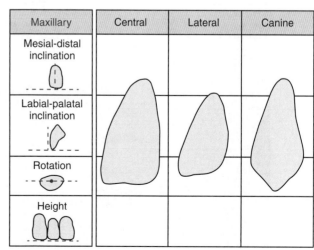

Maxillary	Central	Lateral	Canine
Mesial-distal inclination			
Labial-palatal inclination			
Rotation			
Height			

FIGURE 11-1 Tooth-positioning options for maxillary anterior teeth.

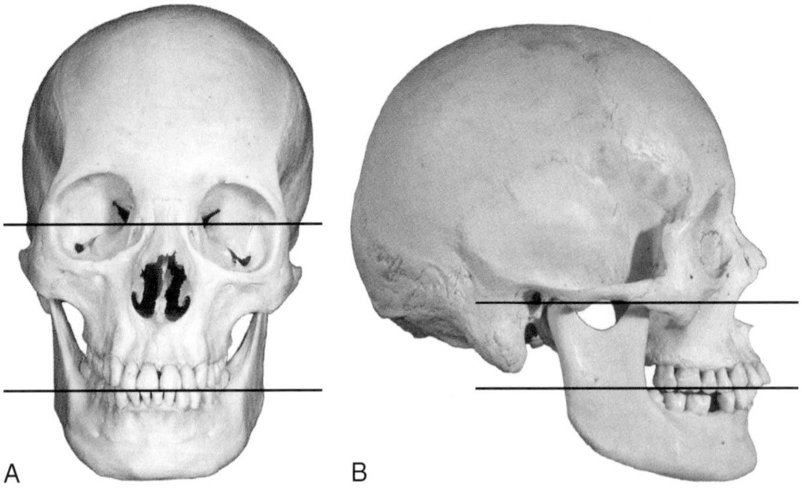

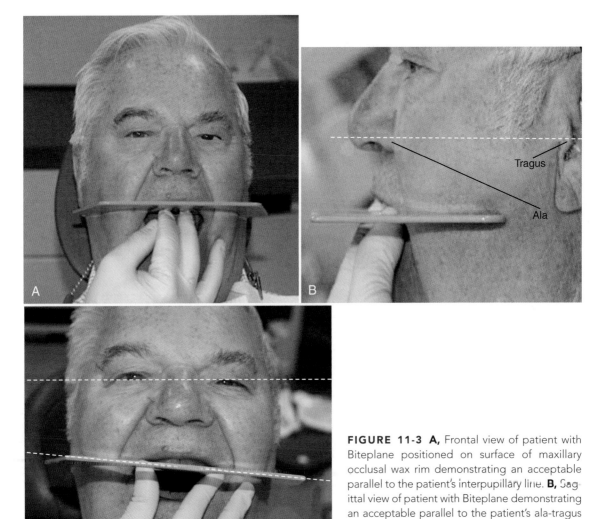

FIGURE 11-2 The ideal occlusal plane viewed in the frontal (**A**) and sagittal (**B**) planes is described as the Esthetic Reference Plane (ERP). (Adapted from Liebgott B: *The anatomical basis of dentistry*, ed 3, St. Louis, 2011, Mosby.)

Tragus

Ala

FIGURE 11-3 A, Frontal view of patient with Biteplane positioned on surface of maxillary occlusal wax rim demonstrating an acceptable parallel to the patient's interpupillary line. **B,** Sagittal view of patient with Biteplane demonstrating an acceptable parallel to the patient's ala-tragus line (Camper's plane). **C,** Biteplane demonstrating that the surface of the maxillary occlusal wax rim is not parallel to patient's interpupillary line.

If the incisal and/or occlusal surfaces are not in harmony with the patient's ERP (Fig. 11-3C), the wax rim is corrected by either removing or adding wax.

Once the wax occlusion rim is determined to be acceptable, it then becomes the prescription to the dental lab concerning the midline, length, and facial position of the maxillary anterior teeth as well as being representative of the patient's ERP.

RELATING THE ERP TO THE ARTICULATOR

There are several ways to communicate this information to the dental laboratory. In this technique a flat mounting table (Ivoclar Vivadent) (Fig. 11-4A,B) is used. The table has pre-marked average value positions that will facilitate the positioning and mounting of the maxillary cast to an average value relationship to the condyles of the articulator.

For the edentulous patient the wax rim is positioned so that the incisal edge rests on the premarked position and the midline (obtained from the patient) corresponds to the midline of the table (see Fig. 11-4A)

The maxillary cast is then mounted to the upper member of the articulator and the surface of the flat mounting table is now representative of the patient's ERP (Fig. 11-4C,D). The surface of the table also serves as a plane of reference for tooth positioning.

Tooth Position Options

There are four positions in which to set anterior teeth: mesiodistal inclination, labiopalatal inclination, rotation, and length (see Fig. 11-1). Mesiodistal inclination is viewed from the frontal plane. When the incisal edges are flush to the ERP the mesiodistal inclination is typically perpendicular to the ERP and is considered to have no inclination (Fig. 11-5A). If the tooth is inclined toward the mesial, it is described as having mesial inclination (Fig. 11-5B) If the tooth is inclined toward the distal, it is described as having mesial inclination (Fig. 11-5C).

Labiopalatal Inclination. Labiopalatal inclination is viewed from the sagittal plane. The facial surface of maxillary anterior teeth is divided into two planes. The incisal plane follows the coronal two thirds of the tooth and the cervical plane follows the apical third of the tooth (Fig. 11-6A). If the

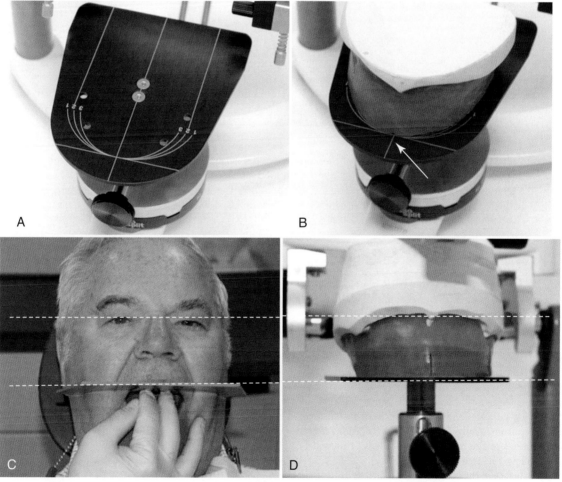

FIGURE 11-4 A, The flat mounting table has etchings that facilitate the average value mounting of the maxillary cast and individual arch form options. **B,** The maxillary occlusal wax rim is positioned to the cross-marks on the flat mounting table matching the clinically marked midline of the maxillary occlusal wax rim to the midline etching of the table. After the maxillary cast is mounted (**C**), the surface of the flat mounting table represents the patient's ERP (**D**).

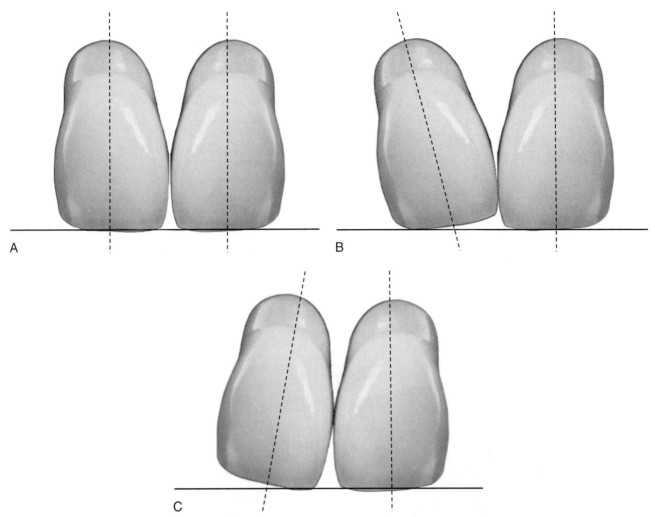

FIGURE 11-5 A, Frontal view of the central incisors illustrating the mesiodistal axes of the teeth in reference to the horizontal plane. The long axes of the centrals in this illustration are perpendicular to the horizontal plane (no inclination). **B,** The long axis of the central incisor on the left is inclined toward the mesial (mesial inclination). **C,** The long axis of the central incisor on the left is inclined toward the distal (distal inclination).

incisal plane is perpendicular to the ERP, the labiopalatal inclination is described as having no inclination (Fig. 11-6B). If the incisal plane of the tooth is inclined toward the labial, it is described as having labial inclination (Fig. 11-6C). If the incisal plane is inclined toward the palate, it is described as palatal inclination (Fig. 11-6D).

Rotation. Rotation is viewed from a perspective perpendicular to the incisal edges of anterior teeth and the cusp tips of posterior teeth and visualizing a center axis line of rotation. If the incisal edge follows the semicircular arch-form, the tooth will automatically have a slight rotation, which positions the mesial of the tooth slightly facially. This will be referred to as follow-the-arch form (Fig. 11-7A).

If the mesial surface of the tooth is rotated facially around the center axis to a degree, which is outside the arch form (i.e., the mesial surface is more prominent) it is considered to have a mesial flare and will accentuate the mesial highlight of the tooth. This will give the tooth a smaller and softer appearance (Fig. 11-7B).

If the distal surface of the tooth is rotated facially around the center axis to a degree that is outside the arch form (i.e., the distal surface is more prominent) it is considered to have a distal flare, which gives the tooth a larger and more bold appearance and the highlight is positioned more toward the center of the tooth (Fig. 11-7C).

Height. The height of a tooth is determined by whether or not it contacts the flat mounting table and is described by the number of millimeters the tooth is elevated from the surface of the table (i.e., the measured space between the incisal edge and the surface of the table) (Fig. 11-8).

RULES OF DENTAL ESTHETICS

Figure 11-9 outlines the four tooth positions previously described and applies them to each maxillary anterior tooth individually. The various esthetic changes that occur are described and illustrated in the rest of the chapter.

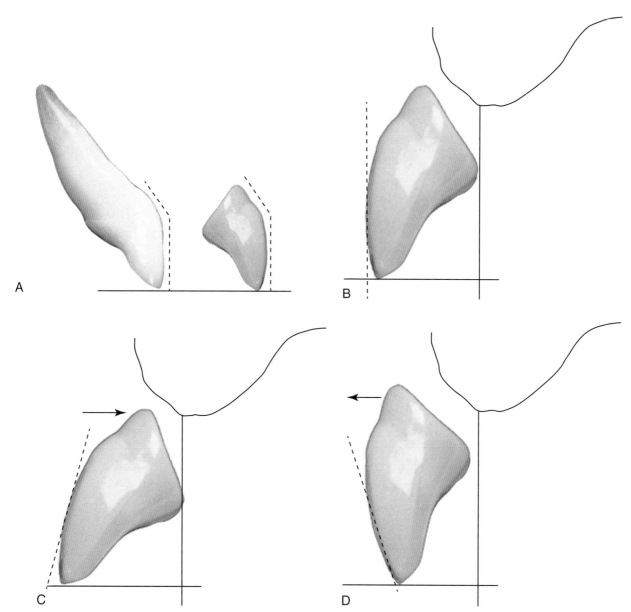

FIGURE 11-6 A, Most denture teeth are designed to match the inclinations of natural teeth. In this illustration both the natural tooth and the artificial denture tooth demonstrate two planes when viewed in the sagittal plane. The coronal two thirds are referred to as the "incisal plane" and the apical third as the "cervical plane." **B,** The incisor tooth is viewed in the sagittal plane using the surface of the flat mounting table as a reference plane. This tooth illustrates that the incisal plane is perpendicular to the reference plane (no inclination). **C,** The incisal plane is inclined toward the labial (labial inclination). **D,** The incisal plane is inclined toward the palate (palatal inclination).

Central Incisors

Mesiodistal Inclination. The central incisors have the most pleasing appearance when they have no mesiodistal inclination and when they are centered to the patient's facial midline. Mesial inclination and/or distal inclination are undesirable and are typically avoided (Fig. 11-10; see Fig. 11-8*B*).

Labiopalatal Inclination. The maxillomandibular relationship influences the labiopalatal inclination (Fig. 11-11*A*-*C*).

The most common Angle's Class 1 maxillomandibular relationship suggests that the incisal plane be perpendicular to the ERP and the maxillary ridge. This position would be considered as having no labiopalatal inclination. A Class 2 maxillomandibular relationship requires some degree of palatal inclination because of the retruded position of the mandible relative to the maxilla and a Class 3 maxillomandibular relationship requires some degree of facial inclination because of the protruded position of the mandible relative to the maxilla.

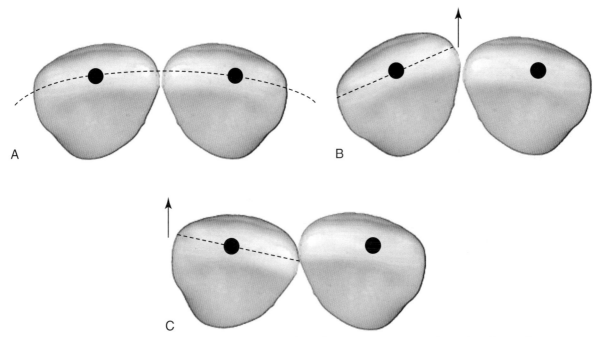

FIGURE 11-7 A, An imaginary center axis line of rotation is represented as a dot. The teeth in this illustration are rotated slightly to the mesial so that the tooth form follows the curvature of the arch, (follow-the-arch-form). **B,** The tooth to the left in this illustration is rotated making the mesial of the tooth most prominent (mesial flare). **C,** The tooth to the left in this illustration is rotated making the distal of the tooth most prominent (distal flare).

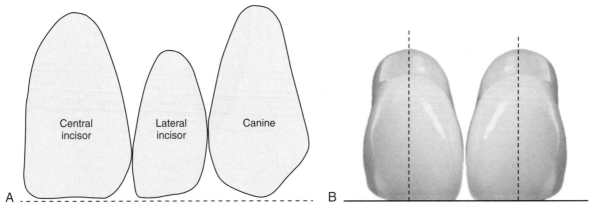

FIGURE 11-8 A, The height of the teeth will be described as the relationship of the incisal edges to the surface of the flat mounting table. If the incisal edges contact the table, the teeth are described as having "no elevation" and if they do not contact the table, they would be described as "elevated." **B,** Incisal edges are set in contact to the surface of the flat mounting table, which automatically sets the mesiodistal long axes of the teeth perpendicular to the table surface (no inclination).

CLINICAL TIP

Regardless of the selected labiopalatal inclination, both central incisors must have the same inclination. If they do not, they may appear to be of different shading. Facial inclination projects reflected light directly back to the viewer and therefore appear lighter (reflection). Palatal inclination projects light downward from the viewer and therefore appears darker (deflection) (Fig. 11-11D).

Rotation. Probably the most dramatic optical effects are produced by rotation. If the incisal edges follow the arch form and therefore have a slight mesial flare the esthetic effect is to soften the appearance (Fig. 11-12A). The soft esthetic effect is primarily caused by the highlight of the teeth that result from the mesial flare rotation (Fig. 11-12B). Having the highlight accentuated on the mesial surface of the tooth also gives the optical perception that the tooth is smaller.

Maxillary	Central	Lateral	Canine
Mesial-distal inclination	No-inclination	**Soft** Mesial **Bold** No **Never** Distal	**Soft** Mesial **Bold** No **Never** Distal
Labial-palatal inclination	**Class 1** none **Class 2** palatal **Class 3** labial **Both centrals same inclination**	**Soft** Labial **Bold** No **Never** Palatal	**Always** Palatal **Never** Labial
Rotation	**Soft** Follow arch-form **Bold** Distal-flare **Never** Mesial flare	**Soft** Follow arch-form **Softer** Mesial flare **Bold** Distal-flare	**Always** Follow arch-form **Never** Distal-flare
Height	No-elevation	**Old** No-elevation **Youth** Degrees of elevation	No-elevation

FIGURE 11-9 The various tooth positions and their esthetic effects for the maxillary anterior teeth.

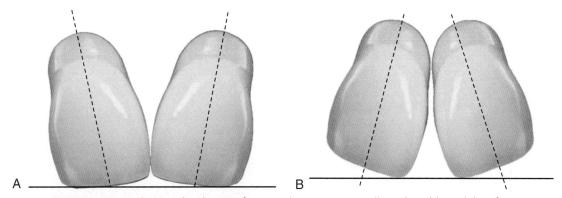

FIGURE 11-10 A, Mesial inclination for central incisors is typically undesirable and therefore not recommended. **B,** Distal inclination for central incisors is typically undesirable and therefore not recommended.

If the incisal edges are set tangentially to the arch form (with no flare), the esthetic effect is to bolden the appearance (Fig. 11-12C,D). The effect of distal flare, which locates the highlights more toward the center of the teeth, produces teeth that appear prominent (bold) and larger.

Excessive mesial flare beyond the arch form creates an unacceptable esthetic appearance (Fig. 11-12E).

Technique for Setting the Central Incisor Denture Teeth

The flat mounting table surface acts as a visual reference and a physical guide to help position the maxillary anterior denture teeth. When the central incisal edges are set in contact with the table surface, the tooth automatically squares itself to the table and assures that there is no mesiodistal inclination (Fig. 11-13A).

When viewing in the sagittal plane the incisal plane of the teeth is easily visualized and adjusted at right angles to the table. Natural teeth also are configured with an incisal plane and cervical plane and when superimposed over denture teeth explains visually why the incisal two thirds of the tooth should be perpendicular to the table surface because of the projection of the root form into the alveolus, which follows the cervical plane of the tooth (Fig. 11-13B,C). A common error is to mistakenly set the central incisors

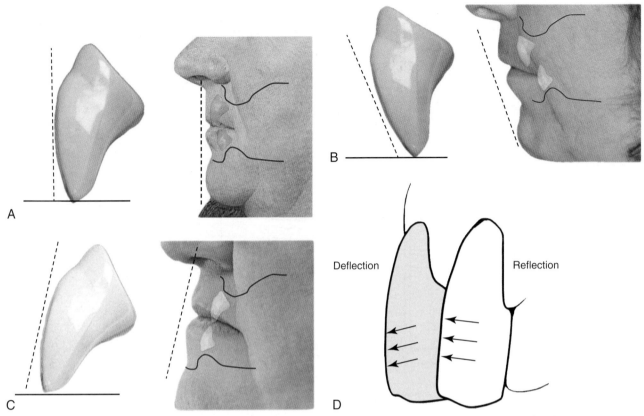

FIGURE 11-11 A, The incisal plane of central incisors are set perpendicular to the occlusal plane for Angle's Class 1 maxillomandibular relationship (no inclination). **B,** The incisal plane of central incisors are set with palatal inclination in reference to the occlusal plane for Angle's Class 2 maxillomandibular relationship. **C,** The incisal plane of central incisors are set with labial inclination in reference to the occlusal plane for Angle's Class 2 maxillomandibular relationship. **D,** It is essential that both central incisors have similar inclinations, otherwise the shades of the teeth may be perceived as different because of differing reflection and deflection of light.

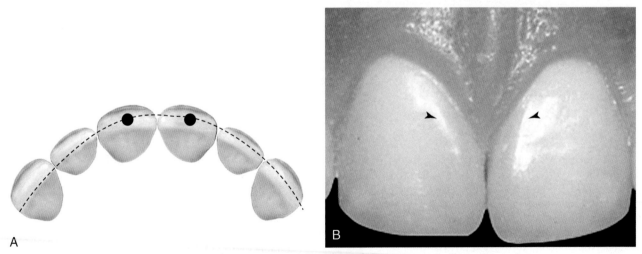

FIGURE 11-12 A, Central incisors set to follow the arch form automatically positions the mesial of the teeth slightly more prominently (mesial flare). This creates a soft effect. **B,** With this arrangement the highlights are most prominent on the mesial surfaces of the teeth.

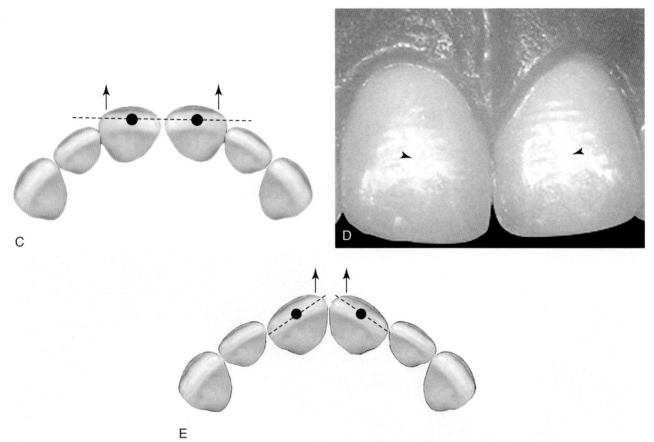

FIGURE 11-12, cont'd **C,** Central incisors positioned with no rotation creating a distal flare and a bold effect. **D,** This arrangement creates highlights that are more toward the center of the tooth. **E,** The central incisors are facially rotated with the mesial surfaces of the teeth more prominent than the arch form (mesial flare) which creating an unesthetic effect.

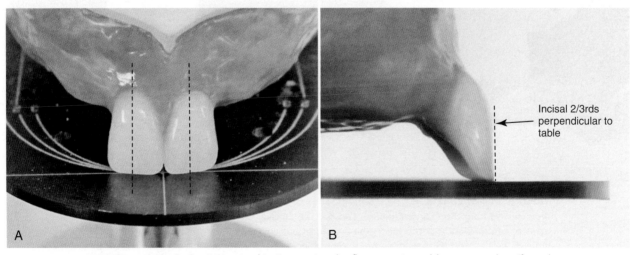

Incisal 2/3rds perpendicular to table

FIGURE 11-13 **A,** Setting central incisors using the flat mounting table as a template (frontal view). **B,** Setting central incisors using flat mounting table as a template (sagittal view).

Continued

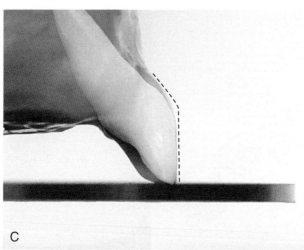

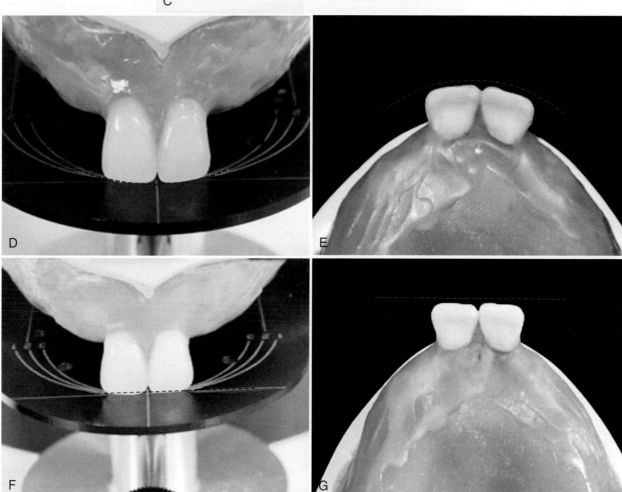

FIGURE 11-13, cont'd C, The superimposition of a natural tooth demonstrates that the root projection is from the "cervical plane" and not the "incisal plane." **D,** Frontal and (**E**) palatal views of central incisors set to follow the arch form pattern on the surface of the flat mounting table. **F,** Frontal and (**G**) palatal views of central incisors set to follow the straight line on the surface of the flat mounting table.

and projecting the root to follow from the incisal plane. This would set the teeth with excessive labial inclination and therefore provide insufficient lip support. Unfortunately, this happens often and can be a dead giveaway that the patient is wearing a denture.

Rotation of the central incisors is guided by the etched arch forms on the surface of the flat mounting table. The appropriate arch form is selected based on the wax rim contour that has been tried in and approved at the time of the wax rim try-in appointment. If the central incisors are set to follow the curve of the arch form, it assures a slight mesial flare, which imparts a soft effect (Fig. 11-13D,E).

If the central incisors are set to follow the straight line on the surface of the flat mounting table, it creates a slight distal-flare, which imparts a bold effect (Fig. 11-13F,G). The length of the central incisors is determined by having the incisal edges set in contact to the surface of the flat mounting table. The incisal length of the wax rim was determined during the wax occlusion rim try-in appointment, and by mounting the wax occlusion rim using the flat mounting table the table surface automatically represents the appropriate incisal length.

Lateral Incisor

The positioning of the lateral incisors is most responsible for establishing a person's esthetic characteristic as soft or bold and/ or young or old. Slight variations in the positioning of lateral incisors give "charm" to the anterior arrangement.

Mesial Inclination. A slight mesial inclination is most common for the lateral incisors and creates a soft effect and gives the illusion that the tooth is smaller due to the location of the highlight confined to the mesial surface of the tooth (Fig. 11-14A,B). The degree of mesial inclination is slight and if projected it would intersect at the patient's navel. No inclination will produce a bold effect (Fig. 11-14C,D)

Distal inclination of lateral incisors creates a highlight that is not in harmony with the central incisor, resulting in an undesirable esthetic effect and is therefore avoided (Fig. 11-14E,F).

Labiopalatal Inclination. Positioning the lateral incisor with a labial inclination greater than that of the central incisors creates a soft effect (Fig. 11-15A,B).

A labiopalatal inclination similar to that of the central incisor creates a bold effect (see Fig. 11-15). Setting the lateral incisor with a more palatal inclination than the central incisor generally creates an undesirable esthetic effect and should be avoided (Fig. 11-15C,D).

Rotation. The rotational position produces the most dramatic changes of soft and bold characteristics. If the lateral incisors are set to follow the curvature of the arch, the mesial surfaces of the teeth are automatically more prominent. This creates a soft perception because the mesial of the tooth will receive the most highlight (Fig. 11-16A).

The softness can be exaggerated by adding more mesial flare (Fig. 11-16B). This effect is especially effective in reducing the perceptual width of the lateral incisors.

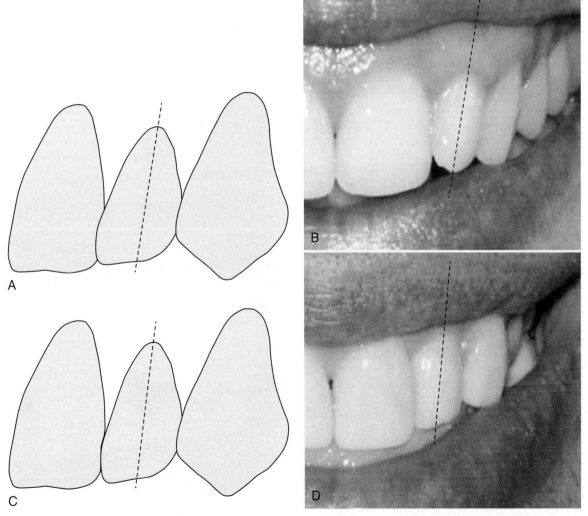

FIGURE 11-14 A, The lateral incisor is set with a mesial inclination creating a soft effect **(B). C,** The lateral incisors are set with no mesiodistal inclination creating a bold effect **(D).**

Continued

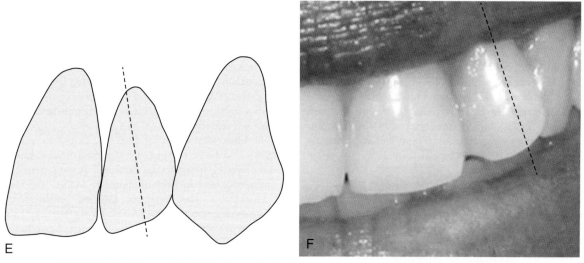

FIGURE 11-14, cont'd E, The lateral incisor is set with a distal inclination creating an undesirable esthetic effect (**F**).

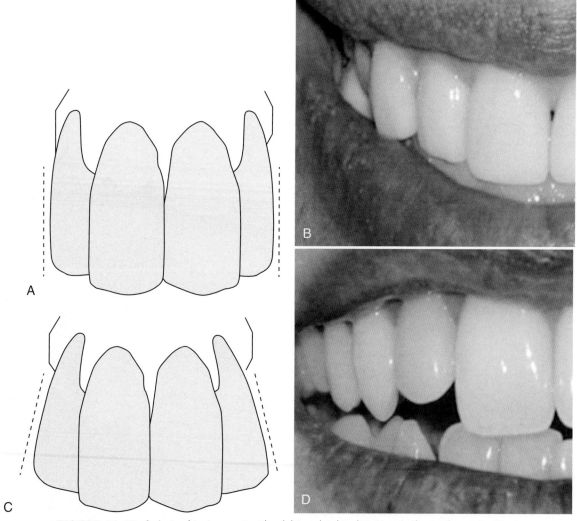

FIGURE 11-15 A, Lateral incisors set with a labiopalatal inclination similar to the central incisors creates a bold effect (**B**). **C,** Lateral incisors set with more labial inclination than the central incisors creating a soft effect (**D**).

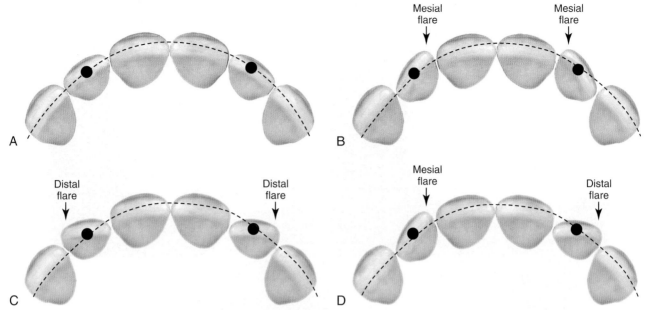

FIGURE 11-16 A, Lateral incisors set to follow the arch form, which automatically places the mesial surfaces of the teeth more prominently and creates a soft effect. **B,** Increasing the mesial flare of the lateral incisors beyond the arch form accentuates the highlights on the mesial surfaces of the teeth and creates a softer effect. **C,** Lateral incisors set with distal flare creating a bold effect. **D,** Lateral incisors are set differently (combination of mesial and distal flares) to create a special esthetic effect.

Distal rotation shifts the highlights to the middle of the tooth and adds a bold characteristic and also gives the perception that the tooth is larger (Fig. 11-16C).

It can be acceptable to set one lateral incisor in a soft position and the other in a bold position, especially if these were the characteristics that the patient exhibited with the natural teeth and if he/she desires those same characteristics to appear in the prosthesis (Fig. 11-16D).

Length. The length of the lateral incisor effects the impression of age. Positioning the incisal edge on the same plane as the central incisor and canine creates an older effect elevating the lateral incisor creates the appearance of various degrees of youth depending on the degree of elevation. The greater the elevation, the younger the appearance (Fig. 11-17).

Technique for Setting the Lateral Incisor Denture Teeth. Setting the desired mesiodistal inclination is facilitated using the table surface as a reference. In addition, the length can be easily set at this time by elevating the incisal edge a predetermined distance from the table surface (Fig. 11-18A,B)

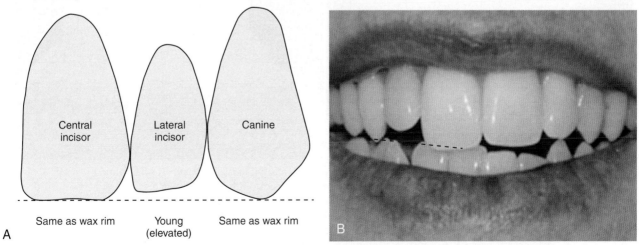

FIGURE 11-17 A, The lateral incisor length in relationship to the central incisor and canine contributes to the perception of age. **B,** The more elevated the lateral incisor, the more youthful the effect.

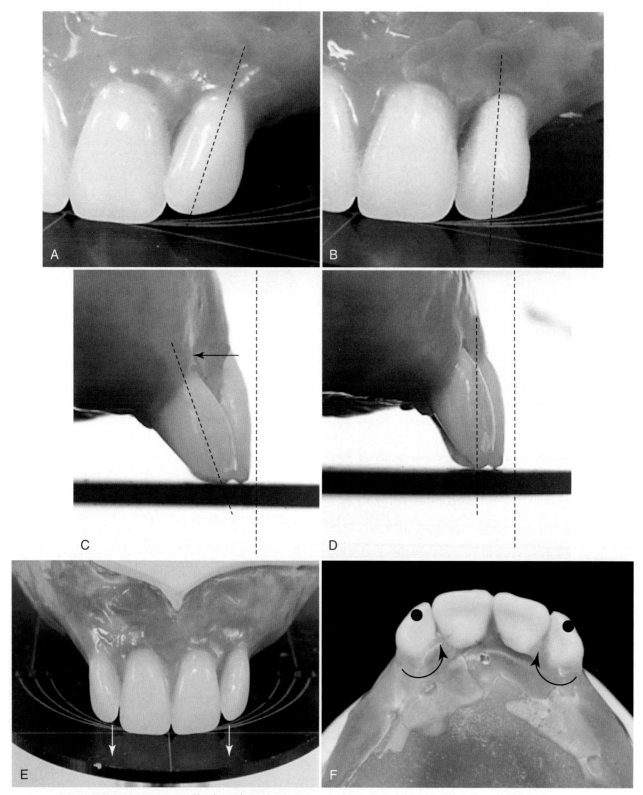

FIGURE 11-18 A, The lateral incisor positioned with a slight mesial inclination and elevation, which creates a soft youthful appearance. **B,** The lateral incisor with no inclination and no elevation, which creates a bold effect. **C,** The labiopalatal inclination is determined by its relationship to the labiopalatal of the lateral incisor inclination of the central incisor and is easily visualized using the surface of the table as a reference plane. **D,** Lateral incisor labiopalatal inclination set similar to central incisor. **E, F,** Lateral incisors set with slight mesial flare accentuating mesial highlights.

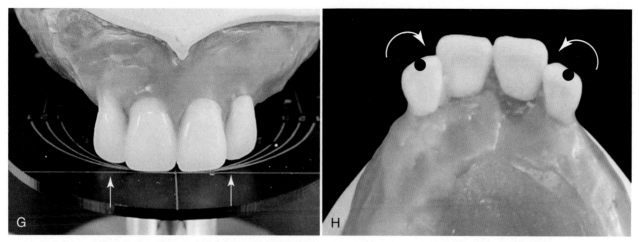

FIGURE 11-18, cont'd G, H, Lateral incisors set with distal-flare accentuatiung highlights toward the center of the teeth.

If the lateral incisor is set with more labial inclination than the central incisor, its effect will be soft (Fig. 11-18C)

If set similar to the inclination of the central incisor the effect is bold (Fig. 11-18D).

If the rotation of the lateral incisor follows the arch form the effect is soft. If the rotation is increased to a mesial flare, the effect is even softer because the highlight becomes more concentrated on the mesial surface of the tooth (Fig. 11-18E,F).

If rotated to have distal-flare, the highlight shifts to the center of the tooth and the effect is bold and gives the perception that the tooth is larger (Fig. 11-18G,H).

Maxillary Canine

The maxillary canine is the cornerstone of the arch and must provide an esthetic transition to the first premolar. Therefore, there are very few characterization options that are esthetically and functionally acceptable.

Mesiodistal Inclination. Similar to the lateral incisor, a slight mesial inclination that projects to the navel provides a slight soft effect which is pleasing and most commonly used for setting canines (Fig. 11-19A).

However, the mesial inclination must be kept to a minimum, otherwise it would be in obvious contrast to the first premolar, which typically is set with no mesiodistal inclination. The bold effect is produced by minimizing or eliminating the mesiodistal inclination (Fig. 11-19B). This does dramatically embolden the canine and should be used only if this effect is desired. Slight mesial inclination of the canine is generally the default setting used most often.

Distal inclination of the canine produces an unesthetic "fanglike" appearance and is therefore never recommended (Fig. 11-19C).

Labiopalatal Inclination. The canine is considered the cornerstone of the arch and must appear more prominent in the cervical area than the central and lateral incisors. It is recommended that a palatal inclination of approximately 30 degrees will give an acceptable effect of prominence in the arch (Fig. 11-19D).

No inclination or labial inclination creates an unesthetic "squatty" appearance to the canine and prevents it from appearing as the cornerstone of the arch.

Rotation. The canine can be considered to have a mesial incisal edge and a distal incisal edge. The mesial incisal edge

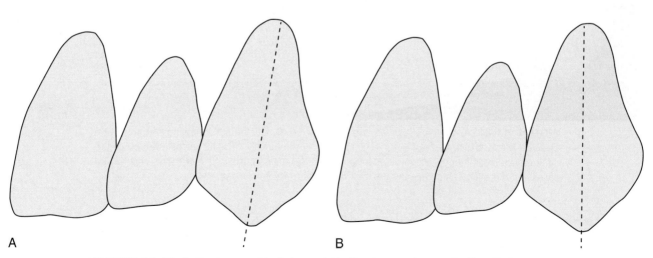

FIGURE 11-19 A, Canine set with slight mesial inclination creating a soft effect. **B,** Canine set with no mesiodistal inclination creating a bold effect. *Continued*

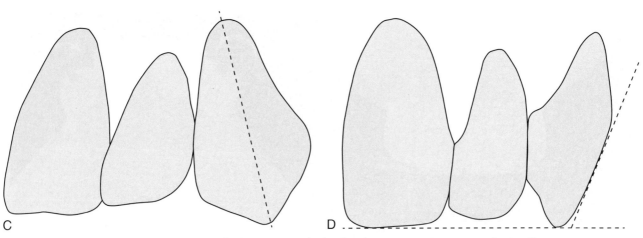

FIGURE 11-19, cont'd C, Canine set with distal inclination creating an unesthetic effect. **D,** Canine is set with approximately a 30-degree palatal inclination.

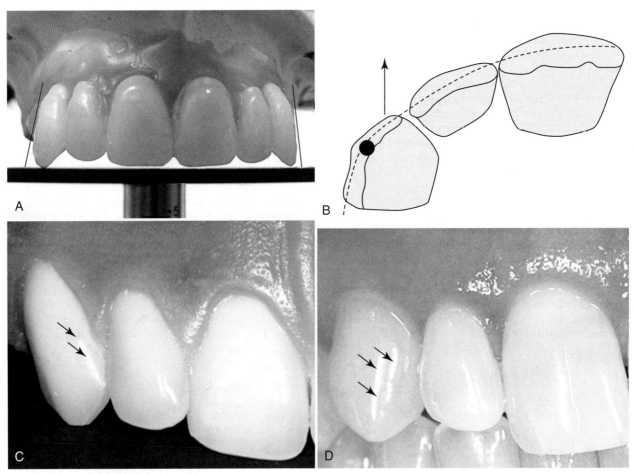

FIGURE 11-20 A, Canines set with labial inclination. **B,** Canine set following the arch form creating a soft effect. **C,** Following the arch form automatically sets the mesial surface of the canine more prominently, accentuates highlight on the mesial surface of the tooth, and should always be done. **D,** The canine is set with a distal flare, which is unesthetic.

should follow the arch form established by the lateral and central incisors. The distal incisal edge projects toward the center of the central fossa of the first premolar (Fig. 11-20A).

The rotational setting of the canine has limited options. The incisal edges of the canine can be divided into a mesial half and a distal half. The mesial half follows the anterior arch form and the distal half aims toward the central fossa of the posterior teeth (Fig. 11-20B). This rotation locates the highlight on the mesial surface of the tooth and gives a desirable appearance for the canine (Fig. 11-20C).

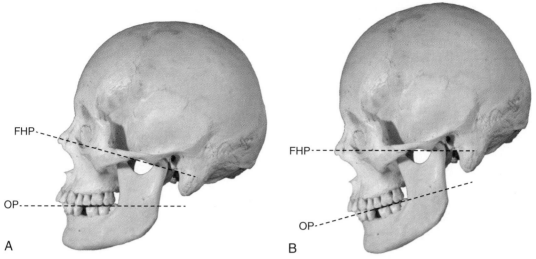

FIGURE 11-21 A, The skull is oriented in a position that has the occlusal plane parallel to the floor. Camper's (ala-tragus) plane similarly would be parallel to the floor. **B,** The skull is oriented in an normal upright postural position. The Frankfort Horizontal is typically parallel to the floor. (Adapted from Liebgott B: *The anatomical basis of dentistry*, ed 3, St. Louis, 2011, Mosby.)

CLINICAL TIP

Any degree of distal flare forces the highlight to be toward the center of the tooth creating a very unesthetic overexposure of the facial surface of the canine. Therefore setting the canine with distal-flare should always be avoided (Fig. 11-20*D*).

Length. Similar to the central incisor the canine is always set into contact with the surface of the flat mounting table.

SMILE LINE ESTHETICS

This technique identifies the occlusal plane (Camper's horizontal plane) from the patient and transfers this plane to the articulator using the flat mounting table. Therefore the orientation of the patient's occlusal plane is parallel to the floor (Fig. 11-21*A*). This is a position of convenience for fabrication of the restoration on the articulator; however, it does not reflect the patient's normal postural position. Typically, when a patient is in a normal upright postural position the Frankfort Horizontal Plane is parallel to the floor and the occlusal plane is approximately 15 degrees elevated posteriorly (Fig. 11-21*B*). Therefore the anterior teeth that were set to the surface of the flat table will assume a smile line elevation when inserted due to the patient's normal postural position. The smile line is plane and not a curve and the appearance of its elevation is related to the patient's posture.

CONCLUSION

Many factors give interpretation to the esthetics of anterior teeth. This chapter outlined several of these criteria and a reliable technique to communicate this information to the dental laboratory.

REFERENCES

1. Frush JP, Fisher RD: Introduction to dentogenic restorations, *J Prosthet Dent* 5: 586-595, 1955.
2. Frush JP, Fisher RD: How dentogenic restorations interpret the sex factor, *J Prosthet Dent* 6:160-172, 1956.
3. Frush JP, Fisher RD: How dentogenics interprets the personality factor, *J Prosthet Dent* 6:441-449, 1956.
4. Frush JP, Fisher RD: The age factor in dentogenics, *J Prosthet Dent* 7:5-13, 1957.
5. Frush JP, Fisher RD: The dynesthetic interpretation of the dentogenic concept, *J Prosthet Dent* 8:558-581, 1958.
6. Frush JP, Fisher RD: Dentogenics: Its practical approach, *J Prosthet Dent* 9:914-921, 1959.
7. The glossary of prosthodontic terms, *J Prosthet Dent* 94(1):10-92, 2005.

12

Luting Agents

Richard D. Trushkowsky

HISTORY

One of the first dental adhesives was conceived by the Mayan Indians to attach semiprecious stones to cavities on the facial surface of anterior teeth. A mixture of bone powder and fruit juice served to etch both the tooth and the stone. Crystals that formed propagated into the etched surface to provide micro-mechanical retention for the stones.[1] In the 1850s the only existing cement was zinc oxide and eugenol,[2] mixed using zinc oxide-based powder and eugenol liquid. The cement had an obtunding effect on pulp but its disadvantages, including a high film thickness, have limited its use. Fifty years ago the selection of cement was relatively easy because there was still little to choose from and gold was the predominant indirect restorative material. Zinc phosphate, a combination of zinc oxide powder and phosphoric acid, was one of the oldest (1879) and most widely used cements. It has the advantages of high compressive strength and a thin film thickness of less than 25 microns. It was acceptable for placement of mechanically retentive metal-constructed restorations but its solubility, low strength, minimal adhesion, and poor esthetics limit its use currently. Zinc polycarboxylate was developed by Dennis Smith in 1968 and was one of the first chemically adhesive formulas (adheres primarily to enamel and to a lesser degree to dentin). This cement is formed when zinc oxide powder is mixed with polyacrylic acid. The advantages of zinc polycarboxylate are its kindness to pulp tissue and its ability to bond to tooth structure. Zinc polycarboxylate may plastically deform resulting in failure after a few years.[3] It has a short working time and greater solubility than other cements.[4] Glass ionomer cements are considered hybrids of silicate cements and polycarboxylate cements. They consist of fluoroalumino-silicate glass and a liquid containing polyacrylic acid, itaconic acid, and water. The development of glass-ionomer cements was first announced by Wilson and Kent. All these cements have two main advantages: they are inexpensive and their chemistry and mode of use are well understood. Appropriate use can still provide excellent results. In 1994 resin modified glass ionomers were introduced, formed by replacing part of the polyacrylic acid in conventional glass ionomer cements with hydrophilic methacrylate monomers.[5] The mechanical properties of all glass ionomers increase with time, which possibly contributes to their clinical success.[6] They can be used with metal and with high strength core materials. Composite resin cements are modified restorative materials and because of this exhibit high strength, excellent adhesion, and minimal solubility and are esthetically pleasing. These attributes are advantageous in their use with weak esthetic restorations such as glass ceramics and indirect composite resins and to increase the retention of a restoration. They also vary in composition (paste-paste, single paste, or powder-liquid).

LUTING AGENT REQUIREMENTS

A luting agent is dental cement that is used to attach indirect restorations to prepared teeth.[7] Luting agents may be classified as definitive or provisional. It has been stated that "no available product satisfies the requirements for an ideal luting agent and comprehensive patient care requires several materials . . . . the best choice is not always easy."[5] Luting agents are intended to maintain an indirect restoration in place for a specific period of time and fill the space at the interface between a tooth and the restoration. Their basic requirements include: not deleterious to tooth or oral tissues, adequate working time to place the restoration, enough flow to seat the restoration completely, able to resist functional forces, radiopacity, and should be insoluble to maintain an intact seal.[8]

Classification

Most cements are created by combining a powder that can release cations into an acid solution (base) and a liquid (acid).

The resulting cations react with acid anions to form a salt. These materials are categorized as AB (acid-base) cements. Resins are formed by the polymerization of macromolecules.[9] Cements have been categorized based on their main ingredient (i.e., zinc phosphate, zinc silicophosphate, zinc oxide-eugenol, zinc polyacrylate, glass-ionomer, and resin),[10] or by matrix type (i.e., phosphate, phenolate, polycarboxylate, resin, and resin-modified glass-ionomer).[11] Cements can be considered active or passive. Active cements such as compomers and composite resin cements involve an interaction with dentin by forming a hybrid layer with the dental material. Cements that mechanically interlock with rough surfaces on tooth structure and the internal aspect of the restoration are considered passive. Although glass ionomers form intermediate layers on dentin they do not bond to materials etched by hydrofluoric acid or treated with silane and are considered passive.

DEFINITIVE (NONPROVISIONAL) LUTING AGENTS

Glass-Ionomer Cements

Glass-ionomer cements (glass polyalkenoate cement). The term *glass-ionomer* is considered generic and includes a larger group of cements with similar compositions[9] that have been very popular due to ease of use, good flow properties, adhesion to tooth structure and base metals, fluoride release, sufficient strength, and moderate cost. Its primary indication is for metal and porcelain fused to metal restorations. The setting reaction for glass ionomers cements is an acid-base reaction with the calcium aluminosilicate (sometimes replaced by strontium or lanthanum) glass reacting with polyalkenoic acids, polyacrylic acid, itaconic acid or maleic acid to develop a hydrogel. The material experiences a sudden set but continues to mature over several months prior to completion.[9] The length of time necessary for a complete set of glass ionomers and its moderate modulus of elasticity may limit its use to single units and fixed partial dentures with a limited span. Post cementation is also not recommended as any vibration would diminish its mechanical retention.[12] To reduce potential postoperative sensitivity, the use of a resin-based sealer, which also enhances retention, has been recommended.[13] Contamination by saliva should be avoided for several minutes to prevent loss of material by erosion caused by early solubility. However, the newer glass ionomer luting cements are fast setting and after 5 minutes are resistant to any water challenge.[14] The bond to tooth structure is significantly reduced when the tooth is excessively dried, which also contributes to postcementation thermal sensitivity.[15]

CLINICAL TIP

Do not desiccate the dentin as this will cause sensitivity. Blot the tooth with a cotton pellet to remove excess moisture. Do not use the cement if the cement surface becomes dull.

Resin-Modified Glass-Ionomer

Resin-modified glass ionomer (resin-modified glass polyalkenoate) was developed in the 1980s to increase the physical properties and minimize water dissolution of glass ionomers. To accomplish this, water soluble or polymerizable resins were added to regular glass ionomers to create a new classification, resin modified glass ionomer cement (RMGI). These materials consist of hydroxymethyl methacrylate and ethylene glycol dimethacrylate and glycidyl methacrylate and Bisphenol A epoxy (Bis-GMA). RMGIs are considered dual hybrids because the setting is both a glass-ionomer reaction and chemical or light activation of the resin component. The initial setting reaction is caused by polymerization of the resin followed by the acid-base reaction that forms a polysalt hydrogel matrix that strengthens the previously formed polymer matrix.[9] The change in composition makes RMGI less susceptible to early erosion during setting, less soluble, and creates higher compressive and tensile strengths than unmodified glass-ionomer luting cement. In addition, when mixed properly and applied to moist dentin little postcementation sensitivity will result.[15]

CLINICAL TIP

Do not desiccate the dentin because this will cause sensitivity. Blot the tooth with a cotton pellet to remove excess moisture. Do not use the cement if the cement surface becomes dull. Avoid contamination with saliva.

Resin Luting Agents

Resin luting agents are distinctive because a polymer matrix forms to fill and seal the space between the tooth and the restoration as opposed to regular cements, which combine a powder and liquid to form a hydrogel.[12] The mechanical properties of resin cements should be considered in addition to their adhesive potential. A higher modulus of elasticity will result in less polymerization shrinkage stress and possibly less microleakage. The elastic modulus measures the ability of a material to resist elastic deformation under load. The elastic modulus is an excellent measure of the capacity of a luting material to transfer a load to a tooth and allow stress distribution.[8] However, the fit of the restoration is also a factor because increased exposure to saliva or other liquids may result in a decline of physical properties. This would increase sensitivity and secondary caries. A strong correlation is also found between the amount of fillers and the mechanical properties. A high modulus material will also enhance then fracture resistance of a ceramic crown. Most resin cements necessitate pretreatment of the dental substrate and often the restoration in order to encourage bonding between the two surfaces.[16] Pretreatment can be etch and rinse, a self-etch dentin adhesive, a self-adhesive resin cement or a dual-affinity adhesive resin. Current resin cements are popular because of their wide range of uses, high compressive and tensile strength, low solubility, and excellent esthetic potential. Disadvantages are the difficulty in removing excess material, technique sensitivity, relative expense, difficulty in removing restorations if needed, and sensitivity to moisture.[12]

Resin cements should be used primarily for their qualities that enhance restorations such as esthetic all-ceramic restorations, lab-processed composite resin restorations, conventional metal ceramic restorations with inadequate retention, resin-bonded fixed partial dentures and for the cementation of either metal or fiber posts. The matrix can form by: mixing two or more components called chemically curing, activating photosensitive molecules of the material with visible light curing, or by combining the two methods (termed *dual curing*). Chemically polymerized materials are gradual and slower setting creating less contraction stress. The main disadvantage is that the reaction cannot be controlled once it is initiated and bubbles may be formed. However, these bubbles, if they form, serve to reduce stress. Visible light is the technique most commonly used for polymerization, but a major concern is delivering sufficient light energy to the entire luting media so that the photoinitiator can begin the polymerization action. The main drawback is polymerization contraction stress occurs more rapidly than with self-curing materials.[8]

Resin bonding to enamel is by micromechanical interlocking into an acid etched surface. Bonding to dentin is also micromechanical but is more complex due to the organic components of dentin. Dentin is a hydrated composite resin material composed of both a collagen based organic matrix in conjunction with mineral reinforcement. Various regions of the dentin react differently to either total etch or self-etch adhesives. Usually bond strengths are higher in superficial dentin compared to deep dentin. In addition, resin bonding in the cervical area is less predictable because of the oblique nature[17] and decreased number of the dentinal tubules.[18] In addition, the different chemical formulations of the three different types of luting resins result in a different morphological appearance of the bonded interface.[19] Total etch luting agents (etch-and-rinse adhesives) involve a preliminary etching step followed by rinsing in order to remove the smear layer and smear plugs. The acid etching will create a dentin demineralization of 3 to 5 μm, allowing collagen fibrils to be exposed with minimal amount of remaining hydroxyapatite. The next step includes the application of a primer with hydrophilic properties followed by a solvent-free adhesive resin applied to the prepared surface and penetration of the hydrophobic monomer into the collagen network and dentin tubules. The primer causes the resin to follow it and they polymerize together. The primer has both hydrophilic and hydrophobic elements to interact with the dentin and the resin. This results in the creation of a hybrid layer.

Two-step adhesives allow the combination of primer and adhesive into one solution. (e.g., RelyX ARC, 3M ESPE) The hydrophilicity of these adhesives makes them more prone to water sorption and possible hydrolyticdegradation. The solvents present in these adhesives are also more difficult to evaporate and may become entrapped in the adhesive layer after polymerization.

Self-etch adhesives contain acid monomers that etch and prime the dentin. Their excessive hydrophilicity allows them to attract moisture from moist dentin and possibly act as semipermeable membranes. This may also contribute to hydrolysis and degradation of the bond. The acidic groups in the unpolymerized layer of these adhesives (due to oxygen) create a competition with the peroxides for aromatic tertiary amines of the luting agent. This creates a problem in the copolymerization between the peroxides and the aromatic amine. To avoid this problem, self-etching primers used with coordinated resin cements contain ternary redox initiators (for example aryl sulphinate salts, ascorbic acid, or barbituric acid salts).[20] This will allow ideal polymerization of the resin cement in either an auto or dual-polymerized method. Without light activation, dual-polymerized cements act as self-polymerize cements. These cements take longer to polymerize, allowing the adhesive to act as a semipermeable membrane. The water can act to increase stress and lead to failure of the adhesive cement. The self-etching primers can be categorized as one-step system (Panavia F,

Kuraray Medical) or two-step system (Bistite II, Tokuyama Corp, Tokyo), which uses an additional resin coating placed over the primed dentin surface prior to application of the dual-polymerized resin cement.[21]

Self-etch cements also create a hybrid layer but it is not as thick as total etch systems. Methacrylates with both hydrophobic and hydrophilic groups promote monomer penetration into suitably prepared dentin. The impregnated monomers become entangled with the collagen fibril of surface demineralized dentin creating a hybrid layer after polymerization.

Self-Adhesive Cements (Self-Etch Cements)

Self-adhesive cements (self-etch cements) are defined as cements that are filled polymer based materials that are capable of adhering to tooth structure without the need for a separate adhesive or etchant. Introduced in the past 10 years, the chief benefit of these materials is their simplicity of use. They combine features of composite resin restoratives, self-etching adhesives, and often dental cements. The additions of acid-functionalized methacrylate or similar molecules are extremely important for these cements to form an effective chemical bond to teeth. This is because a preformed polyalkenoate or one that was established in situ during the curing process requires acidic monomers. These materials are very similar to compomers but they have a different acidic monomer concentration and they also have a lower filler content to improve the cement thickness. The cements are currently two-part adhesives that are mixed by hand, capsule trituration or auto-mix. One component is usually a di-and/or multimethacrylate monomer and an acid-functionalized monomer ([meth]acrylate monomers with carboxylic or phosphoric acid groups)that achieves the demineralization.[22] Resin cements have to be able to bond to a variety of different substrates such as dentin, enamel, porcelain, other ceramic materials, metals, and indirect composite resins. The self-adhesive resin cements are capable of adhesion to the dentin substrate but the acids of the cement do not produce an etch pattern equivalent to that of phosphoric acid. It has been suggested that pre-etching of enamel will increase the bond strength because of the creation of microscopic irregularities on the enamel surface; however, pre-etching the dentin creates a thick collagenous matrix that cannot be penetrated by the cement. Some of these cements are dual polymerized and others such as are self-curing, Multilink, (Ivoclar Vivadent), enabling their use in nearly all clinical situations.

> **CLINICAL TIP**
>
> Etch the enamel surrounding the preparation to decrease staining. Remove excess cement quickly especially in the interproximal areas because set cement can be extremely difficult to remove. When removing excess be careful to avoid pulling material from under the restoration margin.

The placement of indirect restorations requires the proper selection of materials to seal all margins and provide adequate retention of the restoration. The strength, solubility, and adhesion of the luting agent are critical to the longevity of the restoration. The clinician must have adequate knowledge in order to select the appropriate luting material for each clinical situation.

PROVISIONAL CEMENTS

Some of the qualities desirable for provisional cements include the following:[23,24]

+ Easy to dispense, mix, and apply
+ Good retention (adhesion) of the indirect restoration
+ Easy removal of excess from the external surfaces of the restoration after cementation
+ Adequate working and setting time
+ Optimal viscosity and handling properties for ease of application
+ Easy removal of the indirect restoration from the preparation after cementation without damaging the soft tissues, tooth preparation
+ Easy removal of the provisional cement from the tooth preparation, including dentin and enamel, cast core materials (cast metal)
+ Easy removal of the provisional cement from the internal surfaces of the restoration when the restoration needs to be recemented
+ No or minimal reaction to the restorative material
+ Biocompatibility to soft tissues, pulp, and tooth structure
+ Noninterference with adhesion of a definitive cement good shelf life

A provisional cement must protect the pulp and retain the provisional restoration in position in the arch. Once an impression is made, positional stability is extremely important. This relates to both occlusal and proximal contacts. The cement should not interfere with the setting of the impression material. Sometimes the definitive restoration is cemented provisionally to ascertain long-term periodontal and pulpal health.

Originally many of the provisional cements contained zinc-oxide powder and eugenol liquid and many still do. However, the advent of acrylic and composite resin material necessitated the introduction of new materials. The zinc-oxide powder and eugenol-containing cements often interfered with the free radical polymerization in the resins used for provisional restorations and resin-bonded indirect restorations and may soften those restorations.[25-27]

Newer cements may be eugenol free and some do not contain zinc oxide. Some cements contain additives such as fluoride or potassium nitrate for desensitization (e.g., Temp Advantage, GC America, Inc.). This material also contains e chlorhexidine for disinfection. Provisional cements contain polycarboxylate, (e.g., UltraTemp, Ultradent Products, Inc. and HY-Bond Polycarboxylate Temporary Cement, Shofu Dental Company). Temp Advantage (GC America) contains fluoride, chlorhexidine, and potassium. Some manufacturers provide a variety of provisional cements that contain different properties. For example, Temp-Bond (Kerr) contains eugenol, Temp Bond NE (Kerr) has no eugenol and TempBond Clear (Kerr) contains triclosan and is useful in placing a more translucent provisional.

Special implant cements are also a relatively new addition. Ideally, they should provide long-term retention, radiopacity (to verify cement removal), low solubility, easy handling with two-stage set (allows excess cement removal during a gel phase),

a natural appearance, no taste or odor, and the convenience of an automix dual-barrel syringe with disposable tips, which provides a consistent mix and controlled dispensing. (e.g., Premier Implant Cement, Premier Dental Products, Inc.).

CONCLUSION

There are a number of different luting agents available to the clinician. As the definitive component of the restorative process, it is vital that the practitioner have a proper understanding of the indications and limitations of these materials.

REFERENCES

1. Söderholm K-J: Critical evaluation of adhesive test methods used in dentistry, *J Adhes Sci Technol* 23(7,8):973-990, 2009.
2. Anusavice KJ: *Phillips' science of dental materials*, ed 11, St Louis, 2003, Elsevier Science.
3. Smith DC. A new dental cement, *Br Dent J* 124(9):381-384, Nov 5, 1968.
4. Burgess JO, Ghuman T: *A practical guide to the use of luting cements*, Tulsa, OK, 2008, PennWell.
5. Rosenstiel SF, Land MF, Crispin BJ: Dental luting agents: a review of the current literature, *J Prosthet Dent* 80:280-301, 1998.
6. Xu X, Burgess JO: Compressive strength, fluoride release and recharge of fluoride-releasing materials, *Biomaterials* 24:2451-2461, 2003.
7. The Academy of Prosthodontics: The glossary of prosthodontic terms, *J Prosthet Dent* 94(1):21-38, 2005.
8. de la Macorra JC, Pradies G: Conventional and adhesive luting cements, *Clin Oral Investig* 6:198-204, 2002.
9. Wilson AD, Nicholson JW: *Acid-base cements, their biomedical and industrial applications*, New York, 1993, Cambridge University Press.
10. Craig RG, Powers JM: *Restorative dental materials*, ed 11, St Louis, 2002, Mosby.
11. O'Brien W: *Dental materials and their selection*, ed 3, Chicago, 2002, Quintessence.
12. Hill EE, Lott J. A clinically focused discussion of luting materials, *Aust Dent J* 56 Suppl 1:67-76, 2011.
13. Johnson GH, Hazelton LR, Bales DJ, et al: The effect of a resin-based sealer on crown retention for three types of cement, *J Prosthet Dent* 91(5):428-435, 2004.
14. Mount GJ: *An atlas of glass-ionomer cements, a clinicians guide*, ed 3, New York, 2002, Martin Dunitzs.
15. Rosensteil SF, Rashid RG: Post cementation hypersensitivity: scientific data versus dentists' perceptions, *J Prosthodont* 12:73, 2003.
16. Duarte Jr S, Sartori N, Sadan A, Phark J-H: Adhesive resin cements for bonding esthetic restorations: a review, *QDT* 42-65, 2011.
17. Mixson JM, Spencer P, Moore DL, Chappell RP, Adams S: Surface morphology and chemical characterization of abrasion/erosion lesions, *Am J Dent* 8:5-9, 1995.
18. Ferrari M, Cagidiaco MC, Vici A, Mannocci F, Mason PN, Mjor IA: Bonding of all-porcelain crown: structural characteristics of the substrate, *Dent Mater* 17:156-164, 2001.
19. Yang B, Ludwig K, Adelung R, Kern: Micro-tensile bond strength of three luting resins to human regional dentin, *Dent Mater* 22:45-56, 2006.
20. Ikemura K, Endo T: Effect on adhesion of new polymerization initiator systems comprising 5-monosubstituted barbituric acids, aromatic sulphonate amides, and tert-butyl peroxymaleic acid in dental adhesive resin, *J Appl Polym Sci* 72:1655-1668, 1999.
21. Carvalho RM, Pegoraro TA, Pegoraro LF, Tay FR, Silva NR, Pashley DH: Adhesive permeability affects coupling of resin cements that utilize self-etching primers to dentin, *J Dent* 32(1):55-65, 2004.
22. Ferracane JL, Stansbury JW, Burke FJT: Self-adhesive resin cements-chemistry, properties and clinical considerations, *J Oral Rehabil* 38:295-314, 2011.
23. Margeas RC: Temporary cement options, *Inside Dentistry* 7:124-126, 2011.
24. Strassler HE, Morgan RJ: Provisional–temporary cements. Techniques to facilitate placement of provisional restorations, *Inside Dental Assisting* 8:38-43, 2012.
25. Fonseca RB, Martins LR, Quagliatto PS, Soares CJ: Influence of provisional cements on ultimate bond strength of indirect composite resin restorations to dentin, *J Adhes Dent* 7:225-230, 2005.
26. Bagis B, Bagis YH, Hasanreisoğlu U: Bonding effectiveness of a self-adhesive resin-based luting cement to dentin after provisional cement contamination, *J Adhes Dent* 13:543-550, 2011.
27. Grasso CA, Caluori DM, Goldstein GR, Hittelman E: In vivo evaluation of three cleansing techniques for prepared abutment teeth, *J Prosthet Dent* 88:437-441, 2002.

13

Bleaching and Related Agents

Kenneth W. Aschheim

Esthetic improvement of acceptably shaped but discolored teeth by chemical means is highly desirable because of its conservative nature. The chemical agents and specific procedures used depend on a number of factors, including the type, intensity, and location of the discoloration.

HISTORY

A professional response to the unrelenting quest for whiter teeth dates back at least 2000 years. First century Roman physicians maintained that brushing the teeth with urine, particularly Portuguese urine, whitened them.[1] In the 1300s, the most requested dental service, other than extraction, was tooth whitening. After abrading the enamel with coarse metal files, barber-surgeons would apply *aquafortis*, a nitric acid solution, to whiten the teeth. This common practice continued into the eighteenth century.[1]

Early protocols for bleaching of teeth mainly involved nonvital teeth.[2] In the late 1800s, the combination of hydrogen peroxide, ether, and electricity was reported to be an effective method of lightening teeth.[3] In the early 1900s, a pyrozone (ether peroxide) mouthwash was recommended as an effective method of whitening teeth.[4] Pyrozone use continued through the 1960s.[2]

Around 1916 hydrochloric acid was used successfully to treat "Colorado brown stain" (endemic fluorosis).[5] In 1937, the combination of five parts 100% hydrogen peroxide with one part ether and heat was reportedly used as a treatment for this same type of discoloration.[6] Two years later successful bleaching of fluorosis staining using 30% hydrogen peroxide, ether, and heat was described.[7] In 1966, the use of hydrochloric acid combined with hydrogen peroxide was advocated.[8] Not until 1970 was hydrogen peroxide demonstrated to be effective for the treatment of dentinal discoloration as well.[9] In the late 1980s carbamide peroxide (shelf life of 1-2 years) replaced hydrogen peroxide (shelf life of 2 months) as the chemical of choice and has become the most commonly used agent for tooth whitening.[2]

MECHANISM OF ACTION

Chemistry

Carbamide peroxide ($CH_6N_2O_3$), also known as urea peroxide, urea hydrogen peroxide (UHP), or percarbamide spontaneously decomposes into hydrogen peroxide (H_2O_2) and urea ($CO(NH_2)_2$). A 10% carbamide peroxide concentration decomposes into approximately 3.5% concentration hydrogen peroxide of and 6.5% urea.[2] Because of its chemical stability, carbamide peroxide greatly aided the acceptance of bleaching by the dental profession; however, it is the hydrogen peroxide component that accomplishes the bleaching. The exact mechanism by which discoloration is removed by hydrogen peroxide is not entirely understood, but likely it includes oxygen-releasing, mechanical cleansing actions[10] and oxidation or reduction reactions. Hydrogen peroxide is a low-weight molecule and can therefore diffuse easily through the organic matrix of the tooth.[2] It is also capable of denaturing proteins.[11] Depending on conditions, hydrogen peroxide can release free radicals ($H_2O_2 \rightarrow H\cdot + \cdot OOH$ or $H_2O_2 \rightarrow HO\cdot + \cdot OH$); perhydroxyl anions ($H_2O_2 \rightarrow H^+ + :OOH^-$) or a combination of free radicals and anions ($HOO\cdot + OH^- \rightarrow O_2^- \cdot + H_2O$ in a basic solution and $HOO\cdot \rightarrow O_2^- \cdot + H^+$ in an acidic solution).[12] These compounds tend to be attracted to electron-rich alkene double bonds and form unstable epoxides and can form alcohols. It is believed that double bonds can create discoloration; therefore breaking these bonds often eliminates discoloration. The bleaching of tetracycline staining may be through an oxidative degradation of the quinone ring,[13] which converts the molecule to lighter-colored alcohols by adding hydroxyl on tetracycline under types of discoloration (Mechanism, Appearance, and Treatment Considerations discussed later in this chapter). In addition, alcohols are more water-soluble compounds and thus more easily removed.[14] Hydrogen peroxide also increases the permeability of tooth structure, thereby increasing the movement of ions through the tooth.[11]

The peroxide can also join the tetracycline molecule with calcium through a chelation process and a subsequent incorporation into the hydroxylapatite crystal of the tooth during the mineralization stage of development. The mechanisms differ according to the type of discoloration involved and the chemical and physical environment present at the time of action (e.g., pH, temperature, co-catalysts, lighting, and other conditions).[12]

FACTORS AFFECTING VITAL BLEACHING

Surface Cleanliness

All extrinsic stains and surface films must be removed from the tooth surface before bleaching. This will maximize the contact area between the whitening agent and the tooth as well as minimize the chance of diluting the bleaching agent.

Concentration

Higher concentrations of carbamide peroxide produce a more rapid whitening effect[15] as well as increased tooth sensitivity.[2,15] This speed effect is not linear; doubling the concentration does not double the speed.[2] However, the dominant variable obtaining a satisfactory result is time—not the concentration of the bleaching agent.[16]

The Use of a Light

Meta-analysis studies on the use of light during in-office vital bleaching demonstrated that light-activated systems produced better immediate bleaching results than non-light systems when lower concentrations of hydrogen peroxide (15%-20%) were used.[17] At higher concentrations of HP (25%-35%), no differences were noted. In addition, light-activated systems produced a higher percentage of tooth sensitivity than the non-light systems.[17]

Temperature

Higher temperatures increase the rate of oxygen radical release.[18] Although increasing in vitro the temperature of the bleach to 100° C doubled the chemical reaction,[19] the speed of the color change in tooth structure may not be altered and the rise in temperature may lead to additional pulpal sensitivity.[20] This heat-induced increase in chemical reaction rate may explain the increased efficacy of some in-office bleaching lights.[2] To monitor heat-induced sensitivity, local anesthesia should never be used during in-office treatments that produce heat.[20]

Phosphoric Acid

Acid etching agents such as phosphoric acid can alter the tooth surface.[21] The use of 37% phosphoric acid following bleaching can significantly increase the decalcifying effect of the acid on the enamel surface,[22] creating an uneven etched surface,[23] and this greater susceptibility to the action of the acid persisted for at least 1 week after bleaching.[24] The surface changes created by phosphoric acid are far more significant than the changes created by carbamide peroxide.[25-27] Tooth sensitivity can be reduced by using agents with a pH in the range of 7.[2] Studies have shown that the optimal pH for hydrogen peroxide is between 9.5 and 10.8, with the later

producing whitening rates 50% faster than a pH of 9.5[28,29] (see also the section on Non-Vital Bleaching Acid Etching).

Buffering Agents

Carbamide peroxide decomposes into radicals and ions, including hydrogen ions. The hydrogen ions acidify the environment.[30,31] To maintain a more neural pH, buffering agents are added to the gel. These agents protect the pulp and promote the continued production of free radicals, resulting in the breakdown of the large, dark color molecules into ultra-small colorless and white molecules.[32]

Time

The longer the duration of bleach exposure, the greater the degree of whitening. However, extended exposure to bleaching agents increases the likelihood of sensitivity.[33,34]

Gingival Tissue Irritation

Gingival tissues can undergo an acute inflammatory reaction following exposure to even small amounts of carbamide peroxide solution.[35] Higher concentrations will temporarily blanch the gingival soft tissues. Therefore all bleaching procedures should be designed to minimize soft tissue contact. However, carbamide peroxide has been shown to reduce plaque and gingivitis scores[36] and there is some evidence that the extrinsic staining associated with chlorhexidine is reduced when it is combined with carbamide peroxide.[37]

Potassium Nitrate

Potassium nitrate is a common ingredient in desensitizing toothpaste.[38] Its mechanism of action is believed to be caused by an increase in the extracellular potassium ion, which depolarizes nerve fibers and renders them unable to repolarize.[39] However, studies have questioned its effectiveness to reduce sensitivity, particularly when used for a short period of time.[40]

Stability and Potency of Carbamide Peroxide

Carbamide peroxide can be stabilized by both chemical additives and/or thermal stabilization (refrigeration). Cold temperature storage is far more predictable to maintaining the potency, effectiveness, and desired controlled instability of the product.[41-48] In addition, refrigeration reduces the need for chemical stabilizers such as an anhydrous base and "acidifiers,"[43] allowing the whitening gels to be fully aqueous base and at or above pH 7.[49] Carbamide peroxide requires a controlled decomposition into hydrogen peroxide and urea to effectively bleach teeth. Therefore although more inconvenient, thermal stabilization is a far more predictable stabilization method because of the predictability of this decomposition when placed in the warm mouth, than chemical stabilizers, especially if the latter lacks activation agents that will trigger the neutralization of the chemical stabilizer.[48]

Chemical Accelerators

Bleaching effectiveness is directly proportional to the concentration of free radicals (as opposed to non-active oxygen and water), which are produced by the decomposition of carbamide peroxide. Chemical accelerators speed the breakdown of peroxide by both breaking down chemical stabilizers and by producing their own ions and free radicals.[49]

Whitening Gel Viscosity and Solubility

Bleaching trays are open on the periphery; they do not seal in the gel nor prevent the ingress of saliva and sulcular fluid.[45] Therefore the carbamide peroxide gel is combined with a high viscosity, insoluble anhydrous base. Because of the higher concentration, in-office gels are mixed with even higher viscosity base to prevent the gel from running off the teeth. However, high viscosity anhydrous bases exhibit high surface tension, thereby causing less intimate microscopic adaptation of the gel to the tooth surface, which can slow the absorption of gel into the microstructure of the teeth.[49] Therefore bleaching gel formulations must balance the safety of a higher viscosity base with the undesirable diminution of surface wetting.

Sensitivity

Postoperative tooth sensitivity is the most common side effect of tooth bleaching. Some studies using 10% carbamide peroxide agent and various levels of potassium nitrate and sodium fluoride show that almost half the participants exhibiting post-bleaching sensitivity;[50] however, practitioner experiences and other studies report less.[51] The duration of sensitivity, if it occurred, was three or fewer days in 77% of patients.[50] Sensitivity was greatest the first week of bleaching and then declined. The study also suggested that the inclusion of additives such as potassium nitrate and sodium fluoride are effective in reducing tooth sensitivity but not soft tissue irritation.[50]

Types of Sensitivity

Two types of postoperative bleaching sensitivity have been described.[52]

Type 1: Typical Dentinal Hypersensitivity: Generalized tooth discomfort with sensitivity to various stimuli such as hot, cold, or brushing

Type 2: Sharp, Shooting Hypersensitivity: Instantaneous sharp, shooting sensitivity running the length of anterior teeth usually occurring in the absence of external stimulus

Different theories exist for the etiology of each type.[53]

Hydrodynamic Theory of Dentinal Hypersensitivity. Pulpal sensitivity is believed to be mediated by a hydrodynamic mechanism.[54] Smear layer plugs normally block the dentinal tubules reducing the tubular flow;[55] however, peroxide-based whitening systems remove these plugs,[56] which results in a 32-fold increase in hydraulic conductance of dentinal tubular fluid[55,57] and Type 1 sensitivity.[58] The mechanism for this sensitivity involves hyperosmotic-whitening gel contacting tubular fluids, which increases the ability of an irritating stimulus (e.g., temperature, evaporation, osmotic, chemical) to affect the flow of dentinal tubular fluid. This in turn creates pressure on the pulpal odontoblasts, resulting in their deformation and the subsequent stimulation of the cell membranes of A-Delta nerve endings, resulting in the sensation of sensitivity or pain. In addition, once the plugs are removed the tubular fluid continues to be exposed to the oral environment.

Type 2 sensitivity tends to occur more often in incisors and canines. During bleaching, low molecular weight hydrogen peroxide (H_2O_2) may enter the pulp[58] via aberrations in the enamel.[58] The body naturally produces hydrogen peroxide and other oxidative chemicals, which contain free radicals. The body also manufactures antioxidant enzymes such as catalase, superoxide dismutase, hemoxygenase-1, and glutathione peroxidase to protect against these free radicals.[59] The by-products of these reactions are molecular oxygen (O_2) and water (H_2O). Some have theorized that the production of these breakdown products in the confined space of the tooth may also produce pressure on the A-Delta neurons to create the sharp pain sensation.[52]

Safety Issues Relating to the Use of Hydrogen Peroxide in Dentistry

Hydrogen peroxide is an oxidizing agent that liberates oxygen radicals. Localized injury can occur with direct exposure of the radicals to the mucosa, eyes, and the gastrointestinal and respiratory tracts.[60] In levels used in home bleaching, carbamide peroxide can cause mild mucosal irritation to the mucosa, nausea, and vomiting.[60] Eye exposure may result in immediate but generally transient pain.[60] At higher concentrations, dermal and mucosal exposure can cause burning, tingling, and a transient white discoloration of the skin.[60]

CLINICAL TIP

Due to the risk of mucosal exposure with the bleaching gel, the patient must be continuously monitored during in-office bleaching procedures. If tissue contact occurs, the procedure must be stopped and the area rinsed with copious amount of water. Gingival burns appear as whitish areas (Fig. 13-1) and typically disappear after a short time. Patients should be warned of this possibility before treatment.

General Considerations

The efficacy of bleaching teeth with heat and hydrogen peroxide is well documented.[9,61-65] Goldstein observed no known loss of tooth vitality after 30 years of bleaching more than 30,000 vital teeth.[66] Although mild thermal sensitivity is a common sequela

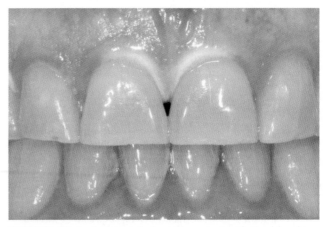

FIGURE 13-1 Accidental gingival contact with the bleaching solution will result in a temporary white discoloration which typically reverts to its original appearance..

of bleaching, clinical studies have failed to demonstrate long-term irreversible pulpal effects.[67]

TREATMENT METHODS

Office treatment (power bleaching) methods generally involve the use of 35% or greater hydrogen peroxide in either liquid or gel form. In the *thermocatalytic* technique, the chemical is heated (see the section on Temperature). High intensity light or laser (*photocatalytic* technique) sometimes combined with heat (*thermophotocatalytic* technique) can also be used to accelerate the chemical reaction.

Power bleaching is also used in combination with home bleaching.[66,67] It has been proposed that a certain segment of the population whose lifestyles are not amenable to home treatment can be treated exclusively by in-office power bleaching.[66]

Restorative Implications

In some cases, discoloration has returned after initial successful or partly successful treatment. Subsequently placed porcelain or composite resin laminate veneers, or any restoration in which the color of the tooth structure will affect the color of the restoration, may not prevent color regression of the underlying tooth structure and the restorative materials may not completely mask the visual display of any such changes. The esthetic effects of such color regression depend on the amount of regression and the degree of translucency of the overlying restoration. This must be considered if discoloration removal therapy is followed by restorative treatment of any kind.

It also has been demonstrated that applying hydrogen peroxide to bovine tooth structure diminishes the bond strength between unfilled resin and acid-etched enamel.[68-70] Presumably oxygen inhibition of resin polymerization and the creation of voids in the resin tags may be caused by residual hydrogen peroxide or peroxide-related substances in the interprismatic enamel areas after bleaching.[69,70] This residual substance apparently is not removed either by a 1-minute water rinse or by thoroughly drying the surface.[70] However, the changes within the tooth structure that cause the diminished bond strength seem to be reversible.[68] The most common recommendation is to postpone placing bonded restorations for 2 to 3 weeks after bleaching.[71-73]

TYPES OF DISCOLORATION: MECHANISM, APPEARANCE, AND TREATMENT

Tetracycline Staining

The broad-spectrum tetracycline group of antibiotics was first introduced in 1948 for use in the treatment of respiratory illnesses. However, tooth discoloration caused by incorporation of systemic tetracycline into tooth structure was not reported until 1956.[74]

Mechanism. The exact mechanism of tetracycline staining is not completely understood. It is hypothesized to occur by the joining of the tetracycline molecule with calcium through a chelation process and a subsequent incorporation into the hydroxylapatite crystal of the tooth during the stage of development.[75-78] A second theory maintains that the discoloration involves a binding of the tetracycline to tooth structure by a metal-organic matrix combination of the tetracycline complex.[79,80] Although some tetracycline accumulates within the enamel, it is primarily deposited in the dentin[81] because of the large surface area of the dentin apatite crystals compared with enamel apatite crystals;[82] however, enamel hypoplasia also can result.[83]

Mode of Action. Extracted tetracycline-stained rat,[84] dog,[85] and primary human teeth[86] darkened when exposed to sunlight. Interestingly, further exposure to various light sources (sunlight, or incandescent or ultraviolet lights) produces a subsequent lightening of the tetracycline stain.[77,84-89] It has been postulated that tetracycline incorporated into hydroxylapatite, when oxidized by light (photo-oxidation), produces the red quinone product 4-α, 12-α anhydro-4-oxo-4-dedimethylaminotetracycline (AODTC).[13,90] Continued photo-oxidation of AODTC photolyzes, or bleaches, the red quinone.[13] Addition of diluted hydrogen peroxide yields an irreversible bleaching of the red quinone as well.[13]

Appearance. Tetracycline discoloration may be yellow, yellow-brown, brown, gray, or blue. The intensity of the staining varies widely. Distribution of discoloration usually is diffuse, and severe cases may exhibit banding. The staining usually is bilateral and affects multiple teeth in both arches.

The hue and severity of tooth discoloration depend on four factors associated with tetracycline administration:

1. Age at the time of administration: Anterior primary teeth are susceptible to discoloration by systemic tetracycline from 4 months in utero through 9 months postpartum. Anterior permanent teeth are susceptible from 3 months postpartum through age 7 years.[91]
2. Duration of administration: The severity of the staining is directly proportional to the length of time the medication was administered.[92,93]
3. Dosage: The severity of the staining is directly proportional to the administered dosage.[91,94,95]
4. Type of tetracycline: Coloration has been correlated with the specific type of tetracycline administered.[96]
   a. Chlortetracycline (Aureomycin): Gray-brown stain
   b. Demethylchlortetracycline (Ledermycin): Yellow stain
   c. Doxycycline (Vibramycin): Does not cause staining
   d. Oxytetracycline (Terramycin): Yellow stain
   e. Tetracycline (Achromycin): Yellow stain

Yellow tetracycline staining slowly darkens to brown or gray-brown when exposed to sunlight. Therefore, the anterior teeth of children often darken first, whereas the posterior teeth, because of reduced exposure to sunlight, darken more slowly.[10] In adults, however, natural photobleaching of the anterior teeth (see the preceding section on Mechanism section under Tetracycline Staining) has been observed, particularly in individuals whose teeth are excessively exposed to sunlight because of maxillary lip insufficiency.[87] Hypocalcified white areas of varying opacity, size, and distribution also may be present.

Tetracycline Staining Categories

A number of different classifications of degrees of tetracycline staining have been suggested.[61] Bleaching success is dependent on the severity and color of the staining. Yellow-brown to brown staining generally responds better to bleaching than blue to blue-gray staining.

1. Mild tetracycline staining. Mild staining can be light yellow, light brown, or light gray and staining is uniform

throughout the clinical crown. No banding is present (Fig. 13-2A).

2. Moderate tetracycline staining. Moderate staining is more intense than mild staining (Fig. 13-2B).

3. Severe tetracycline staining. Severe tetracycline staining is intense, and the clinical crown may exhibit horizontal color banding (Fig. 13-2C). Bleaching generally is not performed because of the time involved and the poor prognosis. However, although less than ideal results are to be expected, the outcome may be esthetically satisfactory to the patient. The yellow-brown to brown component generally responds better than the blue to blue-gray component.

Treatment Considerations. Acid/abrasion techniques are not indicated for the removal of tetracycline stains because the discoloration primarily resides in the dentin. In general the results of bleaching yellow, yellow-brown, and brown stains are more favorable than those with blue-gray to gray stains. When teeth show any combination of yellow, brown, blue, or gray stains, the blue and gray components may remain to some degree despite a more favorable bleaching of the yellow and brown components. In addition, less intense stains have a better prognosis and usually bleach more quickly. Teeth with diffuse staining generally respond better than those with banding.

Ultraviolet Photooxidation. Laboratory evidence that photooxidation is both the cause of and a "cure" for tetracycline staining suggests that light alone is potentially a viable treatment for some tooth discolorations. In vitro ultraviolet (UV) irradiation of tetracycline-stained rat dentin produced complete stain removal after 24 hours of exposure.[87] However, UV light does not penetrate enamel easily. Other sources of higher intensity UV light, such as deuterium arc sources or UV lasers, may overcome this obstacle, but problems such as high temperature generation, skin and mucosal burns, eye damage, potential carcinogenicity, and structural damage to enamel and dentin have not yet been suitably addressed, making this an unacceptable alternative at this time.[87]

Fluorosis

Mechanism. Endemic fluorosis, or mottling, is caused by the presence of excessive systemic fluoride during enamel matrix formation and calcification.[97,98] Fluorosis is actually a form of enamel hypoplasia,[97] hence the white spotting. Darker discoloration occurs through extrinsic staining of the hypoplastic enamel. Thus, the darker stains occur only after tooth eruption.[98] A fluoride concentration of 0.7 to 1.2 parts per million (ppm) in the municipal water supply maximizes the caries-preventive

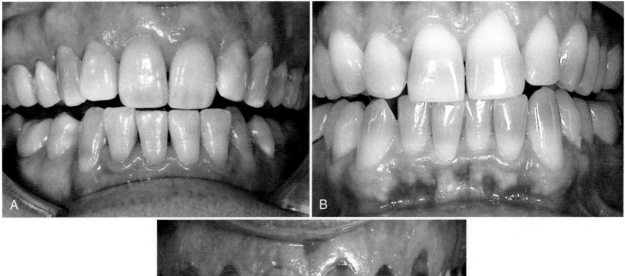

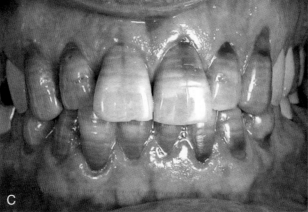

FIGURE 13-2 A, Mild tetracycline staining. **B,** Moderate tetracycline staining. The maxillary arch was previously treated with direct composite resin veneers. **C,** Severe tetracycline staining with typical banding pattern. The blue and gray components remained despite a more favorable bleaching of the yellow and brown components.

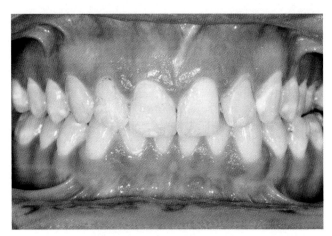

FIGURE 13-3 Fluorosis stains.

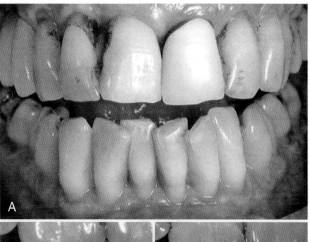

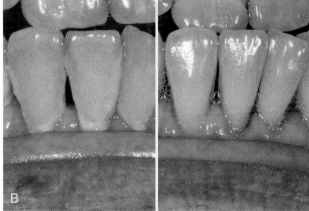

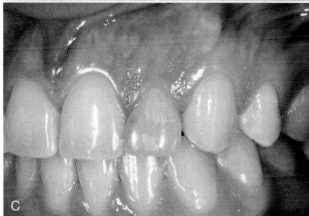

FIGURE 13-4 A, Extrinsic environmental staining. Some extrinsic stains may be eliminated by simple prophylaxis. **C,** Intrinsic staining can result from the deposition of hemorrhagic by-products and decomposition of pulpal tissue into the dentinal tubules after pulpal trauma (see Fig. 13-13A).

benefits of fluoride while minimizing the likelihood of mild dental fluorosis.[99]

Appearance. Staining usually is bilateral and affects multiple teeth in both arches. Fluorosis presents as mild, intermittent white spotting, chalky or opaque areas, yellow or brown staining of varying degrees (Fig. 13-3) and, in the severest cases, surface pitting of the enamel.[99,100]

Treatment Considerations. It has been suggested that bleaching and acid/abrasion systems are effective for treating superficial fluorosis stains.[10,101] It has been proposed that a more conservative approach may be to attempt home bleaching first, followed by selective acid/abrasion if that is still required.[100] It also has been reasoned that treatment time, financial considerations, and the patient's lifestyle may indicate the use of acid/abrasion as the initial treatment, followed by bleaching.[102] (See the section on White Spot Lesions later in this chapter.)

Extrinsic Environmental Stains

Mechanism. Essentially limited to enamel, extrinsic environmental staining is caused by a variety of factors, including food, beverages, and tobacco products.

Appearance. Environmental staining affects multiple teeth and appears as yellow or brown stains of varying intensities (Fig. 13-4A). The staining can be diffuse, but protected areas of the teeth, pits, and other enamel defects may be more intensely stained because of inadequate oral hygiene procedures on these "protected" surfaces

Treatment Considerations. Superficial extrinsic staining often can be removed by proper home care or with routine professional prophylaxis (Fig. 13-4B; see also Fig. 13-4A).

Staining of Pulpal Etiology: Trauma or Necrosis

Mechanism. Intrinsic staining results from the deposition of hemorrhagic by-products into the dentinal tubules after pulpal trauma[103]-105 or necrosis.[105]

Appearance. Discoloration of pulpal origin can be red, yellow, yellow-brown, brown, gray, or black. Obviously, discoloration is limited to the pulpally involved tooth or teeth (Fig. 13-4C).

Treatment Considerations. Acid/abrasion techniques are not indicated for stains of pulpal etiology.

Staining After Endodontic Therapy

Mechanism. Staining that occurs after endodontic therapy can be caused by excessive hemorrhaging during pulp removal or by decomposition of pulpal tissue following incomplete extirpation.[103,106]

Various endodontic medicaments and sealers containing barium, iodine, or silver also may cause discoloration, as can gutta-percha.[103,107-109]

Appearance. Discoloration of pulpal origin can appear red, yellow, yellow-brown, brown, gray, or black. Discoloration from endodontic medicaments and sealers ranges from orange-red to dark red, or gray to black.[106,107] Discoloration obviously is limited to the endodontically treated tooth or teeth (Fig. 13-5B).

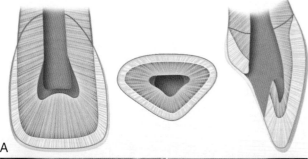

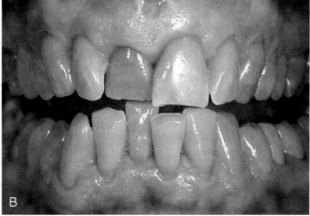

FIGURE 13-5 A, Elusive pulp horns and lateral extensions of the pulp chamber often remain untouched during routine endodontic access preparation. (The access preparation is highlighted in black.) Careful removal of tissue and debris from these areas may help prevent subsequent tooth discoloration. **B,** Intrinsic staining results from the deposition of hemorrhagic by-products and from endodontic medicaments which have filtrated the dentinal tubules.

Treatment Considerations. Acid/abrasion techniques are not indicated for stains of pulpal etiology. The absence of pulp tissue allows for placement of bleaching agents directly into the pulp cavity. Staining caused by medications, sealers, and filling materials generally is less amenable to bleaching than staining resulting from biologic causes.[110] In an in vitro, intracoronal bleaching study in which a combination of sodium perborate and hydrogen peroxide was used in teeth stained with one of seven different sealers, the teeth were markedly improved after bleaching, although some color regression occurred after 6 months.[106]

Staining from Pre-eruption Trauma: Direct and Indirect

Mechanism. Discoloration of a permanent tooth may occur after trauma to its primary counterpart.[111] Blood breakdown products from the traumatized site can infiltrate the developing enamel during the calcification stage.[98] Also, the apex of the primary tooth may directly traumatize the ameloblasts or the enamel matrix. Discoloration of a permanent tooth also may result from jaw fractures associated with the developing dentition, periapical inflammation of a primary tooth, or other infections in the area of a developing tooth bud.[98]

Appearance. Discoloration usually is white or yellow-brown and often sharply demarcated or spotty rather than diffuse.[111] This discoloration can closely mimic that caused by endemic fluorosis or tetracycline ingestion; however, it usually is limited to the facial enamel surface of one or two teeth, usually the maxillary incisors.[112] Enamel defects also may be present if the ameloblasts or the enamel matrix was disturbed.[98]

Treatment Considerations. A normal response to pulp vitality testing can aid in distinguishing between staining induced by developmental trauma and that arising from pulpal etiology.

White Spot Lesions

Mechanism. White spot enamel lesions can be developmental, acquired, or a combination of the two. Developmental lesions result from alterations that occur during the matrix formation or calcification stages of tooth development resulting in surface and subsurface porosities[113] and subsequent optical and physical changes. Endemic fluorosis and trauma are two of the most common causes, but developmental disturbances during this period caused by genetic disorders, febrile and other illnesses, and unknown factors also occur. The same demineralization process can also occur as an adverse side effect of adhesively bonded orthodontic brackets,[114,115] especially in the presence of poor oral hygiene.[112] The term *dysmineralization* has been proposed to refer to these lesions because of the difficulty often encountered in determining the precise nature of these mineralization abnormalities.[116] It has been hypothesized that hypomineralization occurs because of acid production which leads to a loss of calcium ions (Ca^+) and phosphate ions PO_4^- from the tooth enamel.[117] Hypomineralization results in a loss of translucency at the incisal border of the anterior teeth, with concurrent poorly delineated white opacities.[118] Traumatic dental injuries to the developing tooth bud can also cause hypomineralization.[119,120] These areas of hypomineralization are called Striae of Retzius, Hunter Shreger Bands or incremental lines of von Ebner.[121] When they occur in dentin, they are called contour lines of Owen.[115]

Appearance. White spot lesions manifest as discrete areas that are lighter than the surrounding normocalcified enamel (Fig. 13-6A). The intensity of the lesion varies from mildly decreased chroma to opaque chalky white. Size, distribution patterns, and penetration depth vary greatly.

Treatment Considerations. For treatment planning purposes, a tooth with localized white spot lesions can often be considered a mosaic of light areas on a background of normocalcified tooth structure. If the background tooth structure is a desirable color, acid/abrasion techniques may be considered. (See the section on Acid Microabrasion Combined with Resin Infiltration Therapy later in this chapter.) However, if the background color is undesirable, a bleaching system may be appropriate. In this situation, the contrasting white spot lesions may become significantly less noticeable and esthetically more acceptable after a successful bleaching of the normocalcified background area (Fig. 13-6,*B-D*).

(See the general considerations section under Acid Microabrasion Combined with Resin Infiltration Therapy later in this chapter.)

Staining from Silver Amalgam

Mechanism. Tooth discoloration from silver amalgam is caused primarily by the visibility of a restoration through relatively translucent tooth structure. To varying degrees, it also may be caused by direct staining of the tooth structure by the reaction products of intraoral sulfides and the copper or silver ions of the amalgam.

Appearance. Tooth discoloration from silver amalgam is gray to black.

Treatment Considerations. Tooth discoloration from silver amalgam is not routinely amenable to bleaching. Restorative treatment is the usual solution.

Other Discolorations

Numerous other types of discoloration can result from a plethora of causes. Some chromogenic bacteria may cause yellow, orange, brown-black, or green stains.[122,123] Salivary components can cause brown stains.[99] Sulfmethemoglobin, a blood pigment breakdown product, can cause a green coloration to remnants of Nasmyth's membrane.[96,122] Chlorophyll in dental plaque also may cause green stains.[96] The deposition of porphyrin into developing dentin in patients with erythropoietic porphyria, an inborn error of metabolism, may result in a red, purplish brown,

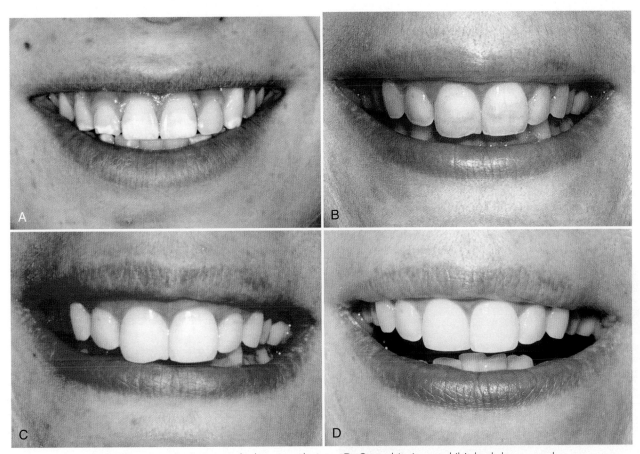

FIGURE 13-6 A, Congenital white spot lesions. **B,** Central incisors exhibit both brown and white developmental discolorations. **C,** Same patient after bleaching with 35% hydrogen peroxide and a bleaching light and (**D**) after cosmetic recontouring.

or brownish discoloration.[33,124] Phenylketonuria, another inborn error of metabolism, can produce brown discolorations.[96] Erythroblastosis fetalis, a syndrome resulting from Rh incompatibility in an infant, is characterized by the hemolysis and breakdown of the infant's blood, producing jaundice. These pigments may produce an intrinsic blue, brown, or green discoloration.[122] Thalassemia and sickle cell anemia may cause similar discolorations.[96] Amelogenesis imperfecta may result in yellow or brown stains.[122] Dentinogenesis imperfecta can cause brownish violet, yellowish, or gray discolorations.[122] Generalized yellow or gray coloration may not result from a pathologic entity but may simply be a variant within the normal range of tooth shade (Fig. 13-7). Some discolorations are of unknown origin.

Discolorations of Unknown Origin

Treatment Considerations. The precise etiology of many stains is not always discernible. This may complicate the generation of a reasonable treatment plan and prognosis. Some discolorations may be treated with routine prophylaxis. Stains resulting from erythropoietic porphyria and erythroblastosis fetalis sometimes can be treated successfully with bleaching agents.[125,126] Treatment of discoloration resulting from amelogenesis imperfecta and other etiologies that interfere with normal matrix formation or calcification of enamel often is less effective.[126] Also treatment often is contraindicated if the current structural integrity of the tooth is sufficiently compromised. The prognosis for the treatment of generalized coloration of nonpathologic origin is highly unpredictable.

TREATMENT MODALITIES

As with any therapeutic treatment, proper diagnosis should be attempted before a course of treatment is promulgated. Although the etiology of a specific tooth discoloration may be difficult to discern, an accurate history and evaluation of the factors discussed earlier (see the section on Discolorations: Mechanism, Appearance, and Treatment Considerations later in this chapter) help in establishing a differential diagnosis. The presence or absence of pulp tissue is also a treatment planning factor. Even with a definitive diagnosis, however, the ultimate outcome can be unpredictable.

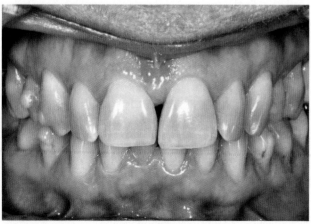

FIGURE 13-7 Generalized yellow/gray coloration of nonpathologic etiology. (Invisalign attachments are present on right side.)

Currently, only four methods of stain removal are available:

- Acid application with mechanical abrasion (acid/abrasion) with or without resin infiltration: Acid/abrasion techniques are enticingly efficient because of the short treatment times. However, because it involves the removal of enamel its application is limited to the most superficial discolorations.
- Resin infiltration therapy: This too involves the use of hydrochloric acid but includes the addition of resin impregnation, which has been successfully used for proximal caries treatment,[127] and has also shown promise for treatment of white spot lesions.[128] It is believed that the resin alters the light refraction behavior of the infiltrated enamel to mimic the surrounding healthy enamel.[129-131]
- Bleaching systems: Bleaching systems can also be used to treat superficial staining and are the only technique available for deeper enamel stains and for staining of the dentin. Repeated treatment applications often are necessary. Vital bleaching is accomplished either completely in the dental office (office or "power" bleaching) or outside of the dental office (home bleaching). (See the sections on Office Bleaching ["Power" Bleaching] and Dentist-Prescribed at Home Bleaching later in this chapter.) Nonvital teeth can be bleached with an intracoronal technique. (See the section on Nonvital Bleaching later in this chapter.)
- Combination therapy: The use of bleaching techniques and acid application/mechanical abrasion consecutively may provide the desired clinical result in some cases. (See the General Considerations section under Acid Application with Mechanical Abrasion [Acid/Abrasion] later in this chapter.)

General Considerations

If the mandibular and maxillary arches are similarly discolored, it may not be necessary to treat the discoloration of the mandibular teeth. In some cases, the lower lip completely hides the mandibular arch during normal function (Fig. 13-8A).

During function, the coloration of the mandibular arch often is obscured because of shadowing from the upper lip, particularly in Angle Class I and Class II horizontal overjet relationships (Fig. 13-8B). The visual perception of the mandibular teeth is further reduced by the continuous motion of the mandible during speaking; the maxillary arch remains relatively stable in space during function. These factors may permit an esthetically acceptable result despite significantly contrasting shades between the maxillary and mandibular arches.

CLINICAL TECHNIQUES

Acid Application with Mechanical Abrasion (Acid/Abrasion)

Acid/abrasion is a relatively simple procedure that removes tooth structure and stain simultaneously. Techniques vary and include at least one commercially produced set of armamentarium.

Hydrochloric Acid. Although hydrochloric acid is not a true bleaching agent, its applications warrant inclusion in any discussion of tooth discoloration treatments.

Hydrochloric acid is a potent decalcification agent. Nonselective in nature, it decalcifies both the tooth structure and the accompanying stains. When hydrochloric acid is used in con-

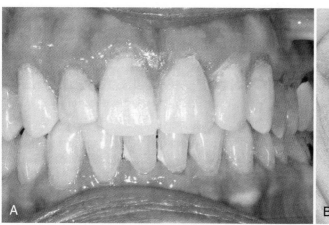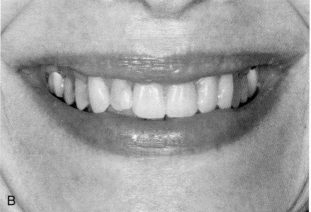

FIGURE 13-8 A, Patient with generalized yellow stained teeth. **B,** A full lower lip hides the mandibular arch during function, precluding the need for mandibular bleaching.

junction with abrasive agents, the affected enamel is completely removed, along with the stain.

In one study, five repetitions of a 5-second acid/pumice application with a wooden stick in vitro removed 112 μm of tooth structure.[132] This resulted in an 11% loss of enamel thickness, assuming a permanent incisor midlabial enamel thickness of approximately 1 mm.[133] It has been suggested that enamel losses of 25%[57] and 30%[134] are clinically acceptable.

It has been postulated that hydrochloric acid applied to the enamel surface does not penetrate the pulpal tissue.[135,136] The acid may form a calcium or phosphorus salt precipitate that limits further penetration of the acid into the dentin. In addition, these salts may further neutralize the acid.[113]

Scanning electron microscopy performed after in vitro treatment with 18% hydrochloric acid and Italian ground pumice revealed a "smeared" enamel surface with tooth structure loss from both chemical erosion and mechanical abrasion.[137] Qualitative elemental analysis of this same enamel surface demonstrated a chemical pattern similar to unetched enamel and an absence of any foreign residue.[115]

General Considerations. Safety considerations include patient cooperation, careful gingival isolation, minimal duration of exposure of the tooth structure to the acid, minimal mechanical abrasion, and meticulous protection of the dentist, patient, and personnel from the acid.

The preponderance of the early literature deals with the use of acid and acid/abrasion techniques for the treatment of superficial brown fluorosis staining.[6,8,112,138-146] Treatment with a commercially available proprietary product has been used for these stains and for white spots and streaks associated with fluorosis, superficial white demineralizations, and many white decalcifications associated with chronic stasis of dental plaque (such as those following orthodontic banding in patients with poor oral hygiene).[147]

Hydrochloric acid treatment of superficial enamel stains resulting from developmental disturbances of the enamel has been suggested,[148] although not for most amelogenesis imperfecta defects.[125] Acid/abrasion techniques are not indicated for stains or discolorations that reside deeper in the enamel or in dentin, for those acquired from food, beverages, or tobacco, or for caries underlying a decalcified region.[125]

If white spot lesions cover significant areas of the labial surface, patients may mistakenly consider the darker, normocalcified areas to be the discoloration, rather than the white spot

lesions. Successful removal of these white spot lesions may result in a darker overall result.[125] It is also possible that deep enamel may be unpredictably removed in areas of hypocalcification.[126] This may necessitate the use of composite resin to restore lost surface contour or to protect exposed dentin. It has been estimated that 50% to 75% of white enamel defects are superficial enough to be removed successfully with acid/abrasion.[125]

It has been proposed that a more conservative approach to the removal of yellow-brown fluorosis staining may be to attempt home bleaching first, followed by selective acid/abrasion if that is still required.[100] It also has been reasoned that treatment time, financial considerations, and the patient's lifestyle may indicate the use of acid/abrasion as the initial treatment, followed by bleaching.[102] (See the section on White Spot Lesions earlier in this chapter.)

Other Abrasion Techniques. Mechanical abrasion using rotary instrumentation without acid and pumice is an alternative approach.[149] However, special care must be taken with this technique to avoid ditching, alteration of labial contours, and excessive enamel reduction.

Acid Abrasion[150]

Armamentarium

- Tinted protective eye glasses with side shields (for patient and operator) (available from dental supply company)
- Shade guide to record shade (e.g., VITA Classic Shade Guide or VITA Easyshade Compact Electronic Shade Guide, (Vident [optional]))
- Rubber Dam Setup (see Appendix B for the complete Armamentarium), including:
  - 6 × 6-inch rubber dam, medium gauge (e.g., Hygienic Flexi Dam Rubber Dam, Non Latex 6X6 Med, Coltene/Whaledent)
  - 6 × 6-inch plastic U-shaped rubber dam frame (e.g., Hygienic Rubber Dam Frame, 6" [Plastic], Coltene/Whaledent)
  - Assorted Rubber Dam clamp
- Copal varnish (e.g., Copalite, Cooley & Cooley, Ltd.)
- 36% Hydrochloric acid USP (available from chemical supply house)
- Two glass dappen dishes (available from dental supply company)
- Distilled water (available from pharmacy)
- Flour of pumice (available from dental supply company)

+ Prophylaxis Cup (Densco Ribbed and Webbed, RA [Latch] Soft Blue Rubber, Water Pik, Inc.)
+ Sodium bicarbonate powder USP (available from dental supply company)
+ Tongue blade (available from dental supply company)
+ Cotton-tipped applicator (available from dental supply company)
+ 1.1% neutral sodium fluoride (e.g., PreviDent, Colgate-Palmolive Company)
+ Fine fluoridated prophylaxis paste (Nupro-Prophy Pastes, Dentsply Professional)
+ Superfine aluminum oxide polishing disc (e.g., Sof-Lex, 3M ESPE)

Clinical Technique

> ### CLINICAL TIP
>
> Pretreatment photographs (see Chapter 22), pretreatment shade determination (see section on Computerized Digital Shade Technology in Chapter 2), and impressions for custom maintenance trays can be performed at this visit.

> ### CLINICAL TIP
>
> WARNING: Protective glasses with side shields must be worn by the patient, dentist, and any auxiliary personnel while working with hydrochloric acid. The dentist and auxiliary personnel should wear rubber gloves, and the patient must be draped. The procedure is contraindicated for uncooperative patients and for teeth that are sensitive to temperature changes or acidic liquids or foods. This technique should not be attempted if the operatory is not equipped with a high-volume evacuation system and a water syringe.

1. Apply a heavy rubber dam to the teeth to be bleached.
2. Seal the labial and lingual (or palatal) rubber dam margins with copal varnish.
3. Prepare an 18% hydrochloric acid solution by mixing equal volumes of 36% hydrochloric acid and distilled water in a dappen dish.

> ### CLINICAL TIP
>
> Always add acid to water; adding water to acid can cause splattering because of the exothermic reaction that occurs upon mixing.

4. Add flour of pumice to the acid solution to make a thick, wet paste.

> ### CLINICAL TIP
>
> WARNING: Hydrochloric acid should never be passed over or held in the region of the patient's face, nor should any mixture containing the acid or any instrument that has come in contact with it.

5. Prepare a thick paste of sodium bicarbonate and water.
6. Place sodium bicarbonate paste on the rubber dam to help neutralize any splashed acid.

7. Apply the acid/pumice mixture to the labial enamel with a wooden tongue blade. Simultaneously use a cotton-tipped applicator to absorb any excess solution.

> ### CLINICAL TIP
>
> The tongue blade can be cut or split to better adapt it to the facial surface.

> ### CLINICAL TIP
>
> WARNING: Rotary instrumentation of any type (e.g., a prophylaxis cup on a slow-speed handpiece) is strictly contraindicated because of the danger of splattering the acid.

8. With firm finger pressure on the tongue blade, grind the mixture into the enamel.

> ### CLINICAL TIP
>
> Total acid contact time should not exceed 5 seconds.

9. Rinse carefully and thoroughly with water for 10 seconds while carefully evacuating with the high-powered suction.
10. Evaluate for excessive enamel wear by viewing, with a mirror, the labial surface from an incisal direction.
11. Wet the tooth with saliva and evaluate for appropriate color change.

> ### CLINICAL TIP
>
> White enamel discoloration usually is more visible on dry tooth structure than when the tooth is wet;[116] thus, color evaluation of dry teeth may result in overtreatment and unnecessary removal of enamel.

12. If the color change is esthetically acceptable, skip to step 14.

> ### CLINICAL TIP
>
> To avoid excessive wear, limit the acid/abrasion application to a maximum of five attempts. However, if no change is observed after the third attempt, discontinue treatment and skip to step 14.

13. If the color change is unacceptable, repeat steps 6 through 13. These steps should not be performed more than five times.
14. Polish with a fine fluoride prophylaxis paste and superfine aluminum oxide composite resin polishing discs.
15. Apply a 1.1% neutral sodium fluoride gel for 4 minutes.

Resin Infiltration Therapy

Recently minimum intervention techniques have been advocated to treat incipient caries.[151] These techniques involved the use the use of phosphoric and hydrochloric acid gels to increase the porosity of the enamel to promote the penetration of a resin infiltration.[151] One of the results of this technique is an alteration of the optical qualities of the infiltrated enamel by the resin which may mask hypocalcified white color.[152,153] Manufacturers (Icon, DMG America) have released a specialized product for performing this technique. Studies on small groups of patients demonstrated complete masking in 22% to 25% of the enamel developmental defect cases,[154,155] and partially masking in 35% of the enamel developmental defect.[152] However, for post-orthodontic decalcification cases 61% were completely masked[152] and 33% were partially masked.[152] The masking remained unchanged after 6 months and 1 year.[152]

Armamentarium
- Tinted protective eye glasses with side shields (for patient and operator) (available from dental supply company)
- Shade guide to record shade (e.g., VITA Classic Shade Guide or VITA Easyshade Compact Electronic Shade Guide , Vident [optional])
- Rubber Dam Setup (See Appendix B for the complete Armamentarium), including:
  - 6 × 6-inch rubber dam, medium gauge (e.g., Hygienic Latex Rubber Dam Non Latex 6X6 Med, Coltene/Whaledent)
  - 6 × 6-inch plastic U-shaped rubber dam frame (e.g., Hygienic Rubber Dam Frame 6" [Plastic], Coltene/Whaledent)
  - Assorted Rubber Dam clamp

> ## CLINICAL TIP
>
> Avoid Non-Latex Dental Dam with this procedure. Some of the materials used in the Icon kit (Icon-Dry) will dissolve the dam.[156]

- Flour of pumice (available from dental supply company)
- Prophylaxis cup (Densco Ribbed and Webbed, RA [Latch] Soft Blue Rubber, Water Pik, Inc.)
- Etching material (e.g., hydrochloric acid, pyrogenic silicic acid, surface-active substance, Icon-Etch, DMG America)
- Drying agent (99% ethanol, e.g., Icon-Dry, DMG America)
- Infiltrating resin (methacrylate-based resin matrix, initiators, additives, e.g., Icon-Infiltrant, DMG America)
- Polishing disks (e.g., EP Esthetic Polishing System, Brassler USA)

Clinical Technique

> ## CLINICAL TIP
>
> WARNING: Protective glasses with side shields must be worn by the patient, dentist, and any auxiliary personnel while working with hydrochloric acid. The dentist and auxiliary personnel should wear rubber gloves, and the patient must be draped. The procedure is contraindicated for uncooperative patients and for teeth that are sensitive to temperature changes or acidic liquids or foods. This technique should not be attempted if the operatory is not equipped with a high-volume evacuation system and a water syringe.

1. Clean the tooth with flour of pumice (Fig. 13-9A,B).
2. Rinse the teeth and air dry (Fig. 13-9C).
3. Apply rubber dam (Fig. 13-9D).
4. Apply Icon-Etch for 2 minutes (Fig. 13-9E,F).

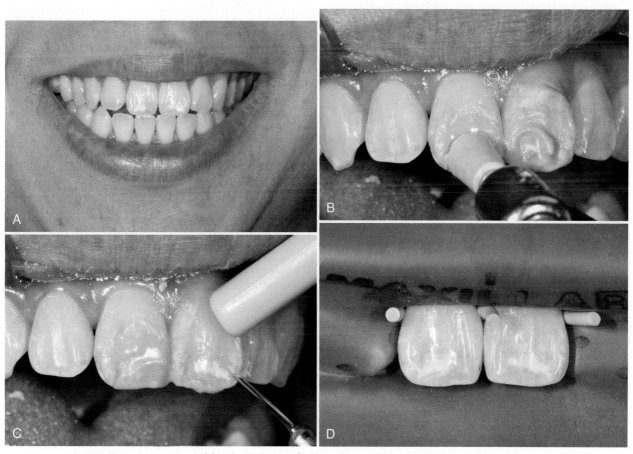

FIGURE 13-9 A, Prebleaching view of white lesions. **B,** The teeth are cleaned with flour of pumice. **C,** The teeth are rinsed with copious amounts of water and air dried. **D,** The teeth are isolated with a rubber dam.   *Continued*

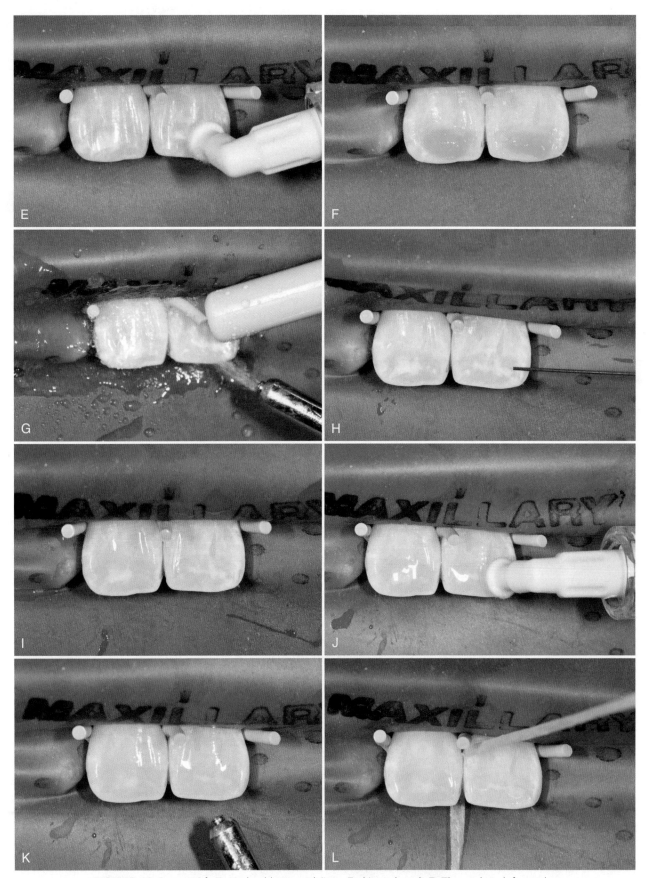

FIGURE 13-9, cont'd E, Hydrochloric acid (Icon-Etch) is placed. **F,** The etch is left on the teeth for 2 minutes. **G,** The teeth are rinsed with copious amounts of water and air dried. **H,** Icon-Dry is placed to preview the effectiveness of acid. **I,** The tooth is dried and inspected for improvement. **J,** Resin (Icon-Infiltrate) is placed on the tooth and allowed to dry for 3 minutes. **K,** Excess material is gently removed. **L,** Dental floss is used to remove any interproximal resin.

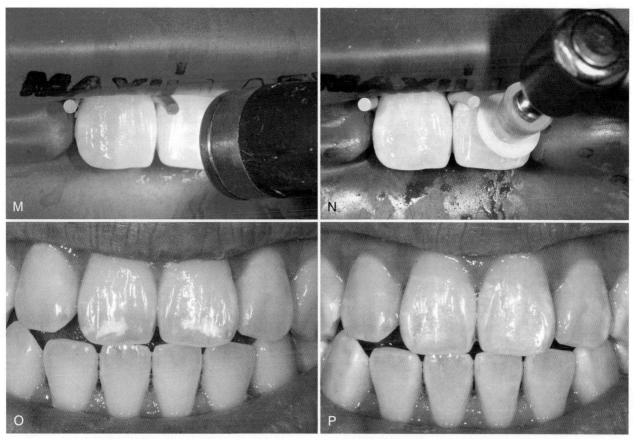

FIGURE 13-9, cont'd M, The material is polymerized for 40 seconds per tooth. **N,** The resin is polished. **O,** Prebleaching and (**P**) postbleaching views of white lesions.

5. Remove the material with water and suction for 30 seconds (Fig. 13-9G).
6. Dry the teeth with the air syringe and suction (see Fig. 13-9G).
7. Apply Icon-Dry and allow it to remain undisturbed for 30 seconds (Fig. 13-9H).
8. Dry the teeth with air and suction and visually inspect the teeth for improvement (Fig. 13-9I).
9. If no or inadequate improvement is observed, repeat steps 4 through 7.
10. Turn off the operatory and overhead lights, apply Icon-Infiltrate, and allow it to remain undisturbed for 3 minutes (Fig. 13-9J).

CLINICAL TIP

To maintain a wet lesion, reapply the resin by occasional twisting the special applicator syringe.

11. Gently air disperse excess resin in the presence of suction (Fig. 13-9K).

CLINICAL TIP

Gently remove excess material with an air syringe and suction before light curing to avoid any abrasion of intact enamel during the subsequent polishing phase.[157]

12. Remove excess resin with floss and suction (Fig. 13-9L).

13. Light polymerize for 40 seconds per tooth (Fig. 13-9M).
14. Reapply resin (Icon-Infiltrate) and allow it to remain undisturbed for 1 minute.

CLINICAL TIP

To maintain a wet lesion, reapply the resin by occasional twisting the special applicator syringe.

17. Gently air disperse excess resin in the presence of suction.
18. Again, remove excess resin with floss and suction.
19. Light polymerize again for 40 seconds per tooth.
20. Evaluate teeth and polish as necessary (Fig. 13-9N, O).

Office Bleaching ("Power" Bleaching)

Bleaching of vital teeth in the dental office (often referred to as "power" bleaching) involves the application of bleaching agents (either 30%-35% hydrogen peroxide or carbamide peroxide concentrations that yield high concentrations of hydrogen peroxide) in liquid or gel form.

Clinical Approaches. Numerous office bleaching products and techniques have been proposed. The American Dental Association (ADA) Seal of Acceptance program includes a category for in-office bleaching. The acceptance program is ongoing, and products are continually added and eliminated.

Stereo headphones playing the patient's choice of music or the use of video often help the patient pass the time pleasantly while bleaching is performed in the office.

Armamentarium

+ Tinted protective eye glasses with side shields (for patient and operator) (available from dental supply company)
+ Shade guide to record shade (e.g., VITA Classic Shade Guide or VITA Easyshade Compact Electronic Shade Guide, Vident [optional])
+ 40% Carbamide Peroxide Gel (e.g., Opalescence Boost/Activator syringes, Ultradent Products, Inc.)
+ Composite based "Rubber Dam" (e.g., OpalDam, Ultradent Products, Inc.)
+ Flour of pumice (available from dental supply company)
+ Prophylaxis Cup (Densco Ribbed and Webbed, RA [Latch] Soft Blue Rubber, Water Pik, Inc.)
+ Bite block/retractor (Isolation Block, Isolation Block LLC)
+ Suction tips (available from dental supply company)
+ Saliva ejectors (available from dental supply company)
+ Saliva ejectors cushion (optional) (e.g., SE Cushion, Zirc Co.)

Clinical Technique

CLINICAL TIP

Pretreatment photographs (see Chapter 22), pretreatment shade determination (see section on Computerized Digital Shade Technology in Chapter 2) and impressions for custom maintenance trays can be performed at this visit.

1. Position complete eye protection on the patient and all operators.
2. Record the pretreatment shade (Fig. 13-10*A,B*).
3. Clean the teeth with flour of pumice in a prophylaxis cup (Fig. 13-10*C*).

CLINICAL TIP

Petroleum jelly can be applied to the lips for protection (Fig. 13-10*D*). Because petroleum jelly can cause latex to degrade, nitrile gloves should be used.

CLINICAL TIP

Because in-office bleaching times can be long, placement of a protective sleeve over the saliva ejector tip to prevent accidental tissue entrapment on the mucosa of the floor of the mouth is advisable (Fig. 13-10*E*).

CLINICAL TIP

The placement of cotton rolls in the buccal vestibule will elevate the lips away from the teeth and protect the mucosa from the gel (Fig. 13-10*F*). Care must be taken to change the cotton rolls between rinsing stages.

4. Place "liquid rubber dam" over the gingiva (Fig. 13-10*G*) and polymerize with a curing light according to the manufacturer's instruction (Fig. 13-10*H*).

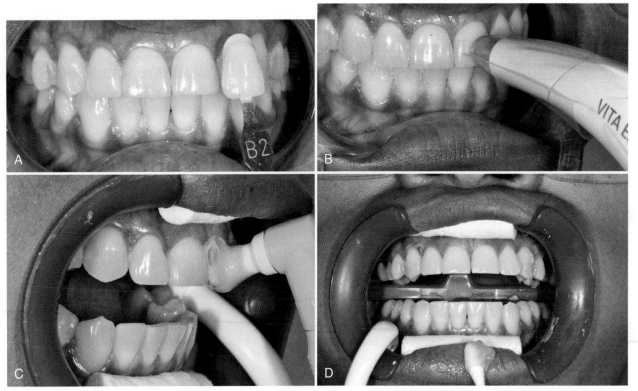

FIGURE 13-10 A, The pretreatment shade is recorded. **B,** An electronic shade guide recorder, such as VITA Easyshade Compact, can be used to make quick and precise measurements. **C,** The teeth are cleaned using flour of pumice **D,**. Petroleum jelly is applied to the lips.

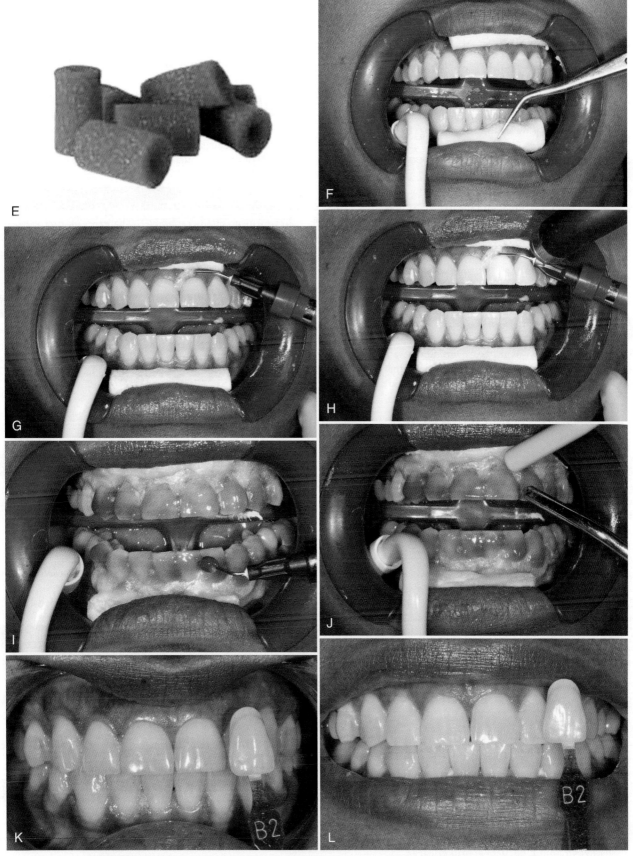

FIGURE 13-10, cont'd E, Protective sleeves to prevent entrapment of tissue by saliva ejector (SE Cushion, Zirc Co.). **F,** Cotton rolls placed in the buccal vestibule to protect then lips and mucosa. **G,** A "liquid rubber dam" is placed over the exposed gingiva. **H,** The "liquid rubber dam" is polymerized with a curing light. **I,** Bleaching agent is applied according to manufacturer's instructions. **J,** Copious amounts of water and suction is used to remove bleaching gel. **K,** Prebleaching appearance. **L,** Postbleaching results following a single treatment.

5. Apply bleaching agent for the time and duration as specified in the manufacturer's instructions (Fig. 13-10*I*).
6. After the appropriate bleaching time remove the gel with copious amounts of water and suction (Fig. 13-10*J*).

7. Repeat the procedure according to the manufacturer's instructions if required.
8. When the procedure is complete, carefully remove the liquid dam and cheek retractors (Fig. 13-10*K,L*).

Laser-Assisted, Ultraviolet-Assisted or White Light–Assisted Bleaching

Bleaching with an argon laser, a carbon dioxide laser, or a combination of the two[67,158] as a light source have been introduced in the past but sufficient long-term or controlled clinical studies of safety and effectiveness currently are lacking.[71,159] Studies have shown that the use of ultraviolet-assisted bleaching did not significantly increase the intrapulpal temperature of teeth when used for the recommended exposure time,[160] although its increased efficacy has been questioned.[161-163] Laser-assisted bleaching also may be no more effective than nonlaser techniques.[67] A white light assisted bleaching regimen was introduced (Zoom WhiteSpeed, Philips Oral Healthcare), which uses white light LED with an light output of 465 nm $\pm$ 15 nm instead of an ultraviolet light "short arc halide lamp."[164] A recent study demonstrated that light increases bleaching effectiveness as compared with no light when using 40% hydrogen peroxide.[165,166]

Light-Assisted Office Bleaching

Armamentarium
+ Light-assisted office bleaching kit (e.g., Zoom WhiteSpeed, Philips Oral Healthcare) (Fig. 13-11*A*), which consists of:
  + Chairside whitening procedure kit
  + Light-activating guide
  + Cheek retractors
  + Retractor covers (face bibs)
  + 2" × 2" gauze squares
  + Surgical suction tips
  + Packet vitamin E oil, 0.43 g, with brush
  + Liquid "rubber dam" (LiquiDam syringes with tips)
  + 25% Hydrogen peroxide (Zoom Chairside Whitening Gel)
+ Shade guide to record shade (e.g., VITA Classic Shade Guide or VITA Easyshade Compact Electronic Shade Guide, Vident [optional])

+ Tinted eye protective glasses with side shields (for patient and operator) protection (see Fig. 13-11*A*)

Clinical Technique
1. Perform a pretreatment consultation with the patient.

2. Use the appropriate manufacturer's recommended protective eyewear (patient and clinician).

3. Record the pretreatment shade (Fig. 13-11*B,C*).
4. Isolate the teeth according to the manufacturer's recommendations (Fig. 13-11*D*).
5. Clean the teeth with non-fluoridate flour pumice (Fig. 13-11*E*).

6. Apply the appropriate skindrape and tissue protection (Fig. 13-11*F,G*).
7. Apply the appropriate gingival protection to the isolated area (Fig. 13-11*H,I*).

8. Place the bleach (Fig. 13-11*J*) and activate the light according to the manufacturer's instructions (Fig. 13-11*K*).
9. Repeat Step 8 according to the manufacturer's recommendations.

10. When the bleaching is completed carefully remove the retractors with water only (not air/water spray) using an air/water syringe and suction (Fig. 13-11L). (Fig. 13-11M,N).

Dentist-Prescribed At-Home Bleaching

Patient self-application of bleaching agents performed at home is perhaps the most popular method of bleaching vital teeth. It is alternately referred to as "home bleaching" or "matrix bleaching."

Carbamide Peroxide. Ten percent carbamide peroxide (also known as hydrogen peroxide carbamide, carbamide urea, urea hydrogen peroxide, urea peroxide, perhydrol urea, and perhydelure) decomposes into approximately 3.5% hydrogen peroxide and 6.5% urea.[167] Carbopol and other thickeners often are incorporated to enhance the material's properties[167] to produce a gel or paste.

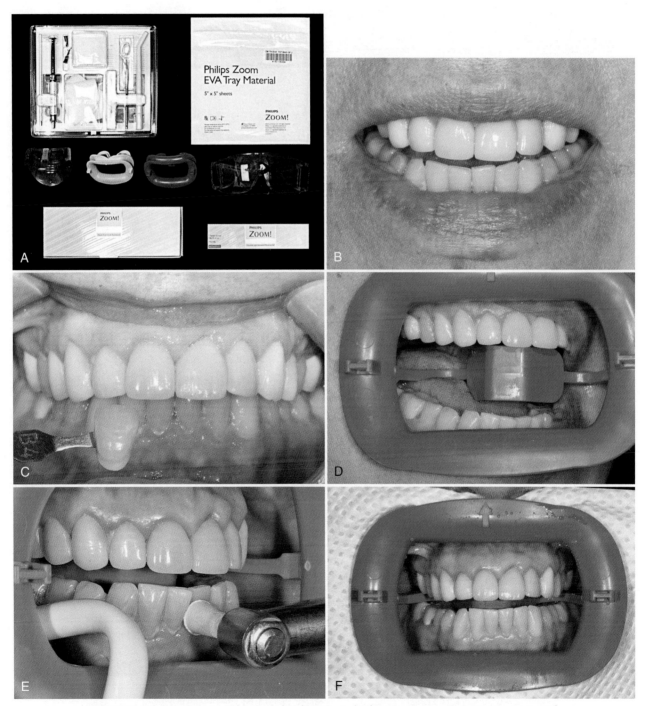

FIGURE 13-11 A, Zoom WhiteSpeed Light-Activated Whitening System. **B,** Pretreatment view of patient with maxillary porcelain laminate veneers who desires bleaching of the mandibular anterior teeth. **C,** The pretreatment shade is recorded. **D,** The teeth are isolated according to the manufacturer's instructions. **E,** The teeth are cleaned with nonfluoridate flour pumice. **F,** The appropriate skin drape is placed.

Continued

FIGURE 13-11, cont'd G, Cotton rolls are placed into the mucobuccal folds. **H,** Place the LiquidDam material. **I,** The isolated area. **J,** The bleach is placed. **K,** The bleach is activated with the light. **L,** The bleaching agent is carefully removed with copious amount of water. **M,** Pretreatment view of patient with maxillary porcelain laminate veneers that were placed ten years prior. **(N)** Post-treatment images demonstrating bleaching of the mandibular teeth. The shade of the maxillary teeth serves a comparative control for evaluating the effectiveness of the mandibular bleaching.

General Considerations. The bleaching agent is held against the teeth by means of a custom-fabricated tray. Techniques vary as to the frequency, timing, number of applications, and duration of treatment.

The retention of bleaching material within the custom tray when the tray is worn overnight was initially questioned.[168,169] However, a later study with a newer generation material reported a retention of greater than 60% of active material after more than 4 hours of use.[167]

The ADA Seal of Acceptance is given to a product that meets the program's criteria for safety and effectiveness.[170] Acceptance of a dentist-prescribed at-home bleaching product includes a review of the instructions provided with the product.[170] The acceptance program is ongoing, and products are continually added and eliminated.

The mutagenic potential[171] of the free radicals released by hydrogen peroxide, as well as their ability to potentiate the effects of known carcinogens, have also been reported.[172] Therefore the use of any known carcinogen, such as tobacco or alcohol, is a consideration. (At the time of the preparation of this manuscript, the American Dental Association was in the process of updating the specific recommendations regarding tobacco and alcohol use in relation to bleaching and should be consulted in this regard.) In addition, this technique should not be used by pregnant women.[173] Calculus should be removed,[173] and if the prophylaxis traumatizes the tissues, bleaching should be delayed 1 to 2 weeks.[173] Teeth to be bleached should be free of caries and have no defective restorations.

The patient should be informed that existing restorations will not whiten. Restorations matched to teeth after bleaching may become esthetically unacceptable if post-bleaching color regression occurs in the surrounding natural tooth structure.

Patients should be instructed to discontinue treatment and to contact the dentist if sensitivity of the teeth or gingiva occurs.[173] Other precautions may exist as well, some of which may be discussed in the manufacturer's instructions and enclosures.

Custom Tray Fabrication. The current ADA Seal of Acceptance program for dentist-prescribed at-home bleaching products includes acceptance of the instructions for use. (The acceptance covers a specific product; acceptance of similar products by the same manufacturer should not be inferred.) Although these instructions differ among specific manufacturers, many of the basic concepts behind these procedures are similar in nature. The step-by-step technique that follows, although adapted from only one product, is helpful in demonstrating the implementation of some of these concepts. Historically, spacers have been placed on the labial surface of the casts to create reservoirs in bleaching trays so that a greater volume of bleaching material will come into contact with the teeth. Recent studies have questioned the efficacy of reservoirs and it appears that the addition of blockout spacers to create reservoirs does not increase the success of home bleaching.[174]

Clinical Approach. This technique was adapted from the instructions for the use of Opalescence (Ultradent Products, Inc.).

> ### CLINICAL TIP
>
> The specific current manufacturer's instructions and enclosures (including patient use instructions) for products adhering to the ADA acceptance program may be updated periodically and therefore should be consulted. Instructions for products from other manufacturers will be different and should be consulted.

Armamentarium

- Fast-set plaster or dental stone (available from dental supply company)
- Model trimmer (e.g., Buffalo Dental Model Trimmers, Buffalo Dental Manufacturing Co., Inc.)
- Tray material (Sof-Tray 0.035 inch, Ultradent Products, Inc.)
- Vacuum former unit (Ultra-Form or EconoForm, Ultradent Products, Inc.)
- Small tactile scissors (Ultra-Trim scissors, Ultradent Products, Inc.)
- Serrated plastic trimmers (Utility Cutters, Ultradent Products, Inc.)
- Portable torch (Blazer Micro Torch, Ultradent Products, Inc.)
- Block-out material (e.g., LC Block-Out Resin, Ultradent Products, Inc.)

Clinical Technique

> ### CLINICAL TIP
>
> Pretreatment photographs (see Chapter 22), pretreatment shade determination (see section on Computerized Digital Shade Technology in Chapter 2) and impressions for custom maintenance trays can be performed at this visit.

> ### CLINICAL TIP
>
> WARNING: Before bleaching is begun, teeth should be free of caries and defective restorations.

1. Pour the impression of the arch with fast-set plaster or dental stone. Irreversible hydrocolloid must be poured shortly after making the impression to ensure accuracy.

> ### CLINICAL TIP
>
> The cast base ultimately is reduced to within a few millimeters of the gingival margins. To save time, use only the minimum amount of stone necessary to ensure removal of the set stone from the impression without fracture.

2. Trim the base of the cast parallel to the occlusal table on a model trimmer to within a few millimeters of the gingival margins. The palate and tongue areas are removed (Fig. 13-12A).
3. Allow the cast to dry for 2 hours.
4. If recommended by manufacturer, apply approximately 0.5-mm thickness of block-out material to the desired labial surfaces to provide reservoir spaces in the tray as follows:
   a. Approximately 1.5 mm from the gingival line
   b. *Do not* extend onto the incisal edges and occlusal surfaces (Fig. 13-12B).

CLINICAL TIP

Extending the block-out material onto the incisal edges or occlusal surfaces can cause the margins of the tray to open upon occluding and/or the tray to impinge on the soft tissues. Patients may experience less tooth discomfort from tray pressures with reservoirs because of reduced "orthodontic" pressures.

5. If block-out material was recommended by the manufacturer, cure the block-out material for approximately 2 minutes (Ultra-Lume). A hand-held intraoral light can be used, and each tooth is exposed for approximately 20 to 40 seconds. Wipe off the oxygen-inhibited layer.
6. Heat the tray material on the vacuum former unit until it sags approximately 2½ inches (Fig. 13-12C). Activate the vacuum and adapt the softened tray material over the cast. Cool and remove the cast.

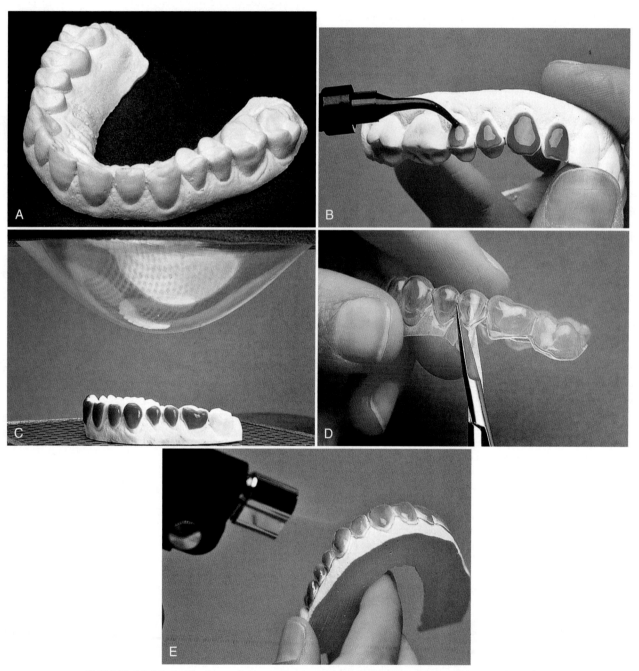

FIGURE 13-12 A, The base of the cast is trimmed parallel to the occlusal table to within a few millimeters of the gingival margins. The palate and tongue areas are removed. **B,** Spacing for reservoirs is created on the cast. **C,** The tray material is heated on a vacuum former unit. **D,** The tray material is trimmed. **E,** The tray is flamed to facilitate adaptation to the cast. (Courtesy Ultradent Products, Inc., South Jordan, UT.)

CLINICAL TIP

Use a serrated plastic trimmer to initially remove the bulk of the tray material. This facilitates the final precise trimming with the small tactile scissors.

7. Trim the tray material carefully and precisely 0.25 to 0.33 mm occlusal from the gingival margin with small tactile scissors. Scallop around the interdental papilla (Fig. 13-12D).
8. Place the tray on the cast and check the tray extensions. Gently flame polish the edges one quadrant at a time with the torch (Fig. 13-12E).
9. While still warm, hold the periphery of each segment firmly against the cast for 3 seconds with a water-moistened finger.

CLINICAL TIP

If an area is short of the desired length, gently heat and push the tray material to the desired location. If the material becomes too thin, a new tray should be fabricated.

Restorative Implications. For a discussion of restorative implications, see the section on Office Bleaching ("Power" Bleaching) earlier in this chapter.

Over-the-Counter Unsupervised At-Home Bleaching

Many home bleaching products are available over the counter or through mail order, print, radio, internet, and television advertisements. Because the dentist often has little knowledge of the composition of these products, their use, overuse, and abuse are a concern.[71] The patient should be told of these risks and the dentists should realize the potential liabilities if they recommend any of these products.

Nonvital Tooth Bleaching

The agents traditionally involved in the lightening of discolored nonvital teeth are sodium perborate and 30% to 35% hydrogen peroxide used alone or in combination.[175] The most commonly used agent has been reported to be 30% hydrogen peroxide.[176] The techniques commonly used include the thermocatalytic technique, in which the bleaching solution is heated from within the pulp chamber with a hot instrument,[175] heated externally with a floodlight apparatus, or a combination of the two; and the "walking bleach" technique, in which the materials are sealed within the pulp chamber for 3 to 7 days.[175] These techniques are repeated until an appropriate result is achieved.[175]

External Cervical Root Resorption. External root resorption is a possible sequela of internal bleaching. Hydrogen peroxide occasionally has been associated with this development.[175] The exact cause or causes of this response are still not entirely understood, although a number of mechanisms have been postulated:

1. In 10% of all teeth, the cementoenamel junction is defective or absent, resulting in a portion of the tooth being devoid of cementum coverage.[177] Thirty-five percent hydrogen peroxide may denature the dentin, invoking a foreign body response by elements in the approximating gingival tissue, which may result in cervical resorption.[178]

2. Internally applied 35% hydrogen peroxide may directly contact the periodontal membrane by passing through patent dentinal tubules[179] or through lateral root canals or accessory foramina.[180] This may elicit an inflammatory reaction, ultimately resulting in cervical resorption.
3. Bleaching agents may infiltrate between the gutta-percha and the root canal walls. They could then communicate with the periodontal membrane through the dentinal tubules, lateral canals, or apex. This may invoke a resorptive process anywhere along the root area, including the apical regions.
4. Heat application during treatment may invoke a resorptive process.[179]
5. Thirty-five percent hydrogen peroxide mixed with sodium perborate can lower the pH in the periodontal membrane area,[180] which may increase the likelihood of cervical resorption.

It also has been demonstrated in vitro that when heat is combined with 35% hydrogen peroxide/sodium perborate paste during an internal bleaching technique, not only is the crown bleached, but also the entire root surface. Significantly, less of the root surface is bleached when the heat is omitted.[181] This may suggest that heat facilitates the permeation of bleaching agent, in all directions, thus possibly increasing the likelihood of external cervical root resorption through some of the discussed mechanisms.

Tooth discoloration often is the result of a traumatic injury to the tooth, and resorption may be a sequela of the original trauma. Resorption also can be caused by orthodontic treatment or surgery, particularly when involving the cementoenamel junction area.[182]

Bleaching Materials and Technique. The literature is equivocal about the efficacy of the various techniques. Two in vitro studies have found intracoronal placement of 30% to 35% hydrogen peroxide (Superoxol, Sultan Healthcare) in combination with sodium perborate provided, after two applications, results that were superior to a sodium perborate/water combination,[104,183] although one of these studies showed equal results after three applications.[183] Another in vitro study found equal results after two applications.[184] In an in vitro study, the success rates for teeth treated intracoronally with a sodium perborate/30% hydrogen peroxide combination, a sodium perborate/3% hydrogen peroxide combination, and a sodium perborate/water combination were found to be essentially equal after 1 year.[185]

It has been stated, however, that the traditional thermocatalytic technique with 30% hydrogen peroxide is faster and more effective.[186] The thermocatalytic method has been described as when the "walking bleach" technique is unsuccessful.[187] In a 1995 literature review of external resorption following intracoronal placement of hydrogen peroxide (thermocatalytic method in most cases), none included the prior placement of a protective base, and many reported previous dental trauma.[187] Sodium perborate/30% hydrogen peroxide combinations are also described.[188] However, cemental exposure to 30% to 35% hydrogen peroxide, especially in combination with high heat, increasingly is being discouraged for dentists performing intracoronal bleaching to reduce the potential for external root resorption.[167] Sodium perborate mixed with water is potentially safer.[167]

An in vitro quantitative analysis of bleaching materials disclosed that after 3 days, further color change was minimal. It was concluded that the interval between bleaching visits could be reduced to reflect this finding.[176]

Acid Etching. In an in vitro study, the removal of the smear layer with phosphoric acid did not significantly change the efficacy of intracoronal bleaching with a sodium perborate/water combination (37% phosphoric acid) or a 35% hydrogen peroxide/sodium perborate combination (37% phosphoric acid).[189] Another in vitro study with a 30% hydrogen peroxide/sodium perborate combination (50% phosphoric acid) had similar results.[190]

Calcium Hydroxide. The literature is equivocal on whether calcium hydroxide placed within the pulp chamber can raise the pH of the microenvironment of the external tooth surface,[180,191] or whether it has no effect.[192] Increasing the alkalinity of the external root surface may be advantageous because polymorphonuclear leukocytes and osteoclasts function best at a slightly acidic pH, elaborating acid hydrolases, which leads to demineralization of hard tissue components and prevents formation of new hard tissue.[180] It has been suggested that if this pH change occurred in the periodontal membrane, external root resorption could result.[180] The mechanism of the recalcification and the role of calcium hydroxide are not completely understood.[193] Calcium hydroxide placed intracoronally has effectively treated cervical root resorption[193,194] but it has also been reported to be ineffective.[195,196] Intracoronal placement of calcium hydroxide following bleaching has been suggested.[180,193]

Protective Base. A 2- to 2.5-mm protective base[197] should be placed over the gutta-percha root canal obliteration; however, the literature is equivocal about the material of choice, its exact positioning and design, and even about its ultimate efficacy in preventing external cervical root resorption.

The dentinal tubules terminate at the external root surface at a point incisal to the level at which they leave the pulp chamber. The dentinal tubules progress in a slightly incisal direction from their point of origin at the pulp chamber to their point of termination at the external root surface. Some have advocated, therefore, that the protective base be placed at a point 1 mm apical to the level of the cementoenamel junction,[104] slightly apical to the gingival margin,[188] or 1 mm incisal to the incisal extent of the epithelial attachment.[198] It has also been proposed that the base extend to a point corresponding to the level of the cementoenamel junction, and that if further cervical bleaching is necessary, the base outline can be gradually repositioned and bleaching can be continued with bleaching materials milder than 30% hydrogen peroxide.[199] It would seem reasonable, therefore, that the more coronally the base is placed, the less may be the chance of external cervical root resorption, but the greater the chance of esthetic compromise.[197] The practitioner must use clinical judgment on this point.

If the patient's lip covers a portion of the tooth during all functions, the base can be positioned even more coronally than the preceding landmarks.

CLINICAL TIP

If the gingival portion of the clinical crown is not visible during function or maximum smiling, the incisal termination of the base can be appropriately positioned to further reduce the chance of external cervical root resorption. Explaining this advantage may help the patient overcome psychological ambivalence about possibly leaving a segment of the tooth unbleached. However, see the next Clinical Tip.

CLINICAL TIP

The position of the lip during maximum smiling (the high lip line) may be deceptive. Patients with unattractive smiles often habitually adapt a high lip line position that is significantly less revealing of tooth structure than is anatomically possible. After cosmetic improvement, the high lip line may significantly elevate because the psychological barriers inhibiting full smiling have been removed.

The vertical height of the cementoenamel junction, the epithelial attachment, and the marginal gingiva at the interproximal area generally is coronal to the level on the labial and lingual surfaces. The protective base should follow the outline of these incisogingival contours. It should extend to a level coronal to the marginal gingiva and cementoenamel junction on the lingual or palatal aspect because this surface need not be bleached. A method of creating a base with a coronal contour that follows a specific design has been described.[198] The base resembles a bobsled tunnel mesiodistally and a ski slope buccolingually.[198] Glass ionomer cement[119] and polycarboxylate cement[119] have been suggested as protective base materials.

Other Considerations. Macrophages may play a role in external root resorption. It has been postulated that external root resorption is found infrequently when only sodium perborate and water are used because sodium perborate has an inhibitory effect on macrophage adhesion.[200]

Proper Endodontic Treatment. A properly sealed endodontic filling is a prerequisite for bleaching. Silver points may be dislodged during the preparatory stages and must be replaced with gutta-percha before bleaching.

Possible Alternative Materials. A material containing the enzymes amylase, lipase, and trypsin with disodium edetate was found to be 40% as effective as hydrogen peroxide in lightening bloodstained teeth in vitro.[176]

Armamentarium
- Orabase Plain (Colgate-Palmolive Company)
- Tinted protective eye glasses with side shields (for patient and operator) (available from dental supply company)
- Rubber dam setup (see Appendix B for the complete Armamentarium), including
    - 6 × 6-inch rubber dam, medium gauge (e.g., Hygienic Flexi Dam Rubber Dam Non Latex 6X6 Med, Coltene/Whaledent)
    - 6 × 6-inch plastic U-shaped rubber dam frame (e.g., Hygienic Rubber Dam Frame 6" [Plastic], Coltene/Whaledent)
    - Assorted rubber dam clamp
- Waxed dental floss
- Glass slab (available from dental supply company)
- Cement spatula (available from dental supply company)
- Periodontal probe (e.g., Periodontal probe, Hu-Friedy Mfg. Co.)
- Flat-ended "plastic" instrument (e.g., Plastic Instrument, Hu-Friedy Mfg. Co.)
- Sodium perborate powder USP (Sultan Healthcare; also available at some local pharmacies)
- Temporary restorative material (e.g., Cavit, 3M ESPE; Provit, Harald Nordin SA)
- Calcium hydroxide powder USP (Eli Lilly & Co.)

- Sterile water
- Material for protective base (e.g., polycarboxylate cement, glass ionomer cement)
- Toothbrush and toothpaste

Clinical Technique
1. Evaluate the high smile line.

CLINICAL TIP

The position of the lip during maximum smiling (the high lip line) may be deceptive. Patients with unattractive smiles often habitually adapt a high lip line position, which is significantly less revealing of tooth structure than is anatomically possible. After cosmetic improvement, the high lip line may significantly elevate because the psychological barriers inhibiting full smiling have been removed.

2. If the cervical area of the tooth remains hidden by the lip during maximum smiling and functioning, consult with the patient about bleaching only the visible portions of the crown.

CLINICAL TIP

If the gingival portion of the clinical crown is not visible during function or maximum smiling, the incisal termination of the base should be appropriately positioned to further reduce the chance of external cervical root resorption. Explaining this advantage may help the patient overcome psychological ambivalence about leaving a segment of the tooth unbleached.

3. Position the protective glasses over the patient's eyes.
4. Apply Orabase Plain to the labial and lingual (or palatal) gingiva.
5. Isolate the tooth with a rubber dam (Fig. 13-13*A,B*).
6. Apply additional Orabase Plain to the rubber dam and the tooth margin.
7. Remove the access restoration and any remaining pulp tissue from the crown. Leave a slight undercut in the access opening to retain the temporary restorative material that will be placed later.

CLINICAL TIP

When performing initial endodontic therapy, carefully remove all tissue, debris, endodontic sealers, and filling materials from the sometimes elusive pulp horns and lateral extensions of the pulp chamber. This may help prevent subsequent tooth discoloration (see Fig. 13-5*A*).

8. Remove excess gutta-percha and endodontic sealer. Remove gutta-percha to 2 to 2.5 mm gingival to the gingival-most point on the coronal extension of the planned base. (See the section on Protective Base earlier in this chapter.)

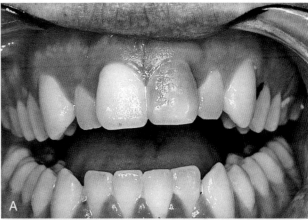
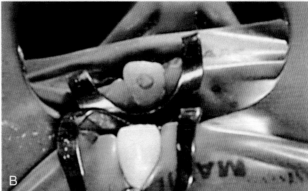
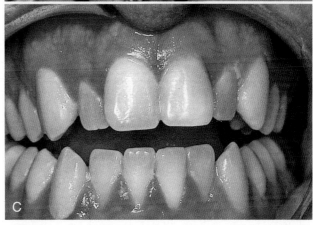

FIGURE 13-13 A, Preoperative view of staining caused by the deposition of hemorrhagic by-products into the dentinal tubules following pulpal trauma. **B,** Tooth after rubber dam isolation and placement of Orabase Plain. **C,** 6 months postbleaching.

CLINICAL TIP

Select the landmark on the labial surface of the tooth that will determine the gingival-most point of the coronal surface of the planned base. Use a periodontal probe to measure the length on the labial surface of the tooth from the above point to a reference point on the incisal tip. Add a minimum of 2 mm to this measurement. Use this final measurement and incisal reference point intracoronally to determine the precise amount of gutta-percha to remove.

9. Place a 2- to 2.5-mm thick protective base that conforms to the predetermined design and location (see the section on Protective Base earlier in this chapter) as follows:
   a. Measure the distance between a reference point on the incisal edge and the desired labial landmark (see the section on Protective Base earlier in the chapter).
   b. Transfer this measurement intracoronally to determine the corresponding coronal positioning of the base.
   c. Repeat steps (a) and (b) for locations between the midlabial and lateral extremes to create a base that conforms to the contour of the desired landmarks (see the section on Protective Base earlier in the chapter).
   d. The palatal (lingual) extension of the base should be coronal to the corresponding palatal cementoenamel junction and gingival margin (see the section on Protective Base earlier in the chapter).
   e. The base should resemble a bobsled tunnel mesiodistally and a ski slope buccolingually.[198]

CLINICAL TIP

Because only the labial portion of the tooth must be bleached, extend the lingual and proximal portions of the base as coronally as possible. This may further reduce the chance of external cervical root resorption.

10. Mix a thick paste of sodium perborate and sterile water on a glass slab and place the mixture into the tooth.
11. Tamp the mixture into place with a moist cotton pellet so that appropriate space is provided for the temporary restorative material.

CLINICAL TIP

To ensure an intimate seal of the temporary restorative material, be certain that the walls of the access opening have been cleared of bleaching material.

12. Seal the access with temporary restorative material.
13. Schedule the next appointment for the patient for 3 days later.
14. If a successful result is achieved after 3 days, skip to step 16.
15. Isolate the tooth with rubber dam, remove the temporary filling, and carefully wash the internal tooth chamber with water. If a successful result has not been achieved after 3 days, repeat steps 10 through 14. After three attempts, the likelihood of further whitening generally is minimal.
16. Isolate the tooth with rubber dam, remove the temporary filling, and carefully wash the internal tooth chamber with water. Mix a thick paste of calcium hydroxide powder and sterile water and place the mixture into the tooth.
17. Tamp the paste into place with a moist cotton pellet so that appropriate space is provided for the temporary restorative material.
18. Seal the access with temporary restorative material.
19. Schedule the next appointment for the patient for 7 to 14 days later.
20. After 7 to 14 days, remove the calcium hydroxide paste and restore the tooth. Figure 13-13C shows the results of the bleaching procedure 6 months after treatment.

(See the section on restorative implications under Office Bleaching ["Power" Bleaching] earlier in this chapter.)

Restorative Implications. For a discussion of restorative implications, see the section on restorative implications under Office Bleaching ("Power" Bleaching) earlier in this chapter.

Postoperative Complications. Because external cervical root resorption may occur even years after bleaching,[179] periodic follow-up radiographs are necessary. Cervical resorption has been treated with calcium hydroxide therapy,[193,194] although it has been suggested that this technique will be ineffective if there is communication between the oral cavity and the resorptive lesion.[193] It has also been suggested that calcium hydroxide therapy is ineffective (see the section on Calcium Hydroxide earlier in the chapter). Resorption also has been treated with surgical repair,[115] orthodontic extrusion,[115] and surgical crown lengthening.[193]

CONCLUSION

Bleaching agents or acid/abrasion techniques are effective and conservative approaches to the removal of unesthetic discolorations from vital and nonvital teeth. As with all types of therapeutic modalities, proper diagnosis, and treatment planning are essential.

ACKNOWLEDGMENT

The author wishes to acknowledge the generous help of Dr. Ilan Rotstein, Professor and Acting Chairman, Department of Endodontics, The Hebrew University–Hadassah School Of Dental Medicine, Jerusalem, Israel, in the preparation of a previous edition of this chapter.

REFERENCES

1. Panati C: *Panati's extraordinary origins of everyday things*, New York, 1987, Harper & Row.
2. Perdigão J: Dental whitening—revisiting the myths, *Northwest Dent* 89(6):19-21, 23-26, 2010.
3. Westlake A: Bleaching teeth by electricity, *Am J Dent Sci* 29:101, 1895.
4. Atkinson CB: Hints, queries and comments: pyrozone, *Dent Cosmos* 35:330-332, 1893.
5. Adams TC: Enamel color modifications by controlled hydrochloric acid pumice abrasion: a review with case summaries, *Indiana Dent Assoc J* 66(5):23-26, 1987.
6. Ames JW: Removing stains from mottled enamel, *J Am Dent Assoc* 24:1674-1677, 1937.
7. Younger HB: Bleaching fluorine stain from mottled enamel, *Texas Dent J* 57:380-382, 1939.
8. McInnes J: Removing brown stain from teeth, *Ariz Dent J* 12(4):13-15, 1966.
9. Cohen BA, Parkins FM: Bleaching tetracycline-stained vital teeth, *Oral Surg Oral Med Oral Pathol* 29:465, 1970.
10. McEvoy SA: Chemical agents for removing intrinsic stains from vital teeth, II: current techniques and their clinical application, *Quintessence Int* 20(6):379-384, 1989.
11. Arwill T, Myrberg N, Söremark R: Penetration of radioactive isotopes through the enamel and dentine, II. transfer of ^{22} Na in fresh and chemically treated dental tissues, *Odontol Revy* 20(1):47-54, 1969.
12. Feinman RA, Madray G, Yarborough D: Chemical, optical, and physiologic mechanisms of bleaching products: a review, *Pract Periodontics Aesthet Dent* 3(2):32-36, 1991.
13. Davies AK, McKellar JF, Phillips GO, Reid AG: Photochemical oxidation of tetracycline in aqueous solution, *J Chem Soc Perkin Trans* 2:369-375, 1979.
14. Loudon GM: *Organic chemistry*, Reading, MA, 1984, Addison-Wesley.
15. Matis BA, Wang Y, Jiang T, Eckert GJ: Extended at-home bleaching of tetracycline-stained teeth with different concentrations of carbamide peroxide, *Quintessence Int* 33(9):645-655, 2002.
16. Sulieman M, MacDonald E, Rees JS, Newcombe RG, Addy M: Tooth bleaching by different concentrations of carbamide peroxide and hydrogen peroxide whitening strips: an in vitro study, *J Esthet Restor Dent* 18(2):93-100, 2006.
17. He LB, Shao MY, Tan K, Xu X, Li JY: The effects of light on bleaching and tooth sensitivity during in-office vital bleaching: a systematic review and meta-analysis, *J Dent* 40(8):644-653, 2012.
18. Fasanaro TS: Bleaching teeth: history, chemicals, and methods used for common tooth discolorations, *J Esthet Dent* 4(3):71-78, 1992.

19. Seale NS, McIntosh JE, Taylor AN: Pulpal reaction to bleaching of teeth in dogs, *J Dent Res* 60(5):948-953, 1981.

20. Goldstein RE, Garber DA: *Complete dental bleaching*, Hanover Park, IL, 1995, Quintessence Publishing, pp. 15, 60.

21. Tong LS, Pang MK, Mok NY, King NM, Wei SH: The effects of etching, micro-abrasion, and bleaching on surface enamel, *J Dent Res* 72(1):67-71, 1993.

22. Torres-Rodríguez C, González-López S, Bolaños-Carmona V, Sánchez-Sánchez P, Rodríguez-Navarro A, Attin T: Demineralization effects of phosphoric acid on surface and subsurface bovine enamel bleached with in-office hydrogen peroxide, *J Adhes Dent* 13(4):315-321, 2011.

23. Yurdukoru B, Akören AC, Unsal MK: Alterations in human enamel surface morphology following the use of an office bleaching agent and consecutive application of 37% phosphoric acid in vivo, *J Clin Dent* 14(4):103-107, 2003.

24. de Medeiros CL, González-Lápez S, Bolaños-Carmona V, Sánchez-Sánchez P, Bolaños-Carmona J: Effects of phosphoric acid on bovine enamel bleached with carbamide peroxide, *Eur J Oral Sci* 116(1):66-71, 2008.

25. Ben-Amar A, Liberman R, Gorfil C, Bernstein Y: Effect of mouthguard bleaching on enamel surface, *Am J Dent* 8:29-32, 1995.

26. Bitter NC, Sanders JL: The effect of four bleaching agents on the enamel surface: a scanning electron microscopic study, *Quintessence Int* 24:817-824, 1993.

27. Shannon H, Spencer P, Gross K, Tira D: Characterization of enamel exposed to 10% carbamide peroxide bleaching agents, *Quintessence Int* 24:39-44, 1993.

28. Zaragoza VMT: Bleaching of vital teeth: technique, *Estomodeo* 9:7-30, 1984.

29. Frysh H, Bowles WH, Baker F, et al: Effect of pH on bleaching efficiency agents, *J Esthet Dent* 7(3):130-133, 1995.

30. Jiménez-Rubio A, Segura JJ: The effect of the bleaching agent sodium perborate on macrophage adhesion in vitro: implications in external cervical root resorption, *J Endod* 24(4):229-232, 1998.

31. Dahl J, Pallesen U: Tooth bleaching—a critical review of the biological aspects, *Crit Rev Oral Biol Med* 14(4):292-304, 2003.

32. Delfino CS, Chinelatti MA, Carrasco-Guerisoli LD, Batista AR, Fröner IC, Palma-Dibb RG: Effectiveness of home bleaching agents in discolored teeth and influence on enamel microhardness, *J Appl Oral Sci* 17(4):284-288, 2009.

33. Haywood VB, Leonard RH, Dickinson GL: Efficacy of six months of nightguard vital bleaching of tetracycline-stained teeth, *J Esthet Dent* 9(1):13-19, 1997.

34. Li Y: Peroxide-containing tooth whiteners: an update, *Compend Contin Educ Dent* 28(suppl):S4-S9, 2000.

35. Martin JH, Bishop JG, Guentherman RH, Dorman HL: Cellular response of gingiva to prolonged application of dilute hydrogen peroxide, *J Periodontol* 39:208-210, 1968.

36. Tam L: The safety of home bleaching techniques, *J Can Dent Assoc* 65(8):453-455, 1999.

37. van Maanen-Schakel NW, Slot DE, Bakker EW, Van der Weijden GA: The effect of an oxygenating agent on chlorhexidine-induced extrinsic tooth staining: a systematic review, *Int J Dent Hyg* 10(3):198-208, 2012.

38. Poulsen S, Errboe M, Lescay Mevil Y, Glenny AM: Potassium containing toothpastes for dentine hypersensitivity, *Cochrane Database Syst Rev* (3):CD001476, 2006.

39. Kim S: Hypersensitive teeth: desensitization of pulpal sensory nerves, *J Endod* 12(10):482-485, 1986.

40. Gallo JR, Burgess JO, Ripps AH, Bell MJ, Mercante DE, Davidson JM: Evaluation of 30% carbamide peroxide at-home bleaching gels with and without potassium nitrate—a pilot study, *Quintessence Int* 40(4):e1-6, 2009.

41. Christensen G: Tooth bleaching, state-of-art '97, *Clin Res Assoc Newsl* 21(4), 1997.

42. McCaslin AJ, Haywood VB, Potter BJ, Dickinson GL, Russell CM: Assessing dentin color changes from nightguard vital bleaching, *J Am Dent Assoc* 130(10):1485-1490, 1999.

43. Freire A, Archegas LR, de Souza EM, Vieira S: Effect of storage temperature on pH of in-office and at-home dental bleaching agents, *Acta Odontol Latinoam* 22(1):27-31, 2009.

44. Scientific Committee on Consumer Products (SCCP): *Preliminary opinion on hydrogen peroxide in tooth whitening products.* Document No. SCCP/0844/04. http://ec.europa.eu/health/ph_risk/committees/04_sccp/docs/sccp_cons_01_en.pdf.

45. Margeas RC: *New advances in tooth whitening and dental cleaning technology*, Tulsa, OK, 2013, PennWell Corp. A peer-reviewed continuing education article. http://www.ineedce.com/courses/1464/pdf/newadvancesintooth.pdf. Accessed November 18, 2013.

46. Greenwall L: *Bleaching techniques in restorative dentistry: an illustrated guide*, Valley Stream, NY, 2001, Martin Dunitz.

47. Chang R: *Quimica*, Lisbon, 1994, McGraw-Hill.

48. Howe-Grant M, editor: *Encyclopedia of chemical technology*, ed 4, vol. 13. New York, 1992, Wiley.

49. Kurthy R: Why we see problems with teeth whitening: the science of whitening, part I, *Dentaltown Mag* 92-99, 2012

50. Browning WD, Blalock JS, Frazier KB, Downey MC, Myers ML: Duration and timing of sensitivity related to bleaching, *J Esthet Restor Dent* 19(5):256-264, 2007.

51. da Costa JB, McPharlin R, Hilton T, Ferracane JL, Wang M: Comparison of two at-home whitening products of similar peroxide concentration and different delivery methods, *Oper Dent* 37(4):333-339, 2012. doi:10.2341/11-053-C.

52. Kurthy R: Why we see problems with teeth whitening: the science of whitening, part III: whitening sensitivity, *Dentaltown Mag* 96-100, 2013.

53. Markowitz K: Pretty painful: why does tooth bleaching hurt?, *Med Hypotheses* 74(5):835-840, 2010.

54. Brännström M: A hydrodynamic mechanism in the transmission of pain-produced stimuli through the dentine. In Anderson DJ, editor: *Sensory mechanisms in dentine: proceedings of a symposium held at the Royal Society of Medicine, London, September 24, 1962*. Elmsford, NY, 1963, Pergamon Press, pp. 73-79.

55. Absi EG, Addy M, Adams D: Dentine hypersensitivity. A study of the patency of dentinal tubules in sensitive and non-sensitive cervical dentine, *J Clin Periodontol* 14(5):280-284, 1987.

56. Strassler H: *The science and art of tooth whitening*, Tulsa, OK, 2013, PennWell Corp. http://www.ineedce.com/courses/1698/PDF/TheScienceandArtWhitening.pdf. Accessed November 18, 2013.

57. Reeder OW Jr, Walton RE, Livingston MJ, Pashley DH: Dentin permeability: determinants of hydraulic conductance, *J Dent Res* 57(2):187-193, 1978.

58. Pashley DH, Tay FR, Haywood VB, Collins MA, Drisko CL: Dentin hypersensitivity: consensus-based recommendations for the diagnosis and management of dentin hypersensitivity, *Inside Dent* 4(9 special issue):1-37, 2008.

59. Esposito P, Varvara G, Murmura G, Terlizzi A, Caputi S: Ability of healthy and inflamed human dental pulp to reduce hydrogen peroxide, *Eur J Oral Sci* 111(5):454-456, 2003.

60. Eldridge D, Holstege CP: Hydrogen peroxide. In Anderson B, de Peyster A, Gad S, et al, editors: *Encyclopedia of toxicology*, ed 2, Waltham, MA, 2005, Academic Press.

61. Jordan RE, Boksman L: Conservative vital bleaching treatment of discolored dentition, *Compend Contin Educ Dent* 5(10):803-805, 807, 1984.

62. Christensen GJ: Bleaching vital tetracycline-stained teeth, *Quintessence Int Dent Dig* 9(6):13-19, 1978.

63. Ingle JI, Taintor JF: *Endodontics*, ed 3, Philadelphia, 1985, Lea & Febiger.

64. Reid JS, Newman P: A suggested method of bleaching tetracycline-stained vital teeth, *Br Dent J* 142(8):261, 1977.

65. Wilson CF, Seale NS: Color change following vital bleaching of tetracycline-stained teeth, *Pediatr Dent* 7(3):205-208, 1985.

66. Goldstein RE: In-office bleaching: where we came from, where we are today, *J Am Dent Assoc* 128(suppl):11S-15S, 1997.

67. Garber DA: Dentist-monitored bleaching: a discussion of combination and laser bleaching, *J Am Dent Assoc* 128(suppl):26S-30S, 1997.

68. Titley KC, Torneck CD, Smith DC, Adibfar A: Adhesion of composite resin to bleached and unbleached bovine enamel [published correction appears in *J Dent Res* 68(2), 1989:inside back cover]. *J Dent Res* 67(12):1523-1528, 1988.

69. Titley KC, Torneck CD, Smith DC, Chernecky R, Adibfar A: Scanning electron microscopy observations on the penetration and structure of resin tags in bleached and unbleached bovine enamel, *J Endod* 17(2):72-75, 1991.

70. Torneck CD, Titley KC, Smith DC, Adibfar A: The influence of time of hydrogen peroxide exposure on the adhesion of composite resin to bleached bovine enamel, *J Endod* 16(3):123-128, 1990.

71. Heymann H: Nonrestorative treatment of discolored teeth: reports from an international symposium, *J Am Dent Assoc* 128(6):710-711, 1997.

72. Swift EJ Jr: Restorative considerations with vital tooth bleaching, *J Am Dent Assoc* 128(suppl):60S-64S, 1997.

73. Swift EJ Jr, Perdigão J: Effects of bleaching on teeth and restorations, *Compend Contin Educ Dent* 19(8):815-820, 1998.

74. Schwachman H, Schuster A: The tetracyclines: applied pharmacology, *Pediatr Clin North Am* 3:295, 1956.

75. Albert A, Rees CW: Avidity of the tetracyclines for the cations of metals, *Nature* 177(4505):433-434, 1956.

76. Finerman GAM, Milch RA: In vitro binding of tetracyclines to calcium, *Nature* 198:486, 1963.

77. Stewart DJ: The effects of tetracyclines upon the dentition, *Br J Dermatol* 76:374-378, 1964.

78. Weinstein L: Antimicrobial agents. In Goodman LS, Gilman A, editors: *The pharmacologic basis of therapeutics*, New York, 1975, Macmillan.

79. Sayegh FS, Gassner E: Sites of tetracycline deposition in rat dentin, *J Dent Res* 46(6):1474, 1967.

80. Sayegh FS: H³-proline and tetracycline as marking agents in the study of reparative dentine formation, *Oral Surg Oral Med Oral Pathol* 23(2):221-229, 1967.

81. Milch RA, Rall DP, Tobie JE: Bone localization of the tetracycline, *J Natl Cancer Inst* 19(1):87-93, 1957.

82. Urist M, Ibsen K: Chemical reactivity of mineralized tissue with oxytetracycline, *Arch Pathol* 76:484-496, 1963.

83. Martin NO, Barnard PD: The prevalence of tetracycline staining in erupted teeth, *Med J Aust* 1(25):1286-1289, 1969.

84. Bridges JB, Owens PDA, Stewart DJ: Tetracycline and teeth: an experimental investigation into five types in the rat, *Br Dent J* 126(7):306-311, 1969.

85. Walton RE, O'Dell NL, Myers DL, Lake FT, Shimp RG: External bleaching of tetracycline stained teeth in dogs, *J Endod* 8(12):536-542, 1982.

86. Stewart DJ: Teeth discoloured by tetracycline bleaching following exposure to daylight, *Dent Pract Dent Rec* 20(9):309-310, 1970.

87. Lin LC, Pitts DL, Burgess LW Jr: An investigation into the feasibility of photobleaching tetracycline-stained teeth, *J Endod* 14(6):293-299, 1988.

88. Ibsen KH, Urist MR, Sognnaes RF: Differences among tetracyclines with respect to the staining of teeth, *J Pediatr* 67:459-462, 1965.

89. Wallman IS, Hilton HB: Teeth pigmented by tetracycline, *Lancet* 1(7234):827-829, 1962.

90. Davies AK, Cundall RB, Dandiker Y, Slifkin MA: Photo-oxidation of tetracycline adsorbed on hydroxyapatite in relation to the light-induced staining of teeth, *J Dent Res* 64(6):936-939, 1985.

91. Moffitt JM, Cooley RO, Olsen NH, Hefferren JJ: Prediction of tetracycline-induced tooth discoloration, *J Am Dent Assoc* 88(3):547-552, 1974.

92. Genot MT, Golan HP, Porter PJ, Kass EH: Effects of administration of tetracycline in pregnancy on the primary dentition of the offspring, *J Oral Med* 25(3):75-79, 1970.

93. Swallow JN: Discoloration of primary dentition after maternal tetracycline ingestion in pregnancy, *Lancet* 2(7360):611-612, 1964.

94. Grossman ER, Walchek A, Freedman H: Tetracycline and permanent teeth: the relation between dose and tooth color, *Pediatrics* 47(3):567-570, 1971.

95. Wehman J, Porteous JR: Tetracycline staining of teeth: a report of clinical material, *J Dent Res* 42:1111, 1963.

96. Eisenberg E: Anomalies of the teeth with stains and discolorations, *J Prev Dent* 2(1):7-14, 16-20, 1975.

97. Stewart RE, Barber TK, Troutman KC, Wei SHY, eds: *Pediatric dentistry: scientific foundations and clinical practice*, St Louis, 1982, Mosby p. 87.

98. Swift EJ Jr: A method for bleaching discolored vital teeth, *Quintessence Int* 19(9):607-612, 1988.

99. US Department of Health and Human Services, Public Health Service: *Review of fluoride: benefits and risks*, Report of the Ad Hoc Subcommittee on Fluoride, Washington, DC, February 1991.

100. Dunn JR: Dentist-prescribed home bleaching: current status, *Compend Contin Educ Dent* 18:760, 1998.

101. McEvoy SA: Chemical agents for removing intrinsic stains from vital teeth. I. Technique development, *Quintessence Int* 20:323, 1989.

102. McEvoy SA: Combining chemical agents and technique to remove intrinsic stains from vital teeth, *Gen Dent* 46:168, 1998.

103. Grossman LI, Oliet S, del Rio CE, eds: *Endodontic practice*, ed 11, Philadelphia, 1988, Lea & Febiger.

104. Ho S, Goerig AC: An in vitro comparison of different bleaching agents in the discolored tooth, *J Endod* 15:106, 1989.

105. Imber S, Gorfil C: A one visit bleaching technique for the endodontically treated tooth, *Refuat Hoshinayim* 4:7, 1986.

106. Van der Burgt TP, Plasschaert AJM: Bleaching of tooth discoloration caused by endodontic sealers, *J Endod* 12:231, 1986.

107. Crane DL: The walking bleach technique for endodontically treated teeth, *Chi Dent Soc Rev* 77:49, 1984.

108. Gutierrez J, Guzman M: Tooth discoloration in endodontic procedures, *Oral Surg* 26:706, 1968.

109. Nutting EB, Poe GS: Chemical bleaching of discolored endodontically treated teeth, *Dent Clin North Am* 11:655, 1967.

110. Sommer FS, Ostrander FD, Crowley MC: *Clinical endodontics*, ed 3, Philadelphia, 1966, Saunders.

111. Andreasen JO, Sundstrom B, Ravn JJ: The effect of traumatic injuries to the primary teeth on their permanent successors: a clinical and histologic study of 117 injured permanent teeth, *Scand J Dent Res* 79:219, 1971.

112. McEvoy SA: Bleaching stains related to trauma or periapical inflammation, *Compend Contin Educ Dent* 7:420, 1986.

113. Thylstrup A, Fejerskov O: Clinical appearance of dental fluorosis in permanent teeth in relation to histologic changes, *Commun Dent Oral Epidemiol* 6:315-328, 1978.

114. Gorelick L, Geiger AM, Gwinnett AJ: Incidence of white spot formation after bonding and banding, *Am J Orthod* 81:93-98, 1982.

115. Staudt CB, Lussi A, Jacquet J, Kiliaridis S: White spot lesions around brackets: in vitro detection by laser fluorescence, *Eur J Oral Sci* 112:237-243, 2004.

116. Croll TP: Enamel microabrasion for removal of superficial dysmineralization and decalcification defects, *J Am Dent Assoc* 120:411, 1990.

117. Cohn EC: ICON treatment of post orthodontic white spot lesions, *Oral Health J* 143:31-41, 2013.

118. Riordan PJ: Perceptions of dental fluorosis, *J Dent Res* 72:1268-1274, 1993.

119. de Amorim Lde F, Estrela C, da Costa LR: Effects of traumatic dental injuries to primary teeth on permanent teeth—a clinical follow-up study, *Dent Traumatol* 27:117-121, 2011.

120. Muñoz MA, Arana-Gordillo LA, Gomes GM, et al: Alternative esthetic management of fluorosis and hypoplasia stains: blending effect obtained with resin infiltration techniques, *J Esthet Restor Dent* 25(1):32-39, 2013.

121. Molnar S, Ward SC: Mineral metabolism and microstructural defects in primate teeth, *Am J Phys Anthropol* 43(1):3-17, 1975.

122. Shafer WG, Hine MK, Levy BM: *A textbook of oral pathology*, ed 3, Philadelphia, 1974, Saunders.

123. Finn SB: *Clinical pedodontics*, ed 4, Philadelphia, 1973, Saunders.

124. Faunce F: Management of discolored teeth, *Dent Clin North Am* 27:657, 1983.

125. Feinman RA, Goldstein RE, Garber DA: *Bleaching teeth*, Chicago, 1987, Quintessence.

126. Goldstein RE: Bleaching teeth: new materials, new role, *J Am Dent Assoc* 115:44E, 1987.

127. Altarabulsi MB, Alkilzy M, Splieth CH: Clinical applicability of resin infiltration for proximal caries, *Quintessence Int* 44(2):97-104, 2013.

128. Lee, SS Kwon, SR Arambula M, Yang H, et al: Assessment of whitening efficacy of two in-office professional bleaching regimens, *J Dent Res* 92(Spec Iss A):1139, 2013.

129. Torres CRG, dos Santos, MG, Borges AB, et al: A micro-invasive approach to treat and mask post-orthodontic white spot lesions, *Dent Pract* May 2011. http://content.yudu.com/Library/A1rzhq/DentalPracticeMay201/resources/20.htm. Accessed November 2013.

130. Shivanna V, Shivakumar B: Novel treatment of white spot lesions: a report of two cases, *J Conserv Dent* 14(4):423-426, 2011.

131. Paris S, Schwendicke F, Keltsch J, Därfer C, Meyer-Lueckel H: Masking of white spot lesions by resin infiltration in vitro, *J Dent* 2013.

132. Waggonner WF, Johnston WM, Schumann S, Schikowski E: Microabrasion of human enamel in vitro using hydrochloric acid and pumice, *Pediatr Dent* 11:319, 1989.

133. Croll TP, Cavanaugh RR: Enamel color modification by controlled hydrochloric acid–pumice abrasion. II. Further examples, *Quintessence Int* 17:157, 1986.

134. Bailey RW, Christen AG: Effects of a bleaching technique on the labial enamel of human teeth stained with endemic dental fluorosis, *J Dent Res* 49:168, 1970.

135. Griffin RE Jr, Grower MF, Ayer WA: Effects of solutions used to treat dental fluorosis on permeability of teeth, *J Endod* 3:139, 1977.

136. Baumgartner JC, Reid DE, Pickett AB: Human pulpal reaction to the modified McInnes bleaching technique, *J Endod* 9:527, 1983.

137. Olin PS, Lehner CR, Hilton JA: Enamel surface modification in vitro using hydrochloric acid pumice: an SEM investigation, *Quintessence Int* 19:733, 1988.

138. Bailey RW, Christen AG: Bleaching of vital teeth stained with endemic dental fluorosis, *Oral Surg Oral Med Oral Pathol* 26:871, 1968.

139. Colon PG Jr: Improving the appearance of severely fluorosed teeth, *J Am Dent Assoc* 86:1329, 1973.

140. Colon PG Jr: Removing fluorosis stain from teeth, *Quintessence Int* 2:89, 1971.

141. Douglas WA: *History of dentistry in Colorado, 1859-1959*, Denver, 1959, Colorado State Dental Association.

142. McCloskey RJ: A technique for removal of fluorosis stains, *J Am Dent Assoc* 109:63, 1984.

143. McMurray CA: Removal of stains from mottled enamel of teeth, *Texas Dent J* 59:293, 1941.

144. Raper HR, Manser JG: Removal of brown stain from fluorine mottled teeth, *Dent Digest* 47:390, 1941.

145. Smith HV, McInnes JW: Further studies on methods of removing brown stain from mottled teeth, *J Am Dent Assoc* 29:571, 1942.

146. Wayman BE, Cooley RL: Vital bleaching technique for treatment of endemic fluorosis, *Gen Dent* 29:424, 1981.

147. Croll TP: Enamel microabrasion: observations after 10 years, *J Am Dent Assoc* (suppl) 128:45S, 1997.

148. McEvoy SA: Removing intrinsic stains from vital teeth by microabrasion and bleaching, *J Esthet Dent* 7:1006, 1995.

149. Coll JA, Jackson P, Strassler HE: Comparison of enamel microabrasion techniques: Prema Compound versus a 12-fluted finishing bur, *J Esthet Dent* 3:180, 1991.

150. Croll TP, Cavanaugh RR: Enamel color modification by controlled hydrochloric acid–pumice abrasion. I. Technique and examples, *Quintessence Int* 17:81, 1986.

151. Meyer-Lueckel H, Paris S, Kielbassa AM: Surface layer erosion of natural caries lesions with phosphoric and hydrochloric acid gels in preparation for resin infiltration, *Caries Res* 41(3):223-230, 2007.

152. Paris S, Meyer-Lueckel H: Masking of labial enamel white spot lesions by resin infiltration—a clinical report, *Quintessence Int* 40(9):713-718, 2009.

153. Vasundhara S, Shivakumar B: Novel treatment of white spot lesions: a report of two cases, *J Conserv Dent* 14(4):423-426, 2011.

154. Feng CH, Chu XY: Efficacy of one year treatment of icon infiltration resin on post-orthodontic white spots, *Beijing Da Xue Xue Bao* 45(1):40-43, 2013. (abstract only; article in Chinese)

155. Kim S, Kim EY, Jeong TS, Kim JW: The evaluation of resin infiltration for masking labial enamel white spot lesions, *Int J Paediatr Dent* 21(4):241-248, 2011. doi: 10.1111/j.1365-263X.2011.01126.x. Epub March 14, 2011.

156. Aschheim K, unpublished data.

157. Yang F, Mueller J, Kielbassa AM: Surface substance loss of subsurface bovine enamel lesions after different steps of the resinous infiltration technique: a 3D topography analysis, *Odontology* 100(2):172-180, 2012. doi: 10.1007/s10266-011-0031-4. Epub June 16, 2011.

158. Cassoni A, Rodrigues JA: Argon laser: a light source alternative for photopolymerization and in-office tooth bleaching, *Gen Dent* 55(5):416-419, 2007.

159. American Dental Association: *Tooth whitening/bleaching: treatment considerations for dentists and their patients.* ADA Council on Scientific Affairs September 2009. (revised November 2010)

160. Yazici AR, Khanbodaghi A, Kugel G: Effects of an in-office bleaching system (ZOOM) on pulp chamber temperature in vitro, *J Contemp Dent Pract* 8(4):19-26, 2007.

161. Carrasco LD, Guerisoli DM, Rocha MJ, et al: Efficacy of intracoronal bleaching techniques with different light activation sources, *Int Endod J* 40:204-208, 2007.

162. Dietschi D, Rossier S, Krejci I: In vitro colorimetric evaluation of the efficacy of various bleaching methods and products, *Quintessence Int* 37:515-526, 2006.

163. Personal communication with manufacturer (Phillips Inc.) April 2013.

164. Li Y, Lee S, Kwon SR, Arambula M, Yang H, Li J, et al: A randomized, parallel-design clinical trial to assess tooth bleaching efficacy and safety of light versus non-light activated chairside whitening in vivo study.

165. Data on file, 2012.

166. Lee SS, Kwon SR, Arambula M, Yang H, Delaurenti M, Li J, et al: Assessment of whitening efficacy of two in-office professional bleaching regimens, *J Dent Res* 92(Spec Iss A):1139, 2013

167. Haywood V: Nightguard vital bleaching: current concepts and research, *J Am Dent Assoc* (suppl)128:19S, 1997.

168. Tooth bleaching, home use products: update report, *Clin Res Assoc Newsl* 13(12), 1989.

169. Ploeger BJ et al: Quantitative in vivo comparison of five carbamide peroxide bleach gels, Abstract No 889, *J Dent Res* 70:376, 1991.

170. Burrell KH: ADA supports vital tooth bleaching—but look for the seal, *J Am Dent Assoc* (supplement)128:3S, 1997.

171. Berry JH: What about whiteners? Safety concerns explored, *J Am Dent Assoc* 121:223, 1990.

172. Weitzman SA, Weitberg AB, Stossel TP, et al: Effects of hydrogen peroxide on oral carcinogenesis in hamsters, *J Periodontol* 57:685, 1986.

173. Instructions for use of Opalescence, Ultradent, Inc. (product received American Dental Association Seal of Acceptance), South Jordan, UT.

174. Janis JN, Javaheri DS: The efficacy of reservoirs in bleaching trays, *Oper Dent* 25(3):149-151, 2000.

175. Rotstein I, Lehr Z, Gedalia I: Effect of bleaching agents on inorganic components of human dentin and cementum, *J Endod* 18:290, 1992.

176. Marin PD, Heithersay GS, Bridges TE: A quantitative comparison of traditional and nonperoxide bleaching agents, *Endod Dent Traumatol* 14:64, 1998.

177. Bhaskar SN, editor: *Orban's oral histology and embryology*, ed 11, St Louis, 1999, Mosby.

178. Lado EA, Stanley HR, Weisman MI: Cervical resorption in bleached teeth, *Oral Surg* 55:78, 1983.

179. Harrington GW, Natkin E: External resorption associated with bleaching of pulpless teeth, *J Endod* 5:344, 1979.
180. Kehoe JC: pH reversal following in vitro bleaching of pulpless teeth, *J Endod* 13:6, 1987.
181. Freccia WF, Peters DD, Lorton L, Bernier WE: An in vitro comparison of nonvital bleaching techniques in the discolored tooth, *J Endod* 8:70, 1982.
182. Heithersay GS: Invasive cervical resorption: an analysis of potential predisposing factors, *Quintessence Int* 30:83, 1999.
183. Rotstein I, Zalkind M, Mor C et al: In vitro efficacy of sodium perborate preparations used for intracoronal bleaching of discolored nonvital teeth, *Endod Dent Traumatol* 7:177, 1991.
184. Weiger R, Kuhn A, Lost C: In vitro comparison of various types of sodium perborate used for intracoronal bleaching of discolored teeth, *J Endod* 20:338, 1994.
185. Rotstein I, Mor C, Friedman S: Prognosis of intracoronal bleaching with sodium perborate preparation in vitro: 1-year study, *J Endod* 19:10, 1993.
186. Rotstein I, Friedman S, Mor C, et al: Histological characterization of bleaching-induced external resorption in dogs, *J Endod* 17:436, 1991.
187. Baratieri LN, Ritter AV, Monteiro S Jr et al. Nonvital tooth bleaching: guidelines for the clinician, *Quintessence Int* 26:597, 1995.
188. Abbott PV: Aesthetic considerations in endodontics: internal bleaching, *Pract Periodontol Aesthet Dent* 9:833, 1997.
189. Horn DJ, Hicks ML, Bulan-Brady J: Effect of smear layer removal on bleaching of human teeth in vitro, *J Endod* 24:791, 1998.
190. Casey LJ, Schindler WG, Murata SM, Burgess JO: The use of dentinal etching with endodontic bleaching procedures, *J Endod* 15:535, 1989.
191. Tronstad L, Andreasen JO, Hasselgren G, et al: pH changes in dental tissues after root canal filling with calcium hydroxide, *J Endod* 2:17, 1981.
192. Fuss Z, Szajkis S, Tagger M: Tubular permeability to calcium hydroxide and to bleaching agents, *J Endod* 15:362, 1989.
193. Gimlin DR, Schindler G: The management of postbleaching cervical resorption, *J Endod* 16:292, 1990.
194. Montgomery S: External cervical resorption after bleaching a pulpless tooth, *Oral Surg Oral Med Oral Pathol* 57:203, 1984.
195. Latcham NL: Postbleaching cervical resorption, *J Endod* 12:262, 1986.
196. Friedman S: Surgical-restorative treatment of bleaching-related external root resorption, *Endod Dent Traumatol* 5:63, 1989.
197. Rotstein I: Personal communication, e-mail, July 22, 1999.
198. Steiner DR, West JD: A method to determine the location and shape of an intracoronal bleach barrier, *J Endod* 20:304, 1994.
199. Rotstein I, Zyskind D, Lewinstein I, Bamberger N: Effect of different protective base materials on hydrogen peroxide leakage during intracoronal bleaching in vitro, *J Endod* 18:114, 1992.
200. Jimenez-Rubio A, Segura JJ: The effect of the bleaching agent sodium perborate on macrophage adhesion in vitro: implications in external cervical root resorption, *J Endod* 24:229, 1998.

Part 4

Esthetics and Other Clinical Applications

14

Esthetics and Periodontics

Edwin S. Rosenberg and James Torosian

Periodontal therapy plays an important role in esthetics, although the images invoked regarding conventional periodontal therapy (ugly spaces, gingival recession, tooth sensitivity) are anything but beautiful. The introduction of new surgical techniques and the adaptation of traditional periodontal procedures have led to a heightened esthetic awareness in periodontology. In addition, the recognition of the etiology and complicating factors underlying an esthetic periodontal problem is crucial. Often this identification alters or dictates the definitive treatment plan.

PERIODONTAL ALVEOLAR BONE DEFECTS

Differential Diagnosis

Traditional periodontal pocket elimination therapy causes unaesthetic results, including large interdental spaces and long clinical crowns. However, without adequate access to deep lesions, a healthy periodontal environment is unachievable. Several surgical solutions exist for this dilemma, depending on whether the defect is anteriorly or posteriorly located.

Treatment Options

Retained Papilla. The retained papilla technique is an ideal treatment alternative for periodontal defects. The procedure provides adequate access to the root surfaces and bone defects allowing for thorough surgical debridement of the area while maintaining the position of the free gingival margin. This technique is used almost exclusively in the maxillary anterior sextant. Access is achieved by including the entire interproximal tissue mass in the surgical flap. A straight-line incision is made in the palate and the papilla reflected buccally with the flap. Full access is provided for thorough debridement of the defect and root surfaces. After performing any treatment to the roots and/or bone (such as grafting, palatal ramping, and regenerative procedures, when indicated), the flaps are sutured to their original positions. By including the papillary tissues (as opposed

to removing them as with conventional pocket elimination), interproximal tissue height is maintained and little or no apical shrinkage occurs. Thus the physiologic needs of the periodontium are satisfied along with the esthetic demands of the patient.

The decision to use the retained papillae technique is, obviously, made before the time of the procedure. However, the decision as how to manage those defects (the grafting and regeneration as stated in the preceding) can be made before or during the procedure.

Guided Tissue Regeneration. The goal of guided tissue regeneration (GTR) is pocket elimination through reformation of the periodontal connective tissue attachment. It is applicable to both anterior and posterior defects. Exclusion of the rapidly proliferating epithelial tissues from the defect allows regeneration of the connective tissue attachment by cells of the periodontal ligament. This epithelial exclusion is achieved by placing a semipermeable membrane between the periodontal defect and the flap, thus allowing nutrients to reach the flap while preventing the formation of a long junctional epithelium. Membranes can be either nonresorbable (e.g., Gore-Tex, W. L. Gore & Associates, Inc.) or resorbable (e.g., BIO-GIDE, Geistlich Pharma North America, Inc.), with the primary difference being that the former requires removal (and a second surgical entry), whereas the latter does not. The choice of membrane is based on the preference of the surgeon and the clinical situation. For example, a resorbable barrier might be indicated when a patient's medical history requires minimizing the number of procedures that are performed.

The site is accessed with a full thickness flap to reveal the defect. Thorough debridement of the roots and bone defect are performed using hand, ultrasonic, and rotary instruments. The membrane is cut so that it fits over the defect with the margins resting on healthy bone. The barrier is then sutured in place and the flaps adapted to achieve primary closure. If a non-resorbable barrier is used, removal with a simple gingival flap procedure can be accomplished after 4 to 5 weeks, revealing a dense connective tissue fill of the defect that may or may not be accompanied with bone regeneration. The same healing process occurs with resorbable barriers; however, it is not visualized because there is no second entry procedure.

Alveolar bone reformation is not always necessary to achieve pocket closure, because the dense connective tissue attachment to the root surface can provide fill for the defect with resultant pocket reduction. Not all defects are amenable to this type of procedure with Class II furcation defects (buccal or lingual), interproximal craters and deep, narrow three-walled defects offering the best prognosis. In wider defects with fewer bony walls, Class II interproximal and Class III furcation defects, the results are not completely predictable.

Osseous Grafting. Osseous grafting is another alternative for the treatment of deep angular defects and, as with GTR, it is applicable to both anterior and posterior defects. The goal of bone grafting is to reform the alveolar bone and attachment in the defect. However, this is not always achieved, with some defects healing via a combination of new bone formation and dense connective tissue repair (with a resultant long junctional epithelial attachment). Both types of healing result in sustainable pocket reduction as long as the area is kept free of inflammation. In either instance, the esthetic goals (maintenance of the tissue height) and functional needs (creation of a cleansable area) are achieved.

The primary types of bone grafts used in periodontal surgery fall into three categories; allografts, xenografts and alloplastic grafts. Allografts are cadaveric in origin and can be either cortical or cancellous (e.g., Puros, Zimmer Dental Inc.). Bovine bone (Bio-Oss, Geistlich Pharma North America, Inc.) and equine bone (Equimatrix, Osteohealth Co.) are examples of xenografts. Alloplastic grafts are biocompatible, synthetic materials (e.g., Bone Ceramic, Straumann USA LLC). The selection of which material to use is based on a number of factors, including defect type, intended goal of the procedure and patient preference. Allografts have the ability to promote new bone formation by stimulating osteoprogenitor cells (osteoinduction) and acting as a scaffold for peripheral bone growth into the defect (osteoconduction). Xenografts and alloplasts are osteoconductive only.

Surgical access to the defect is accomplished with a flap designed to maintain the marginal tissues. Once the defects have been thoroughly debrided, the graft material is placed into the defect to the level of the surrounding bone; defects should not be overfilled to avoid problems with flap healing. The flaps are replaced to cover the graft material and to achieve primary closure and sutured in place. The result is clinical pocket closure with maintenance of the free gingival margin.

As with guided tissue regeneration, the results are not completely predictable and depend on defect type and morphology. Bone grafts are best used in Class II furcations, three-walled defects, and craters (two-walled defects with the buccal and lingual plates intact). In interproximal craters with small interradicular distance, a bone graft is the procedure of choice because of the ease of placement. As with the guided tissue regeneration procedure, the success rate decreases with two- and one-walled alveolar defects and with lingual and buccal plate defects.

Another factor potentially affecting success is the ability to achieve primary closure of the flap margins. Membrane exposure often leads to postoperative infection and failure. The same is true with bone grafts, with the additional problem of graft material dislodging from the defect if it does not remain covered with the membrane. Patient factors must also be considered. Using a resorbable membrane or a bone graft would be preferable in situations in which a second surgery is either not desired or contraindicated (e.g., difficult access, medical complications, patient cooperation).

Palatal or Lingual Ramping. Another esthetic option in the posterior sextant is palatal or lingual ramping of alveolar defects without involvement of the buccal bone. Ostectomy is done to remove the palatal or lingual wall of a crater-type defect. This results in an increased crown length on the palatal or lingual aspect of the teeth, with the gingival tissues angled palatally or lingually. The buccal height of tissue remains relatively intact because the buccal bone is spared.

Open Debridement with Buccal Ostectomy. Although the aforementioned procedures are designed to maintain buccal bone height, buccal ostectomy is sometimes necessary, such as in situations of a markedly uneven buccal bony profile. When this type of situation occurs, blending of the buccal alveolar crests is needed to ensure proper soft tissue healing and pocket closure. The patient must be made aware that despite best efforts to satisfy esthetic needs, physiologic demands may unfavorably affect the esthetics.

Clinical Case: Retained Papilla Technique

A 52-year-old man presented with persistent deep periodontal pocketing of the anterior maxillary teeth 6 weeks after completing initial periodontal therapy consisting of scaling and root planing (Fig. 14-1A,B).

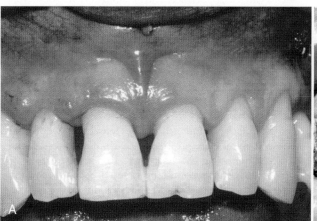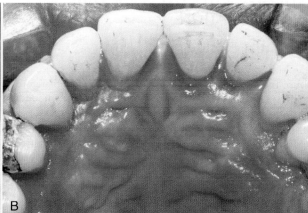

FIGURE 14-1 Facial (**A**) and palatal (**B**) views following initial therapy response in a 52-year-old patient with deep periodontal pocketing.

Continued

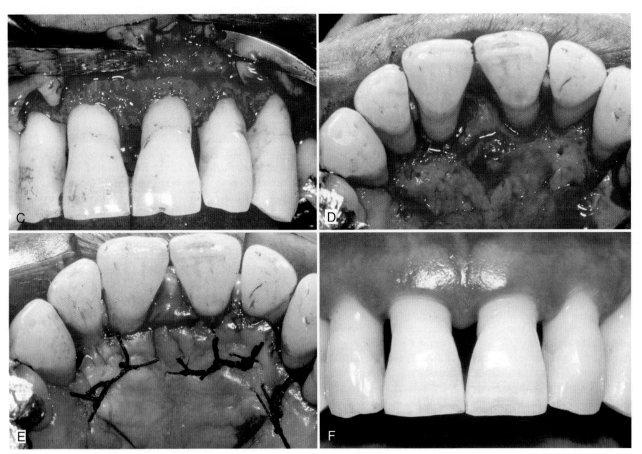

FIGURE 14-1, cont'd C, A full-thickness flap was raised with complete retention of the papillae in the facial flap. **D,** The osseous defects were exposed for thorough debridement. **E,** The flaps were repositioned and sutured in place. **F,** Six months after surgery, pocket elimination has been achieved along with maintenance of the original tissue height.

His medical history was noncontributory. A full-thickness flap procedure was performed using the retained papilla technique (Fig. 14-1C,D). The interproximal tissues were kept in the buccal flap. After thorough debridement of the defects, the papillae were reattached with sutures through the tissue, not over the interproximal space (Fig. 14-1E). Healing resulted in pocket reduction with maintenance of the gingival margin (Fig. 14-1F).

INADEQUATE TOOTH STRUCTURE FOR RESTORATION

Differential Etiology

1. *Caries.* Many patients are unaware of subgingival caries because the lesion is hidden under the gingiva and therefore they do not present for treatment until significant amounts of tooth structure have been destroyed.
2. *Trauma.* With traumatic injuries the patient is keenly aware of the problem. Teeth can be obliquely sheared, leaving margins below the alveolar crest. When the root fracture is horizontal or oblique, the longer the apical segment is, the better the prognosis. Vertical fracture usually requires extraction.
   Biologic Width. Proper margin placement of any type of restoration requires respect for the physiologic principle of biologic width: 1 mm of supracrestal connective tissue, 1 mm of junctional epithelium, and 1 to 2 mm of healthy sulcus. When

a restoration is placed on a tooth in violation of this principle, a chronic inflammatory response occurs. The body is attempting to restore the dimensions required for periodontal health in the supracrestal attachment and sulcus. Histologically, crestal resorption is seen with apical migration of the connective tissue and junctional epithelium. Clinically, gingival redness, swelling, bleeding, and discomfort are present. Even the most natural-looking restoration will fall short of the desired esthetic goals with such a gingival appearance. The inflammatory response will cease only when the biologic width has been re-established, a process that may take years. This inflammation is not bacterial in origin and will not respond to periodontal scaling or antibiotic therapy. Attempting to subgingivally "bury" a restoration margin in the hope of avoiding further treatment will only result in failure.

Treatment Options

Surgical Crown Lengthening. Surgical crown lengthening involves apical flap positioning with ostectomy around the involved tooth and the adjacent teeth. At least 3 to 4 mm of sound root structure must be exposed below the most apical extent of the proposed restoration. In addition, the alveolar crest of the adjacent teeth must be blended in with the involved tooth; otherwise an uneven, unesthetic gingival profile will result.

Forced Eruption with Fiberotomy. When ostectomy will result in extremely long clinical crowns and significantly weakened periodontal support (as with oblique fractures significantly apical to the alveolar crest), or when a surgical procedure is medically contraindicated, orthodontic forced eruption with a sulcular fiberotomy may be performed. Orthodontic force is applied to the involved tooth in an occlusal direction, whereas the supracrestal connective tissue fibers are severed with fiberotomies every 4 days. The periodontal ligament fibers dictate alveolar bone formation and position. Therefore severing these fibers as the tooth rapidly erupts out of the socket results in the exposure of sound tooth structure without changing the position of the alveolar crest or free gingival margin. The crown-to-root ratio of the adjacent teeth remains intact, whereas the crown-to-root ratio of the erupted tooth slightly increases, thus improving the long-term periodontal prognosis compared with performing surgical crown lengthening with bone removal.

To effect the desired movement, a stainless steel eyelet (made from 0.036" orthodontic wire) is cemented into the canal of the tooth and an elastic cord is tied to the eyelet. Because these teeth will eventually require a post and core, the post preparation must be thinner than the definitive post size and the eyelet must be retrievable without causing damage to the tooth structure. Conservative removal of the gutta percha to provide only sufficient retention for the eyelet to function and the choice of cement used to secure the eyelet should be based on these requirements.

CLINICAL TIP

Polycarboxylate cements (e.g., Durelon, 3M ESPE) satisfy both of these requirements. This type of cement will also soften in the presence of warmth (cleavability) facilitating its removal; patients can rinse with warm water before removing the eyelet. Newer generation cements (adhesively bonded or self-adhesive resins) should not be used as they would make eyelet removal extremely difficult.

Armamentarium
- Standard dental setup:
  - Explorer
  - Mouth mirror
  - Periodontal probe
  - Low-speed handpiece
- Orthodontic brackets (optional), stainless steel, or clear plastic edgewise brackets (3M Unitek, 3M ESPE)
- 0.036-inch orthodontic wire to fabricate the eyelet (3M Unitek, 3M ESPE)
- 0.20-inch rectangular arch wire
- Polycarboxylate cement (e.g., Durelon, 3M ESPE)
- Medium- or heavy-gauge orthodontic elastic or thread (3M Unitek Corp.)
- No. 15 surgical scalpel
  - Bird beak orthodontic pliers (Hu-Friedy Mfg. Co.)
  - Small diameter Gates Glidden bur (Dentsply Tulsa Dental Specialties)

Clinical Technique
1. Prepare a post preparation in the canal just wide enough to accept the wire eyelet using the Gates Glidden bur in a low speed handpiece to remove the gutta percha from the canal. The preparation should not be as wide or as long as the eventual post preparation for the core build-up but provide just enough retention for the eyelet to be secured.
2. Cement a 0.036-inch wire with an eyelet (made using the orthodontic pliers) into the preparation (see Fig. 14-4A).

CLINICAL TIP

Add a small amount of water to the cement while mixing. This will allow for easier removal of the eyelet without damaging the internal walls of the canal while providing enough retentive strength to apply the eruptive force.

3. When using orthodontic brackets, etch the teeth to be bracketed and apply orthodontic bonding resin to the bracket pad. Place the bracket on the tooth. When using bonded arch wire (without brackets), bond a heavy gauge wire (0.030- to 0.040-inch) across a portion of the facial surface near the incisal edges of the anterior teeth or occlusal surface of the posterior teeth.

CLINICAL TIP

A clear acrylic is the luting material of choice for the incisal wire. Acrylic is strong enough to retain the wire under function and is easier to remove than composite resin.

For posterior amalgam restorations, prepare the occlusal slots as for intracoronal splints (A-splint) and bond the wire in the slots. The arch wire must be positioned directly over the root to be extruded.
4. Adapt a heavy (0.020-inch) rectangular arch wire in the bracket slots and across the root to be erupted and position it directly over the root to be extruded (see Fig. 14-4C,D).
5. Thread a medium or heavy elastic through the eyelet and wrap it around the anchoring wire. Activate the elastic by pulling it taut and tying it (see Fig. 14-4C,D).
6. Perform an initial fiberotomy with a No. 15 scalpel blade (see Fig. 14-4C).
   a. Anesthetize the area.
   b. Run the scalpel circumferentially in the sulcus around the root. This severs the supracrestal connective tissue fiber attachment.
7. Repeat the fiberotomy every 4 days to prevent the connective tissue fibers from reforming and to prevent coronal reformation of the alveolar bone. Generally eruption is accomplished at a rate of 0.5 to 1.0 mm per week. However, movement as slow as 1.0 mm per month may be observed.
8. When the desired eruption is accomplished, stabilize the tooth for 2 to 3 months before fabricating the definitive restoration (see Fig. 14-4).

Clinical Case: Surgical Crown Lengthening

A 42-year-old woman presented with a provisional restoration from the maxillary right canine to the maxillary left canine. Her medical history was noncontributory. Although the restoration was physiologically acceptable, the varied heights of the restored teeth were esthetically unacceptable (Fig. 14-2A). Surgical crown lengthening was performed to correct this situation. A submarginal incision was made at the desired height of the gingival margin (Fig. 14-2B) and a full-thickness flap reflected (Fig. 14-2C). The disparity in the abutment crown length could

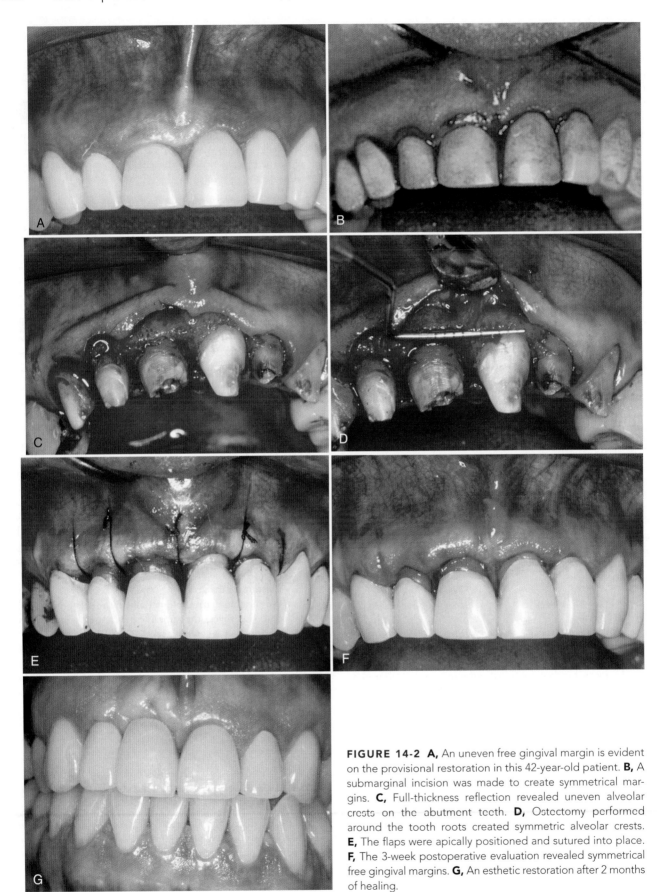

FIGURE 14-2 **A,** An uneven free gingival margin is evident on the provisional restoration in this 42-year-old patient. **B,** A submarginal incision was made to create symmetrical margins. **C,** Full-thickness reflection revealed uneven alveolar crests on the abutment teeth. **D,** Ostectomy performed around the tooth roots created symmetric alveolar crests. **E,** The flaps were apically positioned and sutured into place. **F,** The 3-week postoperative evaluation revealed symmetrical free gingival margins. **G,** An esthetic restoration after 2 months of healing.

be seen after reflection. Following the removal of some supporting bone, a more symmetric appearance was achieved (Fig. 14-2D). The flaps were apically positioned and sutured into place (Fig. 14-2E). This symmetry is reflected by the gingival margins of the definitive restoration (Figs. 14-2F,G).

Clinical Case: Developmental Defect

A 43-year-old female was referred for crown lengthening and presented with asymptomatic subgingival caries on both maxillary central incisors (Fig. 14-3A). Her medical history was noncontributory. A full-thickness flap was reflected using bilateral vertical incisions to avoid involvement of the adjacent papilla. The gingival margin discrepancies at the mesial line angles of the central incisors were corrected using a slight submarginal incision (Fig. 14-3B).

Minor ostectomy was performed to expose the lesions (Fig. 14-3C). However, after some removal of bone, developmental defects (pronounced grooves in the dentin at the mesiofacial line angles) were noted on the root surfaces of both incisors extending apically. The caries at the cementoenamel junction of both teeth was apparently a result of the defects.

Since the root/bone interface on the direct facial aspect of both teeth was healthy and intact, a direct restoration of the lesions was performed. A self-etching primer (Transbond Plus Self Etching Primer, 3M Unitek) was applied (preferable in areas more difficult to isolate) and a hybrid ionomer composite resin (Geristore dual-cure, hydrophilic Bis-GMA, DenMat) was used to restore the cavity and defects (Figs. 14-3D,E). The self-etch primer was chosen for its ease of application and its ability to be used in wet conditions; isolation and moisture control in a surgical field can be difficult to achieve. The restorative material was chosen because of its ability to adhere to enamel, dentin, and cementum and its biocompatibility in a subgingival environment. The restoration was contoured to create a featheredged margin apically (Fig. 14-3F). Approximately 2 mm of apical root surface was not restored to preserve the biological width and allow for proper gingival healing. The flap was repositioned and secured with a small diameter resorbable suture (Fig. 14-3G). A small diameter non-resorbable suture could also have been used in this situation (5° Vicrylm Ethicon, Inc., or 4° Cytoplast, Osteogenics Biomedical, Inc.) with the choice being based on the preference of the surgeon as well as the desires of the patient (avoiding suture removal, if possible).

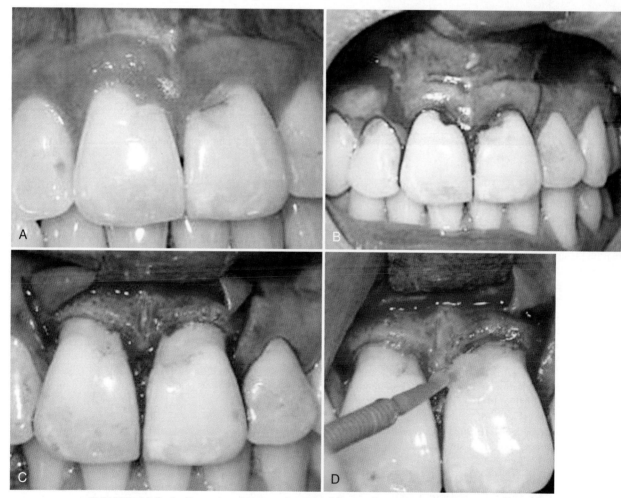

FIGURE 14-3 A, Decay is evident at the mesial line angles of both maxillary central incisors. **B,** The incision design avoids the papillae between the central and lateral incisors and corrects the free gingival margin (FGM) architecture. **C,** Developmental root deformities seen after crown lengthening. **D,** Self-etching primer is applied to the cavity preparations and root surfaces.

Continued

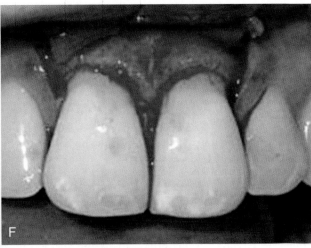

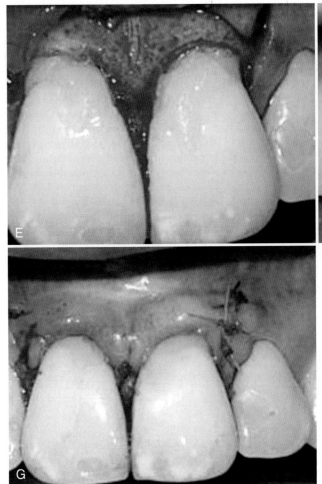

FIGURE 14-3, cont'd E, The composite resin is placed just short of the facial crest of bone. **F,** The material is contoured and featheredged apically. **G,** The flap is replaced and sutured. Note the correction of the free gingival margin profile as a result of the submarginal incision design.

Clinical Case: Forced Eruption with Fiberotomy

A 57-year-old man presented with a maxillary right lateral incisor root that had fractured at the gingival margin as a result of cervical caries. His medical history was noncontributory. The patient desired a tooth replacement but did not wish to have the root extracted. A post preparation was made in the root, and a 0.036-inch wire with an eyelet was cemented into the preparation with polycarboxylate cement. A 0.040-inch orthodontic wire was bonded to the incisal edges of the canine and central incisor over the root to be erupted. This device was then engaged to the arch wire using a heavy elastic tie (Fig. 14-4A,B). A sulcular fiberotomy was performed at the time of activation and every 4 days throughout the time of tooth movement (Fig. 14-4C). The desired eruption was achieved within 3 weeks (Fig. 14-4D,E), at which time a cast post and core was fabricated (Fig. 14-4F) and a provisional restoration was made. This technique produced an excellent esthetic result (Fig. 14-4G).

Clinical Case: Forced Eruption with Surgical Crown Lengthening

A 23-year-old man presented with subgingival caries on his mandibular right second premolar (Fig. 14-5A). His medical history was noncontributory. After caries removal and endodontic therapy

a 0.036-inch orthodontic wire was formed into a loop and cemented into the post preparation (Fig. 14-5B). A straight 0.040-inch orthodontic wire was bonded from the mandibular right first premolar to an occlusal slot prepared in the amalgam of the mandibular right first molar. An elastic thread was used to pull the tooth occlusally (Fig. 14-5C).

Because the patient could come to the office only twice a month, repeated fiberotomy was not possible. As a result, the gingival margin and the underlying attachment moved coronally with the root (Fig. 14-5D). After adequate eruption, apical positioning of the tissues was performed (Fig. 14-5E,F), resulting in adequate tooth structure and an even gingival margin (Fig. 14-5G). Surgery without eruption would have resulted in an uneven gingival margin.

RECESSION

Gingival recession is defined by the American Academy of Periodontology as occurring when the level of the free gingival margin is apical to the cementoenamel junction. Exposure of the root surfaces occurs because there is a loss or lack of facial bone on the tooth root with concomitant apical migration of the soft tissue margin. Different factors may cause recession and the underlying etiology should be identified before determining a course of treatment.

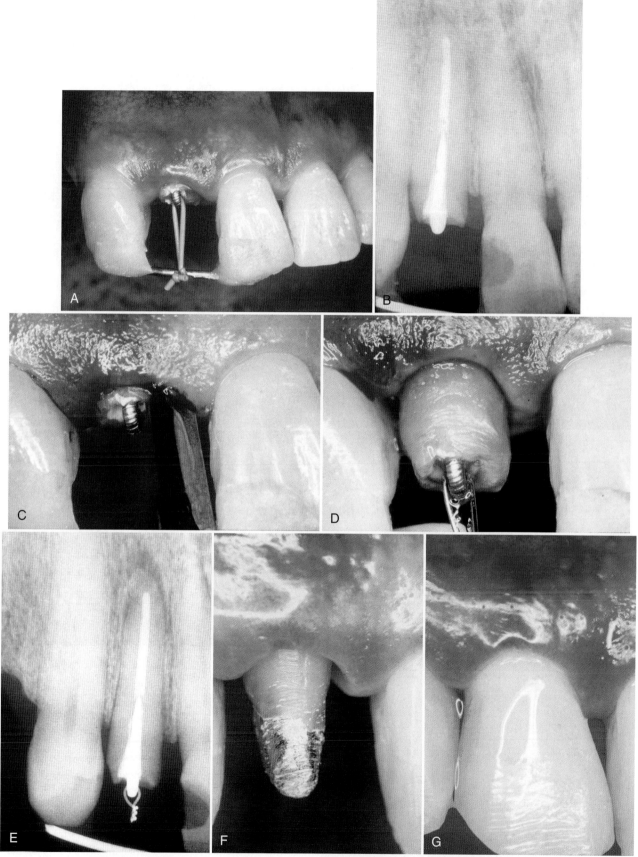

FIGURE 14-4 A, A retained lateral incisor root. **B,** Pre-eruption radiograph of the patient. **C,** A sulcular fiberotomy was performed every 4 days. The elastic tie is removed to provide access for the scalpel blade. **D,** Rapid eruption for 3 weeks exposed adequate root structure. **E,** Postoperative radiograph. **F,** A post and core were fabricated. **G,** An esthetic definitive restoration was placed.

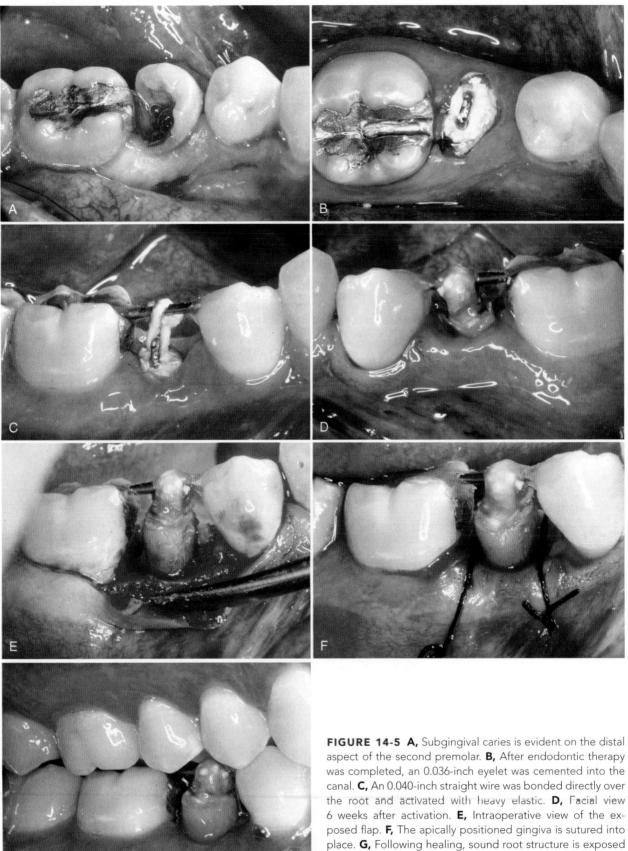

FIGURE 14-5 A, Subgingival caries is evident on the distal aspect of the second premolar. **B,** After endodontic therapy was completed, an 0.036-inch eyelet was cemented into the canal. **C,** An 0.040-inch straight wire was bonded directly over the root and activated with heavy elastic. **D,** Facial view 6 weeks after activation. **E,** Intraoperative view of the exposed flap. **F,** The apically positioned gingiva is sutured into place. **G,** Following healing, sound root structure is exposed while the free gingival margin is restored to a more esthetic level.

Differential Etiology

1. Mechanical factors
   a. The most common mechanical factor is tooth brush abrasion. Overzealous brushing (even with a soft nylon toothbrush) is the predominant cause of mechanically abraded gingiva on a healthy dentogingival complex. The self-diagnosis of "receding gums" is usually made by a patient before presenting to the practitioner. The esthetic imbalance, particularly in the anterior sextants, is a common patient concern.
   b. Intraoral trauma can result in severe defects, depending on the nature of the injury.
   c. Less-frequent mechanical causes of recession include the use of an abrasive dentifrice, iatrogenic flossing, improper use of electric rotary toothbrushes at the highest setting, and intraoral foreign object habits.
2. Inflammatory factors
   a. Periodontal disease and acute periodontal abscesses often destroy buccal attachment, resulting in recession.
   b. Poor oral hygiene also plays a role in recession. Besides leading to inflammatory periodontal breakdown, the progressive accumulation of calcified deposits on the facial surfaces of teeth can directly lead to tissue loss.
   c. Restorations with overhanging or open margins can cause attachment loss and subsequent recession.
   d. Subgingival caries can often result in crestal bone resorption with concomitant recession.
3. Anatomic factors
   a. The presence of high frenal attachments, muscle pulls, a thin periodontium, root prominence, and/or scarring can cause apical migration of the free gingival margin.
   b. Tooth position issues, such as crowding, flaring or severe rotation can also play a role in recession.

Two additional parameters that must be assessed when recession involves the mucogingival junction are the zone of keratinized tissue and the amount of attached gingiva. These two terms are often incorrectly considered synonymous. The zone of gingiva on a tooth is the measurement from the free gingival margin to the mucogingival junction. This describes the amount of keratinized tissue present (alternatively termed *masticatory mucosa*) and is a measure of the amount of gingiva present. An inadequate zone of gingiva or a complete lack of gingiva occurs when there is insufficient or no keratinized tissue present, regardless of whether or not this gingival is attached to the underlying bone and root structure. This situation can contribute to potential recession as described previously.

Attached *gingiva* refers to the amount of the keratinized tissue that is bound down to the underlying bone and root structure. This measurement is arrived at by subtracting the probe depth reading from the amount of keratinized tissue present. For example, a site that has a 5-mm zone of keratinized tissue with a 3-mm probe reading would have 2 mm of attached gingiva. When probing extends beyond the mucogingival junction into the alveolar mucosa, the diagnosis is mucogingival involvement with a lack of attached gingiva. This can occur regardless of the amount of keratinized tissue present.

Once all the parameters are recorded, a diagnosis can be determined. When both conditions exist, the diagnosis is insufficiency of the gingiva and a lack of attached gingiva. However, if an adequate zone of keratinized tissue is present with mucogingival involvement, then the diagnosis would only be a lack of attached gingiva. Although the difference between the two may seem subtle, it plays a role in determining appropriate treatment options.

CLINICAL TIP

An accurate assessment of the patient's mucogingival status must be performed on a healthy dentogingival complex. The tip of the periodontal probe will extend into the gingival connective tissue beyond the junctional epithelium (beyond the mucogingival junction) in the presence of inflammation; this will result in a false indication of the true mucogingival status. Treatment of inflammation (e.g., scaling, root planning, periodontal maintenance, oral hygiene) should be performed, as needed, to restore the integrity of these tissues before the MG assessment or beginning any mucogingival procedures.

Before deciding on what treatment option would be best used in any particular situation, it is important to identify the goal of the procedure. This is best arrived upon through a combination of thorough examination and detailed patient interview. Assessment of the physiologic needs of the situation coupled with the esthetic expectations of the patient gives us the best chance for a successful outcome.

Treatment Options

Three different grafting procedures are discussed for mucogingival reconstruction and esthetic correction: free gingival, lateral pedicle, and connective tissue.

Free Gingival Grafts. Free gingival grafting (FGG) techniques have been used for more than four decades for augmenting the zone of keratinized tissue as well as for root coverage. This technique is highly predictable for the former, but success in covering exposed root surfaces is less predictable and dependent on several factors:
1. The dimension of the root surface to be covered
2. The lateral probing depth
3. The position of the tooth in the arch

Grafts receive their primary nutrient supply from the underlying connective tissue and periosteum of the recipient site, and donor tissue placed over the avascular root surface is fed solely by lateral circulation from the connective tissue bed. Because lateral circulation can maintain the viability of the donor tissue for only a limited distance, areas of narrow recession have better root coverage potential than deeper, wider areas of recession. Some areas that appear to be narrow actually have significant lateral probing depths and therefore have poorer root coverage potential than truly narrow areas.

CLINICAL TIP

Good results are obtained with widths of less than 2 mm and poor results with widths greater than 4 to 5 mm.

In addition, teeth that are prominent in the arch may have little or no buccal bone present, with an underlying dehiscence presenting a major problem. Multiple procedures may be required for optimal results in these situations; however, performing multiple procedures does not guarantee total root coverage. In situations of very wide and deep recession, the purpose of multiple procedures is to achieve as much root coverage as possible. Tooth position and lateral bone support are two factors that could adversely affect the percentage of root coverage achieved.

Free gingival grafting involves three steps:
1. Preparing the recipient site
2. Harvesting the donor tissue
3. Placing the graft

A well-vascularized connective tissue bed must be prepared around the graft site. If the goal is to only augment the zone of keratinized tissue, an incision is made at the mucogingival junction allowing for a partial thickness dissection apically to prepare the recipient bed. This will maintain the existing free gingival margin, preventing possible postsurgical recession and providing a secure coronal border to affix the graft. However, if root coverage is desired, the surface epithelium also needs to be removed peripherally around the area of recession to create a connective tissue bed over which the graft is placed. Laterally the recipient site should extend a distance of at least the width of the area of root to be covered. Apical dissection should be at least 4 to 5 mm. Coronally the existing gingiva must be denuded to a level of the CEJ, minimally. This will provide an adequate blood supply for the donor tissue. If a frenum is present, it is dissected and repositioned at the apical border of the graft bed.

Donor tissue is harvested from the palate. The anterior rugae must not be included in the graft, because they will be visible at the recipient site. A 1- to 2-mm zone of marginal gingiva should be maintained at the donor site to prevent recession. The graft must include the surface epithelium and at least 1.5 mm of underlying connective tissue. A surgical guide should be made for the recipient site and transferred to the palate, thus minimizing and customizing the amount of tissue removed. Once the graft is harvested, a hemostatic dressing is placed in the donor site and a clear acrylic surgical guide is inserted. The surgical guide applies constant pressure for hemostasis and covers the raw palatal tissue during healing to increase patient comfort. The donor tissue is sutured firmly to the recipient bed. Surgical dressing is applied to protect the recipient site. Postoperatively a chlorhexidine rinse may be used for 3 to 4 weeks until proper oral hygiene can be performed without damaging the grafted site. A minimum of 6 weeks of healing is required before resuming or beginning any prosthetic work.

Lateral Pedicle Grafts

Several factors must be considered when a pedicle graft is contemplated:
1. The amount of keratinized tissue adjacent to the recipient site
2. The existence of an adjacent edentulous ridge
3. The existence of frena that could cause excessive pull
4. The width of the recipient root surface
5. The proximity of the apical extent of the defect to the vestibule

When using lateral pedicle grafts, a well-keratinized edentulous ridge or a wide zone of keratinized tissue adjacent to the graft site is ideal. However, if the recipient area to be grafted is wide mesiodistally, excessive pull may occur on the donor tissue, causing strangulation and eventual failure. Bed preparation for lateral grafts is slightly different than for the free graft technique. The recipient site adjacent to the donor site is prepared by creating a 2- to 3-mm band of epithelial denudation. A partial thickness flap of the donor site is elevated into the alveolar mucosa and a single vertical incision is made to release the tension of the flap, allowing for lateral positioning. The primary difference between this procedure and the free gingival graft is that the lateral graft remains attached at its base, which provides additional blood supply. If necessary, a small oblique releasing incision in the alveolar mucosa will eliminate tension of the donor tissue when moved laterally. The flap must be wide enough to cover the root and prepared bed. The graft is then positioned over the root and sutured. The donor area heals by granulation formation.

With the double papilla procedure, a variation of the lateral pedicle procedure, both adjacent papilla are split-thickness dissected and make up the pedicle. Again, the donor site heals by granulation formation. As was the case with free gingival grafts, surgical dressing is placed over the surgical site, although no surgical guide is needed because no palatal tissue is involved. Postoperative care is similar for pedicle graft procedures. A minimum of 6 weeks of healing is needed before prosthetic work can begin.

Subepithelial Connective Tissue Graft. Subepithelial connective tissue grafting (SECT) is indicated when multiple teeth require grafting, although it can also be used for single tooth sites. Similar to a pedicle graft, a partial thickness flap is performed beyond the mucogingival junction overlying the area with placement of a strip of connective tissue (without any surface epithelium) harvested from the palate and placed between the flap and the underlying bed.

The recipient site is prepared using a sulcular incision design with a split-thickness dissection beyond the mucogingival junction; this allows for retention of the epithelium in the flap as well as providing adequate mobility to allow the flap to be advanced coronally. The lateral extension of the flap must be at least one tooth length in either direction to provide for tension-free suturing. An envelope procedure is performed on the palate to obtain the connective tissue. Two parallel horizontal incisions (the length of the site to be grafted) are made 2 to 3 mm apart near the palatal free gingival margin. Sharp dissection is performed vertically in the connective tissue to remove a strip of tissue similar in dimension to the graft site (both in height and width). A hemostatic material (e.g., Collagen Foam, Ace Surgical Supply Co., Inc.) can be placed into the donor site and sutured on the surface.

The harvested donor tissue is a "slab" of connective tissue with the 2- to 3-mm band of epithelium at one edge. The epithelial band is then removed and the strip of connective tissue placed over the exposed root surfaces with the flap positioned over the donor tissue and sutured firmly. Because the initial dissection was performed beyond the mucogingival junction, the flap can be positioned coronally without tension to cover the root surfaces.

Advantages to this type of procedure include no denuded palatal donor site, increased patient comfort during healing, and the double blood supply to the free connective tissue, which is fed by the underlying periosteum and the connective tissue of the flap. Achieving tension-free repositioning of the tissue is necessary to prevent retraction of the flaps and avoid compromising the blood supply. In addition, the connective tissue contains the genetic information that dictates the type of epithelium that will form. Thus areas of the donor tissue that are not completely covered by the flap will form keratinized tissue, thus aiding in healing and providing a much better blend of donor and recipient tissues.

Exogenous or Engineered Donor Tissue

An alternative to an autograft is the use of human connective tissue (AlloDerm Regenerative Tissue Matrix, LifeCell Corp.) or dermal matrices (DynaMatrix and DynaMatrix Plus Extracellular Membrane, Keystone Dental, Inc.). These materials act as a scaffold to support soft tissue regeneration and become integrated into the body's own tissues, unlike typical resorbable membranes that simply act as a barrier (as would be used in guided tissue regeneration). They can be used for the free graft technique; however they are most often used with connective tissue grafting.

Besides the obvious advantage of avoiding a second surgical donor site, the size of the graft is not limited by the size and nature of the palate (thinner and flatter palates limit the amount of connective tissue that can be harvested). Therefore larger areas or multiple sites can be treated at one time. The uniform thickness of these grafts and their ability to be sutured (essential for any type of gingival graft) can provide better surgical handling intraoperatively than autografts.

Regenerative Proteins. Application of certain regenerative proteins can aid in the formation of connective tissue attachment to the root surface. Enamel matrix derivative (Straumann Emdogain, Straumann USA LLC) is an extract of porcine fetal tooth material that can stimulate both soft and hard tissue growth. The material is applied to the denuded root surface and promotes healing via a connective tissue fiber attachment. These materials can be used in conjunction with a graft procedure (FGG or SECT) or with coronal positioning of a flap to cover the roots (if an adequate zone of keratinized tissue already exists).

Prosthetic Gingiva. When interdental spaces are a concern and no cosmetic prosthetic work is anticipated, artificial gingiva is an option. A border molded impression is made of the involved area. The laboratory fabricates a gingival veneer of pink denture acrylic, with the apical extent in the mucobuccal fold and the coronal extent restoring a normal free gingival margin appearance. Disadvantages to using this procedure include inaccurate color matching and instability of the prosthesis. Before embarking on this course of treatment, the patient should see pictures of inserted prostheses and understand their limitations. Only then should fabrication of artificial gingiva begin.

FREE GINGIVAL GRAFT PROCEDURE

Clinical Case: Correction of an Isolated Area of Recession Resulting from Trauma

A 24-year-old man presented with an isolated area of severe recession on the mandibular left central incisor resulting from a traumatic blow sustained during a basketball game. The tooth was monitored for 2 months after the traumatic injury to ensure no additional problems occurred. Ten weeks after the incident, tooth #24 presented with minimal clinical mobility and a vital pulp as determined by electric pulp test and cold tests.

Clinical examination revealed isolated 5-mm facial recession with lateral and apical probing depths of 3 to 4 mm (Fig. 14-6A). His past medical history was unremarkable.

Although loss of the overlying alveolus occurred on tooth #24, none of the adjacent teeth were affected, as demonstrated by minimal clinical probing depth (2-3 mm), lack of clinical mobility, and no radiographic evidence of bone loss. The planned procedure was to place a free gingival graft in conjunction with treating the area with Emdogain regenerative material.

A trapezoidal connective tissue bed was prepared maintaining the gingival tissue attachment on the adjacent incisors (Fig. 14-6B).

The coronal root surface and cementoenamel junction were etched with a 35% phosphoric acid gel for 15 seconds (Fig. 14-6C) and rinsed thoroughly without drying. Emdogain regenerative material was then placed over the root and connective tissue bed (Fig. 14-6D), and the graft sutured intimately with resorbable sutures (Fig. 14-6E). After 1 week, it appeared as if the donor tissue overlying the dehisced root surface had sloughed; however, the tissue was stable and nonretractable (Fig. 14-6F).

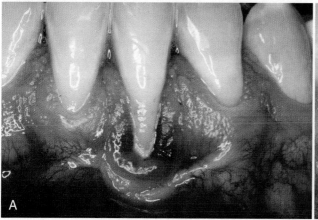
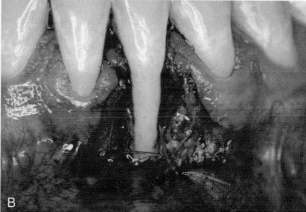

FIGURE 14-6 A, A 24-year-old man with a severe dehiscence on the facial aspect of tooth #24 resulting from a traumatic blow to the site. **B,** Preparation of the connective tissue bed for a free graft revealed 8 mm of exposed root surface with some loss of lateral alveolar bone.

Continued

FIGURE 14-6, cont'd C, The cementoenamel junction and root surface are etched with 35% phosphoric acid for 15 seconds. **D,** Emdogain regenerative material is applied to the root surface and alveolar defect. **E,** The free graft is sutured with 5-0 resorbable sutures. **F,** After 1 week the graft is well attached to the root surface despite its appearance. **G,** Two weeks after surgery. **H,** Root coverage 4 weeks after surgery.

At the 2-week postoperative visit, the graft surface had begun to mature (Fig. 14-6G), with excellent results seen 4 weeks after surgery (Fig. 14-6H).

Clinical Case: Correction of Recession

A 38-year-old woman presented with generalized facial recession in both arches. Her past medical history was noncontributory. The defects on the maxillary central incisors were an esthetic concern because of a high smile line. The clinical examination revealed 2 to 3 mm of facial recession on both central incisors with a 5-mm zone of keratinized tissue on both teeth (Fig. 14-7A). Gingival augmentation was unnecessary and a coronally positioned flap procedure was planned. Before flap elevation, the cementoenamel junction and exposed root dentin were etched for 15 seconds with a 35% phosphoric acid gel (Fig. 14-7B) and rinsed thoroughly. A full-thickness mucoperiosteal flap was elevated on the facial aspect of the four incisors (Fig. 14-7C) to the level of the mucogingival junction with partial thickness dissection approximately 2 to 3 mm beyond the MGJ. This type of flap design releases the tension of

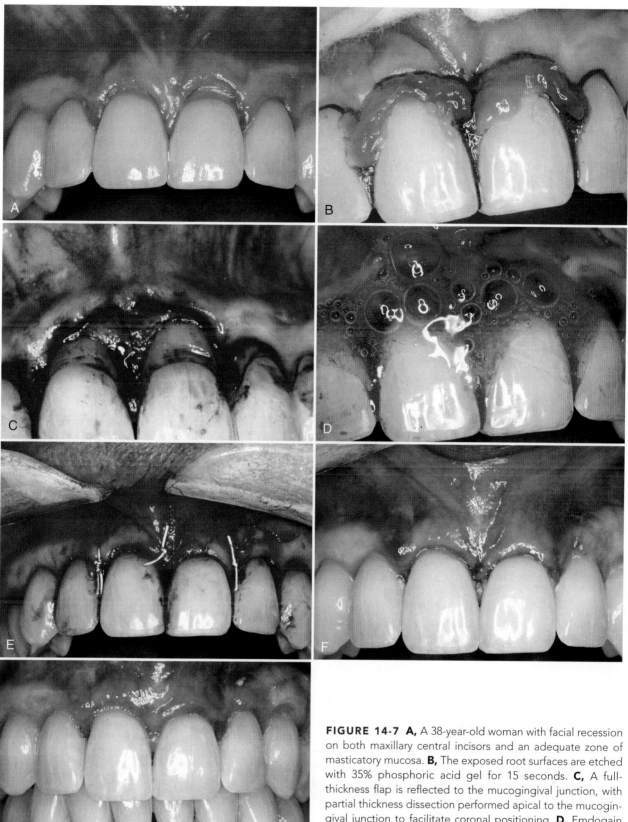

FIGURE 14-7 A, A 38-year-old woman with facial recession on both maxillary central incisors and an adequate zone of masticatory mucosa. **B,** The exposed root surfaces are etched with 35% phosphoric acid gel for 15 seconds. **C,** A full-thickness flap is reflected to the mucogingival junction, with partial thickness dissection performed apical to the mucogingival junction to facilitate coronal positioning. **D,** Emdogain regenerative material is placed over the etched root surfaces. **E,** The flap is coronally positioned to the level of the cementoenamel junction. **F,** Two weeks after surgery. **G,** Four weeks after surgery.

the periosteum (which is tightly adherent to the facial plate of bone) and provides freedom of movement of the flap (provided by the elastic alveolar mucosal connective tissue), thus facilitating coronal advancement of the flap.

The site was treated with Emdogain regenerative material (Fig. 14-7D) and the flap sutured in a coronal position to cover the exposed root surfaces (Fig. 14-7E). The sutures were removed after 2 weeks (Fig. 14-7F). Correction of the defect is seen four weeks after surgery (Fig. 14-7G).

SUBEPITHELIAL CONNECTIVE TISSUE (SECT) GRAFT

Clinical Case: SECT Graft with Coronal Positioning of the Resulting Augmented Gingiva

A 36-year-old woman presented with generalized facial recession in both arches. Her past medical history was unremarkable. The maxillary right second premolar through the maxillary right later incisor, canine, and lateral incisor demonstrated 3 to 5 mm of exposed root surface and probing depth, which extended beyond the mucogingival junction. A minimal band of keratinized tissue was present (mucogingival insufficiency) and there was a lack of attached gingiva (Fig. 14-8A).

A subepithelial connective tissue graft was planned to correct the recession and augment the current zone of gingiva because of the high lip line. Using this technique instead of a free graft would provide better tissue color blending at the site. The exposed root surfaces were etched with 35% phosphoric acid for 15 seconds (Fig. 14-8B), a facial flap elevated, and a subepithelial connective tissue graft placed (Fig. 14-8C,D).

Three months after the procedure, a satisfactory esthetic result was obtained with respect to the gingival augmentation aspect of the procedure, with the increased zone of gingival tissue exhibiting an excellent color match. However, there was some residual recession that remained (Fig. 14-8E).

In an attempt to achieve more root coverage, a coronally positioned, split-thickness flap procedure was performed as a second procedure (Fig. 14-8F,G), resulting in the desired root coverage (Fig. 14-8H), as seen at the end of the first week.

Clinical Case: Correction of Gingival Recession Using Extracellular Dermal Membrane

A 54-year-old woman presented with recession on her maxillary left canine resulting from tooth brush trauma (Fig 14-9A). Her past medical history was noncontributory. The defect noted on the facial aspect of the maxillary left canine resulted from

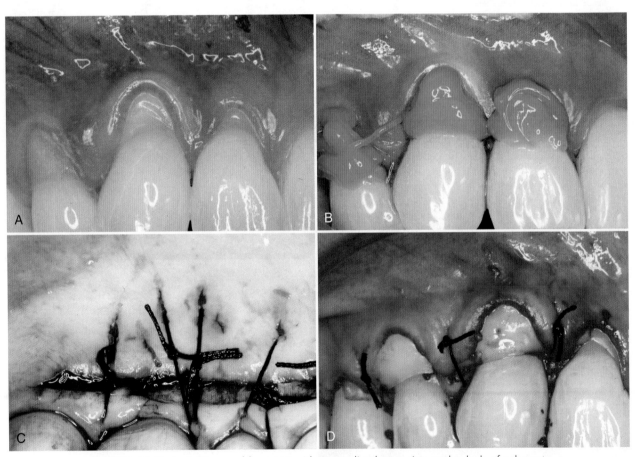

FIGURE 14-8 A, A 36-year-old woman with generalized recession and a lack of adequate masticatory mucosa. **B,** The exposed root surfaces are etched with a 35% phosphoric acid gel for 15 seconds. **C,** A subepithelial connective tissue graft is harvested from the palate. **D,** The connective tissue graft is placed under the full-thickness facial flap and sutured securely.

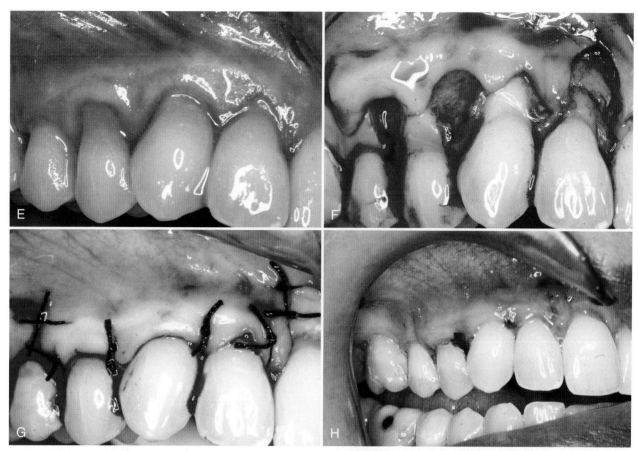

FIGURE 14-8, cont'd E, Reconstruction of the facial gingiva has been achieved with excellent tissue color. **F,** A full-thickness flap is elevated and the periosteum scored apical to the mucogingival junction. **G,** The flap is coronally positioned to cover the exposed root surfaces. **H,** Correction of the recession is seen at the 1-week postsurgical visit

"hitting" the tissue with the hard end of her toothbrush. The defect was isolated to the canine and although there was an adequate zone of keratinized tissue on the canine and the adjacent teeth, a narrower zone was observed on the canine itself. Correction was planned using a combination of a coronally positioned flap and connective tissue graft technique. With the height of the recession and disparity in the zone of gingiva, coronal positioning alone could not correct all aspects of the clinical situation; a graft was necessary. Because of her desire to avoid a second surgical site and a limited ability for postoperative

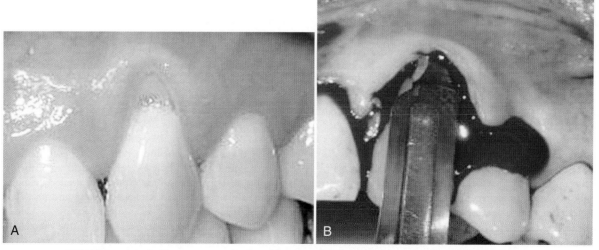

FIGURE 14-9 A, Recession on the facial aspect of the maxillary right canine. **B,** Partial thickness dissection is performed to mobilize the flap.

Continued

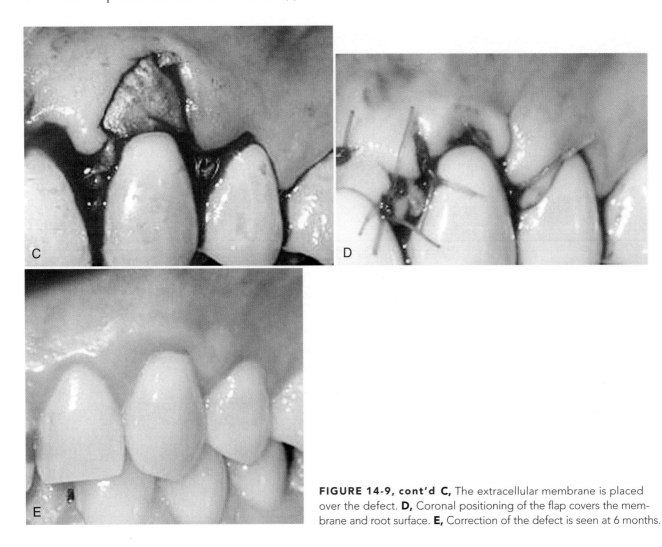

FIGURE 14-9, cont'd C, The extracellular membrane is placed over the defect. **D,** Coronal positioning of the flap covers the membrane and root surface. **E,** Correction of the defect is seen at 6 months.

visits, DynaMatrix (Keystone Dental, Inc.) extracellular membrane was used for the donor tissue.

A partial thickness flap was performed beyond the MGJ of the canine and two adjacent teeth (Fig. 14-9B) to mobilize the flap and facilitate coronal positioning. Because the flap was to be coronally advanced, the measurement between the newly positioned free gingival margin on the facial aspect of the tooth and the peak of the papillae would be reduced. To create the desired gingival architecture, the incision followed the free margin on the tissue adjacent to the direct facial aspects of the teeth, but was placed apical to the peak of the papillae (submarginal) interproximally. This reduced the distance from the height of the papilla to the mid-root FGM of the flap allowing for more esthetic coronal positioning. Any remaining surface epithelium on the papillae was removed to provide the connective tissue bed to which the margins of the graft and flap were sutured. A DynaMatrix membrane was chosen as the allopathic donor because its thinness allowed for optimal coronal positioning and primary closure (less bulk of tissue under the flap). The material was placed between the flap and the canine and the flap sutured coronally at the CEJ (Fig. 14-9C,D).

Restoration of a normal mucogingival complex is seen 6 months postoperatively (Fig. 14-9E).

Clinical Case: Correction of Recession and Mucogingival Reconstruction Using an Extracellular Membrane

A 58-year-old male patient presented with long-standing facial recession with more recent onset of dentinal sensitivity (Fig. 14-10A). Because of the narrow zone of keratinized tissue, the surgical plan involved a combined approach of connective tissue grafting with a coronally positioned flap. DynaMatrix Plus (Keystone Dental, Inc.) extracellular membrane was used as the donor tissue, thus eliminating the large second surgical site, which would have been necessary to harvest the connective tissue needed for the graft.

Partial thickness dissection was performed beyond the mucogingival junction in the surgical site making sure to release any tension on the flap (Fig. 14-10B).

The remaining epithelium on the facial papillae of the surgical site is removed to allow for coronal suturing of the flap. The membrane is trimmed to the dimension needed, hydrated with sterile saline then placed between the flap and underlying bed (Fig. 14-10C-E).

Because of the large area being treated, the membrane is secured to the flap using a 5-degree sling suture (Fig. 14-10F) then the entire complex is sutured in a coronal position (Fig. 14-10G).

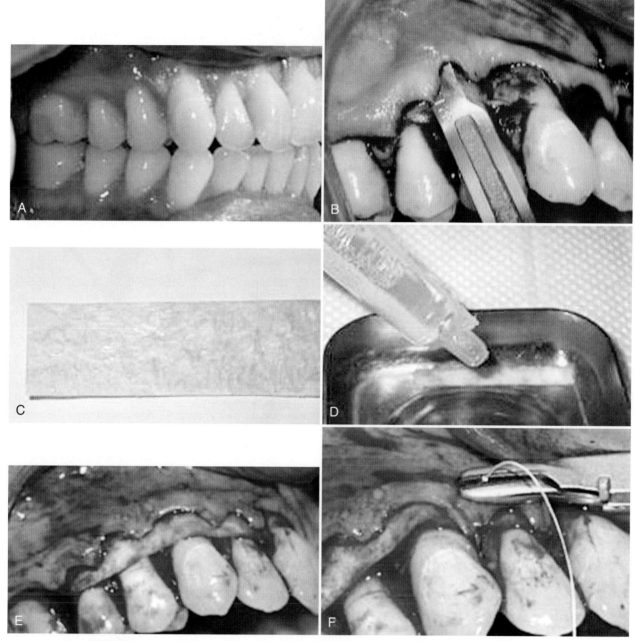

FIGURE 14-10 A, Generalized recession is noted with a narrow zone of masticatory mucosa. **B,** A partial thickness flap is raised in the surgical field. **C,** The extracellular membrane is cut to size. **D,** Hydration of the membrane is done using sterile saline before placement. **E,** The membrane is placed subgingivally over the root surfaces. **F,** The flap is sutured to the underlying membrane with sling sutures to prevent movement.

Continued

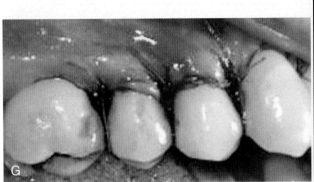
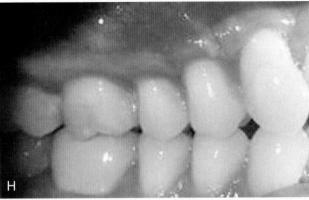

FIGURE 14-10, cont'd G, The entire complex is sutured in a coronal position. **H,** An increase in attached gingiva and root coverage is seen at 18 months.

An increase in the zone of keratinized tissue and reduction in root exposure is seen at the 18-month postoperative visit (Fig. 14-10H).

ESTHETIC MANAGEMENT OF THE COMBINED LESION

Clinical Case: Treatment of External Cervical Root Resorption and Altered Passive Eruption (APE) with Apically Positioned Flap and Surgical Crown Lengthening

A 26-year-old female patient presented with external cervical root resorption on her maxillary right lateral incisor. The clinical examination revealed inflammation of the facial gingiva of tooth #7 with associated bleeding and 5 to 6 mm pocketing. The gingival tissues on the adjacent teeth were within normal limits (Fig. 14-11A). Additionally, the free gingival margins on the maxillary lateral incisor and both central incisors were in a coronal position consistent with altered passive eruption.

The planned surgical procedure was to apically position the facial gingiva and expose the resorptive lesion. The patient's medical history was unremarkable. An internally beveled incision was made in the facial gingiva of teeth #6 through #9, with submarginal placement on teeth #7 through #9 to coincide with the desired marginal position (Fig. 14-11B).

After reflection of the flap, the osseous crest was seen to have a normal relationship with the cementoenamel junction of the involved teeth. A large, ovoid resorptive lesion was seen on the mesiofacial aspect of tooth #7, extending beyond the cementoenamel junction and violating the pulp chamber (Fig. 14-11C).

After degranulation of the surgical site and removal of the resorptive tissue, it was determined that crown lengthening via osteotomy was necessary on the mesial line angle of tooth #7 because of violation of the biologic width (Fig. 14-11D). Crestal bone was removed to expose 3 mm of uninvolved root surface (Fig. 14-11E), and the facial flap was sutured apically (Fig. 14-11F). A composite resin restoration was then placed to seal the resorptive lesion (Fig. 14-11G).

Endodontic treatment was completed on the tooth after initial soft tissue healing (10 days) and an excellent result was noted 1 month after surgery (Fig. 14-11H).

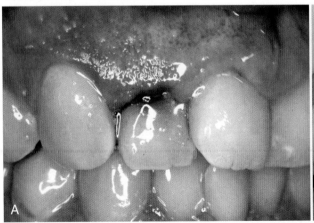
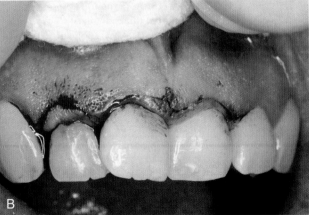

FIGURE 14-11 A, A 26-year-old woman presented with altered passive eruption and external cervical root resorption. **B,** Submarginal incisions have been placed to facilitate apical positioning of the flap.

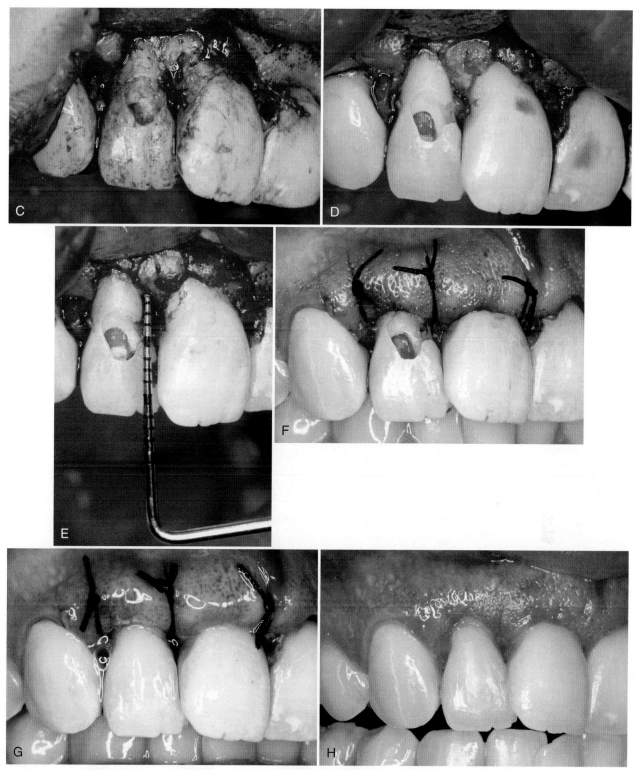

FIGURE 14-11, cont'd C, Full-thickness flap elevation revealed a large resorptive lesion on the mesial aspect of #7 with a normal osseous crest on tooth #6 through tooth #9. **D,** After thorough debridement, violation of the biologic width was seen on the mesial of tooth #7. **E,** The site after ostectomy to expose adequate root structure for the restoration. **F,** Apical positioning of the flap corrected the APE and exposed the resorptive lesion. **G,** A composite resin restoration was placed after suturing of the flap. **H,** Four weeks after surgery.

Clinical Case: The Use of Guided Tissue Regeneration in Enhancing Anterior Esthetics

An 18-year-old woman presented with the chief complaint that the facial recession on her maxillary left central incisor had worsened over the past years. She requested something be done to stabilize the tooth and improve the esthetics.

A review of her past dental history revealed treatment for tooth #9. At age 9, she had a retained tooth #F removed along with a buccally positioned supernumerary incisor apical to #F, as well as exposure of tooth #9, which was horizontally impacted under the anterior nasal spine. Upon completion of orthodontic treatment, #9 was positioned well in the arch. However, because of the loss of adjacent bone (from the extractions and crown exposure) and original position of the tooth high in the facial mucobuccal fold, tooth #9 had no attached gingiva and a wide zone of facial recession extending beyond the facial line angles (Fig. 14-12A).

A free gingival graft was successfully placed to augment the zone of gingiva at age 14, although the esthetics remained unacceptable (Fig. 14-12B). The area remained unchanged until the recent onset of progressive recession and mobility.

The clinical examination at the time of treatment revealed 3 to 5 mm facial probing depth with bleeding upon probing and the detection of subgingival root calculus. Facial recession of 5 mm extended beyond both facial line angles (Fig. 14-12C). Elevation of a full-thickness mucoperiosteal flap was performed in anticipation of coronal positioning; however, complete circumferential bone loss was noted extending apically to the mid-palatal portion of the root (Fig. 14-12D). A decalcified, freeze-dried bone allograft was placed into the defect (Fig. 14-12E) and a wide Gore-Tex membrane affixed around the tooth (Fig. 14-12F) in an attempt to regenerate the lost alveolar bone and provide the needed support for a coronally positioned flap. Vertical releasing incisions were placed laterally, the periosteum scored apical to the mucogingival junction, and the facial gingiva repositioned as coronally as possible (Fig. 14-12G,H). The membrane was removed 3½ months later, revealing a dense connective tissue fill of the entire palatal defect and along the lateral root surface (Fig. 14-12I).

The regenerated tissue provided the needed support and nourishment for the coronally positioned flap to heal and be maintained long term (Fig. 14-12J). Evaluation of the pretreatment and 3-year post treatment radiographs demonstrated excellent, sustained fill of the defect on tooth #8 (Fig. 14-12K,L).

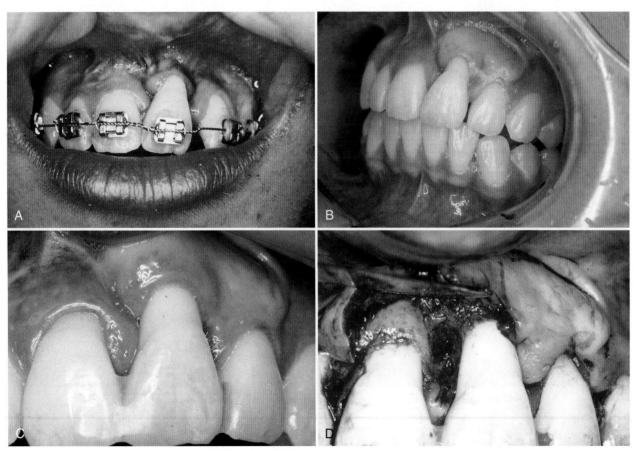

FIGURE 14-12 **A,** A 13-year-old patient before completion of orthodontic therapy. **B,** A free gingival graft was placed apically on tooth #9 to reconstruct the masticatory mucosa; however, no root coverage was achieved. **C,** After 5 years, the patient presented with progressing recession and mobility on tooth #9, with a desire to treat the area functionally and esthetically. **D,** Elevation of a full-thickness flap revealed a 7- to 8-mm alveolar defect involving the entire circumference of the root.

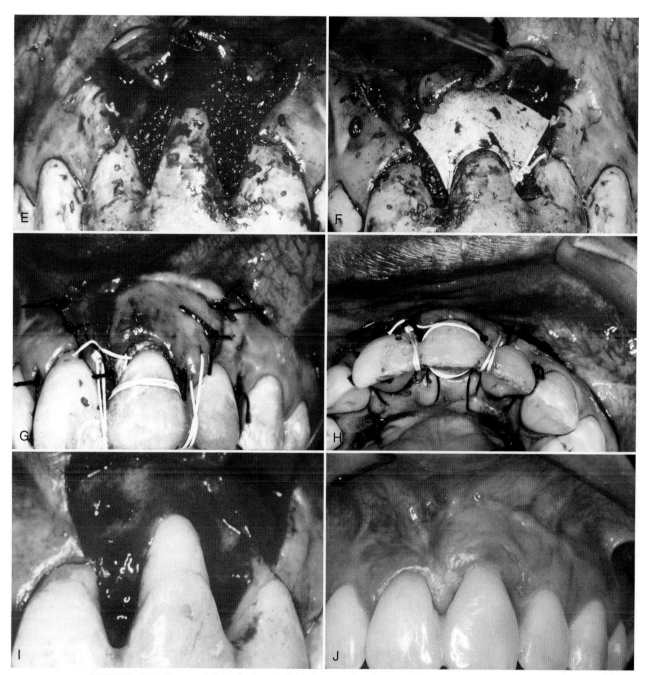

FIGURE 14-12, cont'd E, A decalcified, freeze-dried cortical bone allograft was placed into the defect. **F,** A wide Gore-Tex periodontal membrane was placed over the defect and bone graft. **G,** The facial flap was coronally positioned as far as possible to cover the membrane. **H,** Supraincisal suspensory suturing was used to facilitate apical positioning and stabilize the flap. **I,** After removal of the Gore-Tex membrane, a dense connective tissue fill is seen in the defect palatally and laterally. **J,** The regenerated attachment allowed for the coronally positioned flap to heal in the proper position 3 years after surgery.

Continued

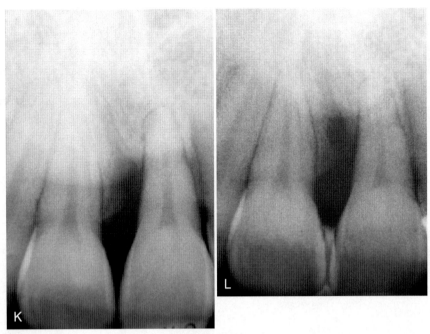

FIGURE 14-12, cont'd K, The preoperative radiograph reveals mesial and circumferential bone loss around tooth #9. **L,** Fill of the palatal and mesial defect 2 years after regeneration.

EDENTULOUS RIDGE DEFORMITIES

Differential Etiology

Trauma. Visible edentulous ridge defects and deformities are particularly challenging to treat both periodontally and prosthetically. The majority of these defects result from facial trauma sustained during motor vehicle accidents, contact sports, work-related accidents, and other mishaps. Violent avulsion of one or more teeth and surrounding buccal or lingual bone segments often occurs. Healing of such injuries results in collapse of the overlying soft tissue into the depression created by the bony loss, leading to a buccolingual or crestal concavity of the edentulous ridge. If the overlying mucosa and connective tissue are also lost at the time of the injury, scarring of the vestibule and gingiva is a further complication.

Periodontitis and Juvenile Periodontitis. Other causes of edentulous ridge deformities include periodontitis and localized juvenile periodontitis (previously termed periodontosis). When advanced periodontal disease affects one or more anterior teeth, a jagged bony topography can be associated with this severe loss of attachment. When these hopeless teeth are extracted, soft tissue healing mimics the alveolar profile, with resultant defects. With localized juvenile periodontitis, severe bone loss often occurs around the central incisors. If extraction is required, similar defects result. When only the buccal plate is lost, the defect created is horizontal (depression or concavity), whereas if the palatal bone is also lost, vertical loss of height occurs.

Classification

Edentulous ridge deformities are classified according to their dimensions:

1. *Buccolingual.* Buccolingual defects manifest as concavities on the buccal surface, brought about by loss of the buccal bone plate. Pontics placed in buccolingual defects appear unnaturally flat or thick.
2. *Occlusoapical.* Occlusoapical defects are the easiest to see because of an obvious discrepancy in the height of the gingival margin. In these situations, the pontics often are longer than the adjacent abutment teeth.
3. *Mesiodistal.* The mesiodistal dimension indicates the width of the area to be reconstructed and aids in determining the number of procedures necessary to correct the problem. (A wide span may involve multiple procedures.) It is not a true classification of a defect type.
4. *Atrophied papilla.* This defect involves loss of the papillae adjacent to an edentulous area. Usually caused by atrophy, this defect is not primarily traumatic or inflammatory in nature. These defects are highly visible and difficult to correct, and in many situations no change can be seen after multiple reconstructive attempts.

Treatment Options

Gingival Onlay Grafts. The primary technique used to correct buccolingual and occlusoapical defects is the gingival onlay graft or soft tissue augmentation procedure, which is an adaptation of the free gingival graft technique to this special situation. Thick palatal donor tissue is used to fill the defect (the minimum thickness is the depth of the defect). The donor tissue is then tightly sutured into the prepared defect site. If a provisional restoration or provisional removable appliance is present, the pontics overlying the grafted site must be adjusted to allow 1 to 2 mm of clearance. This is necessary because the graft will swell during healing, and any excessive pressure can cause necrosis and failure. Once the graft has healed (approximately 6 to 8 weeks), a new provisional restoration can be made and an ovate pontic prepared to create the illusion of natural teeth emerging from their sockets.

Connective Tissue Augmentation. A subperiosteal tunnel can be created under the soft tissue of the defect and a connective tissue graft placed into the tunnel to "plump out" the defect. The connective tissue can be obtained from an area of the palate distant to the defect (free connective tissue augmentation) or adjacent to the defect (connective tissue roll augmentation). This technique attempts to correct the defect by internal augmentation. This procedure can be used for occlusoapical, buccolingual, and papillary defects. Pontics on provisional restorations must be adjusted to allow 1 to 2 mm of clearance over the surgical site during the 6- to 8-week healing period to compensate for postoperative tissue swelling.

Bone Grafts. Bone graft material can also be placed under a ridge to "plump up" the defect. Xenografts or synthetic graft materials are chosen for this procedure because they are not resorbed. They act as scaffolding for connective tissue ingrowth and are not designed to regenerate the lost bone.

Ovate Pontics. Once the desired tissue reconstruction has been achieved, the area can be modified to allow for fabrication of ovate or bullet pontics. The advantage of this type of pontic design is that it creates the illusion of a natural tooth emerging from its socket and provides a more natural appearance to the adjacent "papillae." After adequate maturation of the grafted connective tissue (6-8 weeks), a round depression is placed into the augmented edentulous ridge crest with a coarse round diamond bur, with the dimensions dependent on the tooth to be placed (e.g., a maxillary canine will require a larger preparation than a mandibular incisor). The provisional restoration is then relined so that acrylic material fills the depression and the area heals by epithelialization around the pontic.

The definitive prosthesis thus has apically tapered and rounded pontics that fit intimately into the tissue depression. This esthetic pontic design creates the appearance of a natural tooth emerging from a sulcus; the contours of the gingival aspects of the pontic are round without sharp or abrupt edges. Hygiene is easily performed by flossing under the pontic.

Clinical Considerations

Some shrinkage is involved with these procedures, sometimes necessitating a second procedure. In the situation of occlusoapical and buccolingual defects, several procedures may be needed before the desired result is achieved. The long-term esthetic results are usually well worth the surgical time involved. Papillary reconstruction, unfortunately, is very unpredictable, and the patient should be made aware of the poorer prognosis in these situations.

Clinical Technique: Ovate Pontic.

Armamentarium
- High-speed handpiece
- Course, round diamond bur (#4 or #6)
- Indelible ink marker (e.g., Dr. Thompson's Sanitary Color Transfer Applicators, Great Plains Dental Products Co. Inc.)
- Self-cure acrylic
- Periodontal pack (e.g., Coe-Pack, CG America)

Clinical Technique
1. Anesthetize the area with 2% Lidocaine with 1/50,000 epinephrine (unless medically contraindicated) for hemostasis.

2. Outline the pontic form in indelible marker. The preparation should approximate the desired emergence profile.
3. Using light strokes of the high-speed handpiece and copious irrigation, prepare the tissues to the desired depth using the coarse round diamond. Ideally the diameter of the pontic preparation should mimic that of the desired emergence profile and be 2 to 3 mm deep at the center. The preparation should be parabolic (ovate), not cylindrical, in shape. Take extreme care not to exceed the boundaries of the indelible ink and not to damage or involve the adjacent papillae.
4. Once the depth and lateral dimensions have been achieved, apply pressure with sterile gauze until hemostasis is achieved.
5. Reline the pontic area of the provisional restoration with a self-curing acrylic. Intimate adaptation should be achieved between the relined pontic and the prepared tissue, but no pressure should be placed on the site.

> ### CLINICAL TIP
> A high polish must be placed on the relined surface to ensure optimal healing and minimize patient discomfort.

6. Recement the provisional restoration with provisional cement and place periodontal packing around the surgical site.
7. Epithelialization of the ovate preparation occurs in approximately 3 to 4 weeks. Completion of the definitive restoration can occur at that time (see also Figs. 14-11 to 14-13).

> ### CLINICAL TIP
> The definitive restoration should lie passively on the tissue depression. Pressure may create an abscess with resultant necrosis.

Clinical Case: Connective Tissue Augmentation and Gingivoplasty

A 37-year-old woman presented with a cupped occlusoapical ridge defect resulting from the extraction of the maxillary left central incisor after an endodontic perforation (Fig. 14-13A).

Her medical history was noncontributory. The pontic was reduced in apical height before proceeding with connective tissue augmentation of the edentulous ridge. This revealed the occlusoapical deformity as well as a slight buccal soft tissue concavity (Fig. 14-13B,C).

A partial-thickness palatal flap was reflected (Fig. 14-13D) to allow harvesting of the underlying connective tissue, which was left as a pedicle. This connective tissue roll was placed over the edentulous bony ridge and under the connective tissue of the defect. The graft was sutured through to the buccal mucosa for stability (Fig. 14-13E,F), the provisional restoration was recemented (Fig. 14-13G), and the area was allowed to heal (Fig. 14-13H). After 12 weeks of healing, most of the defect resolved (Fig. 14-13I) and a new provisional fixed partial denture was fabricated (Fig. 14-13J). At that time it was noted that the central incisors had a slightly uneven gingival margin (Fig. 14-13K). A simple gingivoplasty was performed to even the facial margins of the central incisors (see Fig. 14-13L).

The patient was referred for definitive restoration 4 weeks after this second surgery (Fig. 14-13M) and the definitive restoration was fabricated (Fig. 14-13N,O).

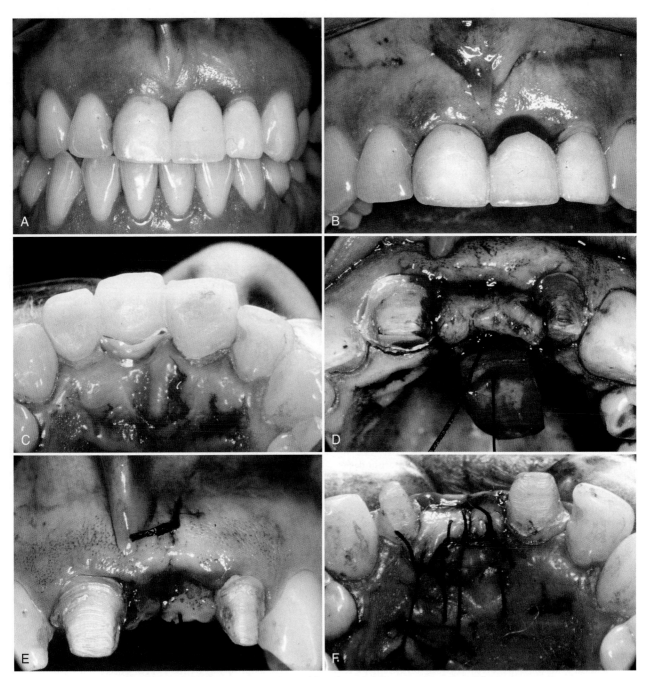

FIGURE 14-13 A, A three-unit provisional fixed partial denture was placed from the maxillary right central incisor to the left lateral incisor 3 months after removal of the left central incisor. **B,** The pontic is reduced in apical height before proceeding with connective tissue augmentation of the edentulous ridge. **C,** Palatal view of the patient. **D,** A partial thickness flap is reflected toward the palate. **E,** The connective tissue pedicle is sutured through to the buccal aspect. **F,** The palatal flap is sutured over the area.

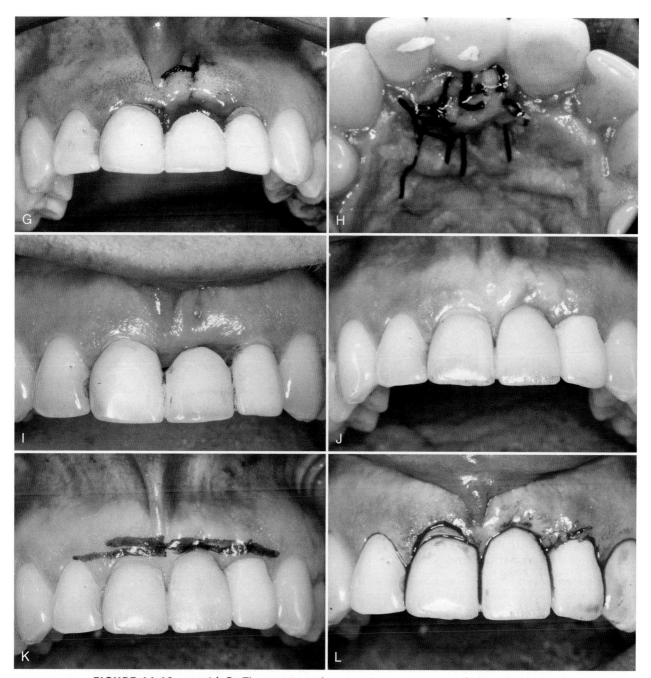

FIGURE 14-13, cont'd G, The provisional restoration is recemented. **H,** Palatal view 10 days after surgery. **I,** Facial view 3 months after surgery. **J,** A new provisional restoration was fabricated. **K,** A discrepancy in the free gingival margins of the central incisors was noted. **L,** A gingivoplasty was performed to create symmetrical margins.
Continued

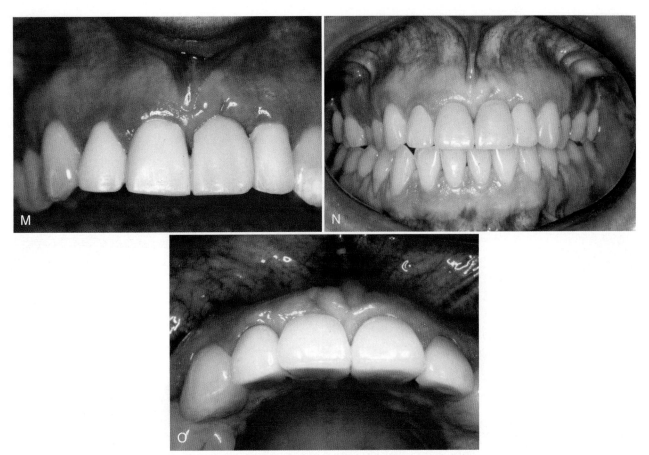

FIGURE 14-13, cont'd M, Facial view after healing. **N,** The definitive restoration was inserted after adequate healing. **O,** The occlusal view demonstrates elimination of the concavity and restoration of a normal buccal soft tissue profile.

Clinical Case: Multiple Free Gingival Grafts and a Synthetic Bone Graft

A 33-year-old woman was involved in an automobile accident, resulting in traumatic avulsion of the maxillary right central incisor (Fig. 14-14A). Her medical history was noncontributory. The significant edentulous ridge defect required a multiple surgical approach.

First the buccolingual aspect was corrected by placing a thick free graft. Only the outer epithelial layer was removed at the recipient site to maintain as much of the connective tissue as possible (Fig. 14-14B).

By removing only the epithelial layer, all existing connective tissue at the recipient site was maintained. Removing some of the connective tissue during bed preparation would result in increasing the dimension of the defect to be grafted. For example, 4 mm thickness of tissue at the recipient site and a 5-mm defect warrant removal of the surface epithelium while maintaining the defect dimensions; however, removal of epithelium and 2 mm of connective tissue would increase the amount of defect to 7 mm.

The graft (Fig. 14-14C) was placed in the recipient site (Fig. 14-14D) and the pontic trimmed (Fig. 14-14E,F) to avoid pressure necrosis. Healing was uneventful (Fig. 14-14G,H). After 2 months, a second procedure was performed to correct the incisoapical defect (Fig. 14-14I). The edentulous ridge was prepared (Fig. 14-14J) and a thick palatal graft, including the fatty tissues (Fig. 14-14K), was sutured over the recipient site (Fig. 14-14L).

The graft was sutured in place and allowed to heal. After 8 weeks this area healed, but a slight depression remained (Fig. 14-14M). To correct this incisoapical defect, a full-thickness flap was reflected (Fig. 14-14N,O) and a synthetic bone graft was placed (Fig. 14-14P). The provisional restoration was recontoured and recemented in place (Fig. 14-14Q). A pleasing esthetic result was thus achieved (Fig. 14-14R,S).

Clinical Case: Papillary Reconstruction via Connective Tissue Augmentation

A 22-year-old man presented with unesthetic replacement of both maxillary lateral incisors. His medical history was noncontributory. He was dissatisfied with the lack of papillae (Fig. 14-15A).

A connective tissue roll was used to "plump" the area (Fig. 14-15B). The graft was taken from the palate directly behind the defect and sutured through the buccal mucosa for stability (Fig. 14-15C). The pontic on the removable appliance was trimmed to prevent excessive pressure (Fig. 14-15D).

After healing, the ridge was prepared to accept an ovate pontic using a course round diamond bur with copious irrigation (Fig. 14-15E,F). After 6 weeks the patient was referred for prosthetic restoration and an acid-etch retained fixed partial denture fabricated (Fig. 14-15G).

Although the entire papilla could not be reconstructed, the patient was satisfied with the results (Fig. 14-15H).

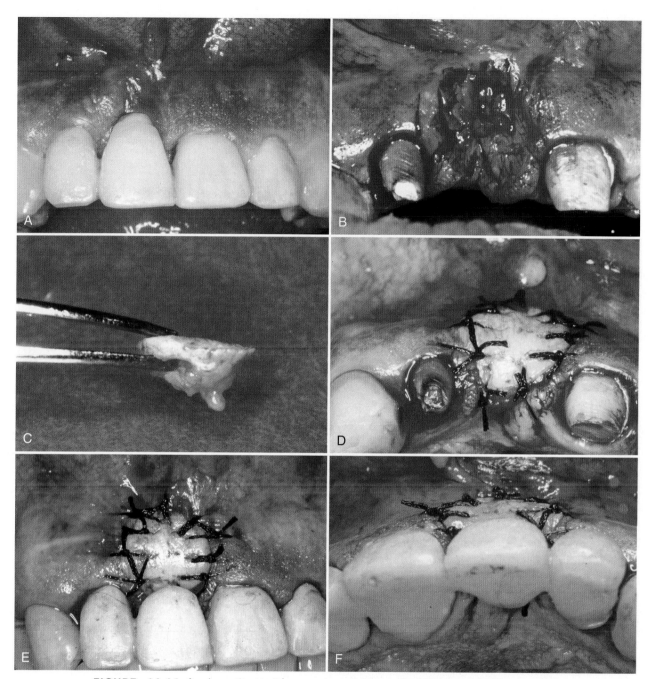

FIGURE 14-14 A, A patient with severe scarring and deformity of the maxillary anterior vestibule. **B,** The first surgical procedure addressed the buccolingual defect. **C,** A thick palatal graft was harvested. **D,** The graft is sutured in the recipient bed. **E,** The pontic is relieved and recemented. **F,** Palatal view of the patient.

Continued

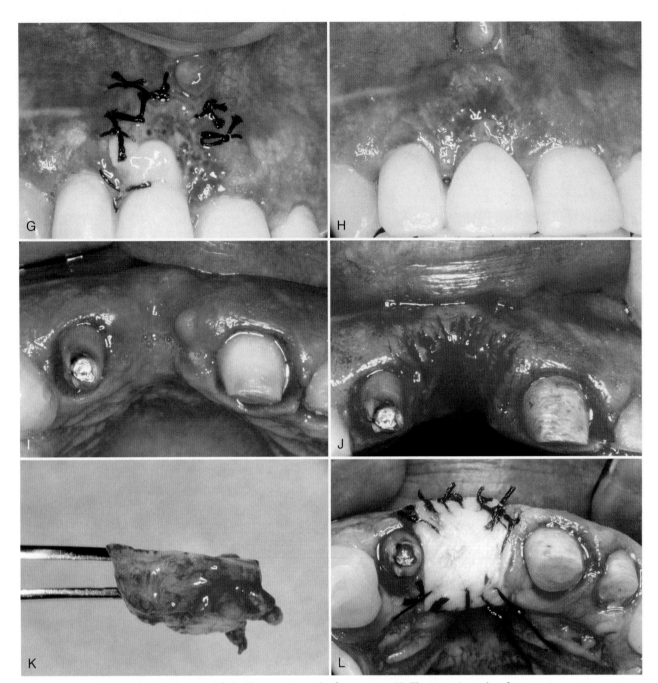

FIGURE 14-14, cont'd G, The area 1 week after surgery. **H,** The area 6 weeks after surgery. **I,** The second surgical phase addressed the incisoapical defect. **J,** The recipient bed is prepared. **K,** A thick piece of donor palatal tissue is removed. **L,** The graft is sutured intimately into the defect.

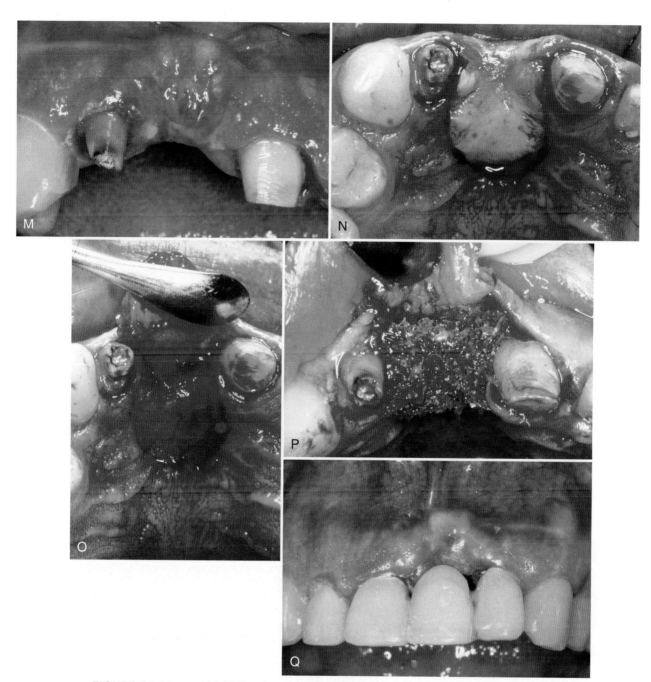

FIGURE 14-14, cont'd M, Despite adequate healing, some residual defect remained. **N,** A third procedure was performed. **O,** The flap is reflected buccally. **P,** A synthetic bone graft is placed beneath the graft to correct the residual defect. **Q,** The area is sutured and the provisional restoration is replaced.

Continued

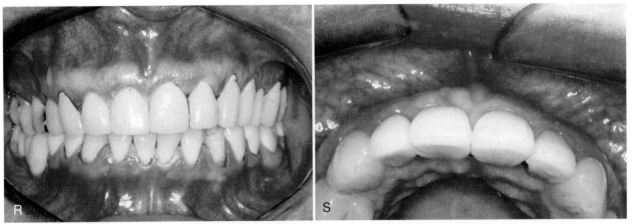

FIGURE 14-14, cont'd R, After restoration of proper buccolingual and incisoapical dimensions apically and interproximally, a definitive restoration was placed. **S,** Palatal view of the patient.

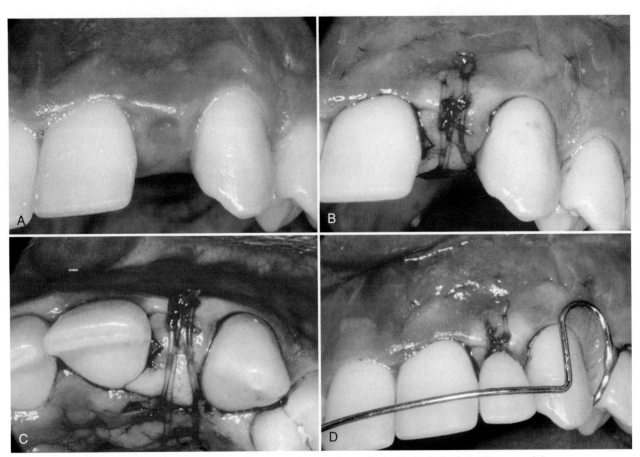

FIGURE 14-15 A, A young male patient who was dissatisfied with the lack of papillae around the missing lateral incisor. **B,** A connective tissue roll was taken from the palate and sutured in place into a subperiosteal tunnel created under the edentulous ridge. **C,** Palatal view of the patient. **D,** The pontic on the removable appliance was trimmed to prevent excessive pressure on the ridge.

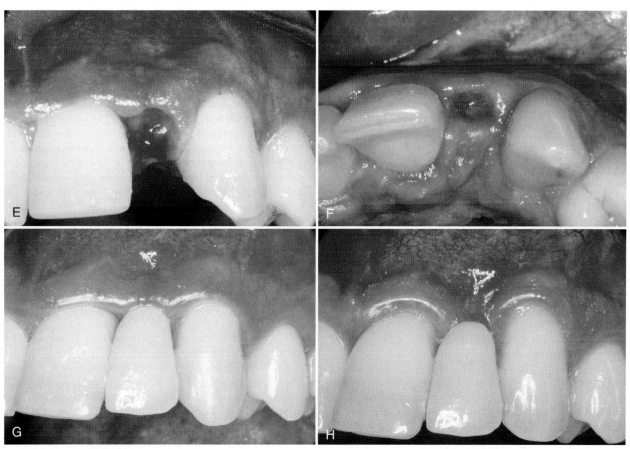

FIGURE 14-15, cont'd E, After healing, an ovate pontic preparation was performed into the augmented edentulous ridge to allow for fabrication of an ovate pontic on the Maryland bridge. **F,** Palatal view of the patient. **G,** Patient at 1 month after insertion of the Maryland bridge. **H,** Although tissue has regressed in the apical region, the interproximal papilla remains stable.

GINGIVAL OVERGROWTH

Patient dissatisfaction with the short appearance of the anterior teeth is commonplace. Identifying the underlying etiology is essential for proper treatment planning and prognosis.

Differential Etiology

1. *Noninflammatory hyperplasia.* Noninflammatory hyperplasia is the most prevalent presentation for both localized and generalized gingival overgrowth. Commonly prescribed medications are often the cause of this phenomenon, with one of the best known being Dilantin. Several other frequently prescribed drugs may cause a similar response (e.g., nifedipine, cyclosporine, Inderal). Such an underlying cause should be discovered during the medical history. The hyperplasia observed may be localized to a sextant or an arch or generalized in both jaws. Another noninflammatory factor is irritation. This is seen with ill-fitting removable partial dentures or overhanging margins of restorations. In these situations, the overgrowth is seen only at the site of the irritation. An uncommon cause is genetic predisposition to gingival overgrowth. This presents as generalized buccal and lingual hyperplasia. These noninflammatory conditions are usually accompanied by an inflammatory component because of the difficulty in performing proper oral hygiene.

2. *Inflammatory hyperplasia.* In some situations gingival hyperplasia is purely inflammatory. This is usually observed in chronic gingivitis or periodontitis with severe gingival involvement. Localized inflammatory hyperplasia is also seen adjacent to caries.

3. *Altered passive eruption.* Altered passive eruption has neither an inflammatory nor an extrinsic noninflammatory etiology. During normal eruption of the permanent dentition, the tooth erupts coronally while the gingiva migrates apically (passive eruption). When insufficient apical migration occurs, the gingival margin appears as gingival overgrowth. Clinically, this appears as short crowns with the free gingival margin in the middle one third of the enamel.

   Histologically, two distinct presentations of altered passive eruption exist. In both situations, the free gingival margin is coronally positioned, but the position of the alveolar crest is different. In the first situation, the alveolar crest is at its normal level of more than 1 mm apical to the cementoenamel junction. In the second situation, the alveolar crest is at or above the cementoenamel junction. Although both situations are clinically identical, the histologic differences dictate different surgical approaches. The differentiation between the two histologic types can be made radiographically only when the alveolar bone can be definitely seen below the cementoenamel junction. Otherwise, it is often impossible to predict the position of the buccal or lingual bone radiographically, and the need for ostectomy can be determined only after flap elevation.

Treatment Options

Plaque Control. Plaque control is paramount in treating inflammatory hyperplasia. Oral hygiene instruction, scaling, and root planing or subgingival curettage should be performed before evaluating the need for surgical correction.

> ### CLINICAL TIP
>
> Often conservative, cause-related therapy will resolve inflammatory hyperplasia.

If the hyperplasia persists, surgical reduction is indicated. The choice of surgical procedure (e.g., gingivectomy vs. apically positioned flap) is determined by any underlying periodontal problems (e.g., pocketing, infrabony lesions) and the status of the tissues (e.g., the amount of gingiva present, severity of inflammation).

Gingivectomy or Gingivoplasty. In situations of noninflammatory gingival hyperplasia, gingivectomy is usually indicated. The incision design for this approach can be either externally beveled (the incised surface of the tissues are visible facially) or internally beveled (submarginal incisions with the incised edge in the sulcus). No flap reflection is performed with either approach. The incision design is based upon the amount of tissue that must be removed, with an externally beveled incision being contraindicated when there is a risk for creating a mucogingival deficit. When there is a wide zone of keratinized tissue, either incision design can be used. With irritation-induced overgrowth, local reduction or excision is performed in conjunction with removal of the irritant. These patients usually respond well, without recurrence. With drug or genetically induced hyperplasia, gingivectomy is still the procedure of choice, although the frequency of recurrence must be considered. Changing the patient's medication often results in eliminating recurrences, although it will not reverse any existing hyperplasia. If change in medication is contraindicated, retreatment of recurrent problems must be evaluated on an individual basis. Recurrence is also common with genetically predisposed hyperplasia. The patient's functional and esthetic needs must be considered in deciding how often to perform surgical reduction.

Apically Positioned Flap with or without Ostectomy. Altered passive eruption is best treated with an apically positioned flap, which accomplishes two objectives: It positions the gingival margin at a normal level and allows the evaluation of the alveolar crest. If the alveolar crest is correctly positioned, only apical positioning of the gingiva will be necessary. However, if the alveolar crest is at or above the cementoenamel junction, ostectomy is required to first achieve a normal physiologic relationship between tooth and bone before apically positioning the soft tissue. The purpose of bone removal is to establish a new biologic width (see the section on inadequate tooth structure for restorations), allowing the gingival margin to reform at an appropriate level. If a gingivectomy alone was performed in this situation, the gingiva would heal to its previous position because the underlying bone dictates gingival margin position.

Clinical Case: Full-Thickness Flap with Ostectomy

A 17-year-old female patient presented for correction of the esthetics of her maxillary anterior teeth. Her medical history was noncontributory. She desired bonding to make the teeth larger and close the spaces between them. Clinically, she had short teeth occlusogingivally and she exhibited multiple diastemata (Fig. 14-16A).

The diagnosis was altered passive eruption and a discrepancy between the tooth and arch size. The situation demanded an integration of periodontal and restorative therapy. Restorative diastema closure would have resulted in unnaturally wide teeth with an apparently over-exaggerated incisal edge. The anatomic crown was exposed with a full-thickness flap (Fig. 14-16B,C).

The alveolar crest was at the level of the cementoenamel junction (Fig. 14-16D), thus requiring ostectomy to allow for establishment of a proper biologic width (see the section on inadequate tooth structure for restorations). The tissue was apically repositioned and sutured into place (Fig. 14-16E,F).

After 3 months of healing, the patient was referred for restorative treatment. A microfilled composite resin was used to close the diastemata. The increased crown length permitted fabrication of an esthetic restoration (Fig. 14-16G).

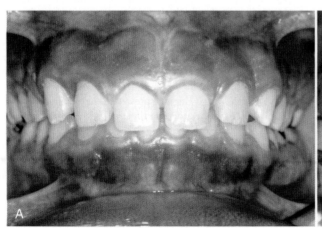
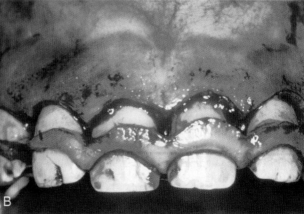

FIGURE 14-16 A, A 17-year-old female patient with altered passive eruption and a discrepancy between the tooth and arch size. **B,** The first phase of treatment required exposure of the anatomic crowns.

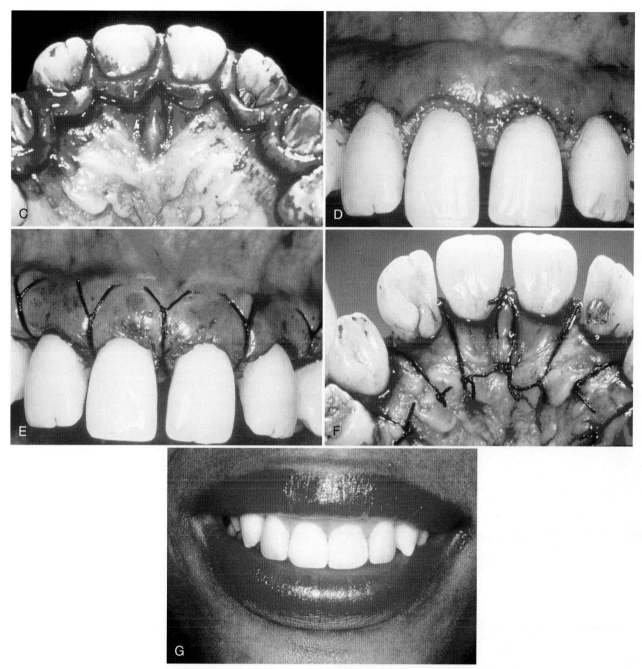

FIGURE 14-16, cont'd C, An additional incision was made on the palatal aspect of the six maxillary anterior teeth. **D,** Reflection of the flap revealed the alveolar crest at the level of the cementoenamel junction. **E,** Minimal ostectomy was performed and the tissues sutured apically to reestablish the biologic width. **F,** Palatal view of the patient. **G,** The teeth were ultimately restored using a microfilled composite resin.

Clinical Case: Correction of Post-Orthodontic Gingival Overgrowth in an Adolescent Patient

Six months after removal of fixed orthodontic hardware, a 14-year-old male patient presented with gingival overgrowth, thickening of the interdental papillae, and a coronally positioned free gingival margin (Fig. 14-17A).

The medical history was noncontributory. A diagnosis of gingival overgrowth with altered passive eruption was made. It is important to consider the potential for further dentoalveolar

growth in younger patients. In this situation, it was determined that position and development of the anterior dentition was complete and correction was indicated. In the posterior sextants no papillary overgrowth was noted, and after conferring with the orthodontist it was decided that further passive gingival eruption was possible, so posterior correction was deferred.

There was an adequate zone of attached gingiva in both anterior sextants; however, the amount of anatomic crown uncovering required ruled out correction by classic gingivectomy because this would have created a mucogingival problem. The surgical treatment plan involved a combination of gingival reduction with apical positioning of the existing tissues. Submarginal incisions were performed (internally beveled gingivectomy) followed by reflection of a full-thickness mucoperiosteal flap, allowing for creation of a normal scalloped FGM profile without causing a mucogingival defect (Fig. 14-17*B*). The sites healed extremely well at 4 weeks with continued monitoring of the posterior sextants on an ongoing basis (Fig. 14-17*C*).

CONCLUSION

Facial esthetics involves the interaction of many elements. The periodontium, which serves as a backdrop for the teeth, determines the environment in which any esthetic rehabilitation is seen. It is essential that periodontal procedures be considered an important part of any comprehensive esthetic treatment plan.

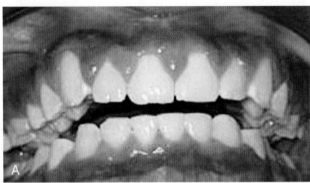
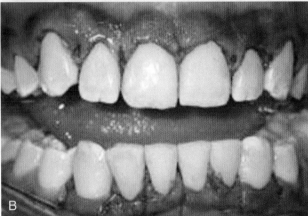
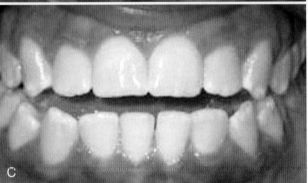

FIGURE 14-17 A, Gingival overgrowth and altered passive eruption in a 14-year-old post-orthodontic patient. **B,** Correction of the overgrowth is seen after an internally beveled gingivectomy and apically positioned flap is performed. **C,** At 4 weeks after surgery a normal dento-gingival relationship is seen.

BIBLIOGRAPHY

AADC Positions Committee: *Parameters of soft tissue grafting: final-position statement,* June 4, 2009.

Abrams L: Augmentation of the deformed residual edentulous ridge for fixed prosthesis, *Compend Contin Educ Dent* 1:205, 1980.

Allen EP: Use of mucogingival surgical procedures to enhance esthetics, *Dent Clin North Am* 32:307, 1988.

Allen EP, Miller PD Jr: Coronal positioning of existing gingiva: short term results in the treatment of shallow marginal tissue recession, *J Periodont* 60:316, 1989.

Becker BE, Becker W: Use of connective tissue autografts for treatment of mucogingival problems, *Int J Periodontics Restorative Dent* 6:88, 1986.

Becker W, Becker BE, Berg L: Repair of intrabony defects as a result of open debridement procedures. Repair of 36 treated cases, Int J Periodontics Restorative Dent 6:8, 1986.

Bernimoulin JP, Luscher B, Muhlemann HR: Coronally repositioned periodontal flap, *J Clin Periodont* 2:1, 1975.

Breault L, Fowler E, Lyons J: *Subgingival restorations with resin-ionomer: a periodontal alternative,* Compendium, 21(9):733-737, 2000.

Clark JW, Weatherford TW, Mann WV Jr: The wire ligature-acrylic splint, *J Periodont* 40:371, 1969.

Cohen DW, Ross SE: The double papillae positioned flap in periodontal therapy, *J Periodont* 39:65, 1968.

deWaal H, Kon S, Ruben MP: The laterally positioned flap (review), *Dent Clin North Am* 32:267, 1988.

Dorfman HS, Kennedy JE, Bird WC: Longitudinal evaluation of free autogenous gingival grafts: a four year report, *J Periodont* 53:349, 1982.

Evans CA, Schaff HA: Acid etch technique adapted for splinting anterior teeth, *Am J Orthodont* 71:317, 1977.

Evian CI, Corn H, Rosenberg ES: Retained interdental papilla procedure for maintaining anterior esthetics, *Compend Contin Educ Dent* 6(1):58, 1985.

Gray JL, Quartlebaum JB: Correction of localized alveolar ridge defects utilizing hydroxyapatite and a "tunnelling" approach: a case report, *Int J Periodontics Restorative Dent* 8:72, 1988.

Grupe HE, Warren R: Repair of gingival defects by a sliding flap operation, *J Periodont* 27:92, 1956.

Ingber J: Forced eruption: part II. A method of treating non-restorable teeth—periodontal and restorative considerations, *J Periodont* 47:203, 1976.

Kozlovsky A, Tal H, Lieberman M: Forced eruption combined with gingival fiberotomy. A technique for clinical crown lengthening, *J Clin Periodont* 15:534, 1988.

Kurthy R: Use of a resin-ionomer for subgingival restorations (external root resorption): case report, *Dent Today*, 20(2), 2001.

Langer B, Calagna L: The subepithelial connective tissue graft, *J Prosthet Dent* 44:363, 1980.

Langer B, Langer L: Subepithelial connective tissue graft technique for root coverage, *J Periodontol* 56:715, 1985.

Maynard JG Jr, Wilson RDK: Physiologic dimensions of the periodontium significant to the restorative dentist, *J Periodontol* 50:170, 1979.

Mellonig JT et al: Clinical evaluation of freeze-dried bone allografts in periodontal osseous defects, *J Periodontol* 47: 125, 1976.

Mellonig JT: Decalcified freeze-dried bone allografts as an implant material in human periodontal defects, *Int J Periodontics Restorative Dent* 4:41, 1984.

Miller CJ: The smile line as a guide to anterior esthetics, *Dent Clin North Am* 33:157, 1989.

Miller PD Jr: Regenerative and reconstructive periodontal plastic surgery. Mucogingival surgery (review), *Dent Clin North Am* 32:287, 1988.

Miller PD Jr, Binkley LH Jr: Root coverage and ridge augmentation in Class IV recession using a coronally positioned free gingival graft, *J Periodont* 57:360, 1986.

Nelson SW: The sub-pedicle connective tissue graft. A bilaminar reconstructive procedure for the coverage of denuded root surfaces, *J Periodont* 58:95, 1987.

Nevins M: Attached gingiva—mucogingival therapy and restorative dentistry, *Int J Periodontics Restorative Dent* 6:9, 1986.

Nevins M, Nevins ML, Carmelo M, et al: The clinical efficacy of DynaMatrix extracellular membrane in augmenting keratinized tissue, *Int J Periodontics Restorative Dent* 30:150-161, 2010.

Ochsenbein C: A primer for osseous surgery, *Int J Periodontics Restorative Dent* 6:1, 1986.

Ochsenbein C, Bohannan HM: The palatal approach to osseous surgery: part II. Clinical application, *J Periodont* 35:54, 1964.

Pontoriero R et al: Guided tissue regeneration in the treatment of furcation defects in man, *J Clin Periodont* 14:618, 1987.

Pontoriero R et al: Guided tissue regeneration in degree II furcation-involved mandibular molars. A clinical study, *J Clin Periodont* 15:247, 1988.

Pontoriero R et al: Guided tissue regeneration in the treatment of furcation defects in mandibular molars. A clinical study of degree III involvements, *J Clin Periodont* 16:170, 1989.

Pontoriero R, Celenza F Jr, Ricci G, Carnevale G: Rapid extrusion with fiber resection: a combined orthodontic-periodontic treatment modality, *Int J Periodontics Restorative Dent* 7:30, 1987.

Raetzke PB: Covering localized areas of root exposure employing the "envelope" technique, *J Periodont* 56:397, 1985.

Ross SE, Crosetti HW, Gargiulo A, Cohen DW: The double papillae repositioned flap—and alternative. I. Fourteen years in retrospect, *Int J Periodontics Restorative Dent* 6:46, 1986.

Saroff SA et al: Free soft tissue autografts: hemostasis and protection of the palatal donor site with a microfibrillar collagen preparation, *J Periodont* 53:681, 1980.

Seibert JS: Reconstruction of deformed, partially edentulous ridges, using full thickness onlay grafts, *Compend Contin Educ Dent* 15:437, 1983.

Sepe WW et al: Clinical evaluation of freeze-dried bone allografts in periodontal osseous defects. Part II, *J Periodont* 48:9, 1978.

Steinberg AD: Office management of phenytoin-induced gingival overgrowth, *Compend Contin Educ Dent* 16:138, 1985.

Sullivan HC, Atkins JH: The role of free gingival grafts in periodontal therapy, *Dent Clin North Am* 13:133, 1969.

Takei H, Yamada H, Hau T: Maxillary anterior esthetics. Preservation of the interdental papilla, *Dent Clin North Am* 33:263, 1989.

Werbitt M: Decalcified freeze-dried bone allografts: a successful procedure in the reduction of intrabony defects, *Int J Periodontics Restorative Dent* 7:56, 1987.

15

Esthetics and Orthodontics

Gail E. Schupak, Joseph Hung, and Edward C. McNulty

The orthodontist, striving for excellent form and function, not only aligns the dentition and provides for good masticatory function but also produces an esthetically pleasing result. Generalists and specialists in fields other than orthodontics should be capable of diagnosing the need for orthodontic intervention and be competent in performing simple orthodontic corrections. The orthodontist corrects complicated occlusal disharmonies, often using complex orthodontic mechanotherapy.

Before the introduction of more esthetic fixed appliances and removable appliances, patients (especially adults) often refused to accept full appliance mechanotherapy of even the shortest duration. This often compromised the success of the definitive restoration or placed its long-term stability in jeopardy.

RATIONALE FOR ORTHODONTIC INTERVENTION

A treatment plan with a focus on esthetics must take into account whether orthodontic movements will enhance the success or stability of the definitive restorations. Diagnostic determinations should be based on the following principles:

1. Masticatory efficiency. Proper occlusion and the development of proper interdigitation allows for enhanced masticatory efficiency.
2. Periodontal protection. Correct axial inclination of the teeth dissipates the forces of mastication and lessens trauma to the periodontium.
3. Oral hygiene. Corrective alignment of a crowded dentition eliminates food impaction, improves self-cleansing during normal masticatory movements, and permits easier oral hygiene by the patient.
4. Temporomandibular joint protection. Proper occlusion, which permits a good functional relationship between the maxilla and mandible, mitigates strain of the masticatory muscles and the temporomandibular joint.
5. Speech improvement. Proper anatomic relationships between the teeth and the musculature of the orofacial complex enhance proper speech.

6. Esthetics. Orthodontic correction establishes a dentition that is esthetically pleasing and takes into consideration the soft tissue profile of the patient.

THE BIOLOGY OF TOOTH MOVEMENT

A proper understanding of the cellular physiology is crucial before attempting orthodontic therapy. Tooth movement occurs due to remodeling of bone around the roots of the teeth. Two types of cells are primarily responsible for this remodeling, osteoclasts and osteoblasts. Orthodontic forces lead to compression and/or straining (stretching) of the periodontal ligaments sending biochemical mediators that activate osteoclasts and osteoblasts to, respectively, resorb bone on the compression side and produce new bone on the strained (stretched) side. The teeth reposition within the alveolus as this remodeling occurs.

BASIC PREMISES FOR DIAGNOSTIC EVALUATION

Patients often have misconceptions regarding treatment results. The orthodontist should discuss probable results with the patient to build a diagnostic plan on a firm foundation of understanding.

1. There must be a clear pathway for tooth movement to take place when the patient is in maximal intercuspation. Interferences can be removed by selectively grinding the teeth when function or esthetics permits or by opening the vertical dimension of occlusion through fixed or removable appliance therapy. If the latter is attempted, a thorough evaluation of the effects of altering vertical dimension must be considered.
2. Dentofacial harmony can be evaluated only on a personal, subjective basis. The clinician therefore should be prepared to discuss any profile or other facial changes expected to result from treatment with the patient before therapy begins. This is especially important when skeletal disharmonies will be improved by orthognathic surgery.
3. The treated occlusion must be stable. All orthodontic appliance therapy is planned with stability in mind. Overexpansion

of the dental arch commonly results in relapse of crowding after retention is discontinued. Rotational discrepancies should be overcorrected because they also tend to relapse, as do deep bites, open bites, and Class III malocclusions.

4. Adult orthodontic treatment has little effect on facial growth. This applies even to full-banded mechanotherapy performed by an orthodontist. The facial pattern exhibited by the patient should be accepted as the framework in which tooth movement must take place. In the mature adult, growth is negligible. It is possible to produce some orthognathic changes in the maturing maxilla and local changes in the alveolar arches and lips, but facial changes are mostly the result of growth and not treatment. The clinician should be well versed in predicting facial growth in the maturing patient or should refer the patient for an orthodontic consultation. Predictions are based on the current conditions of the face and dental arch presented by the patient, correlated with statistical probabilities. Race, gender, and familial tendencies are also important factors to consider in diagnosis and treatment planning.

5. The mandibular dental arch provides the best starting point for diagnostic analysis and treatment planning, especially for fixed appliance mechanotherapy performed by an orthodontist. Treatment therefore must be planned so the maxilla will conform to the therapeutic result that can be achieved in the mandible. An exception to this premise is Angle Class III malocclusions in which limitations in the treatment of the maxilla take on primary diagnostic and treatment priorities.

DIAGNOSTIC EVALUATIONS

Malocclusions may result from skeletal, dental, or muscular disharmonies or from a combination of these components. The origin of the problem often dictates the treatment modality. The mandible and maxilla should be evaluated separately and in their relationship to each other during differential diagnosis. A general outline is provided here, but the clinician must examine each situation on its own merits and design a treatment plan accordingly.

A patient with a therapeutic problem involving orthodontic principles beyond the scope of the clinician's knowledge should be referred to a specialist for a diagnostic opinion and, if needed, treatment. The orthodontist, in turn, must always consider whether restorative modalities may better serve a patient's needs than complicated orthodontic therapy.

Each situation poses many questions and presents a set of different, self-limiting circumstances, making differential diagnosis easier for the astute clinician.

Assessment of the Skeletal Component

The relationship of the bones of the face may or may not be the cause of a malocclusion. A Class II malocclusion may be caused by a small mandible, a large maxilla, or a combination of both, and a Class III malocclusion may be caused by a large mandible, a small maxilla, or a combination of both. The Class II or Class III malocclusion could also be caused by the dental or muscular component. An Angle Class I bimaxillary protrusion is often seen in certain races and must be evaluated on racial norms and patient preference, not on the clinician's preconceived notion of an orthognathically ideal profile. The orthodontist should determine

whether these skeletal disharmonies are mild enough to be masked by conventional orthodontic treatment or whether a surgical approach should be undertaken. Many Class I bimaxillary protrusions can be treated orthodontically, but if a large open bite is present, surgery may be indicated. Class II malocclusions have been successfully resolved orthodontically; however, the clinician must take care when treating patients with these malocclusions that the midface or chin does not become too prominent. As a rule, Class III relationships that allow the teeth to come into edge-to-edge contact when the mandible is placed in its most retruded position can be successfully treated with conventional orthodontics, but the resulting soft tissue profile must again be considered in evaluating the patient. More severe Class III relationships often require a combined orthognathic surgical approach.

Assessment of the Dental Component

Diastemas or crowded teeth may be evidence of a poor tooth size/arch length ratio. The teeth may be too large or too small for the basal bone present. Other causes, such as early loss of primary teeth with resultant mesial migration of the posterior teeth, must be ruled out. Other concerns are congenitally absent or impacted teeth, whether long standing edentulous areas exhibit bite collapse, and whether the periodontal integrity has been threatened by tipping or crowded teeth.

Assessment of the Muscular Component

Deviation of the mandible laterally, anteriorly, or posteriorly during closure may be caused by muscular imbalances or by cuspal interferences causing the muscles to deflect the mandible. Pernicious habits may exert an undue influence on the dentition.

Evaluation of the Mandibular Arch

The present arch dimensions and any expected growth changes may be adequate to permit alignment of the teeth without expansion or additional space may be required to align the teeth properly. Needed space may be able to be gained by interproximal reduction of the enamel or with the extraction of teeth.

Evaluation of the Maxillary Arch and Its Relationship to the Mandibular Arch

Space requirements may be similar to those in the mandible. In addition, using the mandibular molar position as a guide the maxillary molars may require repositioning to provide a Class I interdigitation (Fig. 15-1).

The mandibular incisor teeth may be used as a guide to determine what anteroposterior and vertical movements are required.

FUNDAMENTALS OF ORTHODONTICS— TYPES OF MOVEMENTS

Types of Appliances

Orthodontic tooth movements may be accomplished with many different types of orthodontic appliances. General dentists

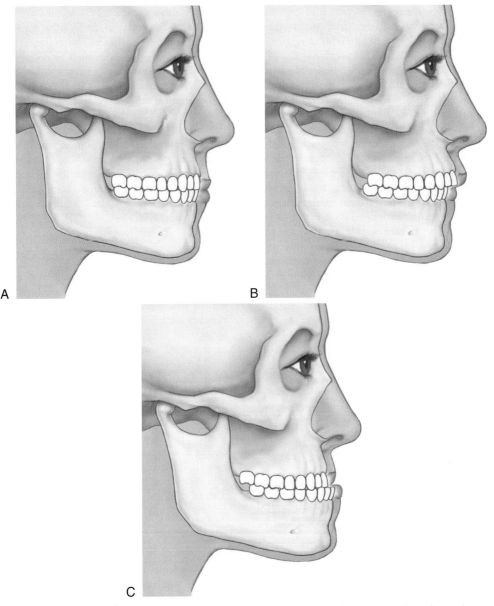

FIGURE 15-1 A, Molar relationship in a normal Angle Class I occlusion. **B,** Molar relationship in an Angle Class II malocclusion. **C,** Molar relationship in an Angle Class III malocclusion. Adapted from Morcos SS, Patel PK. The vocabulary of dentofacial deformities. Clin Plast Surg 34(3):589-99, 2007.

typically use clear aligner therapy, whereas orthodontic specialists have many other appliance choices. Some examples of typical orthodontic appliances are as follows:

1. Anterior ceramic or plastic brackets bonded to the *facial surfaces* of the teeth
2. Metal brackets bonded to the *facial surfaces* of the teeth
3. Lingual appliance—Specially designed metal brackets can be bonded to the lingual surfaces of teeth. Specially designed lingual arch wires must be used and the biomechanics of treatment must be analyzed to use this appliance.
4. Hawley appliance—A removable acrylic and metal wire appliance that can move teeth or can be used as a retainer (Fig. 15-2A).
5. Functional appliances (e.g., Andresen, Bimler, Fränkel, Monobloc)—Removable appliances can fit over the teeth and reposition the maxilla or mandible to stimulate growth of the jaws to obtain the desired occlusion. Some of the

appliances have plastic flanges that fit in the labial vestibule and prevent the buccal and orofacial musculature from contacting the teeth, thereby allowing some expansion of the jaws.
6. Spring aligners are removable appliances that can correct anterior tooth malpositions such as minor crowding or spacing. Anterior teeth are reset in an ideal setup in wax on a stone model. A removable appliance with active springs is fabricated over this ideal setup and the appliance is worn full time until the teeth achieve an acceptable alignment (Figs. 15-2BC). It may then be worn at night as a retainer.
7. Clear aligners—Invisalign (Align Technology, Inc.), Insignia Clearguide (Ormco Corp.), or ClearCorrect (ClearCorrect) PVC vacuum formed appliances. Most clear aligners are sequentially fabricated through a three-dimensional computer technology to improve the position of the teeth incrementally. Essix appliances (Raintree Essix, Dentsply International) can be fabricated by either the clinician or the laboratory technician.

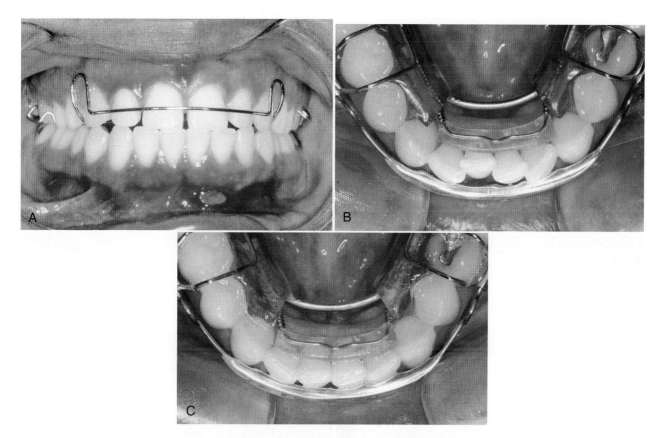

FIGURE 15-2 A, Anterior view of a maxillary Hawley appliance inserted to reduce spacing between anterior teeth. **B,** Preorthodontic view and **(C)** postorthodontic view (6 months of treatment) showing a removable appliance with active springs used to correct anterior crowding.

The most common modality used by general dentists is clear aligners such as the Invisalign System. Clear aligners have made it easier for the generalist to apply orthodontic forces to correct or improve malocclusions without the need for fixed traditional orthodontic therapy. A series of thermoplastic removable aligners achieve predictable movements. After treatment, occlusal stability must be ensured. An adjustment to the occlusion is usually necessary to balance the dentition in maximal intercuspation and all excursive movements. Changes in the occlusion occur during fixed and removable orthodontic treatment and the definitive positions of the teeth must have stability and long-term retention. Relapse can easily result from reoccurring interocclusal interferences during maximal intercuspation and/or excursive movements if the occlusion is not evaluated and adjusted, if necessary, at the end of any active phase of orthodontics. Proper training in this, and any approach to orthodontic therapy, is mandatory.

If Invisalign is used then, treatment begins with a Clin-Check design (Align Technology, Inc.), a web-based software product that creates and analyzes the dentition and creates a staged three-dimensional plan on virtual diagnostic casts. ClinCheck plans that are designed by the company should not to be accepted as a fully accurate representation of what the clinical outcome will be. Because of variability in the amount of time a patient wears the aligners, the fit of the aligners, the elasticity of the aligner material, and an individual's physiologic responses to tooth movement, the proposed treatment plan may produce a treatment outcome that will be quite different than anticipated by the ClinCheck plans. The technicians involved in the treatment plans must be instructed by the dentist as to what the treatment objectives are for each patient. Each step (i.e., aligner change) needs to be evaluated by the doctor, who must predict if this plan will work. Clinicians can be as involved in the design as they wish to be. Some will design their own tooth movement sequences and attachment designs and others will rely on assistance from the laboratory. However, the dentist is ultimately responsible for treatment and results, even if assistance was requested. Treatment should begin only when the clinician is confident with the software-generated plan. Cases with questionable outcomes or questionable mechanics should be referred to an orthodontist.

With any removable device, tooth movement is dependent on proper patient compliance. Intermittent forces from less than ideal compliance result in the inability to attain the definitive treatment goals, which further results in orthodontic relapse, as will interocclusal interferences left unattended at the end of the active phase of orthodontics.

CLINICAL TIP

Long-term compliance with the retainer is critical to maintain correction.

Clear Aligner Attachments

To enhance tooth movement with clear aligner therapy, small bonded shapes are placed on specific teeth with a template as a guide (Fig. 15-3A).

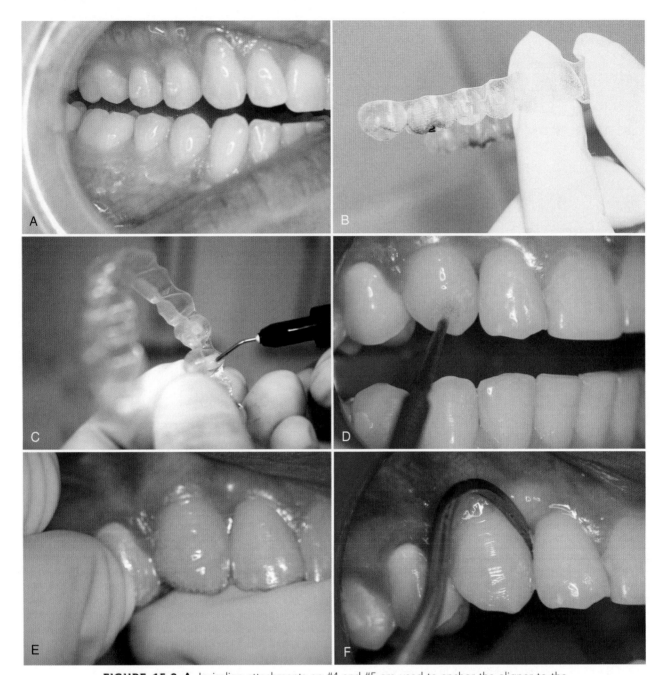

FIGURE 15-3 A, Invisalign attachments on #4 and #5 are used to anchor the aligner to the teeth and control tooth movement. **B,** An Invisalign attachment template will form the shape of the attachment. **C,** Composite is loaded into the Invisalign attachment template to form the shape of the attachment. **D,** The etch and prime are placed on a slightly larger surface area to allow for overflow material. **E,** The composite loaded attachment template is placed over the teeth and light cured. **F,** Excess composite is removed around the finished attachment and rough edges are smoothed.

The attachments help to optimize root control, extrusive movements and help with rotations. Originally, only oval attachments were available to assist the clear aligners with anchorage for tooth movements. Currently there are several types of clear aligner attachment shapes used to achieve specific tooth movements. These attachments not only provide the aligners with a better grip on the teeth, but also deliver a broader pushing surface to achieve a more controlled movement.

CLINICAL TIP

The technicians will help select the best attachment design for the specific movements that are requested. However, clinicians can further customize the attachment design and override a technician's suggestion.

Clear aligner cases that are sequentially fabricated through a three-dimensional computer technology are delivered with an attachment template along with a series of aligners. The attachment template (Fig. 15-3B) is a thinner, passive aligner, which is designed to create the shape of the desired attachments. After etching and priming the teeth, unpolymerized composite resin is placed into the wells of the template, which is then placed onto the maxillary and mandibular arches. The composite resin is light cured through the template plastic, the template is removed, and excess composite resin is eliminated.

CLINICAL TIP

Load the composite resin material into the attachment wells before etching and priming the teeth. The preloaded attachment template can be place in a closed retainer case to prevent the resin from premature curing.

CLINICAL TIP

The entire tooth should not be etched and primed. Use the software used to design the aligners to determine the specific area of the tooth on which the attachment will be placed (Fig. 15-3C). Then etch and prime a slightly larger surface area to allow for overflow material (Fig. 15-3D) to extend slightly beyond the limits of the attachment borders (Fig. 15-3E).

CLINICAL TIP

When loading the attachments into the wells, overload slightly to allow for a little bit of spreading (Fig. 15-3F). This will increase the attachment strength. After removing the excess composite resin, remove any sharp edges along the borders of the composite resin attachments.

Precision cuts serve as hooks in the plastic, which allow for the placement of interarch elastics. Precision cuts serve as hooks in the plastic that allow elastics to be used from maxillary to mandibular arches. The location of the cuts will create a direction of force, which will assist in directing the movements of the teeth. The direction of the elastic pull will determine the movement. The desired effect from the elastics is achieved only if the elastic is stretched in a way that favors the movements of the teeth. To correct a Class II malocclusion, a vector of force can be achieved with elastics stretched from the maxillary anterior teeth to the mandibular molars. A Class III force can be achieved with elastics directed from the mandibular anterior teeth to the maxillary molars. The resultant movement depends on patient compliance with proper wearing of the elastics with the clear aligners.

TREATMENT OF CLINICAL PROBLEMS— GENERAL CONSIDERATIONS

For the sake of simplicity, each type of malocclusion is discussed as a single entity. Often, however, the patient exhibits a combination of disharmonies. The definitive treatment plan must account for all the factors causing a malocclusion, allowing the dentist to select the most appropriate mechanotherapy to treat the particular patient.

Generalized Spacing

Diagnosis. Generalized spacing can be caused by the following:
1. Small teeth
2. A large tongue
3. Generalized spacing is confirmed by measuring the size of the teeth on diagnostic casts.
4. A component of a more severe syndrome
5. A combination of one or more of the above

Generalized spacing is confirmed by measuring the size of the teeth on diagnostic casts. These conditions may be treated successfully with restorations by the general dentist, orthodontic space closure, or a combination of both orthodontics and restorative dentistry

If diastemata are localized, the clinician should suspect sucking or tongue habits. A large tongue that is physiologically active usually has a scalloped edge because of constantly pushing against the teeth. Sucking habits can range from involvement of the thumb to several fingers turned in various positions when placed in the mouth. The fingers that are used in a sucking habit invariably are cleaner than their neighbors and often exhibit a callus where the mandibular incisors contact them.

Treatment. Elimination of pernicious habits is never easy but can be accomplished if the clinician is patient, persistent, and, most importantly, enlists the cooperation of the patient. The first step is to convince the patient that it is his or her responsibility to break the habit and that the doctor only offers assistance. It is helpful to encourage young patients to "give permission" for their parents to remind them that the habit exists. However, parents should not force the patient to stop. Start with small successes and build on them. It is essential to avoid discouraging the patient if small episodes of backsliding occur.

The plethora of devices used to break sucking habits speaks for their lack of singular success. They may be used, but should be considered adjuncts to the primary treatment previously described. Wearing cotton gloves is sometimes successful, as is the use of a bitter substance placed on the finger or fingernail used during the habit. Success can often be obtained by asking the patient to wear an elastic bandage around the elbow during the times the patient is concentrating on breaking the habit (usually at bedtime and reading time and while watching television). The patient's parent should place the bandage so that no pressure occurs when the arm is extended. It should become tight when the elbow is bent. The resultant pressure on the elbow reminds the patient of the desire to stop the sucking habit. Frequent office visits reinforce patient progress. After the habit has been stopped, the spaces may correct by themselves or orthodontic closure may sometimes be necessary.

Diastema Closure via Arch Contracture

In order to treat multiple spacing with contraction of the maxillary arch, the orthodontist must ensure that the mandibular antagonist does not interfere with movement.

The most common generalized spacing situations involve anterior spacing and well aligned, Class I molar and premolar occlusion with tight interproximal contacts. The spaces occur most

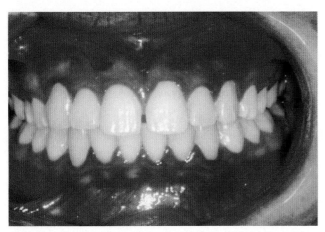

FIGURE 15-4 Anterior view of a patient with a diastema between the maxillary central incisors.

often due to outward tongue pressures against the lingual surfaces of the maxillary and mandibular incisors. The proclination of the incisors also may lead to maxillary and mandibular lip protrusion. The most effective way to eliminate this condition is to retract and intrude both the maxillary and mandibular anterior teeth simultaneously. Although the chief complaint will often refer to maxillary diastemata, the key to the correction is the retraction of the mandibular incisors, which would otherwise interfere with the retraction of the maxillary teeth (Fig. 15-4).

Mandibular spacing often occurs in these situations as well. In some instances, there are either no mandibular anterior spaces or mild crowding, which will then require interproximal reduction (IPR) to reposition the mandibular anterior teeth lingually. Intruding the mandibular anterior teeth during the retraction will help minimize these interferences. An evaluation must be performed for the presence of interferences between the mandibular incisal edges and the palatal and incisal surfaces of the maxillary incisors.

CLINICAL TIP

Sometimes the dentist must specify in the treatment plan that the aligners need to simultaneously intrude and retract the incisors. Since the incisal third of the anterior teeth is so much thinner than the gingival third, if the patient has a deep bite, intrusion will allow for more retraction. Without intrusion, the retraction potential is more limited.

LOCALIZED SPACING—CLINICALLY ABSENT TEETH

Diagnosis. Causes of the clinical absence of teeth include the following:
1. Congenitally missing teeth
2. Unerupted teeth
3. Premature loss of permanent teeth
4. Supernumerary teeth that prevent normal eruption
5. A combination of the above

Overlong retention of primary teeth can cause ectopic impaction of the permanent successors. Congenitally missing lateral incisors are discussed later in this chapter in the section on localized spacing of maxillary central incisors. The diagnosis ultimately is confirmed by examination of the appropriate radiographs.

Prosthetic treatment sometimes is complicated by the mesiodistal drifting of teeth adjacent to the edentulous space. This drifting can occur through tipping or bodily movement. In the latter situation, the crown and the apex of the root move bodily through the bone with the long axis of the tooth remaining perpendicular to the occlusal plane. In the former condition, the crown tips mesially or distally ahead of the apex of the root. Radiographs confirm the type of movement that has occurred.

CLINICAL TIP

A tipped tooth always must be brought upright so that the crown is positioned over the apex. This provides a stable result.

Attempts to correct a mesiodistally drifted tooth with an abnormally proportioned restoration often create periodontal problems. Therefore, teeth should be orthodontically uprighted before prosthetic treatment.

Treatment. Ectopic impaction should be treated by extraction of the primary teeth. If less than half of the root has formed, the permanent tooth usually is delayed in eruption. If more than half of the root is present and the tooth has failed to erupt despite the loss of the primary tooth, surgical exposure of the crown may be required, often followed by mechanical orthodontic therapy to force eruption of the tooth.

Congenitally missing teeth can be treated by prosthetic replacement. However, orthodontic intervention often is necessary if adjacent teeth have shifted mesiodistally.

LOCALIZED SPACING OF MAXILLARY CENTRAL INCISORS

Because of the great esthetic impact of localized spacing of the maxillary central incisors, this condition is described separately. The most common causes of this spacing are as follows:
1. Normal growth
2. Imperfect fusion of the midline
3. Enlarged labial frenum
4. Congenitally missing lateral incisors
5. Supernumerary teeth (mesiodens)
6. Anatomically small clinical crowns

CLINICAL TIP

Clinical examination of the frenum, along with lifting of the maxillary lip to note any blanching of the mucosa on the palate between the central incisors, will confirm an enlarged or malpositioned labial frenum.

Radiographic evidence will confirm a spade-shaped septum when the labial frenum is malpositioned. This radiologic characteristic also is seen in imperfect fusion of the midline, but in such situations no blanching of the frenum occurs when the lip is stretched. Supernumerary teeth and congenitally missing lateral incisors are confirmed with radiographs. Spacing as part of normal growth also can occur in patients with small bony bases and large teeth. The large crowns of the developing and unerupted lateral incisors and canines push the central incisor roots mesially toward each other, causing the central incisor crowns to erupt with a distal inclination and an accompanying diastema. Anatomically small teeth may be confirmed by measurement.

Treatment

Normal Growth. If the spacing is determined to be part of normal growth, observe the patient until the lateral incisors and canines have erupted. In many instances, the diastema closes during the normal eruption process.

Imperfect Fusion of the Midline. In the primary and mixed dentition, imperfect fusion of the midline becomes evident with the eruption of the permanent anterior teeth, including the canines, and should be treated in the permanent dentition stage. Treatment of imperfect fusion of the midline in the permanent dentition consists of moving the teeth together and retaining the positions.

DIASTEMA CLOSURE—REMOVABLE APPLIANCE

Simple closure of a maxillary midline diastema often creates spacing distally. For this reason, restorative dentistry may also be required to achieve proper esthetics (see Fig. 15-12).

The maxillary midline diastema is one of the most common chief complaints. The midline diastema in some patients is accompanied by small maxillary lateral incisors and/or mild mandibular crowding. There is usually a history of the familial maxillary midline diastema with a slow increase in diastema size over time. If restorations for enlargement of the lateral incisors are planned, the maxillary midline diastema can be closed and this space can be distributed distally and evenly between the lateral incisors. If there is no plan to change the dimension of the maxillary lateral incisors, then this situation is treated similarly to the generalized diastemata treatment plan. The goal is to retract and intrude the mandibular anterior teeth followed by maxillary anterior teeth retraction and intrusion. Mild mandibular crowding and/or the absence of anterior diastemata require IPR to allow for the retraction and intrusion of the mandibular incisors.

CLINICAL TIP

Evaluation of the occlusion with articulating paper is necessary following diastema closure. This will ensure stability and help prevent relapse. Use articulating paper to mark incisal edges during centric and protrusive/excursive movements. Once marked, the edges must be reduced carefully to allow for even function among each of the incisors. If there are excessive labially directed forces from an interference with the central incisors, then the diastema will reoccur when the retainer is removed. Closure of the diastema occurs nightly as the retainer is worn. The patient will complain of a "strange bite" in the morning after retainer removal and the inability to touch the posterior teeth together. This will self-correct very soon after the appliance is out of the mouth (Fig. 15-5).

DIASTEMA CLOSURE—FIXED APPLIANCE

Fixed appliances require that the generalist be absolutely familiar with all aspects of fixed orthodontic therapy. Failure to adhere to proper orthodontic technique could have adverse consequences. Because simple closure of a maxillary midline diastema often

creates spacing distally, restorative dentistry may also be required to achieve proper esthetics. To confidently maintain the space closure of the maxillary midline diastema, a fixed bonded retainer is suggested. Place a bonded wire palatally from central incisor to central incisor (Ortho-Flextech 30-inch gold chain [Reliance Orthodontic Products]). The bonded retainer must be out of occlusion or it will debond, causing flaring of the maxillary incisors, or cause unwanted movement of the mandibular incisors.

Enlarged or Malpositioned Frenum

Treatment and retention are identical to those described in the section on Generalized Spacing of maxillary central incisors earlier in this chapter except that a frenectomy is necessary.

Supernumerary Teeth

Supernumerary teeth—for example, a mesiodens—must be extracted. After removal of the supernumerary tooth in the primary or mixed dentition, normal tooth eruption may correct the situation. If spacing, ectopic eruption, or malposition persists, use conventional orthodontic therapy. In the permanent dentition, conventional orthodontic therapy is required.

Congenitally Missing Lateral Incisors

Congenitally missing permanent lateral incisors are not clinically evident in the primary dentition. If the condition is suspected from the family history, radiographs may be taken.

In the mixed dentition, congenitally missing lateral incisors can be clinically distinguished from other causes of localized spacing of the maxillary central incisors by overretention of the primary lateral incisors. Radiographs confirm the diagnosis.

In the permanent dentition, congenitally missing lateral incisors present the clinician with one of the greatest esthetic challenges. If the canines are slender, the spaces may be closed and the canines contoured to resemble the missing lateral incisors. This is often difficult because of the bulkiness of the canine. Several restorative approaches can be taken, dictated by the anatomic relationships present. Consultation and coordination of treatment objectives between the generalist and the orthodontic specialist are essential. The introduction of new esthetic materials has enhanced the resolution of these cases.

Anatomically Small Teeth

Anatomically small teeth are best treated with esthetic restorative materials. Occlusal interferences from the mandibular dentition may cause spacing or prevent attempts at space closure. Both arches must be treated to resolve these situations properly.

LABIOVERSION OF THE MAXILLARY INCISORS

Labioversion of the maxillary incisors is a type of malocclusion usually caused by adverse oral habits such as thumb or finger sucking. The generalist is likely to see these patients first, when palliative treatment of oral habits might prevent the condition from fully developing and reversal may occur. Therefore,

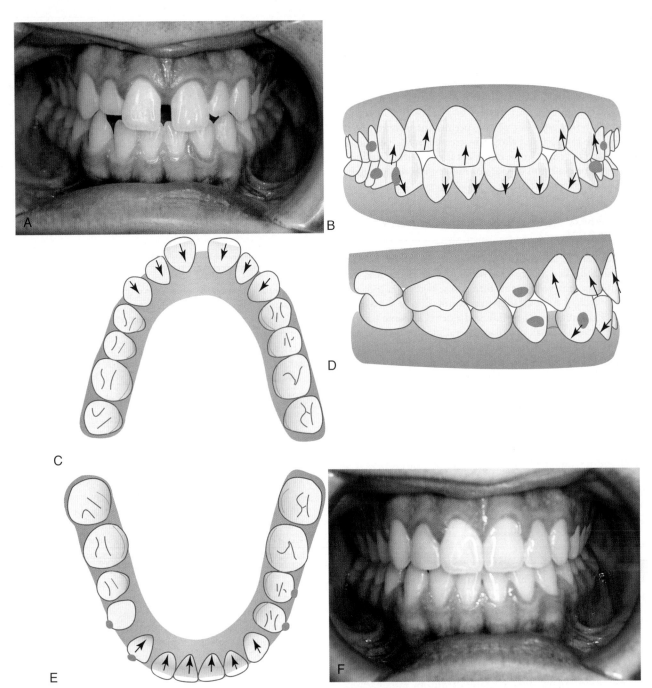

FIGURE 15-5 A, An example of a spacing situation treated with Invisalign. The patient will have veneers placed on both maxillary lateral incisors at the end of orthodontic treatment. **B-E,** The arrows show the direction of force. Retraction and intrusion of the anterior teeth is necessary to close anterior spaces. **F,** This is the clinical outcome from Invisalign space closure with retraction and intrusion of the anterior teeth. Porcelain veneers were placed on the maxillary lateral incisors to maximize the esthetic outcome.

carly diagnosis and treatment or referral is essential. If serial extraction is selected, the clinician is committed to following the patient's treatment through the time of full eruption of the permanent dentition. The patient and the patient's parents should be advised of the extended nature of this type of correction and that treatment may include further fixed appliance therapy. However, such intervention usually tends to simplify and shorten the duration of active orthodontic appliance therapy if it is required.

Diagnosis. Increased horizontal overlap of the maxillary anterior teeth often is combined with a Class I molar relationship. The amount of vertical overlap varies, but a deep curve of Spee is common because the mandibular anterior teeth overerupt when their antagonists' forward position cannot provide a normal occlusal stop. It is important not to confuse this with the situation of a Class II, division 1 malocclusion in which the mandibular molars have moved mesially into a Class I position because of the early loss of the deciduous molars. Although the latter instances also show both increased vertical overlap and horizontal overlap, the mandibular anterior teeth show extreme crowding as well.

Treatment. In the primary dentition, palliative control of oral habits is indicated. In mixed dentition, the elimination of oral habits also is indicated. Removable appliance therapy may be successful at this time. Selected serial extraction of the primary dentition may also influence the eruption pattern of the secondary teeth.

In the permanent dentition, full appliance mechanotherapy is used to open the bite and retract the anterior teeth. Oral habits also must be corrected for treatment to succeed.

LABIOLINGUALLY MALPOSITIONED TEETH

Diagnosis. Teeth may be labiolingually malpositioned for a number of reasons.

Normal Growth. Often no other malocclusion occurs except for a lingually or labially displaced tooth. This can be caused by overretained primary teeth or by the individual growth pattern of the patient. If a simple labiolingual displacement is involved, a removable Hawley appliance is used. If the teeth are rotated or tipped, fixed orthodontic appliance therapy is indicated.

Crowded Teeth. Crowded teeth usually result from teeth that are too large for the dental arch and are one of the most common patient complaints. Crowding is categorized as minor (4 mm or less), moderate (4-8 mm) and severe (more than 8 mm).

Arch Form Expansion. When considering expansion, the shape of the alveolar ridges must be assessed. If the teeth are overexpanded, they can move through the buccal plate of bone, leading to bone loss and recession. An anteroposterior cephalometric radiograph or cone beam scan can provide further information about the limits of the alveolar complex.

Unilateral and bilateral crossbites are often targeted for correction without consideration of the true width of the maxillary alveolar housing. The unilateral posterior crossbite is usually caused by maxillary constriction with an accompanying lateral shift of the mandible to the left or right (Fig. 15-6).

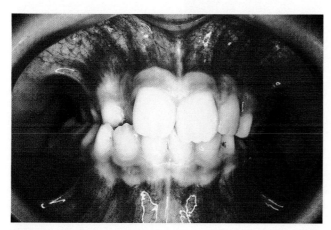

FIGURE 15-6 Frontal view showing a midline shift of the mandibular anterior teeth, which indicates that the maxilla is narrowed bilaterally and that the patient shifts to the right side into a "bite of convenience."

If the maxillary alveolar width is not considered, correction of the narrow arch with expansion without maxillary surgery to expand the alveolar housing will result in loss of buccal bone and recession from the lateral repositioning of the teeth. If a significant amount of expansion is planned, it is prudent to consult an oral surgeon to review the possible need for surgically assisted expansion. Consultation with a periodontist may also be considered to prevent recession and creation of dehiscences.

Proclination. Proclining anterior teeth can be an easy way to create space and is the same as arch expansion; however, it occurs in the anterior region. The limits of the anterior alveolar bone must be accessed prior to planning proclination, otherwise gingival recession can occur if the teeth are moved beyond the buccal plate of bone. Careful evaluation of the profile and lip posture at rest must be considered before beginning treatment. Definitive lip position will be determined by the definitive positions of the incisors.

Distalization. Distalization is a method of repositioning posterior teeth distally when third molars are not present. This is a vital part of conservative orthodontic treatment. Inadvertent proclination of the anterior teeth is the most common consequence of failing to consider principles of biomechanics. If basic anchorage requirements are not met, the resultant forces will cause the repositioning of the anterior teeth further forward rather than distalizing the posterior teeth.

Extraction. Extraction is often considered to eliminate crowding. The century-long debate over the need for the extraction of teeth to gain alignment is ongoing. Careful planning of space needed for the periodontally healthy alignment of teeth may prevent the need for extractions. Other space-gaining techniques, such as interproximal reduction, rotation corrections, and recontouring restorations, are considered more conservative and should be considered before the extraction option. In moderate to severe crowding conditions, combinations of space-gaining techniques can substitute for extractions. Patient acceptance is obviously higher with nonextraction approaches.

When extractions are planned, it is imperative that the roots of repositioned teeth remain parallel to those of the neighboring teeth. Root parallelism is necessary for masticatory forces to be directed along the long axis of the root of the tooth, thus minimally affecting the surrounding periodontium. This is difficult to accomplish with clear aligners but not impossible by positioning attachments that are oriented vertically. Mesial or distal root torque is important to lead the tip of the root towards the extraction spaces. The addition of the long vertical attachments ensures proper torquing forces. Although attachments are usually placed on the buccal surfaces of teeth, sometimes lingual attachments, which are also long and vertical, can help with root torquing.

CLINICAL TIP

Check the aligners to ensure that the teeth are tracking with the attachments. The term *tracking* refers to the evaluation of the movement of teeth as an aligner is replaced by the succeeding aligner. Insufficient space or insufficient force and patient noncompliance are the most common reason for teeth not tracking properly. The fit of the aligner should be tested and modified throughout the course of treatment. The attachments should be fully seated into the space for them in the aligner. It is imperative that the aligner and long vertical attachments are tracking because if they are not, the crowns will be tipping into the space and the roots will not move in the proper direction. Moving teeth bodily instead of tipping them ensures that the roots will be parallel. This allows for enhanced periodontal health by preventing pseudopockets and improved force application when in occlusion. Torquing forces are lost when the tracking is lost. Adding more attachment material is recommended to at least continue the general torquing direction but full control of the tooth has been lost and a midcourse correction will be needed. New impressions or a new scan as well as photographs need to be sent to the aligner company along with a revised treatment plan. Another way to remedy the problem is to place fixed traditional braces to correct the torque problem and upright the teeth on either side of the extraction space.

Interproximal Reduction. Interproximal reduction (IPR) is the process of removing enamel from the sides of a tooth, thus reducing the overall mesiodistal width. It allows for crowded teeth

to align better and fit over the alveolar bone. Conservative IPR can help eliminate mild to moderate crowding. Invisalign will usually aid in the planning of up to 0.5mm of IPR per tooth to minimize any risk of sensitivity or complications. Three methods of IPR are often used: hand stripping with diamond-coated strips, diamond-coated disks in a slow-speed handpiece, and a fine tip diamond bur on a high-speed handpiece (Fig. 15-7).

Hand Stripping with IPR Strips

Hand stripping with IPR strips (Fig. 15-8A) is the most conservative method. Strips come in many different variations to accommodate specific clinical situations; have varying thicknesses, which allow for varying the size of the space created; and are either single sided or double sided. Single-sided IPR strips allow the operator to reduce one tooth without affecting the adjacent tooth. Double-sided IPR strips allow the operator to simultaneously reduce two adjacent teeth. The level of roughness varies; coarse strips abrade the tooth surface quickly and effectively but leave a rough surface, which must be followed with a smoother finishing strip.

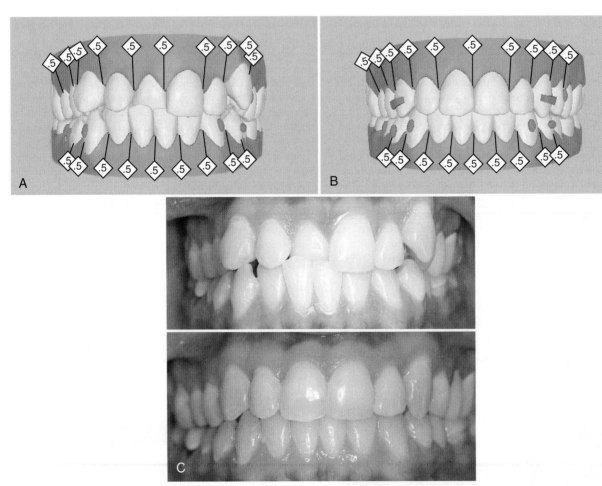

FIGURE 15-7 A, This crossbite and crowding situation was treated with Invisalign. IPR was used to create the space. The IPR amount and location are noted by the numbered flags. **B,** This is the predicted outcome for this situation. Horizontal attachments are to be placed on the maxillary canines to assist in extrusion of the canines. **C,** The clinical outcome is very similar to the predicted outcome from the ClinCheck design. The crossbite and the crowding were both corrected.

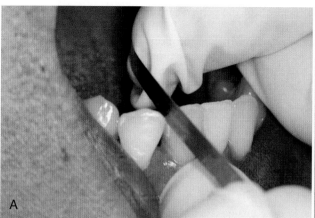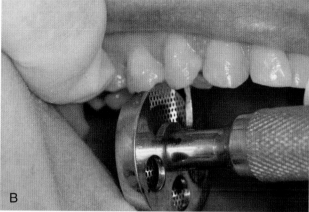

FIGURE 15-8 A, Hand stripping with an IPR strip. **B,** IPR with a disk and guard.

CLINICAL TIP

The finer the grit, the smoother the surface. Smooth surfaces, which are consistent with natural enamel, are the desired result and this can be achieved with finishing strips.

When IPR is performed by hand, the operator holds both sides of the strip and places it in the target area. The strip is manually driven through the contact point with a back-and-forth motion following the contours of the teeth.

CLINICAL TIP

If there is a plan to reduce only one surface, then a single-sided IPR strip is used with the rough side toward the target tooth. Sometimes a hand-stripping tool is used to hold and maintain tension on the strip, which makes it easier for the operator to perform the task. However, this instrument limits the degree to which the strip can follow the contours of the tooth because the amount of the tension along the strip is so high.

Patients will feel a sensation from the stretching of the periodontal ligament as the strip is manually driven through the contact point; however, there is only low-level discomfort and anesthesia is not necessary. Care must be taken because the surrounding soft tissue is easily injured during IPR.

CLINICAL TIP

Care must be taken to avoid accidental laceration and puncturing of the cheeks, lips, gingiva, or tongue. Use the non-working (third, fourth, or fifth) fingers to reflect the cheeks and lips. Constantly observe the location of the entire strip during the procedure. Focusing on stripping the tooth while accidentally disregarding the location of the ends and edges of the strip can lead to unexpected injuries.

Stripping With a Disk and Guard

Performing IPR with a disk and guard (a metal protective covering over the disk; Fig. 15-8B) is a very quick and effective method for creating larger IPR spaces but also can result in the most problems. The ideal clinical situation for using this method is when two teeth are in alignment and a clear path can be visualized from the point of insertion to the final gingival contact area. The entire path of the disk must be planned prior to beginning tooth reduction. . Once the initial cut is made, the angulation of the disk cannot be changed. Changing the path of the disk creates ledges and will leave the IPR space larger than intended. This technique is relatively painless but because of the higher risk of iatrogenic injury, should only be attempted when the dentist has the utmost confidence in the entire path of the disk.

CLINICAL TIP

It is imperative that a guard be used. Accidental cutting of the lip with the disk can easily occur.

Using dental floss to simulate the entire path of the disk will aid in ensuring that the proposed path of the disk is properly evaluated. If the floss must be repositioned as it travels through the proposed path of the disk, then the disk will also need to be similarly repositioned. Because the disk should not be repositioned once the cut is started, the use of a disk in this instance is contraindicated. Angling the disk properly before beginning the cut is crucial. If the entire path cannot be visualized, this technique should not be used. It also should not be used if a large amount of overlapping exists because angled cuts will be created, ultimately resulting in irregular contact points. Using a disk in an area of tooth overlapping or crowding will also significantly increase the chances of creating ledges and/or accidental cutting of adjacent teeth. This can very easily occur in the canine area because the palatal cusp of the first premolar can deflect the disk pathway.

CLINICAL TIP

It is difficult to use the disk in the molar area. The ideal angle of the disk path is inconsistent with the angle that is necessary to allow the disk to reach its depth without the handpiece contacting the patient's anterior teeth or lip. Hand stripping is preferred in this situation. If IPR is performed through a restoration that is to be replaced, the use of a fine-tipped diamond bur is also acceptable.

The use of a finetipped smooth diamond bur in a high-speed handpiece is useful to retain the architecture of the enamel surface. After hand stripping or disking, the resulting sharp edges should be finished with a fine diamond bur. This will ensure proper contact areas when the teeth are aligned. A fine-tipped bur can be used to reduce this surface, but the amount of IPR will be difficult to quantify and must be performed in increments to ensure that the desired amount of reduction is not surpassed (Fig. 15-9).

> ## CLINICAL TIP
>
> Successful treatment of labiolingually malpositioned teeth requires adequate space within which to reposition the malpositioned tooth. If this space is not present or cannot be created, complete orthodontic therapy by a specialist is required.

Rotated Teeth

Diagnosis. When spaces are present, the teeth often not only migrate mesiodistally but also may rotate. In addition, overretention of primary teeth may cause abnormal eruption patterns of the permanent tooth, causing abnormal rotational eruption.

Treatment. In the primary and mixed dentition, early diagnosis of overretained primary teeth is imperative. Extraction of the offending tooth often leads to self-correction. Appliance therapy is not recommended at this time. In the permanent dentition, orthodontic correction is necessary.

Rotations are achievable using Invisalign and other clear aligners with relatively consistent results in the mandibular anterior regions. Maintaining the axis of rotations along the long axis of the root is crucial to rotations. Simultaneously introducing torquing while rotating the tooth is possible with attachments that counteract the intrusive and/or extrusive movements produced.

The maxillary central incisors are among the easier teeth to rotate. The anatomy allows for the plastic aligners to maintain the correct position on the teeth and remain completely seated (i.e.. track properly). Maxillary lateral incisors are harder to rotate. Smaller lateral incisors are hard to control with precision because their shape is difficult for the plastic to hold tightly and effectively. The more a lateral incisor is shaped like a peg, the more difficult it is to control. The broader the tooth is mesiodistally, the easier it is to control. Rotating around the long axis of the tooth is crucial. Rotations of canines differ due to their

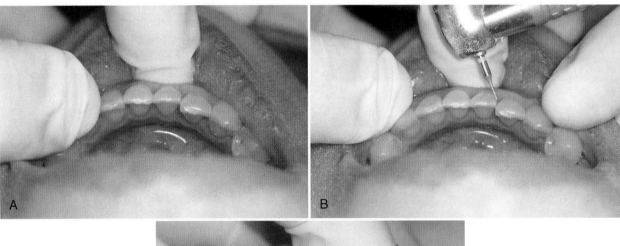

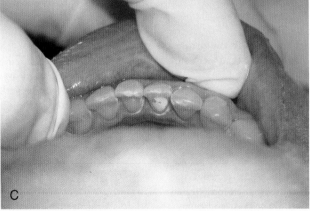

FIGURE 15-9 A, After using an IPR strip between the mandibular right central and lateral incisors, the sides of the teeth have corners that need to be rounded to mimic natural anatomy. **B,** A fine-tipped diamond bur is used to smooth off the corners of the teeth after IPR is performed with either hand stripping or a disk. **C,** Using a fine-tipped diamond bur allows the contours of the teeth to be more anatomically accurate after the hand stripping or IPR with a disk.

shape. The maxillary canines are pointed and the convergent profile and circular shaped circumference leads to easy slippage between the tooth and the aligner. Attachments can aid rotations, especially the new optimized attachments. These attachments have a teardrop shape, which is oriented in a manner that increases the grip of the aligner on the tooth, allowing for more predictable and reproducible rotations. The maxillary premolars are also difficult to control without attachments because of their circular shape as viewed from the occlusal. Buccal and lingual attachments enable rotations using a coupled force to better control the premolar rotation. Maxillary molars are relatively easy to rotate and doing so can create a considerable amount of space. This is often not considered. The rhomboid shape of the molar as viewed from the occlusal allows for relatively predictable rotations.

Rotating mandibular incisors is a relatively predictable movement. The fanlike shapes are easy for the plastic to control. The mandibular canines and premolars are just as difficult as their maxillary counterparts to rotate. Attachments are needed. Mandibular molar rotations are similar to maxillary molar rotations and have reproducible results as long as the degree of rotational discrepancy is relatively minimal and attachments are used.

CLINICAL TIP

Relapse is common after rotational correction of malpositioned teeth. Overcorrection is recommended to compensate for this relapse. Permanent retention can be achieved by bonding the lingual surface of the tooth to the adjacent teeth with a thin orthodontic wire embedded in composite resin.

Extruded Teeth

Diagnosis and Etiology. An extrusion occurs when a tooth has overerupted past the normal plane of occlusion. It is most commonly seen when opposing teeth are absent, have not fully erupted possibly because of ankylosis, or exhibit periodontal involvement.

Treatment. The correction of extrusion is possible with clear aligners if the tooth has an attachment that can maintain tracking with the aligner throughout the entire path of the extrusion. If the aligner is not fully seated, accurate tooth movement is interrupted, the intrusion ceases, and relapse often occurs in a very short period. If interocclusal forces are present on the extruding tooth, it will be forced back to its original position if the aligner ceases to fully seat on the tooth. Compliance is a critical factor. Attachment design must be considered carefully. Horizontal flat surfaces for the attachments that are perpendicular to the direction of the extrusive forces are crucial in producing this movement.

Intruded Teeth

Diagnosis and Etiology. Causes of intrusion of teeth can be ankylosis, habits such as thumb sucking or pipe smoking, or trauma. Teeth intruded because of ankylosis are impossible to move orthodontically and often require prosthetic treatment to correct esthetic problems. Traumatically intruded teeth or teeth that require extrusion because of traumatic loss of the clinical crown can be extruded orthodontically. The principles discussed in the section on Extruded Teeth apply, except that the forces are reversed.

Treatment. Intrusion is a movement that involves pushing a tooth gingivally toward its periodontal housing. Intrusive forces are possible with clear aligners. The degree and accuracy of the intrusive movement depend on the amount of time the force is delivered. With good compliance a tooth can intrude with relatively predictability as long as there is enough space to do so and compliance with the wearing of the aligners is 22 hours per day. If an adjacent tooth interferes with the path of intrusion, IPR might be necessary.

CLINICAL TIP

To achieve predictable intrusion, there is a need for attachments on adjacent teeth, which will serve as an anchor. The tooth that is being intruded does not need an attachment. The force on the incisal edge plastic will move the tooth. If an intruded tooth will eventually become an anchorage unit, an attachment is recommended.

These patients normally can be diagnosed upon clinical examination, but space requirements are easier to determine when diagnostic casts are used.

Crossbite

Diagnosis and Etiology. A crossbite is an aberrant occlusal relationship wherein a maxillary tooth is lingually positioned relative to its ideal position relative to an antagonist tooth (or teeth) or the mandibular tooth is facially positioned relative to its ideal position relative to an antagonist tooth (or teeth). Crossbites can involve a single tooth or multiple teeth, can be bilateral or unilateral, and are often classified as anterior or posterior. Anterior crossbites are typical of Class III skeletal relations (prognathism). Causation can be dental or skeletal.

Treatment. The use of a removable appliance is indicated when space is sufficient. A Hawley appliance with either an acrylic inclined plane or a finger spring to push the tooth into position is used (Fig. 15-10*A*). The finger spring appliance incorporates an occlusal plane to prevent the mandibular incisors from occluding. This type of appliance is used when a true crossbite relationship exists. The inclined plane appliance (Fig. 15-10*B*) is used when the patient can incise in an edge-to-edge relationship when closing into the most retruded mandibular position but the mandible slips anterior into a bite of convenience during mastication. Sometimes, especially when space is insufficient, it is necessary to use full appliance therapy with Class III mechanics to correct the crossbite (Figs. 15-10*C,D*).

The correction of a single-tooth crossbite is very effective with clear aligners due to the ability of the plastic to disocclude the jaws. The plastic shields the tooth from interocclusal forces that create relapse. As the tooth moves toward the corrected position, the opposing tooth is moving in an equal and opposite direction, making the collision heavier as the tooth travel toward the point where the teeth hit edge to edge. Constant shielding of the teeth in crossbite is critical in preventing the relapse during moments the teeth are not covered with the aligner. Once the tooth has passed the edge-to-edge relationship, the interocclusal forces on the crossbite tooth will favor the direction of correction.

Single-tooth crossbite corrections require space and IPR is usually a necessary method to assist the crowded tooth in

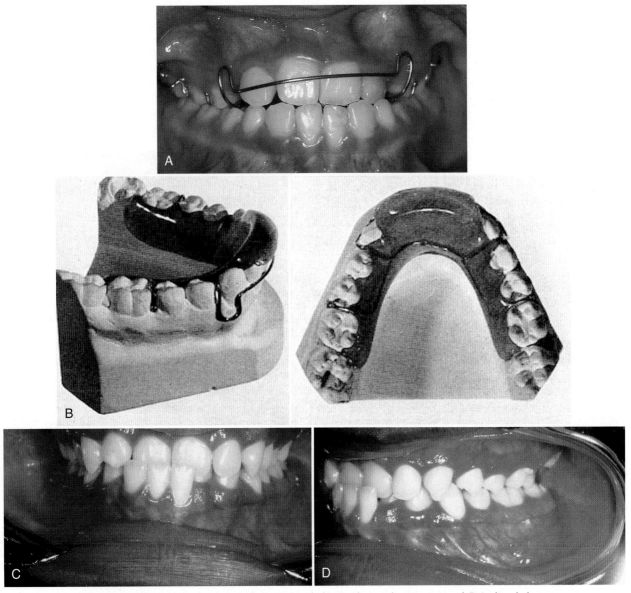

FIGURE 15-10 A, Occlusal view of a patient with the Hawley appliance engaged. **B,** Inclined plane appliance. **C,** Frontal view and (**D**) left labial view of a patient with an anterior crossbite involving the maxillary central incisors and the mandibular right lateral, right central, and left central incisors.

crossbite. Distributing the IPR among several teeth is often needed to overcome larger amounts of crowding around a blocked-out tooth. Single-tooth crossbites can occur in any region of the mouth. It is always necessary to check the occlusion and occlusally and esthetically adjust the tooth once the tooth is out of crossbite. Usually, there are uneven wear patterns on the corrected tooth.

Anterior Open Bite

Diagnosis. An open bite occurs when teeth of the opposing arches do not meet when the teeth are in maximal intercuspal position (Fig. 15-11).

Treatment often is complicated, and diagnosis usually requires clinical evaluation along with examination of diagnostic casts and cephalometric and panoramic radiographs (see Fig. 15-11). Anterior open bites can occur with any type of molar relationship. The

generalist may wish to consult a specialist about these patients. Ankylosed teeth may require alternative treatments.

Diagnosis. Deleterious habits, such as finger, lip, or tongue sucking, are the causes of anterior open bites in children. Constant biting on pencils or on the stem of a pipe can be the cause in adults. Sometimes the problem persists when the tongue fills the void. Gross osseous dysplasia, such as is seen in maxillary micrognathia, mandibular hypertrophy, or rickets, can give rise to an open bite, but this usually is a minor manifestation of the gross discrepancy.

Treatment. Treatment requires elimination of the habit. See the section on Generalized Spacing earlier in this chapter. Conventional orthodontic fixed appliance therapy with vertical elastics may be necessary to close the bite. In extreme situations a surgical orthognathic approach may be indicated. It is important to provide adequate stabilization of the teeth after orthodontic therapy.

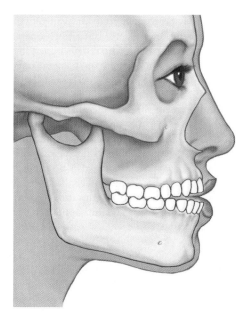

FIGURE 15-11 An anterior open bite.

Posterior Open Bite

Diagnosis. Tongue thrusting often is the suspected cause of a posterior open bite, but it is rarely the primary cause; it merely allows the problem to persist. Abnormal skeletal development is the primary cause of a bilateral posterior open bite. Ankylosis of primary or permanent teeth may also be the cause of a localized posterior open bite.

   Treatment. The etiology of the open bite must be considered when planning treatment.

   Skeletal Cause. A bilateral posterior open bite of skeletal origin must be treated with orthodontic mechanotherapy alone or combined with a orthognathic surgical approach.

   Muscular Cause. Although the tongue is rarely the primary cause of a posterior open bite, an appropriate appliance often must be constructed to keep the tongue from interfering with bite closure.

   Dental Cause. If the posterior open bite is caused by ankylosis of a primary tooth, radiographs must be taken to verify that a permanent tooth is present. Often this occurs when permanent teeth are congenitally absent. If the primary tooth is present, the primary tooth might need to be extracted and the permanent successor might need to be brought into position by an orthodontic specialist. If it is not present, alternative therapy includes attempting to rebuild the primary tooth to proper occlusion or extracting the tooth and placing an implant or fixed partial denture. If a permanent tooth is ankylosed, it cannot be moved orthodontically. The ankylosed tooth must be restored to proper occlusion prosthetically. If the ankylosed tooth cannot be restored, it should be extracted and prosthetically replaced.

Excessive Vertical Overlap

Excessive vertical overlap can occur with all types of molar relationships. Dental factors are often the cause in Class I malocclusions, whereas skeletal factors are often combined with dental factors in Class II or Class III malocclusions. The generalist most commonly works with a specialist to diagnose these patients, with the orthodontist treating the more complicated types.

   Diagnosis. Cephalometric analysis is necessary to confirm whether the problem is skeletal or dental in nature.

   Treatment. Diagnosis often can be made clinically, but it is confirmed with diagnostic casts and radiographic evidence. In the mixed and permanent dentition, if a Class I molar relationship exists, use a bite plate to allow the first molars to erupt and the curve of Spee to decrease. Diagnosis often can be made clinically, but it is confirmed with diagnostic casts and radiographic evidence. Usually seen in adults with any molar relationship, a closed bite is best diagnosed and treated through a team approach. Diagnosis often can be made clinically, but it is confirmed with diagnostic casts and radiographic evidence.

   Diagnosis. In situations involving areas that have been edentulous for a long period, teeth commonly have tipped into a neighboring extraction site or supererupted from the opposing dental arch. A loss of arch length and posterior bite collapse, resulting in a closing or deepening of the bite, results in an exaggerated curve of Spee.

   Treatment. The bite is opened by orthodontic movement of tipped and intruded teeth in preparation for prosthetic rehabilitation. The removal of the orthodontic appliances should occur on the same day as preparation for fixed prosthetic replacements because the provisional restoration acts as a retainer.

LATERAL DISHARMONIES OF THE TEETH AND DENTAL ARCHES

Lateral disharmonies of the teeth and dental arches appear in patients of all ages, without regard to anteroposterior molar relationships. Lateral disharmonies result in excess wearing of the cusps that normally maintain a functional occlusal relationship. Because cuspal wear is generally a function of time, the earlier the treatment is instituted, the more successful and stable the definitive result.

   Diagnosis. Diagnostic casts will show cuspal wear, but a clinical examination is required to determine whether the disharmony is unilateral or bilateral and whether it is caused by a skeletal or muscular deviation from normal development.

   Skeletal Cause. With a skeletal cause, there is a gross disharmony between the bony bases. Unilateral crossbites exhibit a deviation of the midline of the two jaws when the teeth are in occlusion. Bilateral crossbites may have a normal midline relationship or may mimic a unilateral crossbite with a shifted midline. The difference is that this shift is one of convenience and occurs at the last moment of mandibular closure. If the mandible is placed in its most retruded position and slowly closed, the midline will be centered until just before occlusal contact is made.

   Muscular Cause. Occlusal interference develops because of an aberrant muscular closing pattern.

   Dental Cause. In this situation the condition often is the result of lack of space in the dental arch. It usually involves tipped teeth and sometimes is accompanied by a muscular shift.

   Treatment. Treatment of these conditions can be handled by the experienced generalist, especially when dealing with the dental type. Those caused by skeletal or muscular deviations probably should be referred to a specialist for treatment.

   Skeletal Cause. If the crossbite is slight, a maxillary lingual arch may be used to expand the maxilla or a Hawley appliance with an inclined plane may be used if only one or two teeth are involved (see the section on Crossbites earlier in this chapter; modify the appliance to move involved buccal teeth). In more severe situations the treatment of choice would be a palatal expansion appliance, possibly assisted by an orthognathic surgical procedure.

Muscular Cause. In the primary or mixed dentition, occlusal grinding often allows the proper closing pattern to resume. In the permanent dentition, occlusal grinding may allow for a proper closing pattern, but appliance therapy may be necessary.

Dental Cause. Space must be regained for the tooth or teeth to fit into the arch; this is accomplished by expanding the arch or by interproximal stripping.

The crossbite is eliminated by banding or bonding brackets onto the teeth in the opposing arches and having the patient wear through-the-bite elastics attached from buttons or hooks placed on the side of the tooth opposite the direction of desired tooth movement. If an anterior tooth is involved, a Hawley appliance with a finger spring to push the tooth labially and an occlusal plane to prevent the opposing arch from making contact during the time of movement may be used. See the section on Correction of Anterior Crossbites earlier in this chapter.

Class II Distoclusion

A normal relationship, or neutroclusion (Angle Class I), exists when the mesial buccal cusp of the maxillary molar occludes between the mesial and distal buccal cusps of the mandibular first molar (see Fig. 15-1A).

A Class II distoclusion occurs when the mandibular first molar occludes posterior to its normal relationship with the maxillary first molar (see Fig. 15-1B). This is easily ascertained on clinical examination and is well documented on diagnostic casts or cephalometric radiographs. Some simpler situations, especially in young patients, can be treated by a clinician who is well versed in orthodontic treatment procedures; however, referral to an orthodontist usually is indicated.

Diagnosis
Skeletal Cause. These distoclusions are caused by inherent growth patterns within the facial skeleton. Sometimes it is possible to mask these skeletal disharmonies with conventional orthodontic therapy. Occasionally orthognathic surgery is the treatment of choice. Clinically, these patients have a large horizontal overlap of the maxillary anterior teeth.

Muscular Cause. These distoclusions are caused by learned neuromuscular reflexes that can be altered in the primary and mixed dentition. The horizontal overlap usually is slight, and functional appliances are sometimes successful in correcting the malocclusion.

Dental Cause. These distoclusions involve mesial drifting of the teeth in the maxilla. Teeth often show edge-to-edge occlusion with severe crowding in the maxillary arch and distoclusion of the mandibular first molars.

Treatment
Skeletal Cause. In the primary dentition, palliative treatment involves control of deleterious sucking habits and elimination of any tooth interferences that might inhibit mandibular growth. Judicious occlusal equilibration at an early age allows free anterior growth of the mandible if it has been forced distally because of occlusal interferences. Many appliances

and techniques have been advocated for controlling sucking habits, but the most important factor is patient cooperation. No appliance can overcome a patient who is determined to continue a pernicious habit. See the section on Generalized Spacing earlier in this chapter.

Palliative treatment of distoclusion in a mixed dentition usually is beyond the scope of the generalist. However, the following procedures are normally undertaken by the orthodontist. If there is a good tooth size/arch length ratio, headgear will allow growth of the mandible while keeping the maxilla in place. A functional appliance may also be used. Many of these patients require full appliance mechanotherapy. If there is an unfavorable tooth size/arch length ratio, the patient may require the extraction of teeth and full appliance therapy. In the permanent dentition, comprehensive orthodontic therapy usually is necessary.

Muscular Cause. In the primary dentition, treatment involves elimination of cuspal interferences. This often can be accomplished by the generalist, and it allows the jaw to assume its normal occlusal position. If a patient requires treatment by an orthodontist, a Bionator, Activator, or Frankel functional appliance could be used successfully at this stage of development.

The same therapeutic measures are used for treatment of distoclusion in the mixed dentition as in the primary dentition. Because the harmful habits are now longer standing, they are harder to correct.

In the permanent dentition, the distoclusion has commonly progressed to a locked-in bite; therefore full orthodontic appliance therapy is usually needed.

Dental Cause. Distoclusion is rarely seen in the primary dentition because there has not been time for mesial drifting of the teeth to take place.

In the mixed dentition of persistent thumb or finger suckers, all the maxillary teeth are tipped forward. Treatment, usually undertaken by the orthodontist, first necessitates elimination of the harmful habit. A fixed or removable habit breaker may be used and this is usually followed by full fixed appliances. Headgear usually is used in the treatment of these patients.

Distoclusion in the permanent dentition is more difficult to treat because all growth potential has been lost. Often full orthodontic appliance therapy is necessary.

SPECIAL CONSIDERATIONS FOR CLASS II MALOCCLUSIONS

Certain situations can affect the prognosis of a Class II case and may require treatment by a specialist.

Tooth size/alveolar arch length ratio. Large teeth may require therapeutic extractions, making the situation more difficult to treat.

Nasorespiratory function. Poor nasal breathing habits result in a narrow, underdeveloped palate, often rendering treatment and retention more difficult.

Parental and patient interest in treatment. Enthusiastic cooperation is essential for good results.

ANGLE CLASS III MESIOCLUSION

The mandibular first molars are mesial of their normal occlusal relationship in an Angle Class III malocclusion (see Fig. 15-1C). Although true Class III cases represent only about 3% of the malocclusions seen in the United States, they are among the most difficult to treat. Referral to a specialist for diagnosis and therapy is indicated. When the cause is skeletal, it can be due to either a micromaxilla or mandibular hypertrophy. If the cause is functional in nature, tooth interferences cause the mandible to be moved forward of its normal position. This also is called an apparent or pseudo Class III occlusion. If the cause is dental in nature, linguoversion of the maxillary anterior teeth exists with a Class I molar relationship. See the section on Correction of Anterior Crossbites earlier in this chapter.

Diagnosis. A differential diagnosis requires cephalometric radiographs, diagnostic casts, and clinical examination of the patient both at rest and during function.

Skeletal (True Class III) Cause. A differential diagnosis requires cephalometric radiographs, diagnostic casts, and clinical examination of the patient both at rest and during function. The characteristics of the skeletal or true Class III malocclusion follow.

Profile. The mandible is dominant and cannot be retruded (Fig. 15-12).

This can be caused by either a large mandible or a small maxilla. The patient will have a "dished in" appearance of the midface, especially in situations caused by a small maxilla.

Mandibular Angle. The mandibular angle is 130 to 140 degrees.

Mandibular Incisal Angle. The mandibular incisors often are crowded and in linguoversion.

Mandibular Closing Pattern. An even closing pattern occurs (not a "hit and slide" pattern because of cuspal prematurities).

Molar Relationship. The molars will always be in a Class III relationship when the teeth are in maximum intercuspation.

Dental (Pseudo Class III) Cause. The characteristics of the dental or pseudo Class III malocclusion follow.

Profile. The mandible is in a Class I relationship posturally at rest but shows the full Class III face when the teeth are in occlusal contact.

Mandibular Angle. The mandibular angle is close to 120 degrees.

Mandibular Incisal Angle. The mandibular incisors are vertical or slightly in labioversion.

Mandibular Closing Pattern. When closing into maximal intercuspation, the mandible slides anteriorly because of cuspal interference.

Molar Relationship. The pseudo Class III relationship sometimes demonstrates molars in either a Class I or Class III alignment, with the mandible in maximum intercuspation and postural rest positions; therefore the clinician cannot rely solely on the molar position for the diagnosis. In some situations a shift from a Class I to a Class III relationship occurs on closing of the mandible.

Treatment. The etiology of the malocclusion must be considered when planning treatment.

Skeletal (True Class III) Cause. Referral to a specialist is indicated in true Class III malocclusions. Active intervention with full appliance mechanotherapy often is delayed until the permanent teeth are present. It may be necessary to include a orthognathic surgical approach (Fig. 15-13).

Dental (Pseudo Class III) Cause. In the primary or mixed dentition, it is sometimes possible to correct the bite by removing any tooth interferences. This could be accomplished in the primary or mixed dentition phase with a mandibular Hawley appliance that has an anterior inclined plane (see the section on Correction of Anterior Crossbites earlier in this chapter, but modify the appliance to move the inclined plane in the opposite direction because the appliance is now on the mandible). Fixed orthodontic appliances may be used in some instances, with the use of Class III elastics to encourage a new closing pattern. In the permanent dentition, this is always treated with full appliances and often requires orthognathic surgery.

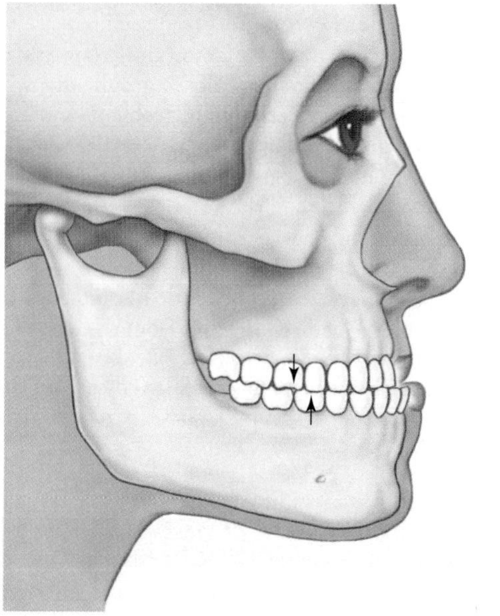

FIGURE 15-12 A true Angle Class III skeletal relationship. Adapted from Morcos SS, Patel PK. The vocabulary of dentofacial deformities. Clin Plast Surg 34(3):589-99, 2007.

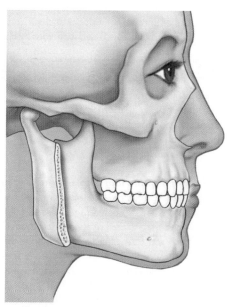

FIGURE 15-13 Surgical correction of a true Angle Class III skeletal relationship.

BIMAXILLARY PROGNATHISM

In bimaxillary prognathism, the molars are in an Angle Class I relationship. Careful evaluation of the cephalometric radiograph and diagnostic casts to determine the true nature of the problem is essential. Careful evaluation of the cephalometric radiograph and diagnostic casts to determine the true nature of the problem is essential. The three types of bimaxillary prognathism follow.

Skeletal Bimaxillary Prognathism. In these situations both the mandible and the maxilla are anterior to the cranial base. Usually this is a hereditary growth pattern. It is more commonly seen in individuals of Australian, African, or Asian descent.

Dental Bimaxillary Prognathism. In these situations the maxillary and mandibular teeth are positioned anteriorly in their bony bases. This growth pattern is seen in patients with large teeth.

Combined Bimaxillary Prognathism. In these situations the mandible, maxilla, and teeth are anteriorly positioned.

Treatment. The etiology of the malocclusion must be considered when planning treatment.

Skeletal Bimaxillary Prognathism. Treatment planning is complicated in these situations because it is difficult to predict growth. Maxillary growth ceases at approximately 12 years of age, but mandibular growth continues into young adulthood. These patients are difficult to treat, despite extractions, using conventional orthodontic appliances. An orthognathic surgical approach is often indicated.

Dental Bimaxillary Prognathism. These patients are difficult to treat during growth. Treatment is not possible during the primary or early mixed dentition stages because all the first premolars have not yet erupted. These patients can be treated in the late mixed dentition stage once the first premolars have erupted because these teeth must be extracted. The teeth usually are mesially inclined on their bony bases; therefore treatment is successful in young adults with the extraction of four first bicuspid teeth and the use of conventional fixed appliance mechanotherapy.

Combined Bimaxillary Prognathism. Treatment of these patients consists of correcting both the skeletal and dental components of the prognathism (discussed earlier in the chapter).

CLINICAL TIP

The clinician's personal esthetic preferences must not be imposed in situations of bimaxillary prognathism. Genetic and racial factors must be respected, and the wishes of the patient must be solicited and taken into consideration.

Although a wide variety of facial dysplasias may be encountered in association with congenital deformities, only two are seen frequently enough to be discussed in this chapter. All gross facial deformities should be referred to specialists for treatment.

Mandibular Prognathism. In this condition the mandible is proportionately too large for the rest of the face. It may be caused by mandibular hypertrophy, midface deficiency, or a combination of the two. Clinical examination is sufficient to diagnose the condition, but radiographs and diagnostic casts are necessary to ascertain the cause and the preferred method of treatment. The diagnosis of cleft lip and palate is made at birth when the lip is involved. Situations involving only the hard or soft palate are discovered later and may be brought to the dentist for diagnosis. There are several popular approaches to treatment, and much research is being carried out at several centers that focus on this condition. Referral is indicated.

OCCLUSAL ADJUSTMENT

Occlusal adjustments are needed in almost every orthodontic treatment, even if the movement is limited to a single tooth. Imbalances in the local force system are inevitable with any orthodontic treatment. Evaluation of interferences is necessary. Interferences may occur in centric relationship and protrusive and excursive movements. The chance of creating an anterior interference is extremely high and contributes to claims of posterior tooth intrusion from the plastic thickness. Posterior teeth contact is usually achievable at the end of orthodontic treatment if simple evaluation and adjustment of anterior interferences is performed during functional movements. If the posterior occlusion is open at the end of treatment, attachments in the posterior can be used for interarch elastics to establish contact between the maxillary and mandibular teeth. Using fixed traditional braces for a short period is a predictable solution if the bite is not corrected. The length of time needed in fixed braces is usually minimal compared with the treatment time when clear aligners are used. Cutting the clear aligners to encourage slight posterior extrusion of the uncovered teeth also assists in closing down a posterior open bite.

Retention

Rotations can be a particular relapse problem and retention is advised. Fixed lingual arches may be placed; removable Hawley appliances, Essix retainers, or a positioner may be used, depending on the requirements of the situation. Most cases are retained for more than a year and many cases require lifetime retention. The necessity for and method of retention should be reviewed with the patient prior to the decision to undergo orthodontic therapies. Changes in local pressures and forces can lead to shifting tooth positions over time. Fixed retainers are useful in situations where compliance is a factor and relapse is a significant risk. Fixed retainers increase flossing difficulty, which can lead to the development of periodontal problems and caries over longer periods of time. Patients may have a false sense of security because fixed retainers can fail at one of the bonded areas, which can lead to migration of the anterior teeth. Those patients can relapse unless an overlay thermoplastic retainer is also worn simultaneously with the fixed retention.

Removable thermoplastic retainers do not interfere with oral hygiene efforts and provide protection from the effects of bruxism and clenching. If a retainer is lost or broken, relapse can occur before a replacement can be fabricated. Patients should be advised that the sooner the replacement of a lost retainer, the less the chance of relapse.

CLINICAL TIP

Advise patients that retainers and aligners are commonly lost when wrapped in a napkin and left behind on lunch trays and countertops. Providing patients with duplicate retainers is useful in this regard.

CONCLUSION

The goal of the dentist is to provide a stable and maintainable occlusion. An occlusion that cannot be maintained and is unstable will fail.[2] If restorations can be avoided by moving the teeth into a correct relationship, orthodontics is the method of choice.[3] Collaboration between the general dentist, the orthodontist, the periodontist, or any appropriate specialist is essential.[4]

Orthodontic treatment traditionally has been limited to correcting malocclusions in children or adolescents. Advances in esthetic appliance design have made adult esthetic orthodontic care feasible and commonplace.[5]

Removable appliances may be used in some situations, but fixed appliances can offer more predictable and faster results.[6]

With an enlightened introduction to modern orthodontic treatment, adults will happily accept it as part of their restorative plan.

REFERENCES

1. Ward HL, Simring M: *Manual of clinical periodontology*, ed 2, St. Louis, 1978, Mosby.
2. LaSota EP: Orthodontic considerations in prosthetic and restorative dentistry, *Dent Clin North Am* 32:447, 1988.
3. Dawson PE: *Evaluation, diagnosis, and treatment of occlusal problems*, St. Louis, 1974, Mosby.
4. Baker IA, Stewart AV: Adult orthodontics services, *J Am Coll Dent* 57:16, 1990.
5. McNulty EC: Appliance selection, *Dent Clin North Am* 32:571, 1988.
6. DeAngelis V: Integration of orthodontics with prosthodontics and reconstructive dentistry, *J Mass Dent Soc* 30:130, 1981.

Some color figures courtesy of Joy Hudecz, D.D.S., Assistant Clinical Professor of Dentistry, and Malcolm E. Meistrell, Jr. D.D.S., Clinical Professor of Dentistry, Orthodontic Department, Columbia School of Dental and Oral Surgery, New York, NY.

16

Esthetics and Implant Surgery

James Torosian and Edwin S. Rosenberg

Implants are a major component of the armamentarium of the dental provider, offering the ability to deliver a predictable esthetic and functional end result for patients. Case success is predicated on formulating and executing a sound plan based on accurate information and an understanding of the biology of the treatment options.

DIAGNOSIS

Clinical Examination

An accurate diagnosis and assessment is critical for any clinical situation, but particularly for those involving the esthetic zone. The patient's esthetic expectations should be ascertained and the anticipated treatment time, the possibility of multiple procedures, and other contributing factors (such as orthodontic, occlusal, periodontal, restorative or endodontic needs) should be discussed. At this point a comprehensive examination should be performed that includes a detailed restorative and periodontal charting, occlusal evaluation, alveolar ridge evaluation, appropriate radiographs, and study casts. Successful treatment outcome is predicated on satisfying the functional needs of the case and the cosmetic expectations of the patient. A successful outcome cannot be achieved if these factors are mutually exclusive,

---

CLINICAL TIP

The patient's expectations must not be beyond what is surgically and restoratively possible.

It is at this point that the treatment plan can be formulated. Based on this information and in conjunction with the clinical examination, a determination should be made if three-dimensional (3-D) imaging is indicated.

Radiographic Assessment

Often 3-D imaging using computer-assisted tomography or cone-beam volumetric tomography (CBCT) is a vital part in formulating both the surgical and restorative aspects of the treatment plan. Fixture placement is a 3-D endeavor, occurring in the occlusoapical, mesiodistal, and buccolingual planes, with each having their separate requirements. The information obtained with scans will allow the surgeon to determine the optimal location and size of the fixture(s) to be placed in order to satisfy surgical and prosthetic needs. This is true for both the single implant restoration and the multiple-fixture–supported prosthesis.

These images allow the surgeon to identify anatomic structures that might influence the location that a fixture can be placed as well as any change or divergence from normal ridge anatomy that could affect the treatment outcome. Adequate bone for healing and stability of the fixture is necessary and the cross-sectional slices of the scan provide this information. While conventional radiographs may provide an idea of the amount of bone that is present, only the 3-D image will provide specifics. This is particularly true for the buccolingual dimension of the bone.

CLINICAL TIP

Ridges that appear perfectly adequate on periapical films may be very narrow when scanned.

This is especially true in the maxilla where thicker gingival connective tissue can visually appear to cover a wide bony ridge even if the underlying alveolar ridge is knife-edged. Scans can reveal ridge concavities that may cause the fixture to perforate the cortical plates. In these cases, augmentation may become necessary either before or during fixture placement (Fig. 16-1).

The location of certain bony landmarks is important in the planning stage as well. These include the proximity of the floor of the nose in the anterior maxilla, prominent maxillary

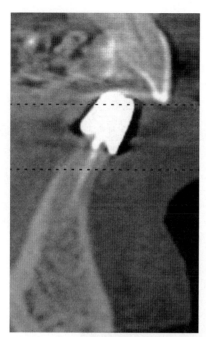

FIGURE 16-1 A cross-sectional slice of a 3-D scan showing a dehiscence and severe undercut on the facial aspect of #26 that will require grafting before fixture placement.

incisive foramen or mandibular genial tubercles, or a more anteriorly positioned maxillary antrum for a maxillary canine or first premolar clinical situation. Modification of the surgical plan may become necessary based on the findings on the scan.

Additionally, any pathology found on the scan must be identified and factored into treatment. If the clinician does not feel she/he has the expertise to fully interpret image data, it should be referred to a specialist.

Anything that is identified on the scan that may alter or modify the treatment plan must be discussed by all members of the treatment team as well as with the patient. This may involve simple changes (such as from screw to cement retention for the crown), or much more significant modifications (such as a change in the number of or location of fixtures as well as preimplant reconstructive procedures).

CLINICAL TIP

All involved individuals must understand and accept the treatment plan before treatment begins.

TREATMENT PLANNING

Treatment planning includes the number of teeth that will be replaced, the number and location of implant fixtures (determined by the scan results), whether site development is required and what type of procedures are necessary to achieve this (determined from both the clinical examination and the radiographic assessment), whether teeth will be removed, if fixture(s) will be placed immediately or delayed and if the restoration will be screw-retained or cemented.

Radiographic/Surgical G

A properly designed guide stent is often crucial for esthetic situations. The stent should be anatomically correct and represent the size, shape, and position of the planned restoration. The stent can be made of hard acrylic (such as a night guard designed with pontics) or with rigid tray material (formed on a wax-up of the case) (Fig. 16-2A). (See the section on Stents in Chapter 17). When there is a posterior edentulous distal extension, the stent should be secured on the adjacent teeth anterior to the planned implant site(s). For cases with only posterior teeth in one sextant (anterior and unilateral posterior edentulous ridge), the stent must extend far enough posteriorly on the edentulous side so it rests on the crestal gingiva *beyond* the extent of the incision. Often the stent will serve a dual role, being both a radiographic and surgical guide

When used during scanning, radiopaque markers are placed to show the location of the planned restoration in relation to the underlying bone. If a single tooth is being replaced, then markers are put on the stent in that location only. If multiple teeth are missing, then the markers need to be placed for each tooth in the restoration regardless of how many fixtures are considered, thus allowing for identification of the most ideal sites.

Marking the stent can be achieved in different ways. A radiopaque material can be applied on the surface of the teeth on the stent (such as barium powder or a piece of lead foil from a conventional x-ray film) which will provide an outline of the planned restoration on the scan image. Another method is to place a 2- to 3-mm diameter hole in the center of the occlusal table (for posterior teeth) or cingulum (for anterior teeth) to mimic the screw access hole of the fixture (Fig. 16-2B).

The hole in the stent is filled with gutta percha that will be displayed radiographically as a white vertical line over the scanned ridge (Fig. 16-2C). In both instances, the markers will allow the surgeon and restorative dentist to see the location of the bone in relation to the planned restoration.

CLINICAL TIP

Lead foil can be placed over the pontic(s) of an existing provisional bridge to act as a radiographic stent. This can also be done on a "flipper" pontic if it has no wires (which interfere with the image).

With this information the surgeon can relay to the restorative team member the size options for the fixture, such as length and diameter ranges, and the location the fixture can occupy in the ridge. This also allows the restorative dentist to convey a fixture location preference. In the case of multiple fixtures, this information can be used to identify the best location for the fixtures supporting the restoration. At this time the stent can be adjusted to represent the endpoint of this collaboration. Repositioning of the guide hole of the radiographic stent can be accomplished, thus converting it into the surgical stent.

Gathering as much initial pertinent information as possible and maintaining good communication between all team members can eliminate most, if not all, potential future problems.

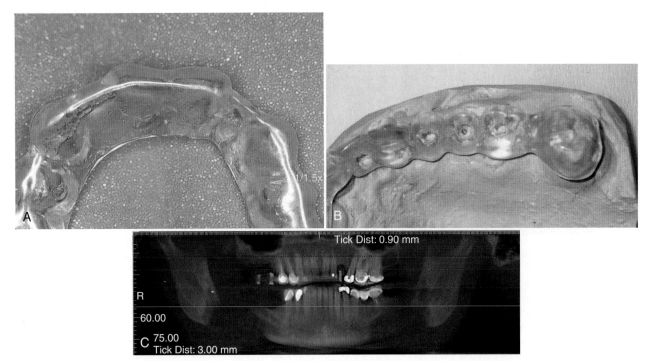

FIGURE 16-2 A, Radiographic/surgical stent for #10 has been made of a rigid tray material. **B,** A hard acrylic stent with guide holes placed in the planned implant sites. **C,** The panoramic reconstruction of the CBCT scan displays the gutta percha markers for the planned implants in the maxillary right posterior sextant and maxillary left canine.

SURGICAL PLANNING

Surgical treatment planning the single tooth case may appear to be quite simple. However, the basic principles of surgical preparation and placement apply regardless of the number of implant fixtures that will be placed. The single implant situation is unique because there are usually two natural teeth adjacent to the fixture location and the relationship between the position of the fixture and the interdental bone between the approximating teeth is critical to the outcome of treatment.

One of the major esthetic challenges is the creation of a normal peri-implant gingival complex mimicking that of a natural tooth. The fixture platform must be positioned sufficiently apical to allow formation of a proper restoration subgingival emergence profile. In the non-periodontally involved case (no crestal bone loss) this requires the platform to be at least 2 to 3 mm apical to the level of the facial cementoenamel junction (CEJ) of the adjacent teeth (Fig. 16-3A). In a restored dentition, the facial restoration margins (crowns, veneers, etc.) of the adjacent teeth are used as the landmark instead of the CEJ. If restoration of the adjacent teeth is anticipated, the final position of the soft tissue margins need to be determined (with provisional restorations or a diagnostic wax-up) before fixture placement. These guidelines apply to implants placed into a healed edentulous ridge or for immediate placement at time of extraction. When immediate placement is performed, the platform will be apical to the interproximal bone height, and radiographically this will show the implant platform being apical to the interproximal bone (Fig. 16-3B). Therefore only hard tissue landmarks can be used when assessing platform position radiographically. Clinical observation is needed to assess platform position in relation to the soft tissue margins.

When the diameter of the fixture is less than that of the tooth root that was extracted, this apical placement is necessary in order to create a natural sub-gingival flare (emergence profile) which will mimic the shape of a natural tooth. Without this submarginal space, it may be impossible for the dental laboratory to provide a naturally appearing crown. If the platform is positioned too coronally, there is also a risk that the crown-fixture interface could become visible.

CLINICAL TIP

The lateral borders of the fixture must be at least 1.5 mm away from the roots of the adjacent teeth (the mesiodistal dimension) and is necessary in order to achieve proper osseointegration.

Violation of the periodontal ligament space of an adjacent tooth would result in damage to the natural dentition as well as create a fixture-to-periodontal ligament (PDL) fiber contact. The latter would interfere with osseointegration and result in fibroencapsulation of the implant (Fig. 16-3C) placed too close to the adjacent canine violating the PDL space. The fixture ultimately failed.

In addition, if the platform is too close to the approximating teeth, there will be insufficient lateral space to create the appropriate tooth shape.

The center of the fixture should be palatal to the position of the incisal edge or at the cingulum (the buccolingual dimension) of the final planned restoration. For proper surgical healing sufficient thickness of the buccal plate is required in order to maintain the integrity of the facial crest. The closer the fixture

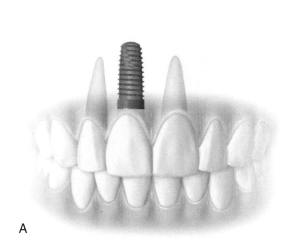

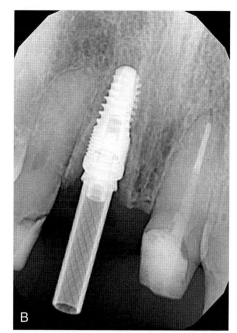

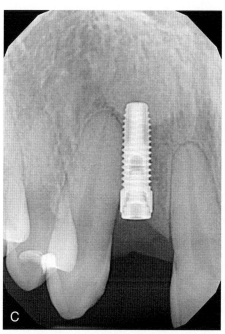

FIGURE 16-3 A, The location of the fixture platform in relation to the adjacent teeth. Note the apical positioning to the cementoenamel junction and marginal gingival height. **B,** A post-placement radiograph of an immediate fixture, showing platform location in relation to the adjacent teeth and interproximal bone, which will allow for proper gingival tissue height. A temporary cylinder is attached to the fixture in preparation for immediate provisionalization. **C,** A submerged fixture that has been placed too close to the adjacent canine violating the PDL space. The fixture ultimately failed.

is positioned to the buccal plate, the greater the likelihood of a dehiscence and apical shrinkage of the soft tissues. Improperly angled placement could also result in perforation of the facial plate, with the fixture apex being beyond the confines of the bony housing.

Palatal positioning is a necessity for the screw-retained restoration. The long axis of the implant must provide sufficient space for the laboratory to add material to the body and incisal edge of the restoration while leaving adequate space for the insertion of driver tips within the screw access hole (Fig. 16-4A).

The angulation of insertion of the fixture is also crucial for the screw retained restoration. Using the platform level as the fulcrum of rotation, the angle of insertion can affect the type of retention for the restoration.

If a cement retained restoration is planned, the long axis of the screw path should be no farther facial than the incisal edge to

allow for proper abutment design (Fig. 16-4B). With this type of restoration, more flexibility is present regarding platform positioning. The long axis of the fixture should ideally be in line with the incisal edge of the planned restoration.

The angulation of insertion of the fixture is also crucial for the screw retained restoration. Using the platform level as the fulcrum of rotation, the angle of insertion can affect the type of retention for the restoration (Fig. 16-4C). If the platform is positioned too far buccally, then the proper height of contour and emergence profile of the restoration cannot be achieved regardless of whether the restoration is screw or cement retained.

The maintenance or creation of interdental papillae and avoiding "black triangles" is one of the most crucial aspects of success in the esthetic zone. To achieve this requires an understanding of the biology as it applies to both the surgical and prosthetic aspects of single tooth replacement.

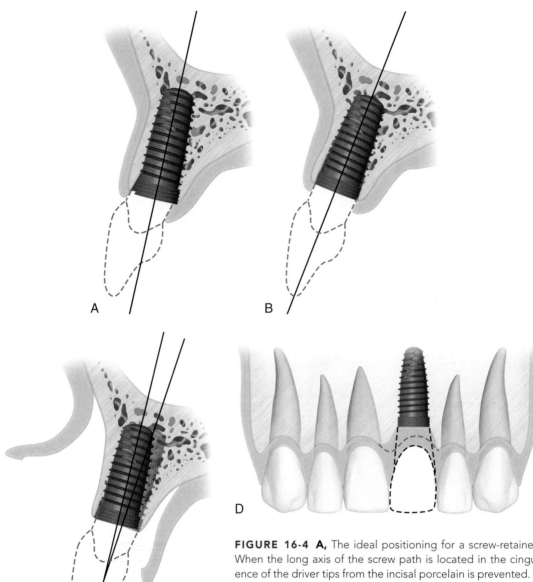

FIGURE 16-4 A, The ideal positioning for a screw-retained restoration. When the long axis of the screw path is located in the cingulum, interference of the driver tips from the incisal porcelain is prevented. **B,** If a cement retained restoration is planned the long axis of the fixture should ideally be in line with the incisal edge of the planned restoration. **C,** By slightly angulating a fixture using the platform as a fulcrum, the correct path of insertion for a screw-retained restoration can be achieved. **D,** Papillae form is driven by the bone on the natural dentition.

CLINICAL TIP

For the presence of a papilla, the bone level on the tooth side is the determining factor, not the implant fixture side (Fig. 16-4D)

The fixture must have proper 3-D placement (particularly occlusoapically and mesiodistally) to allow the restorative dentist to create proper restoration contours to support the papilla.

CLINICAL TIP

The distance between the crest of the bone on the tooth adjacent to the implant fixture and the interproximal contact area of this tooth (virgin or restored) should be 5 mm or less in order to maintain papillary height. Even if the distance between the crest of bone on the implant fixture and the interproximal contact area of the implant crown is greater than 5 mm, a papilla should be able to be maintained if the adjacent tooth interproximal contact area to adjacent tooth crest of bone is 5 mm or less; the bone to interproximal contact area distance on the tooth adjacent to the implant is the determining factor.

Clinical Case: Maintaining the Papillae

A 33-year old woman presented with a fractured maxillary right first premolar (Fig. 16-5A,B) that was not restorable. After atraumatic extraction (Fig. 16-5C), fixture placement the site revealed an intact socket with good interproximal crestal bone (Fig. 16-5D).

An immediate implant fixture was placed and after healing (Fig. 16-5E) and provisionalization (Fig. 16-5F), an excellent soft tissue result was achieved.

The same considerations regarding single tooth implants apply to multiple tooth edentulous areas; however, there are additional factors to consider other than the volume of bone. From the soft tissue standpoint, when single implants are placed between two teeth, the bone and PDL fibers on the natural tooth determine papilla position. When placing two adjacent implants, this is no longer the case. Without the root surface and PDL fibers to maintain bone height, the interimplant bone is more prone to resorption and cannot support the soft tissues. For the low esthetic risk patient (low lip line, thick, flat gingival biotype

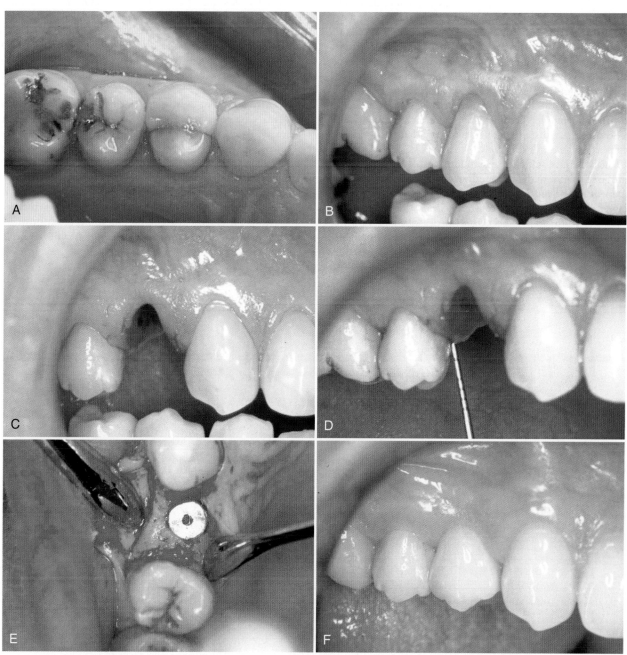

FIGURE 16-5 A, This 33-year-old female presented with a complete mesiodistal fracture of the maxillary right first premolar, which rendered it non-restorable. **B,** The facial papillae are intact at the site. **C,** After atraumatic extraction, the soft and hard tissues were favorable for immediate placement. **D,** Probing of the adjacent teeth revealed intact bone levels. **E,** Excellent healing of the site is noted three months after fixture placement. **F,** With favorable interproximal bone and proper fixture placement, the papillae could be maintained.

and/or wide alveolar ridge mesiodistally) or a patient without any cosmetic expectations, placing individual fixtures could be acceptable. Many patients present with a thinner, scalloped gingival biotype with considerable esthetic display of gingiva, whereby placement of a fixture to replace each missing tooth runs a higher risk of failing to achieve esthetic expectations.

The minimum distance requirements are slightly different when placing adjacent fixtures as compared with a single fixture. Although the 1.5 mm distance requirement from the adjacent teeth does not change, there must be at least 3 mm between each fixture (discussed below) in order to maintain bone and tissue height. This effectively increases the amount of mesiodistal edentulous ridge length necessary to successfully place individual fixtures for a cosmetic end result. This concept applies to placement in the immediate socket as well as the healed ridge. These situations occur most often in the maxillary lateral incisor positions as well as with all mandibular incisors, where the size of the teeth and the amount of interradicular bone is typically narrow. In the case of the mandibular incisors, avoiding adjacent fixture placement often becomes a functional necessity (e.g., lack of adequate mesiodistal length to place two fixtures), but the esthetic considerations still apply.

When there is sufficient edentulous span length and adequate bone volume in the two tooth span, then individual fixture placement can be considered, with the most common situation being two missing maxillary central incisors. Where narrower mesiodistal restorative space exists (as described previously), placing adjacent fixtures should be avoided whenever possible,

particularly in the anterior maxilla. When a two tooth edentulous space is treated, it is preferable to place a single fixture for the larger of the two teeth being replaced (such as the central incisor/lateral incisor or canine/lateral incisor situation) with the final restoration, being an implant-supported two-unit cantilevered bridge (Fig. 16-6). This provides a better ability to manipulate the soft tissue (e.g., papillae and facial gingiva) and minimize the negative effects adjacent fixtures have on the soft tissue frame.

Treating a two tooth span with one fixture provides more restorative flexibility, particularly with soft tissue considerations. The absence of a second fixture eliminates constraints on the shape of the pontic. Emergence contours (buccolingually and mesiodistally) and interproximal contact area location and length can be manipulated to maximize the esthetic results. Ovate pontics can create the illusion of a papilla more predictably than when two fixtures are placed in adjacent tooth locations.

When developing ovate pontic form in the immediate extraction case, the apical portion of the pontic must extend into the extraction socket beyond the soft tissue margin by approximately 2 to 3 mm. This will allow circumferential healing around the bullet-shaped underside of the pontic. Care must be taken that the restoration does not extend beyond 3 mm. into the socket, which will interfere with proper healing. This type of soft tissue development can be performed whether or not the site is grafted. As the gingiva matures, modifications of the provisional restoration can be performed to guide the healing as needed;

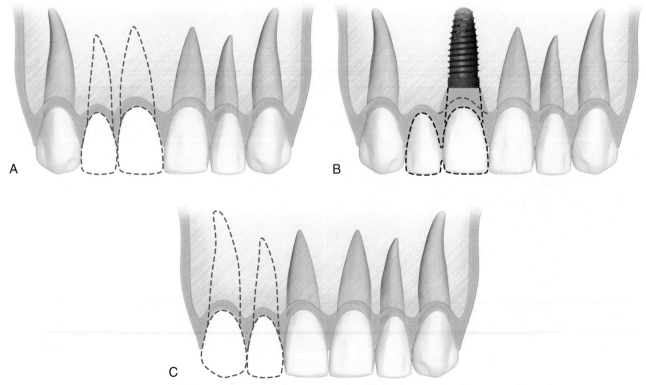

FIGURE 16-6 A, Two tooth span involving a central and lateral incisor. **B,** Placement of a single central incisor fixture in this two tooth span allows for proper functional restoration with a favorable esthetic result using an ovate pontic form for the lateral incisor. **C,** A two tooth span with the canine and lateral incisor.

material can be added or subtracted depending upon the needs of the individual situation. This is especially helpful when performing immediate provisionalization in cases demonstrating a thin, scalloped gingival biotype.

CLINICAL TIP

A high polish must be placed on the ovate pontic in order to allow the tissues to heal without irritation from the provisional material.

If implant placement is performed in the healed edentulous ridge, conventional ovate pontic preparation (as described in Chapter 14) should be accomplished. Adequate volume and dimension of keratinized soft tissue (height and width) must exist at the ovate pontic site in order to reasonably consider this option. The ovate pontic preparation must be neither too shallow nor too deep. Underpreparation can result in flattening of the tissue profile with exposure of the underside of the pontic. Overpreparation can result in an uncleansible pontic area or cause pressure necrosis with both soft tissue and bone loss. Making a 2- to 3-mm deep preparation into the gingival connective tissue of the pontic site is appropriate. As with immediate placement situations, modification of the underside of the pontic can be performed at any time to guide the desired soft tissue healing. The patient should remain with a provisional restoration in place until full healing has occurred (minimum of 8 weeks) before proceeding to the definitive restoration.

The practice of using a cantilever as part of any implant supported prosthesis is usually discouraged because of the off-axis forces that are placed on the restoration. This is true for a posterior case where the forces of mastication are stronger. Even vertically directed force on a cantilever can create an eccentric vector on the fixture/abutment interface. However, in the anterior dentition the strength and direction of forces differ from that in the posterior region which allows the use of cantilevers in certain situations. In the mandible, either the central or lateral incisor site can be considered, though only the lateral incisor site in the maxilla is a good candidate. Contact in maximal intercuspal position on the pontic from the opposing arch must be lighter than on the adjacent anterior teeth and implant. Lateral and protrusive excursive movements must be on the natural teeth and implants, with minimal to no contact on the pontic. The use of an occlusal appliance is also highly recommended to control nocturnal parafunction. Situations in which cantilevers would be contraindicated include patients with severe parafunctional habits (even if an appliance is used), those with a deeper bite greater than 50%) or with anterior malocclusion (Class II - Division 2 or Class III relationships), severe crowding, and/or rotation.

For the three and four tooth spans, placing a single fixture next to the adjacent teeth and restoring as a three or four unit implant-supported bridge is preferred over replacing each tooth position with a separate implant. Good papilla form can be maintained or created in the presence of adequate bone on the adjacent natural teeth and by using ovate pontics (Fig. 16-7).

Another option for replacing four missing maxillary incisors is the placement of two central incisor fixtures with two lateral incisor pontics. This is preferred when the bone volume is greater in the central incisor locations as opposed to the lateral incisor locations or if there is a deficiency at the lateral incisor sites.

If the need arises to place two adjacent implants, there must be at least 3 mm between fixtures in order to preserve the crestal bone, which in turn supports the papilla (note that this is different than the 1.5-mm minimum distance between implants and adjacent teeth). Even if some bone remodeling occurs around the restorative platform of the fixture, interproximal crestal loss is kept to a minimum if the correct distance between fixtures is satisfied, Fixtures placed too close to each other will result in horizontal crestal resorption, which will lead to a flat gingival profile without creating the desired scalloped architecture. Slight subcrestal placement can be considered to create a higher interfixture peak of bone to support a papilla.

CLINICAL TIP

When placing two adjacent implants, the minimum distance between the initial osteotomy pilot holes must be the sum of the diameter of the largest fixture placed plus 3 mm (diameter + 3) (Fig. 16-8). If this distance is less, then correcting the spacing of the osteotomies must be done before enlarging the holes.

SURGICAL PLACEMENT

Flap Design

The placement of incisions for implants in the esthetic zone should provide adequate access to perform the procedure and be as conservative as possible so as not to create changes in the tissue architecture of the implant site and the adjacent teeth. Obviously, adequate reflection of the tissues is required to assure proper positioning as well as provide the ability to perform any adjunctive procedures (such as bone and/or soft tissue grafting at the time of placement). Presurgical planning is crucial (see the sections on diagnosis, treatment planning, and surgical planning earlier in this chapter).

When adequate buccolingual width of the ridge exists, a papillae preserving incision design should be employed, particularly in the maxillary esthetic zone. Two vertical incisions are placed at the base of the adjacent papilla and connected with a horizontal incision paracrestally (toward the palate). The buccal extent of the vertical incisions will be predicated upon the amount of reflection that is necessary for placement of the fixture (Fig. 16-9A,B).

If the incision must be extended buccally near or beyond the mucogingival junction, there should be slight divergence apically. If the base of the flap is wide, the blood supply is not compromised. Once placed, the fixture can either be buried (two-stage approach) or a healing abutment or provisional restoration can be attached (one-stage approach) (Fig. 16-9C,D).

Minor mucogingival issues can often be corrected at the time of placement with buccal positioning of the flap if adequate reflection is achieved.

If full access to the edentulous ridge is required, the entire body of the papilla should be included in the buccal flap using the paracrestal incision design (Fig. 16-10A). Vertical incisions for this approach should be kept to a minimum. If placed, they should be at the line angles of the teeth adjacent to the implant site to provide access. If significant buccal reflection is needed, conservative vertical releases can be performed away from the

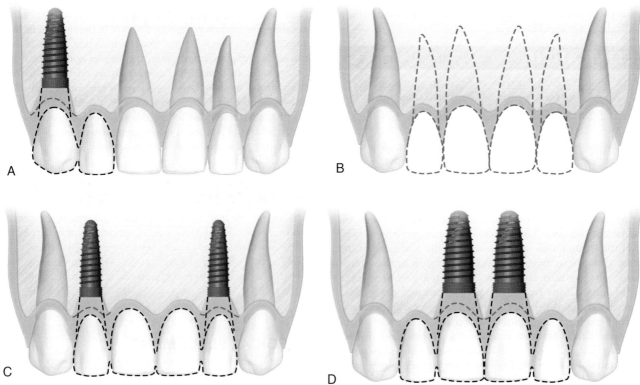

FIGURE 16-7 A, A similar plan as the two incisor situation satisfies the functional and esthetic requirements using a single canine implant. **B,** The four maxillary incisor situation has requirements that are similar to a two tooth span. **C,** A conventional four-unit implant-supported bridge can be fabricated using two central incisor ovate pontics. With bilateral support, it is not as critical to use the larger central incisor sites. **D,** If the lateral incisor locations are not favorable for fixture placement, then two central incisor implants can be placed with the restoration being either bilateral two-unit bridges or a single, splinted four-unit bridge with cantilevered ovate pontics at the lateral incisor positions.

implant site or an envelope flap design can be used. With either choice, buccal access is achieved while maintaining the blood supply and integrity of the papillae that have been included in the flap. Using these types of incision designs, a two-stage procedure should be performed and the flap should be replaced to its original position covering the fixture. The papillae-preserving flap design (discussed earlier in this section) can be used when uncovering the fixtures after integration.

CLINICAL TIP

Use a smaller sized scalpel blade to make the initial incisions in narrower spaces (such as a 15c). Reflection of the flap can be performed with a narrow-edged periosteal elevator (such as a Buser periosteal elevator) or a gingivectomy knife (Goldman-Fox #7 or #11), taking care not to perforate the flap.

Implant Fixture Placement

The contours of the anterior ridge receiving a fixture will often have a rounded profile as opposed to the flatter, plateau-type appearance of a posterior ridge. Assuming adequate width of

bone is present to place the fixture; this type of ridge shape does not preclude implantation, but presents the challenge of ensuring that the initial pilot preparation is properly positioned. Using a precision point twist drill or a small round burr allows the creation of a small pilot hole or dimple in the ridge, thus providing the surgeon with a positive seating location to begin the drilling sequence (Fig. 16-10B). If an initial twist drill (typically 2 mm in diameter) were to be used first, the tip can sometimes move or "skip" on the surface of the ridge. If a positive entry point is made, this occurrence is minimized. A stent is used for this initial osteotomy preparation, with the drills placed directly through the guide hole.

During surgery, the stent guides the placement of the initial osteotomy preparation in the edentulous ridge. The stent must be secure on the adjacent teeth in order to provide for accurate placement of the osteotomy (Fig. 16-10C).

When designed properly the stent allows for accurate positioning of the fixture in both the buccolingual and mesiodistal dimensions, all of which were predetermined in the planning phase. Use of the stent to confirm proper positioning when widening the osteotomy site should be accomplished by checking the angulation using surgical guide pins (Fig. 16-10D).

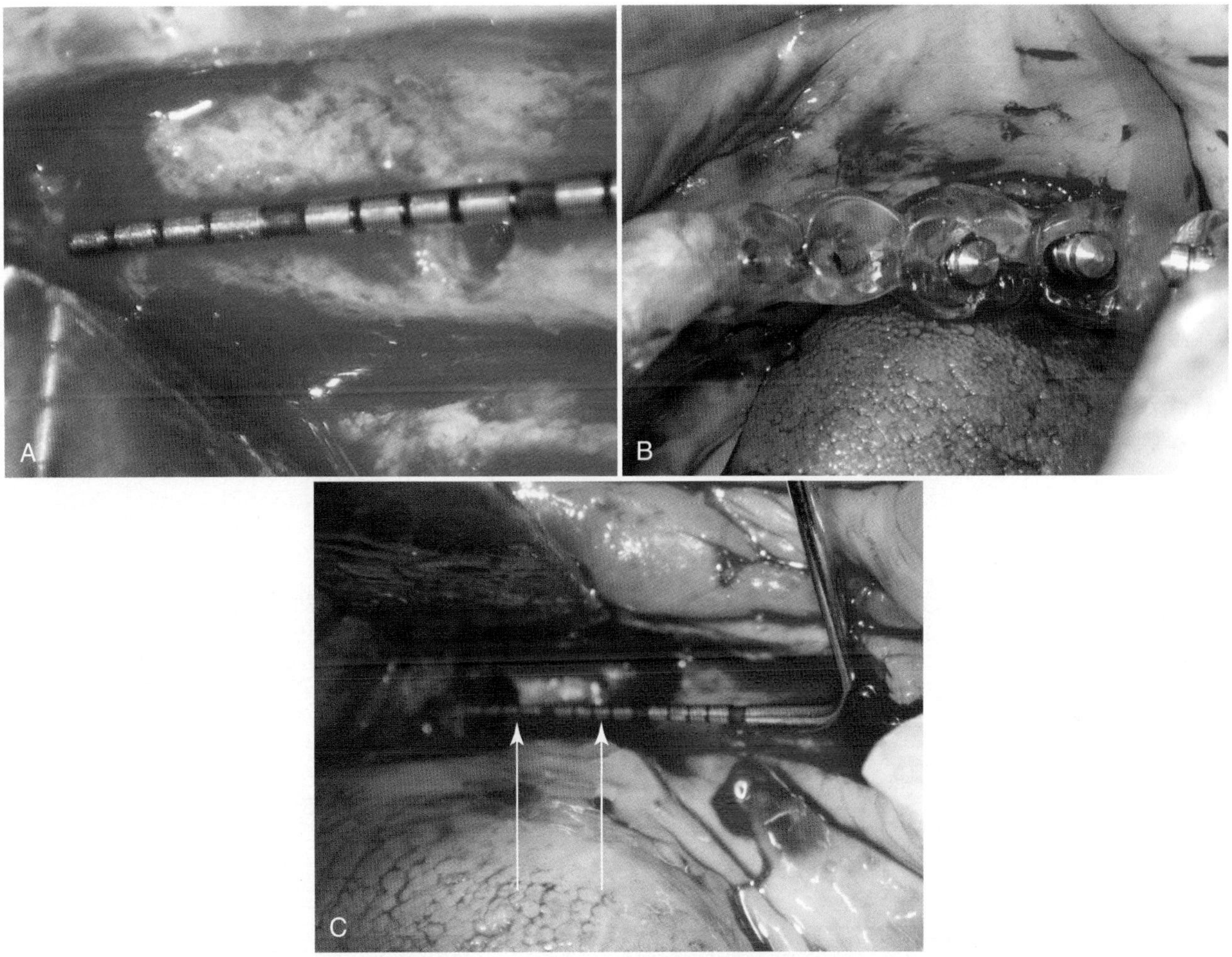

FIGURE 16-8 A, This site was planned for the placement of two 5-mm diameter fixtures. The initial pilot preparations were made 9.5 mm apart to allow for adequate interfixture spacing (*arrows* indicate location of pilot holes). **B,** Proper positioning of the initial osteotomy site is confirmed using the guide stent. **C,** After final preparation of the osteotomies, the interfixture bone distance is 4.5 mm (*arrows*), satisfying the inter-implant distance metric.

With proper initial placement, minor angulation differences with subsequently larger diameter twist drills can occur. By using the stent in this manner, the surgeon can insure proper placement. This is particularly important when placing more than one fixture because the greater the distance between implants, the greater the chance that buccolingual and mesiodistal errors can occur.

A check radiograph should be taken to ensure that the direction of the initial osteotomy is correct in the body of the alveolar bone. Surgical guide pins can be placed into the osteotomy site positioned through the access hole in the stent, with a radiograph showing the angulation in relation to the adjacent roots of the natural dentition. The osteotomy preparation should be equidistant from the adjacent roots on the surface and not converge too closely to either of the roots as the site is prepared apically to avoid violating the 1.5-mm root-implant minimum distance requirement. Before enlargement of the osteotomy any correction should be made so as to avoid buccal or lingual plate perforation as well as violation of the implant/tooth or implant/-implant distance requirements (Figs. 16-10E,F).

The final osteotomy site should leave at least 1.5 mm of interproximal bone between the fixture and each of the roots of the two adjacent teeth (or 3.0 mm of bone between adjacent implants), maintain approximately 1.5 mm of intact facial and lingual/palatal plate of bone and have proper platform positioning, as described earlier, in an apical location in relation to the adjacent teeth. Platform height should be assessed as the osteotomy is enlarged with increased diameter drills because as an osteotomy site is widened, the height of the buccal or lingual crest may move apically (many anterior ridges are rounded and not flat). It may be necessary to use a shorter fixture or deepen the preparation if this occurs.

Surgical Site Closure

Closure of the surgical site will be predicated upon how the internal screw access of the implant is covered. If a cover screw or internal closure screw is placed, then primary closure is preferable. Proceeding in this manner will require a second stage uncovering procedure once the fixture has integrated. Regardless

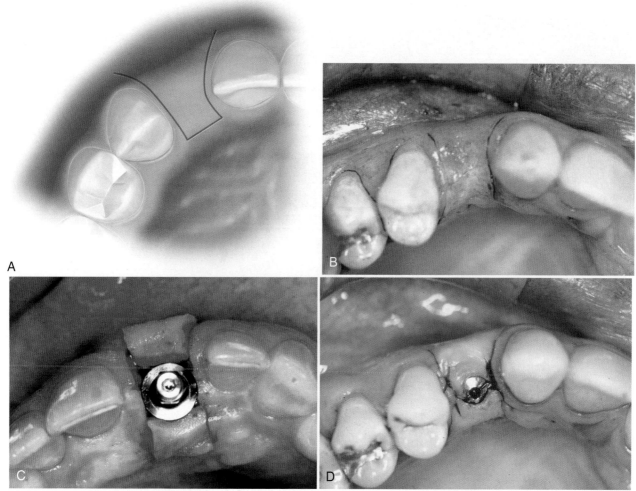

FIGURE 16-9 A, The diagram shows incision placement for conservative flap elevation. Note the paracrestal incision on the palate and the wider base of the flap buccally. **B,** A papillae sparing incision is made for single fixture placement. **C,** After placing the fixture, the buccal tissues can be positioned facially. **D,** The healing abutment provides additional stability for flap replacement in addition to suturing.

of the reason for performing a two-stage approach (such as minor grafting of the site), any endeavors toward guiding the soft tissue emergence profile must be performed at the second stage. If the patient has a transitional restoration, whether fixed (resin bonded bridge or acrylic provisional bridge) or removable ("flipper"), relief of the pontic tooth is necessary in order to avoid pressure on the flaps.

When primary closure is not necessary, closure of the surgical site should attempt to create the desired soft tissue profile in preparation for the final restoration whenever possible. This can be accomplished with a healing abutment or provisional crown. An immediately placed provisional crown should exactly mimic the contours of the definitive restoration and guide soft tissue healing. Once adequate stability of the implant occurs (approximately 6 weeks), the provisional restoration can be removed and the shape adjusted if needed.

If a healing abutment is used, the contours should approximate those of the final restoration, taking into account the selections available from each implant manufacturer. Both methods can be used even when minor bone grafting is performed (Fig. 16-11).

CLINICAL TIP

If a provisional restoration is placed on an immediate fixture requiring grafting, the contouring, finishing and polishing of the restoration should be accomplished before placing the graft. A high polish is necessary to avoid plaque accumulation or tissue irritation.

When securing the provisional crown, it is crucial that light force is used with a hand driver when tightening the abutment screw while simultaneously holding the crown/implant unit with finger stabilization. Even though the fixture may seem extremely stable, it is purely a mechanical phenomenon. Using a torque driver or heavy finger pressure at this point could cause eccentric force to be applied to the fixture and could possibly interfere with successful osseointegration. Using light force at initial placement will also allow for easier removal of the provisional restoration when making any modifications or changes that may be desired after the initial 6 weeks of healing.

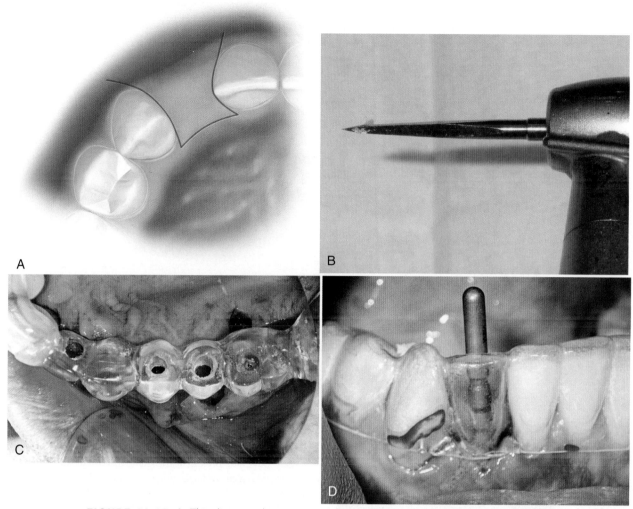

FIGURE 16-10 A, This diagram shows incision design for full site access. Notice that the full body of the papillae are included in the flap with the rest of the incisions located in the same position as shown in Fig. 16-9A. **B,** This precision point bur allows for accurate and stable positioning during initial osteotomy preparation. Markings on the bur assist in preparing to the proper depth. **C,** A hard acrylic stent supported by the adjacent teeth with guide holes over the planned implant sites. Given the long edentulous span, this type of stent is preferred to eliminate distortion during placement. **D,** Using a clear stent, confirmation of buccolingual positioning (by placement in the cingulum holes) and mesiodistally (by visual assessment) can be confirmed before enlarging the osteotomy site.

Continued

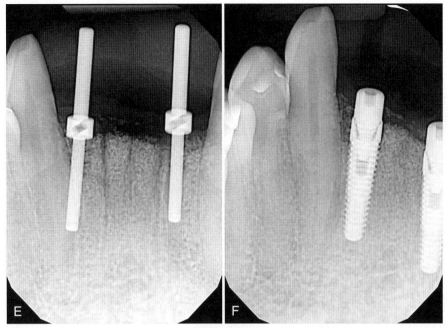

FIGURE 16-10, cont'd E, A radiographic check film reveals off-angled positioning of the initial osteotomy for the right lateral incisor. **F,** Proper placement of the fixture is accomplished after correcting the angle of the osteotomy.

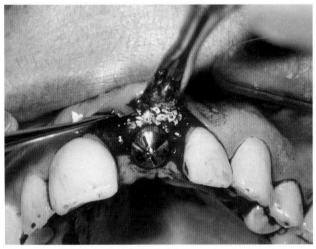

FIGURE 16-11 A bone graft for buccal contouring is performed at the time of fixture placement.

If vertical incisions are placed beyond the mucogingival junction or an envelope flap is extended laterally, buccal positioning of the flap is possible, with the abutment maintaining this surgical augmentation The height of the abutment must be considered if a transitional restoration is being used because it could interfere with full seating. Relining of a removable appliance or adjustment of a fixed provisional restoration must be accomplished post placement. A limiting factor with healing abutments is that they have a round profile (less of a factor for incisors). However, by placing a provisional restoration after healing, any minor discrepancies are easily corrected.

Clinical Case: Single Tooth with Soft Tissue Guidance

A 29-year-old man presented for a single implant in the maxillary right central incisor position. Adequate bone volume of the edentulous ridge was present for implant placement, but there was a sloping deficit of the facial gingiva (Fig. 16-12A). Papillae-sparing incisions were made and the flap was reflected (Fig. 16-12B).

After placing the implant, a healing abutment was placed on the fixture. This allowed for facial positioning of the keratinized tissue of the flap (Fig. 16-12C) which created a normal facial gingival profile (Fig. 16-12D). With the provisional restoration in place, an esthetic free marginal contour and emergence profile could be created (Fig. 16-12E).

Immediate provisionalization should create an emergence profile and height of contour mimicking that of the planned restoration. The provisional restoration can be constructed from a laboratory fabricated shell (based on the ideal contours of a presurgical wax-up) or a stock polycarbonate temporary shell (Figs. 16-12F-I). Another option is the conversion of an existing crown of the extracted tooth with contours created at chairside. For all of these options, screw retention is desired to allow for easy access to modify the provisional restoration and to eliminate any possibility of cement adversely affecting the surgical wound. The margins and underside of the provisional restoration must be highly polished in order to avoid any tissue irritation.

If a cement retained provisional restoration is placed the cement line should not extend more than 1 to 2 mm subgingivally, otherwise contamination of the surgical site could occur.

CLINICAL TIP

If possible, cement removal should be accomplished before closing the flap.

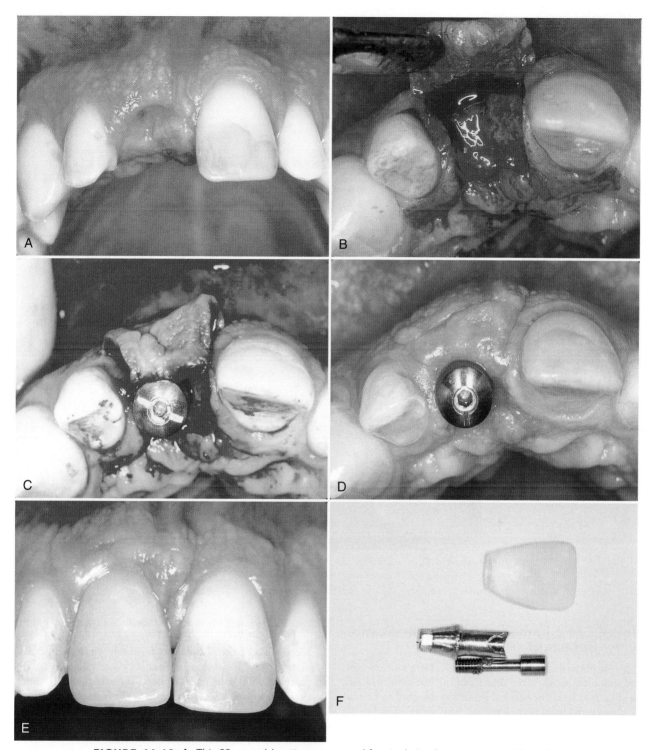

FIGURE 16-12 A, This 29-year-old patient presented for single implant restoration. Note the soft tissue depression on the facial aspect of the edentulous site. **B,** A papillae sparing incision is performed with reflection revealing a favorable ridge for fixture placement. **C,** After the fixture is placed, a healing abutment is affixed and the flap tissues positioned facially to "plump up" the soft tissue defect. **D,** Six weeks postoperatively, proper implant positioning with correction of the soft tissue deficit is evident. **E,** The additional facial tissue allowed for a provisional restoration with excellent esthetics. **F,** A laboratory processed provisional shell with temporary restorative components.

Continued

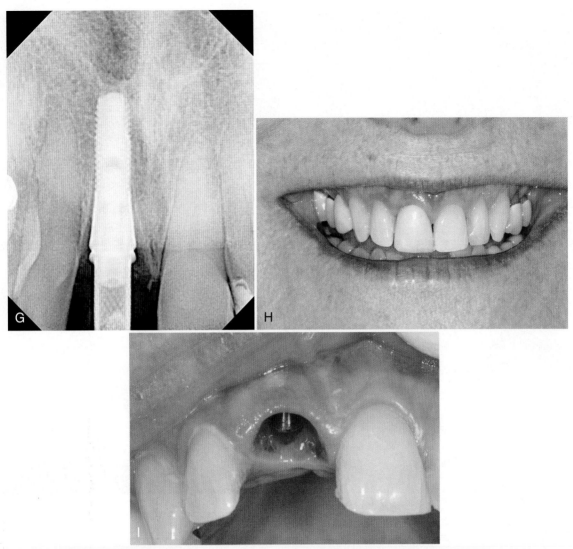

FIGURE 16-12, cont'd **G,** A radiograph of the provisional restoration on the newly inserted fixture. **H,** A good esthetic result is achieved, despite the high smile line. **I,** An excellent peri-implant soft tissue response from the use of an immediate provisional restoration.

Clinical Case: Immediate Provisionalization (Screw Retained)

A 56-year-old male was treatment planned for a four-unit implant-supported fixed partial denture in the mandibular incisor area (Fig. 16-13A). The surgical guide was designed to be converted to a provisional restoration and had "wings" placed in the canine positions to stabilize it during surgery (Fig. 16-13B). Two fixtures were placed in the lateral incisor positions and the guide modified to allow it to fit over the temporary abutment sleeves (Fig. 16-13C-F).

Composite material was then applied to the cylinders (Fig. 16-13G) and the provisional restoration before seating (Fig. 16-13H). Once the cylinders were secured to the provisional restorations, the voids were filled extraorally and the provisional restoration was seated for final contouring and adjustment (Figs. 16-13I,J). This type of restoration provides an excellent functional and esthetic result (Fig. 16-13K).

IMMEDIATE FIXTURE PLACEMENT

Placing an implant fixture at the time of tooth extraction will minimize the number of surgical procedures and overall treatment time. However, this cannot always be accomplished and the circumstances must be favorable in order to have a successful outcome. The most favorable situations for immediate fixture placement are maxillary lateral and mandibular central and lateral incisor sites. The narrower diameter of these sites often allows for the osteotomy preparation to be as large as (if not larger than) the socket itself, eliminating any bone-fixture gaps. However, any site can be a potential candidate as long as favorable conditions exist.

Immediate placement should only be considered when the soft tissue is present on the facial aspect and there is an intact buccal plate (Type I socket). In these situations, our only concern is proper placement of the fixture without the complications of having to reconstruct the hard or soft tissue in the vertical (occlusogingival) dimension (Fig. 16-14A,B). With a Type II socket (intact facial gingiva with loss of buccal plate) or Type III socket (loss of both facial gingiva and buccal plate), site development should be performed before fixture placement. Even with the predictability of regenerative therapy, it is not always possible to predict the exact final location of the hard and soft tissues. If a fixture was placed at the time of augmentation and the desired end result does not meet the predicted expectations, exposure of the fixture could occur.

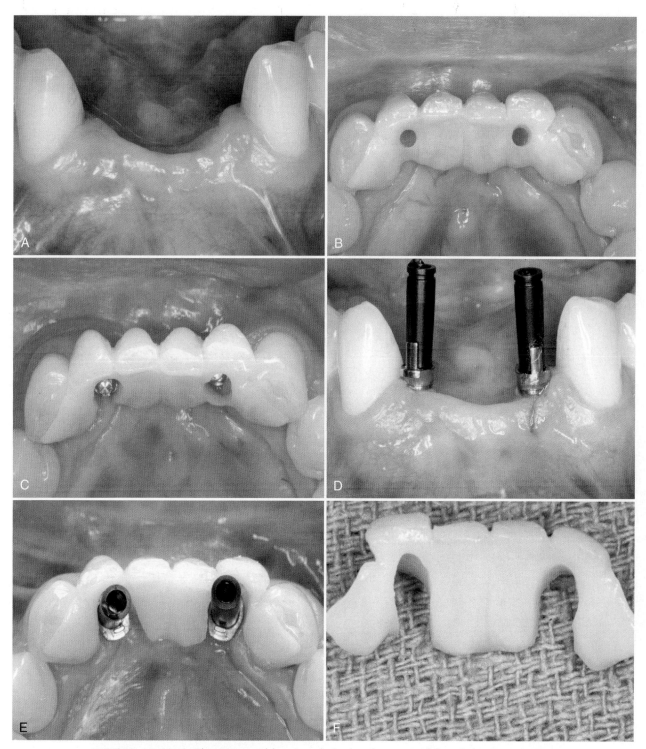

FIGURE 16-13 A, This-56-year-old patient desired replacement of the missing lower incisors with an implant supported fixed partial denture. **B,** The surgical guide was designed to allow proper positioning for two lateral incisor fixtures and to be converted into a provisional restoration. Note the stabilizing "wings" on the lingual aspects of the canines. **C,** The guide confirms the correct positioning of the two fixtures. **D,** Temporary abutment sleeves placed on the two fixtures. **E,** The guide is positioned over the cylinders and is still supported by the canine "wings." **F,** The additional cut-outs were necessary to accommodate the temporary cylinders.
Continued

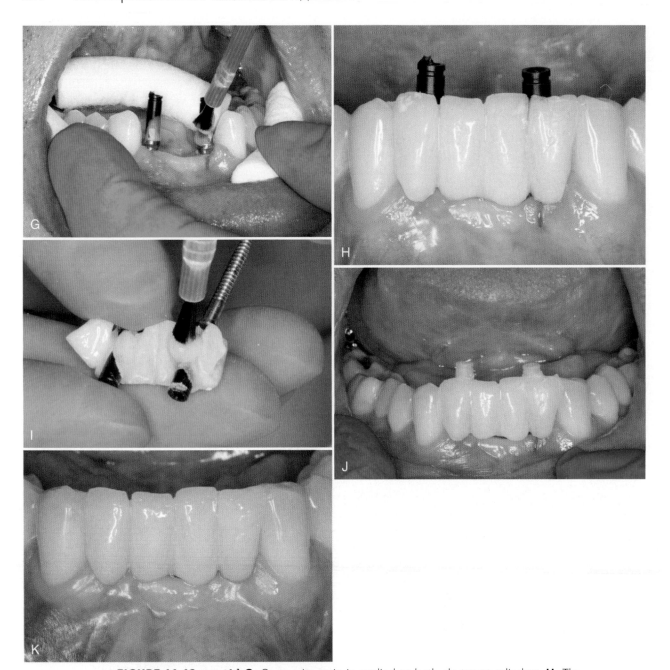

FIGURE 16-13, cont'd G, Composite resin is applied to both abutment cylinders. **H,** The provisional restoration is seated and additional composite resin material is added to secure the temporary cylinders to the restoration. **I,** Final luting is performed extraorally. **J,** Final adjustments are done intraorally to establish the occlusion. Note the white plastic "block-out" posts that protect the lingual screw access holes during final modification and contouring. **K,** The provisional restoration in place.

Although the decision to place an implant at the time of extraction can be made intraoperatively, it is far better to have as much diagnostic information before surgery, with a 3-D image being a critical planning tool. Besides assessing the status of the buccal bone, the cross-sectional images obtained can also provide information regarding the buccolingual dimension of the ridge, the angulation of the socket, as well as the presence of bony undercuts. If there is inadequate

buccolingual dimension for the planned fixture (which could result in dehiscence of the facial bone) or angulation or anatomic issues (which could result in perforation of the facial plate by the apex of the fixture), then the chances of success are significantly reduced.

Apical infection (such as endodontic involvement with a large radiolucency) or lateral infection (as could be the case with a root fracture or post perforation) associated with the

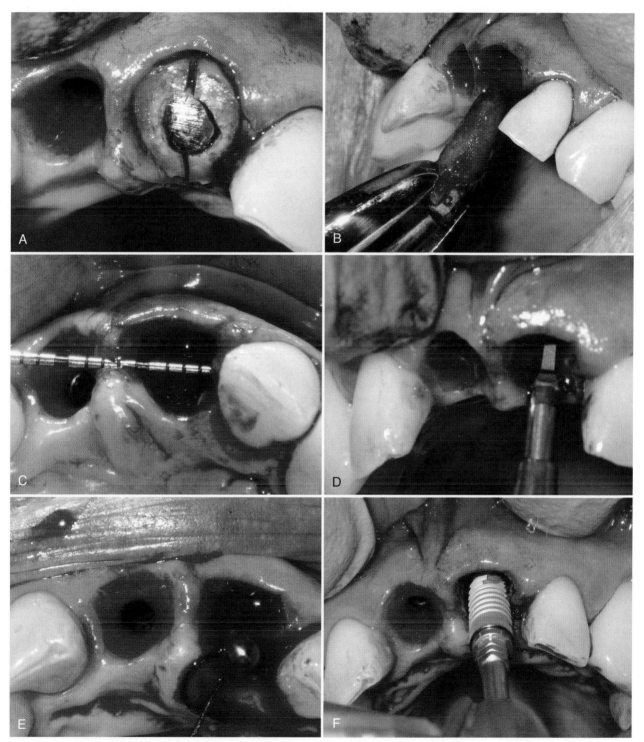

FIGURE 16-14 A, The maxillary left central incisor presented with a complete vertical fracture. The right central incisor site was previously restored with a provisional implant crown. **B,** The incisor was removed atraumatically revealing a Type I socket. **C,** The intact socket walls and soft tissue height coupled with adequate distance from the adjacent implant allowed for predictable placement of an immediate fixture. **D,** A spear point pilot drill was used to make the initial osteotomy preparation in the palatal socket wall to an adequate depth to allow the use of conventional twist drills without experiencing eccentric movement. **E,** A guide pin was placed into the osteotomy site during preparation to confirm positioning. **F,** The implant was installed engaging the palatal wall of bone. Bidigital support of the site aids in keeping the path of insertion true.

tooth to be extracted could possibly preclude proceeding with immediate fixture placement. In these situations the size of the lesion is the determining factor. If complete bone debridement is accomplished, immediate placement can be considered as long as the final osteotomy preparation will extend beyond the lesion and primary stability of the fixture can be achieved. If, however, any of these parameters are not met, socket grafting with delayed placement of the fixture is indicated. In situations in which acute infection is present, immediate placement should be avoided.

When immediate placement is performed, the same principles described earlier hold true, though there are some special considerations. When placing the initial osteotomy the necessary angulation for the fixture and the angulation of the extraction socket are often different.

Using the socket as a "guide" could result in apical perforation (buccally or palatally), improper angulation for the final restoration (especially if screw retention in planned), or placing the fixture outside the buccal contour of the arch. The initial entry point must often be on the hard, sloping palatal cortical wall of the socket in order to properly position the fixture. This can be difficult. Patience and precision are required given the hardness of the socket wall and the tendency for any bur to "skip" along the sloped wall. Great care must be taken to insure that the entry point is in the correct position. Using a small round bur or a precision point drill is a necessity to avoid misplacement of the preparation (Figs. 16-14C,D).

Enlargement of the osteotomy proceeds in a similar manner as describe earlier using stents, guide pins, and check radiographs throughout the process. The position of the implant must not deviate from the intended path of insertion during placement (Fig. 16-14E). Because there is usually a gap between the buccal wall and the fixture, it is very common that the implant can be inadvertently "pushed" facially as it is inserted owing to the denseness of the palatal wall of bone, even in a tapped osteotomy preparation. The handpiece must be kept steady and the insertion angle much be checked to ensure that the fixture is positioned in a proper palatal location (Fig. 16-14F).

After the fixture is placed (usually engaging the palatal wall of bone) it is necessary to assess any gaps (mesiodistally and buccolingually) between the fixture and the coronal confines of the socket (Fig. 16-15A) with the critical distance in deciding whether a bone graft is needed being 2 mm. If proper 3-D placement is accomplished and the gap is less than 2 mm, bone will fill in the void. Clinical situations wherein this distance is greater than 2 mm require grafting (Fig. 16-15B,C).

A provisional restoration or healing abutment can be place on the fixture even if grafting the bone-fixture gap is performed (Fig. 16-15D) as long as the soft tissue can cover the graft. If coverage of the graft cannot be achieved, then a membrane must be placed over the grafted site. This can be accomplished even when a healing abutment is in place (Fig. 16-15E,F).

When there is graft material inside the socket, this clinical situation is treated the same as if placement were into a healed edentulous ridge. However, if augmentation outside the socket area is performed, primary closure is preferable (such as connective tissue or bone grafting for contouring purposes only).

CLINICAL TIP

If a provisional restoration is placed on an immediate fixture requiring grafting, the contouring, finishing and polishing of the restoration should be accomplished before placing the graft. A high polish is necessary to avoid plaque accumulation or tissue irritation.

Clinical Case: Immediate Placement and Provisional Fabrication (Cement Retained)

A 33-year-old woman presented with a history of trauma to #8 at age 21. She had been asymptomatic since the incident, but recently developed percussion sensitivity. A horizontal root fracture was found and the tooth was deemed nonrestorable. Her medical history was unremarkable. The treatment plan was to extract the tooth, place an immediate implant, and fabricate an immediate screw-retained provisional crown.

After atraumatic removal of the tooth, the socket walls were found to be intact. The initial osteotomy preparation was made in the palatal wall of the socket using a precision point drill. The long axis of the initial preparation was positioned over the cingulum in preparation for a screw-retained provisional (Fig. 16-16A,B).

During enlargement of the osteotomy site, there was concern that the apical portion of the preparation might perforate the buccal plate, so slight re-angulation was performed. When the fixture was inserted, it was centered mesiodistally (Fig. 16-16C) but the buccolingual position was now coincident with the incisal edge (Fig. 16-16D-F). This slight re-angulation required the fabrication of a cementable provisional crown

A nonrotational abutment was placed on the fixture (Fig. 16-16G) using a hand driver and light finger pressure. After determining the necessary amount of reduction, the abutment was placed on an abutment holder and prepared extraorally (Fig. 16-16H). The abutment was transferred back to the implant several times during the preparation to check for proper clearance and to ensure that the chamfer margin was located approximately 1 mm subgingivally. The prepared abutment was affixed to the implant and the access hole sealed with PTFE tape and Cavit (Fig. 16-16I).

A lab processed shell was relined using acrylic resin material. The acrylic was added using a brush to minimize any voids on the inside of the provisional restoration (Fig. 16-16J). A hole was placed in the cingulum of the provisional restoration to prevent excess material from being hydraulically forced under the tissues. Excess subgingival material mechanically engaging an undercut could cause difficulty in removing the provisional restoration. The acrylic could also be pushed into the socket and possibly "wick" on the threads of the fixture itself, which would have disastrous consequences in terms of healing.

After final trimming of the provisional restoration, it was tried-in without cement and the occlusion checked to ensure that there were no contacts maximal intercuspation and in any excursions. With the occlusion established, the provisional restoration was cemented using a noneugenol provisional cement. The contours of the provisional restoration maintained the soft tissue profile (Fig. 16-16K). Complete cement removal was able to be achieved because of the shallow subgingival margin.

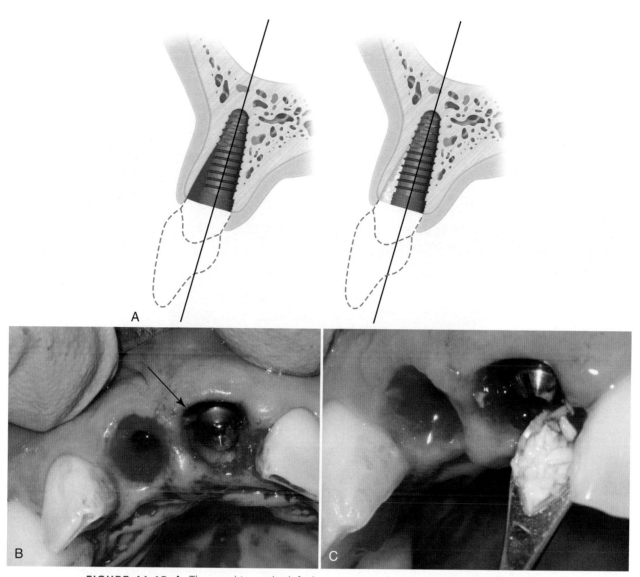

FIGURE 16-15 A, The graphic on the left shows an immediately placed fixture with a bone-fixture gap buccally. The one on the right demonstrates grafting of the gap. **B,** With the cover screw in place, proper positioning of the implant can be observed against the palatal wall of the socket. The gap between the buccal plate and the implant was greater than 2 mm, necessitating grafting (*arrow*). **C,** The gap was grafted using a cortical allograft. A healing abutment had been placed to help support the soft tissue.

Continued

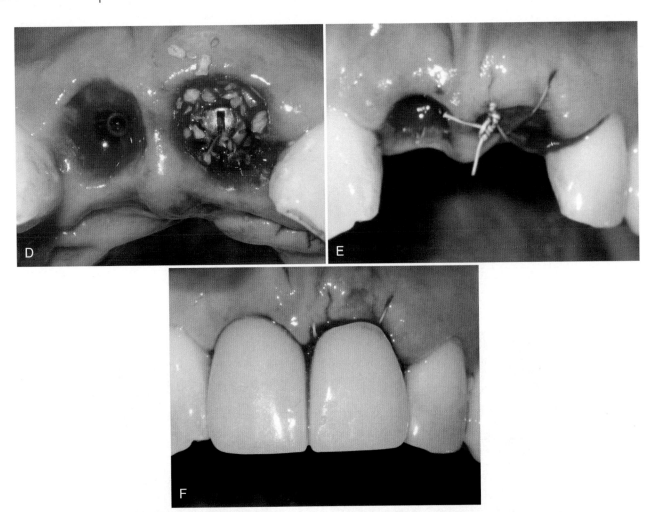

FIGURE 16-15, cont'd D, The site was filled with graft material slightly above the bony crest of the socket. The coronal diameter of the socket precluded coverage of the graft, with membrane placement being indicated. **E,** A collagen matrix was adapted over the site, tucked under the buccal and palatal flaps and sutured using a small diameter polytetrafluoroethylene (PTFE) suture. **F,** A screw-retained provisional restoration was placed engaging the healed fixture in the maxillary right central incisor position. The pontic was contoured to mimic the desired marginal shape to help guide soft tissue healing. No contact was made with the underlying socket and a high polish was placed on the pontic.

SITE DEVELOPMENT

Not every implant site presents with ideal or favorable soft and hard tissues. It is often necessary to correct deficits, caused by pathology, atrophy, trauma, or other anatomical considerations such as a lack of keratinized tissue, aberrant frenal attachments, ridge concavities (occlusoapically, buccolingually or both), or loss of papillae. With more involved defects, a combination of soft and hard tissue procedures may be indicated.

Soft Tissue Defects

Soft tissue corrections involve the same surgical principles and procedures used in nonimplant periodontal clinical situations (see Chapter 14) including free grafts, connective tissue grafts, and pedicle grafts using either an autograft or an alloplastic substitute. The timing of these procedures is determined by individual case requirements. A frenectomy with free grafting or buccal augmentation can usually be done at any point in treatment, and is often performed in conjunction with either fixture placement or second stage surgery. Correction of a mucogingival junction disparity at the implant site can be accomplished using a buccally positioned flap and a provisional restoration or healing abutment to maintain the tissue in the corrected position and can be performed in both the one and two stage approaches. This also applies for sites with multiple missing teeth receiving two or more implants; however, sometimes it becomes necessary for soft tissue grafting to be done before implant placement in order to create adequate keratinized tissue for proper flap management. In all of the clinical situations mentioned, the underlying bone must be adequate.

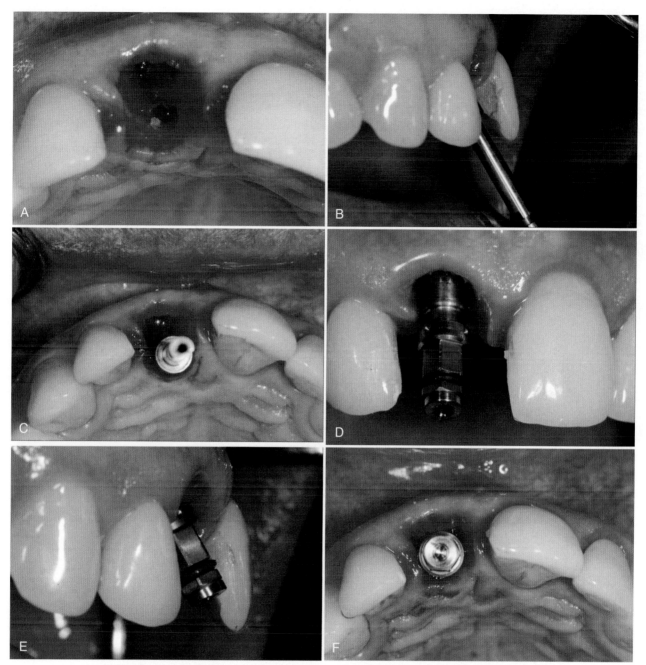

FIGURE 16-16 A, Proper osteotomy preparation required placing the initial entry point on palatal wall of this Type I immediate extraction socket. **B,** The long axis of the preparation was favorable for screw retention after using the initial 2.0-mm twist drill. **C,** The pathway of the guide is coincident with the location of the cingulum. **D,** The implant is ideally positioned in the center of the edentulous ridge. **E,** Because slight re-angulation was necessary to avoid perforation of the buccal plate, the final position of the fixture was now in line with the incisal edge of the adjacent teeth, requiring the use of a cementable provisional restoration. **F,** From the occlusal view, the long axis is seen to be in line with the incisal edges of the natural dentition.

Continued

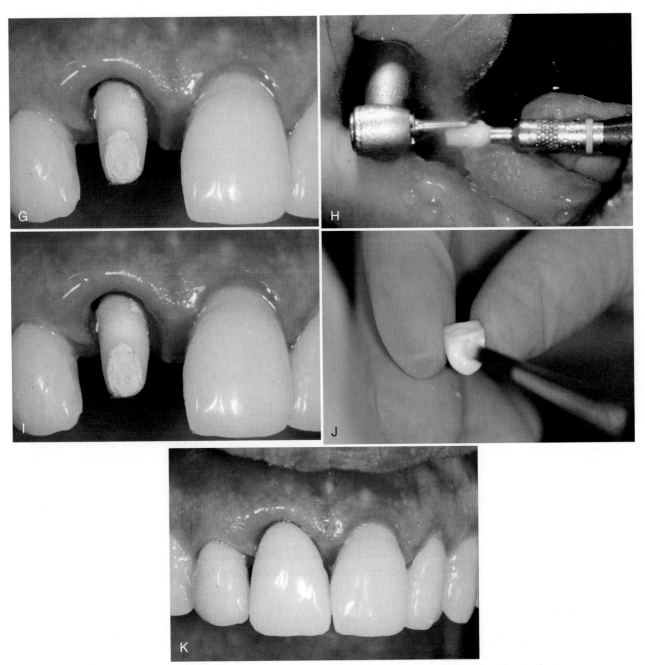

FIGURE 16-16, cont'd **G,** A non-rotational provisional abutment was placed on the implant and the amount of incisal and gingival reduction determined. **H,** Preparation of the abutment is performed extraorally using a high speed diamond bur. An abutment holder should be used to stabilize the abutment during preparation. **I,** After finishing the preparation, the abutment is affixed to the implant and sealed with PTFE tape and Cavit (3M ESPE). Note the slight subgingival chamfered finish line. **J,** Acrylic is added using a brush to minimize any internal voids in the provisional restoration. **K,** The final provisional restoration

Ridge Augmentation

Correcting bony defects or deficits presents one of the greatest challenges in implant treatment. Adequate hard tissue is an absolute requirement for case success. Generally, all significant site development should be performed before fixture placement in the esthetic zone. There are some exceptions such as immediate fixture placement with socket grafting or augmentation of a buccal concavity for cosmetic reasons where adequate ridge dimensions already exist.

CLINICAL TIP

If there is insufficient bone for placement in any dimension, augmentation procedures must be performed before fixture placement.

Guided bone regeneration is the primary method for hard tissue site development, and is based upon the principles of guided tissue regeneration (see Chapter 14). Bone, growth factors and barrier membranes are used to reconstruct the edentulous ridge as well as maintain the integrity of the immediate extraction socket. The primary difference is that the regeneration involves bone only without the presence of a tooth. Before performing any regenerative site development, the surgeon must identify the goals and expected outcome of the procedures using the clinical and radiographic information previously obtained.

Augmentation in the horizontal (buccolingual) dimension is predictable. For the edentulous ridge, a full thickness mucoperiosteal flap is reflected to provide total access to the defect. The initial incisions are typically paracrestal in the ridge and are biased toward the lingual or palatal. Adequate lateral flap reflection, usually involving at least 1½ or 2 teeth on either side of the ridge, allows for access without tissue tearing. If vertical incisions are used, they must be sufficiently distant from the planned graft area to avoid closure near any graft or membrane.

After thorough debridement of the soft tissue in the defect, the cortical bone in the regenerative site is decorticated using a round bur. This should be performed at a very low rotational speed (such as with the implant drilling unit) using copious irrigation. This step in the procedure creates a bleeding base for perfusion of the graft, as the cortical surface is relatively avascular. Damage to any of the roots adjacent to the graft site must be carefully avoided. The graft material is then placed and adapted to rebuild the ridge dimensions. When multiple implants are planned, the interimplant bone should be overbuilt. This will provide the ability to create crestal scalloping when the implants are eventually placed, thus allowing for a more esthetic final restoration.

The choice of graft material is based upon the surgical requirement and the surgeon's and patient's preferences and includes human allografts (Puros Allograft, Zimmer Dental Inc.), xenografts (Endobon, BioMet 3i), bone blocks (Bio-Oss Collagen, Geistlich Pharma North America, Inc.) and synthetics (Straumann Bone Ceramic, Straumann USA). If hydration of the graft is necessary, sterile saline or blood should be used. If growth factors in liquid form are being added to the graft, hydration is not necessary (Gem-21, Osteohealth; Emdogain, Straumann USA).

A membrane or barrier must be placed over the graft with the lateral and apical borders resting on ungrafted bone beyond the material itself. Resorbable membranes (Bio Mend, Zimmer Dental Inc. and DynaMatrix—Keystone Dental, Inc.), nonresorbable membranes (Cytoplast PTFE, Osteogenics Biomedical) and/or titanium reinforced membranes or perforated titanium meshes can be used. The choice of material is based upon the volume of defect that is to be regenerated. For smaller defects, a resorbable barrier draped over the graft is preferred. Fixation tacks are sometimes indicated to secure the membrane and prevent movement. For larger defects, a more rigid barrier must be used. These membranes are pliable enough to be bent and cut, allowing for adaptation to the ridge, yet are strong enough to maintain their shape throughout the healing process (Figs. 16-17A,B). Fixation screws are necessary to secure the mesh to prevent any movement (Fig. 16-17C) and are removed during re-entry.

If a perforated mesh is used, a resorbable barrier must be placed between the mesh and the flap before closure. This protects the flap from irritation by the mesh and satisfies soft tissue exclusion at the graft site (Fig. 16-17D).

With this procedure, primary closure is imperative to avoid slough of the flap. Passivity of the flap is crucial. The flap must be released to allow for coronal and palatal/lingual positioning and advancement because the size and volume of the ridge is

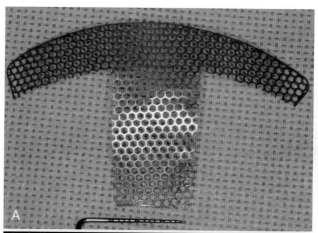
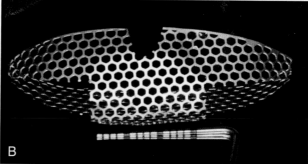
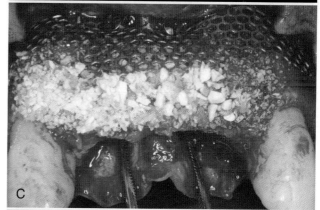
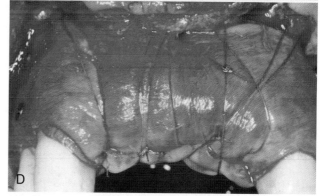

FIGURE 16-17 A, Titanium mesh is trimmed to the dimensions needed for the guided bone regeneration (GBR) procedure. **B,** The body of the mesh has been shaped to fit over the edentulous ridge and provides space for the pending graft. Note the cut-outs for the anterior nasal spine. **C,** A mesh positioned and secured with fixation screws before graft placement. **D,** A resorbable membrane placed over the mesh and secured with connective tissue suturing.

being expanded from its original dimensions. This is accomplished using a combination of submucous dissection, subperiosteal release, and vertical incisions. If vertical incisions are placed, they must be positioned distant from the membrane so as not to interfere with achieving primary closure. It the incisions are placed too close to the regenerative site, they could potentially open causing infection and failure of the procedure.

If a removable provisional restoration is used, it must be supported by the natural dentition and have no contact with the surgical site. In order to accomplish this, the adjusted removable provisional restoration must be inserted immediately after surgery is completed. This can confine subsequent swelling at the site to the space between the flap and underside of the appliance, thus enabling the patient to continue wearing the appliance. Patients must wear their appliance 24 hours a day during the initial healing time except for cleaning and oral hygiene. If, however, the patient were to remove the appliance for an extended period of time and then replace it intraorally, or were to not wear the appliance immediately after surgery is completed, and the tissues were to swell to a greater extent than the space created in the appliance at the time of surgery, wearing the appliance at this time would put detrimental pressure on the graft. Similarly, the undersides of fixed provisional pontics must be adequately trimmed to avoid placing pressure on the healing wound. After 1 week the soft tissue should have healed adequately, so as to allow for relining either type of restoration; however, this needs to be assessed at the first postoperative visit because healing times can vary.

Clinical Case: Guided Bone Regeneration

A 61-year-old woman presented requesting to have implants placed to restore her anterior maxilla (Fig. 16-18A). Clinical and radiographic evaluation determined that inadequate bone width existed and guided bone regeneration was indicated. After reflecting a full thickness flap (Fig. 16-18B) a narrow ridge was evident in the incisor region. Given the size of the area and volume of bone that required regeneration, a titanium mesh with a cortical bovine bone (xenograft) graft was used. The titanium mesh was adapted to the site, allowing adequate space for building out the bone, and then secured with surgical screws (Fig. 16-18C). Care was taken to insure that the mesh did not touch the roots of the adjacent natural teeth. Decortication of the graft site was performed (Fig. 16-18D), the graft placed (Fig. 16-18E), and the mesh adapted over the site (Fig. 16-18F). A resorbable membrane was then placed over the mesh and sutured to the flap before closing the site (Fig. 16-18G,H).

The lack of buccal keratinized tissue was noted in the initial workup and was treatment planned for correction at the time of membrane removal (Fig. 16-18I). A full thickness flap was reflected to gain access to the fixation screws (Fig. 16-18J) with a substantial increase in buccolingual ridge dimension observed (Fig. 16-18K). A connective tissue graft was harvested

from the posterior palate and placed over the site before closure (Fig. 16-18L) with adequate soft tissue reconstruction evident postoperatively (Fig. 16-18M-O).

A post-graft CT scan demonstrated a significant increase in the width the buccal bone compared to the preoperative image (Fig. 16-19A-D). Two implants were subsequently placed in the central incisor positions and provisionalized to aid in guiding soft tissue development (Figs. 16-19E,F). Proper implant location and platform positioning are evident in the radiograph at the time of prosthesis insertion (Fig. 16-19G). Some pink porcelain was used to avoid creating an overly lengthy contact point (even with favorable implant location and bone height, the soft tissues remained relatively flat) with the desired esthetic goals being achieved with the definitive restoration (Fig. 16-19H).

Ridge Preservation

Ridge preservation or socket preservation is performed when delayed fixture placement is planned. This procedure follows the same guidelines as regeneration for the edentulous ridge, except for the presence of an immediate extraction socket. After atraumatic removal of the tooth, the need for flap reflection is determined. If a flap is reflected, the graft material is placed into the socket and covered with a barrier. The choices of barrier material include both resorbable and nonresorbable membranes.

Site closure is accomplished using simple sutures.

In the flapless approach, the graft material can be covered by the patient's own tissues with a free gingival "plug" being used (Fig. 16-19I). When a deficit is noted in the bone (such as a narrow dehiscence buccally), a resorbable membrane can be trimmed to allow it to cover the defect on the inside of the socket and to provide coverage of the graft at the crest. For this technique, an "ice cream cone" shaped barrier satisfies these requirements. The membrane must be placed inside the socket before the bone graft. Site closure is achieved using simple suturing.

Clinical Case: Socket Preservation

A 23-year-old woman presented with a fracture of her maxillary left central incisor (Fig. 16-20A,B). After removal of the root fragment, a dehiscence of the facial plate was observed. A closed socket graft was indicated. After thorough debridement, a resorbable membrane was trimmed to allow coverage of the dehiscence and the occlusal portion of the socket (Fig. 16-20C). The membrane was placed into the socket followed by graft placement (Fig. 16-20D,E). The wider portion of the membrane was then tucked under the palatal tissues and sutured in place (Fig. 16-20F,G).

As with the ridge augmentation procedure, the underside of the transitional restoration must be contoured to avoid pressure on the site. If there is concern regarding movement of the barrier, this can be controlled by suturing the membrane to the

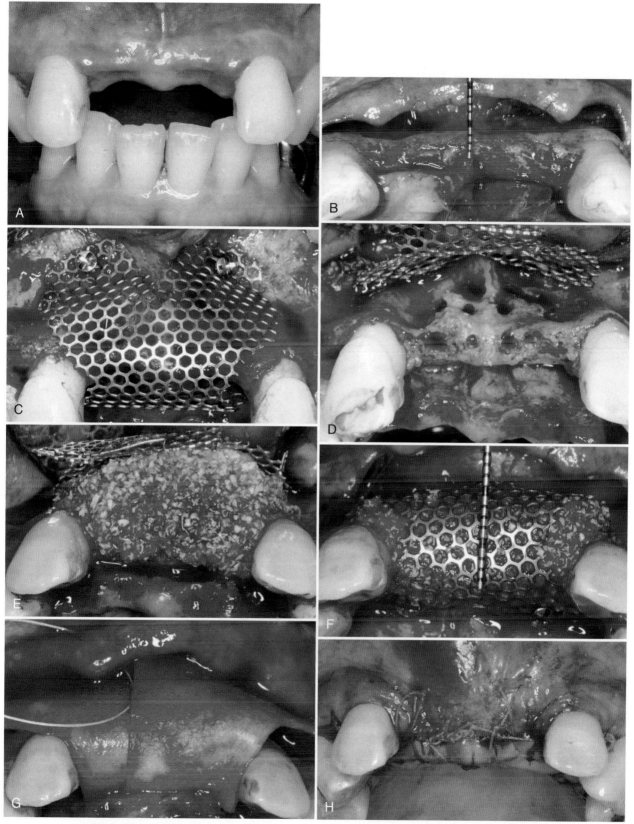

FIGURE 16-18 A, A 61-year-old patient with a resorbed anterior maxillary edentulous ridge. **B,** After reflection of a full thickness flap, a very narrow bony ridge is noted. **C,** A titanium mesh is adapted and secured to the site with apical fixation screws. Space is created for the graft material. **D,** Perforation of the cortical plate is done using a round bur. **E,** The bone graft is placed building up the dimensions of the ridge. **F,** The mesh is adapted over the graft. **G,** A resorbable membrane is placed over the mesh and sutured to the underlying connective tissue and the flap. **H,** Primary closure of the site is achieved.

Continued

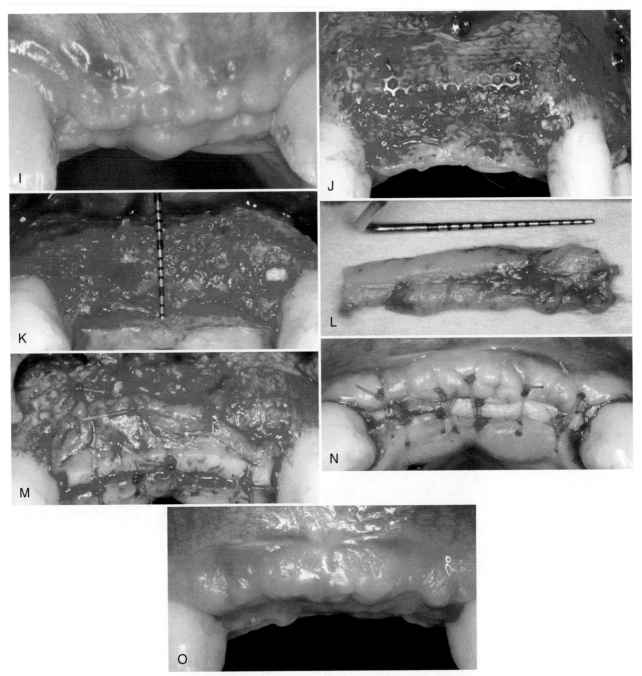

FIGURE 16-18, cont'd I, The site 4 months post grafting. The lack of buccal masticatory mucosa was preplanned for correction at the time of membrane removal. J, The mesh was exposed after full thickness flap reflection. K, After removing the mesh a significant increase in the B-L dimension of bone is evident. L, A thick connective tissue graft was harvested from the posterior palate with some of the epithelium purposely attached. M, The connective tissue portion of the graft was placed buccally with the epithelial portion abutted against the palatal margin. N, Primary closure of the site showing the position of the connective tissue graft. O, Six weeks postoperatively adequate augmentation of the gingival tissues is evident.

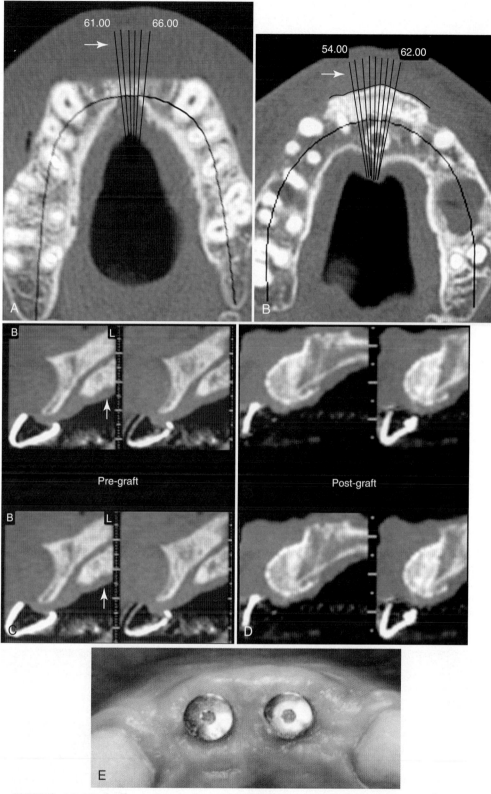

FIGURE 16-19 A, The pretreatment coronal scan view revealing the deficiency of anterior bone. **B,** The post-graft coronal scan view revealing the amount of bone augmentation. **C,** Cross-sectional slices of the pregrafted anterior maxilla. Note the severe deficiency of the bone in relation to the outline of the teeth on the stent. **D,** The scan after the graft shows formation of adequate bone for fixture placement. The barium outline of the stent is visible over the sites. **E,** Two central incisor fixtures with healing abutments.

Continued

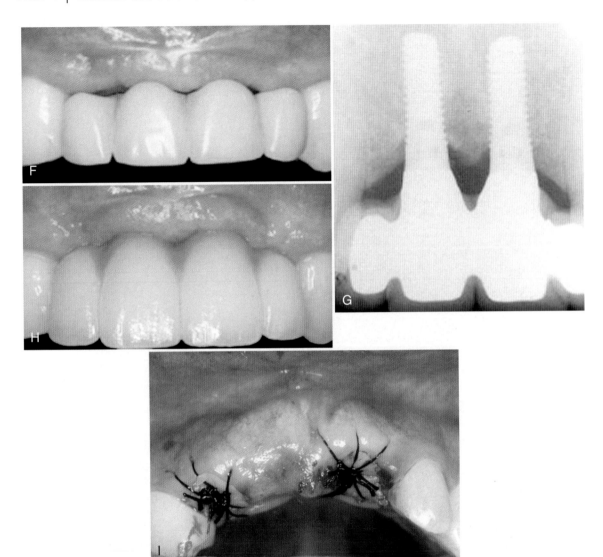

FIGURE 16-19, cont'd **F,** The provisional restoration in place. **G,** A radiograph of the definitive restoration demonstrates maintenance of the midline crestal peak of bone necessary for papillae formation. **H,** The final restoration demonstrates a good esthetic result. Pink porcelain was used to create the appearance of proper tooth shape and contour. **I,** Circular free gingival grafts are used to cover these two bone grafted extraction sockets.

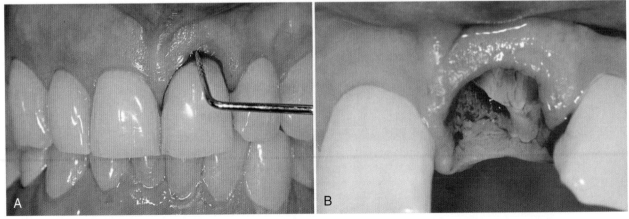

FIGURE 16-20 **A,** 23-year-old patient presented with a fracture of her maxillary left central incisor associated with significant mid-facial probing depth. **B,** Removal of the coronal segment revealed oblique subcrestal involvement with an associated dehiscence.

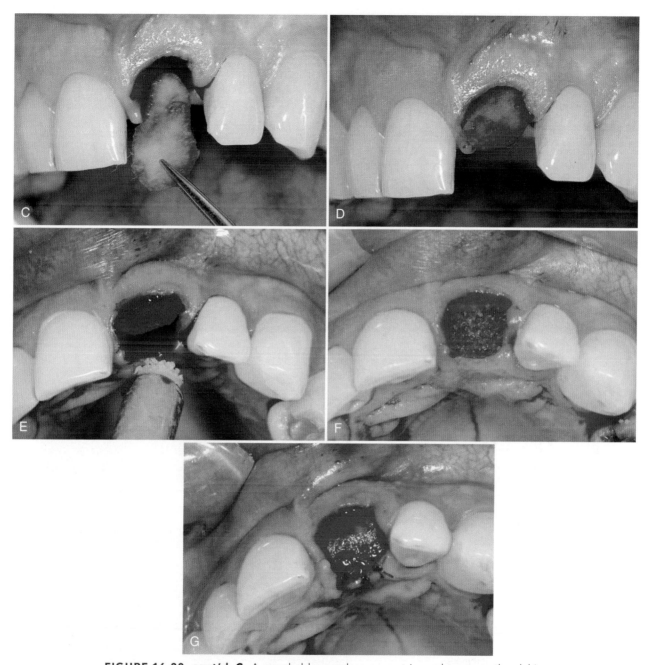

FIGURE 16-20, cont'd C, A resorbable membrane was trimmed to cover the dehiscence internally and allow for coverage of the graft. **D,** The membrane is placed into the socket before graft placement. **E,** Bone is placed into the socket with a bone syringe. **F,** The socket filled with graft material before covering with the membrane. **G,** The edge of the membrane is secured to the palatal tissues using small diameter resorbable sutures.

margin of the flap with a small diameter suture. For both ridge augmentation and preservation procedures, approximately 4 to 6 months are required for healing and maturation of the bone to occur before fixture placement. Patients usually wish to proceed more quickly with treatment; however; the time necessary for wound healing must be respected.

TOOTH MOVEMENT

When considerable vertical defects are present on the natural teeth, orthodontic forced eruption can be a solution. If the attachment levels on the adjacent teeth are favorable and peri-gingival inflammation is controlled, the hard and soft tissues can be improved before fixture placement.

CLINICAL TIP

When forced eruption is performed under controlled conditions, both the soft and hard tissue attachments will move coronally with the tooth (Fig. 16-21A,B).

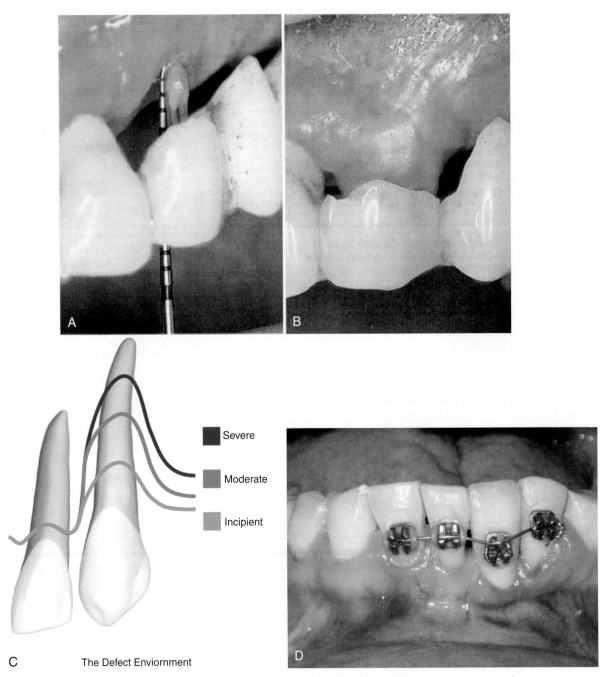

C　　　The Defect Enviornment

FIGURE 16-21 A, Retained lateral incisor root is engaged through an opening prepared in a provisional fixed partial denture for eruption to modify the bone and tissue before fixture placement. **B,** With controlled force, the soft tissue attachment and underlying bone can be greatly modified. **C,** The severity of the defect will determine how much ridge modification can be achieved as long as the attachment on the adjacent teeth is good. **D,** This patient presented with an unaesthetic crown with gingival marginal discrepancy. Brackets were placed to effect eruption to modify the soft and hard tissues.

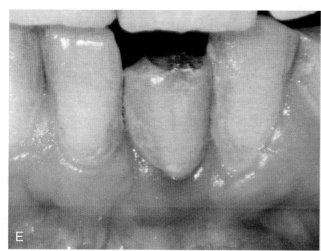

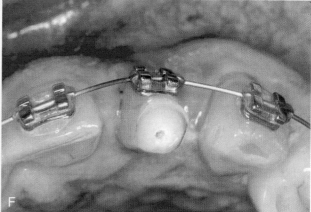

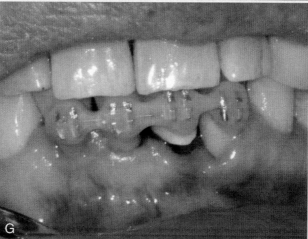

FIGURE 16-21, cont'd E, Occlusal adjustment has been performed during eruption to prevent traumatic occlusion. **F,** Exposure of the pulp canal has occurred after eruption of this lateral incisor. **G,** Correction of the defect after 4 months with a composite resin splint on the brackets. Note the more apical level of the tissue on the distal of the mandibular left central incisor which was driven by the lower attachment level on the mandibular left lateral incisor before treatment.

This is true for even the most severe defect (Fig. 16-21C). Teeth that are erupted in the absence of inflammation maintain the level of the underlying gingival connective tissue fibers (the biological width) on the root surface, which allows for coronal movement of the soft tissue.

This, in turn, allows coronal bone deposition to occur as the tooth erupts. Unlike forced eruption for crown lengthening (see Chapter 17) wherein the goal is to pull part of the root out of the bone, the goal here is to use a hopeless tooth in order to modify the local defect environment.

From the periodontal standpoint, the vertical bony dimension of the site can be predictably increased and the adjacent papillae predictably preserved, thus providing a favorable ridge-tooth relationship for esthetic implant placement. From the restorative standpoint, a more ideal supragingival restorative space can be created allowing for an optimally esthetic restoration to be fabricated.

The number of teeth to be erupted and the periodontal status of the surrounding dentition will determine the extent of the bracketing necessary to achieve the desired end result. If a single tooth is to be erupted, then a quadrant or sextant can suffice for anchorage. If multiple teeth crossing the midline are involved, full arch banding may be indicated. Bracket placement on the tooth being moved should be apical to that of the other teeth. Depending upon the amount of eruption planned, brackets may need to be repositioned during treatment. A smaller gauge flexible wire (such as .012 titanium or stainless steel) should be used that fits passively in the brackets of the anchor teeth and only engages the tooth being moved (Fig. 16-21D).

This provides the ability to control the amount of force used.

CLINICAL TIP

Slow eruption is necessary in order to ensure that the attachment will be erupted along with the tooth: the use of excessive force could result in orthodontic extraction.

Periodic occlusal adjustment is necessary as the tooth erupts to prevent trauma as well as to create room for further movement (Figs. 16-21E). Pulpal extirpation may become necessary depending upon how much vertical movement is needed; the greater the planned distance of eruption, the higher the likelihood that the pulp chamber will be exposed.

CLINICAL TIP

If pulp exposure occurs during forced eruption, the root canal can be filled with calcium hydroxide and sealed after pulpal extirpation: final endodontic obturation is usually not necessary (Fig. 16-21F).

When the tooth is in the desired position, the movement apparatus must be fixated to allow maturation of the newly formed coronal attachment. This can be achieved by connecting all of the brackets with a stainless steel ligature wire or by placing a composite material over each bracket (Fig. 16-21G). In either case, the bone requires time to heal before fixture placement.

Once the site has healed, fixture placement can proceed as described earlier with the same rules applied regarding surgical case planning, site development, and surgical placement.

Clinical Case: Orthodontic Eruption for Site Development

A 57-year-old man presented with advanced attachment loss and severe recession on the maxillary left lateral incisor (Fig. 16-22A). Given the severe soft and hard tissue discrepancy between this tooth and the adjacent incisor and canine, orthodontic eruption for site development was planned. Brackets were placed and the lateral incisor was engaged with a .014 Ti wire (Fig. 16-22B). As the tooth erupted, a second bracket was affixed to the lateral incisor (Fig. 16-22C); this allowed it to be engaged to the arch wire before removing the more coronally positioned bracket owing to its mobility. Occlusal adjustment was performed throughout movement, with pulpal extirpation becoming necessary.

Once the desired amount of movement was achieved, the lateral incisor was splinted to the two adjacent teeth using a composite resin material (Fig. 16-22D), allowing maturation of the newly formed bone. At the time of extraction, immediate fixture placement was performed given the small amount of root remaining in the bone (Fig. 16-22E,F). Even with the eruption of the free gingival margin, there was still a narrow zone of keratinized tissue present, so a two-stage procedure was planned.

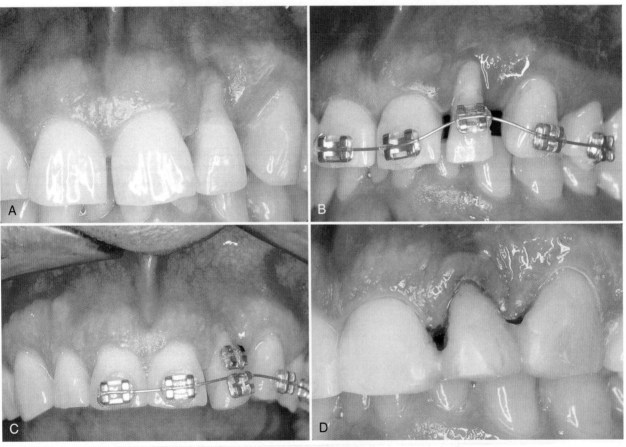

FIGURE 16-22 A, Mucogingival insufficiency, root dehiscence and lack of bone are present on the lateral incisor of this 57 year old patient. **B,** Brackets are placed on the two adjacent teeth, bilaterally and in a more apical position on the lateral incisor. A light gauge wire is placed to begin eruption. **C,** As the tooth erupts, a second bracket is placed more apically. This will allow for more control of the movement as well as stabilizing the tooth when the original bracket is removed. **D,** An extra-coronal composite resin splint is placed to stabilize the tooth after eruption is complete.

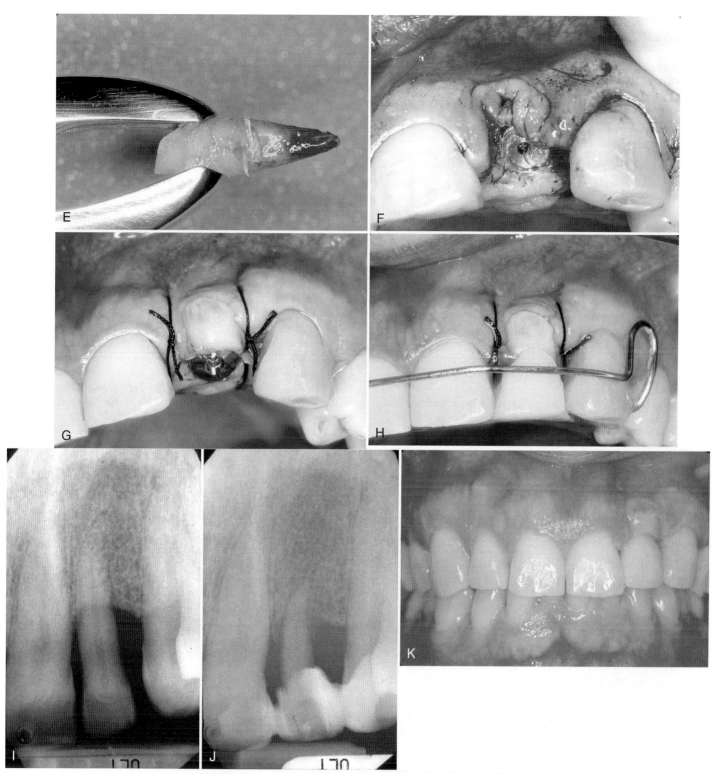

FIGURE 16-22, cont'd E, At the time of fixture placement, the tooth is removed. Note the small amount of attachment at the apex of the tooth. **F,** An immediate fixture is able to be placed because of the amount of bone gained and the small size of the root socket. **G,** Buccal positioning of the flap performed at second stage surgery with the healing abutment helping to keep the tissue in place. **H,** The transitional appliance is adjusted to eliminate pressure at the surgical site. **I,** The pre-treatment periapical radiograph. **J,** The post-eruption radiograph at the time of debracketing demonstrating the vertical gain in bone height. Note the position of the healing bone on the root of the lateral incisor. **K,** The provisional restoration in place after soft tissue healing.

After integration of the fixture, a healing abutment was placed using a paracrestal incision design, which allowed for buccal positioning of the flap to increase the zone of masticatory mucosa (Fig. 16-22G,H). The initial and pre-extraction radiographs reveal the leveling of the crestal bone and the amount of eruption (Figs. 16-22I,J). After soft tissue healing, a provisional restoration was placed (Fig. 16-22K).

Clinical Case: Combined Site Development for a Multiple Tooth Edentulous Span

A 47-year-old woman with failing restorations on both maxillary central incisors presented for implant replacement. Given the deficiency of bone in the buccolingual and occlusoapical dimensions, a combined approach was planned for ridge reconstruction; forced eruption to modify the occlusoapical deficiency, and guided bone regeneration (GBR) to correct the buccolingual defect. Initially the maxillary arch was bracketed in preparation for orthodontic eruption of both central incisors (Fig. 16-23A). Because multiple teeth were to be erupted that crossed the midline, full arch bracketing was indicated. After tooth movement was completed, the central incisors were splinted (Fig. 16-23B). The post-eruption radiograph demonstrates positioning of the crestal bone of the incisors is coronal to the adjacent lateral incisors (Fig. 16-23C).

Despite the gain in bone and soft tissue, a buccolingual deficiency remained. However, given the gains from the eruption (soft and hard tissue), guided bone regeneration became a more predictable endeavor. After reflection of a full thickness flap, the edentulous site was prepared for bone graft and membrane placement and primary closure achieved (Fig. 16-23D-G). A resorbable collagen pad was placed between the sutured site and the removable appliance, with the patient instructed to wear it without removal for the first several postoperative days (Fig. 16-23H,I); this provided both hemostasis and prevented swelling beyond the contours of the provisional appliance. After healing, a favorable interarch relationship was created (Fig. 16-23J), which allowed for placing two fixtures in the central incisor positions. Proper interfixture distance was confirmed during osteotomy preparation (Figs. 16-23K,L). A provisional restoration was placed on both fixtures (Fig. 16-23M) to guide the marginal tissue and papillary healing.

Clinical Case: Implant Problem Solving

A 72-year-old woman presented complaining about her maxillary right central incisor crown. Her past history revealed that the maxillary right central incisor had been extracted and replaced with a larger diameter immediate fixture. The platform location and buccal positioning led to an unacceptable esthetic outcome (Fig. 16-24A). Removal of the existing implant was necessary along with GBR correction of the mucogingival issues in order to satisfy the patient's cosmetic desires. After crown removal and full thickness flap reflection, it was observed that the fixture was positioned too far apically and buccally (Fig. 16-24B). The fixture was immobile when torqued or when lateral force was applied. Therefore a trephine was used, taking care not to damage the buccal plate (Fig. 16-24C-F).

A cortical bone allograft was placed into the explant socket and over the ridge, covered with a dermal matrix membrane and closed primarily (Fig. 16-24G-I). After 4 months

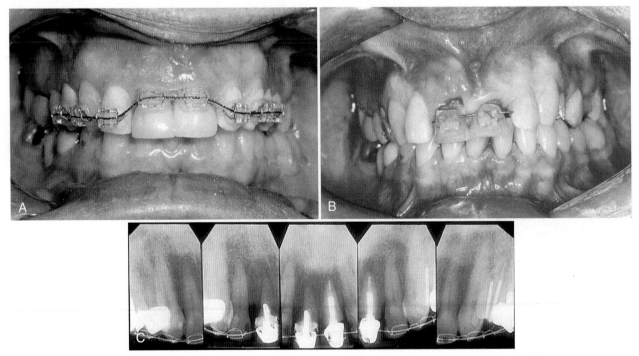

FIGURE 16-23 A, 47-year-old patient with failing central incisor crowns. Full arch brackets were placed for eruption of the incisors. **B,** The free gingival margin is at a more coronal position in relationship to the adjacent teeth after eruption. **C,** A periapical film during eruption reveals the failed restorations and the reverse bony architecture resulting from the eruption.

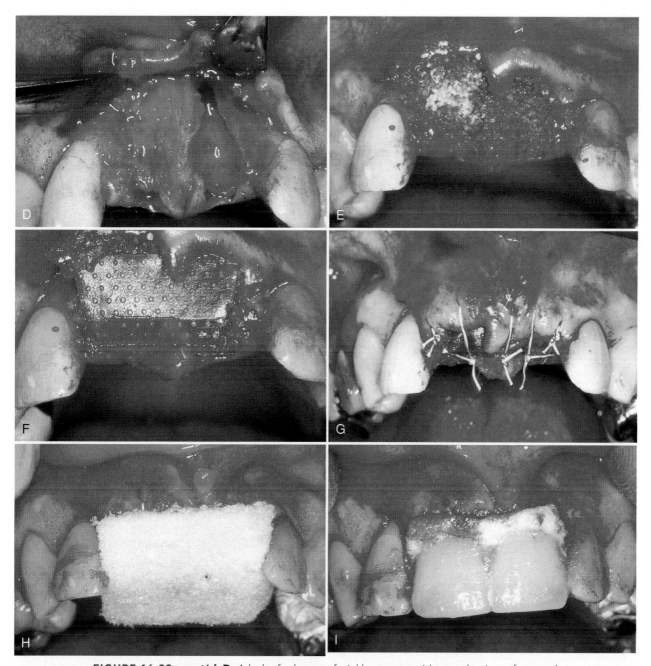

FIGURE 16-23, cont'd D, A lack of adequate facial bone was evident at the time of removal of both teeth. The palatal aspect of the ridge was intact, allowing for GBR to be performed. **E,** A bone graft was placed into the defect to create the desired ridge contours. **F,** A resorbable barrier was adapted over the graft and tucked under the palatal flap. **G,** Primary closure was achieved over most of the site. **H,** A collagen sponge was placed over the sutured wound. **I,** The provisional appliance was inserted with the instructions that it be worn 72 to 96 hours for hemostasis and control of swelling.

Continued

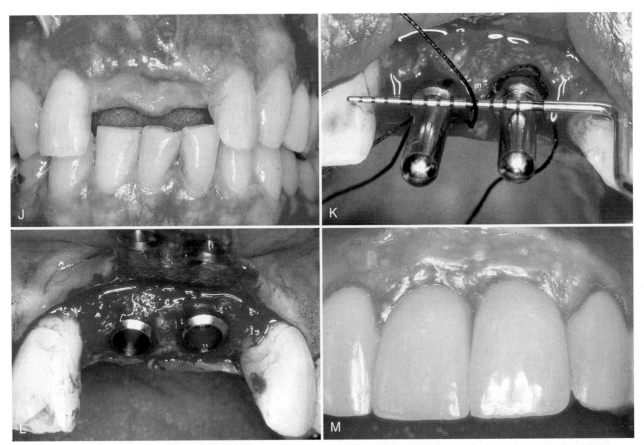

FIGURE 16-23, cont'd J, Good ridge and interarch dimensions are obtained post-surgically. **K,** The guide pins demonstrate adequate distance between the two osteotomy sites. **L,** The two fixtures are shown properly positioned in relation to each other and the adjacent teeth. **M,** The provisional restoration inserted at the time of fixture placement demonstrates a good soft tissue profile at the site.

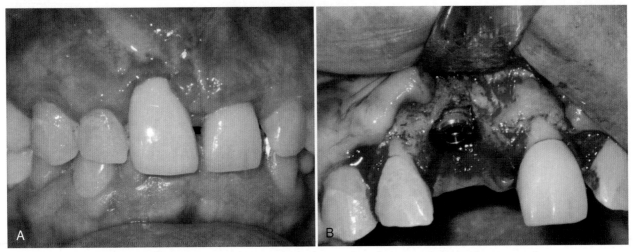

FIGURE 16-24 A, 72-year-old patient wanted correction of an unaesthetic implant restoration in the maxillary right central incisor position. The crown is overcontoured in all dimensions. **B,** The fixture can be seen improperly positioned after flap reflection.

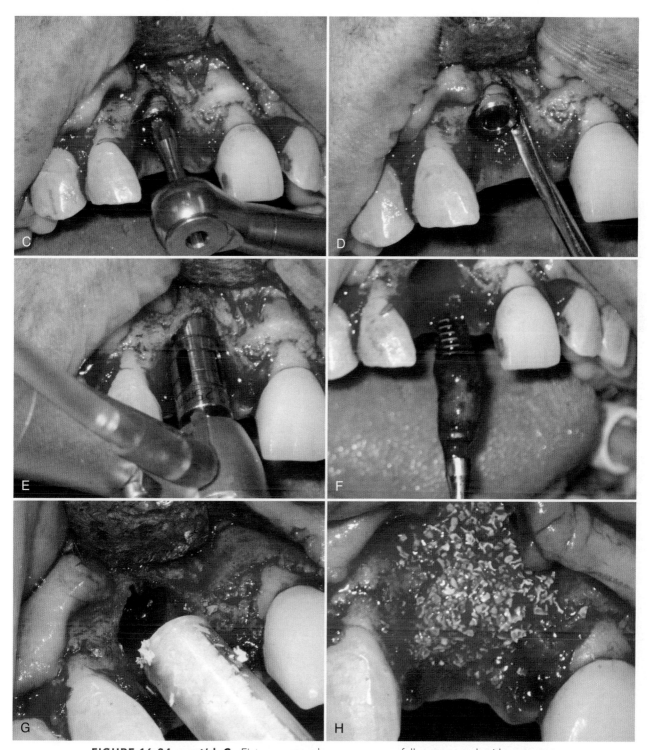

FIGURE 16-24, cont'd C, Fixture removal was unsuccessfully attempted with a torque wrench. **D,** Use of a small elevator revealed no movement on the fixture. **E,** A 5.25-mm ID trephine was used to core out the fixture using very slow speed and copious irrigation. Care was taken to not damage the buccal plate of bone. **F,** The fixture was able to be removed atraumatically without disturbing the buccal plate. **G,** A bone graft was placed into the socket using a bone syringe. **H,** Additional graft material was placed over the ridge and socket before placing a resorbable dermal membrane.

Continued

FIGURE 16-24, cont'd I, Primary closure of the site was achieved. **J,** The patient's "flipper" in place. **K,** A hole is placed in the cingulum of the "flipper" which was used as the guide stent. **L,** The position of the initial osteotomy is confirmed using a guide pin placed through the cingulum hole in the "flipper" and into the preparation. **M,** After fixture placement, a soft tissue graft was performed to increase the zone of masticatory mucosa using a collagen matrix as the graft. **N,** The 2-week postoperative view reveals proper positioning of the fixture and the creation of sufficient facial gingiva to create an esthetic emergence profile.

adequate healing occurred, allowing the placement of a new fixture. The patient approved the shape and position of the pontic tooth on the "flipper" (Fig. 16-24J), which also served as the guide stent by preparing a hole in the cingulum for placement of the initial osteotomy and confirmation of positioning. (Fig. 16-24K,L).

After the fixture was placed, a 4-mm height, small diameter healing abutment was placed to facilitate primary closure. A free graft using a collagen matrix was placed in the midline to create an even, free gingival margin profile and favorable vestibular depth (Fig. 16-24M). Postoperatively, the fixture is centered in the edentulous ridge and placed sufficiently palatally to allow the creation of an esthetic restoration (Fig. 16-24N).

The restorative dentist requested a narrower healing abutment to be placed at second stage (uncovering) surgery in order to maintain as much height of the gingival tissues as possible. This provided adequate subgingival depth to guide the soft tissue profile with the emergence contours of the provisional crown (the greater the "bulge" facially of the height of contour of the gingival third of the facial surface of the provisional restoration, the more the free gingival margin will be forced apically). In other words, when the gingival contour is stretched in a facial direction, there is a concomitant apical repositioning of the gingival height. Had a wider healing abutment been used, the free gingival margin would have become positioned more apically, creating less space for the development of the soft tissues with the provisional crown.

CONCLUSION

Many factors affect the outcome of esthetic implant treatment, but successful results can occur if specific guidelines are carefully followed. Fixture placement is a three-dimensional process. Before any treatment, adequate diagnostic information must be ascertained. All significant site development should be accomplished before fixture placement. Papillae preserving techniques should be used whenever possible. Proper communication between all members of the treatment team is essential.

The esthetic zone implant situation presents some of the greatest challenges faced by clinicians. Planning and executing treatment based upon sound biologic principles can result in an outcome that will be satisfying for both clinician's patients.

ACKNOWLEDGMENT

The authors wish to thank Dr. David Silver and Dr. Jagdeep Singh for their assistance in preparing this chapter.

BIBLIOGRAPHY

GENERAL

2010 Guidelines of the Academy of Osseointegration for the provision of dental implants and associated patient care, *Int J Oral Max Impl* 25:3 620-627, 2010.

Adell R, Eriksson B, Lekholm U, Branemark P-I, Jemt T: A long-term follow-up study of osseointegrated implants in the treatment of totally edentulous jaws, Int J Oral Max Impl 5:347, 1990.

Almog D et al: Comparison between planned prosthetic trajectory and residual bone trajectory using surgical guides and tomography—a pilot study, *J Oral Implantol* 21:275, 1995.

Anderegg CR et al: Clinical evaluation of the use of decalcified freeze-dried bone allograft with guided tissue regeneration in the treatment of molar furcation invasions, *J Periodontol* 62:264-268, 1991.

Avivi-ArberL, Zarb G: Clinical effectiveness of implant-supported single-tooth replacement: the Toronto Study, *Int J Oral Max Impl* 11:311, 1996.

Babbush CA, Kent JN, Misiek DJ: Titanium plasma-sprayed (TPS) screw implants for the reconstruction of the edentulous mandible, *J Oral Maxillofac Surg* 44:274, 1986.

Becker W et al: Guided tissue regeneration for implants placed into extraction sockets: a study in dogs, *J Periodontol* 62:703-709, 1991.

Becker W, Becker BE: Guided tissue regeneration for implants placed into extraction sockets and for implant dehiscence surgical technique and case reports, *Int J Periodont Rest Dent* 10(5):377-391, 1990.

Becker W et al: Bone formation of dehisced dental implant sites treated with implant augmentation material: a pilot study in dog, *Int J Periodont Rest Dent* 10(2):93-102, 1990.

Buser D, Martin W, Belser UC: Optimizing esthetics for implant restorations in the anterior maxilla: anatomic and surgical considerations, *Int J Oral Max Impl* 19 Suppl:43-61, 2004.

Buser D et al: Localized ridge augmentation using guided bone regeneration. I. Surgical procedure in the maxilla, *Int J Periodont Rest Dent* 13:29-45, 1993.

Buser D, Weber HP, Bragger U, Balsiger C: Tissue integration of one-stage ITI implants: 3-year results of a longitudinal study with hollow cylinder and hollow-screw implants, *Int J Oral Max Impl* 6:405, 1991.

Carter L, Farman AG, Geist J, et al; American Academy of Oral and Maxillofacial Radiology. American Academy of Oral and Maxillofacial Radiology: Executive opinion statement on performing and interpreting diagnostic cone beam computed tomography, *Oral Surg Oral Med Oral Pathol Oral Radiol Endod*, 106(4):561-562, 2008.

Caudill RF, Meffert RM: Histologic analysis of the osseointegration of endosseous implants in simulated extraction sockets with and without e-PTFE barriers. Part I. Preliminary findings, *Int J Periodont Rest Dent* 11(3) 207-215, 1991.

Choquet V, Hermans M, Adriaenssens P, Daelemans P, Tarnow DP, Malevez C: Clinical and radiographic evaluation of the papilla level adjacent to single-tooth dental implants. A retrospective study in the maxillary anterior region, *J Periodontol* 72(10):1364-1371, 2001.

Cochran DL, Nummikoski PV, Higginbottom FL, Hermann JS, Makins SR, Buser D: Evaluation of an endosseous titanium implant with a sandblasted and acid-etched surface in the canine mandible: radiographic results, *Clin Oral Imp Res* 7:240-252, 1996.

Cosyn J, Eghbali A, De Bruyn H, Collys K, Cleymaet R, De Rouck T: Immediate single-tooth implants in the anterior maxilla: 3-year results of a case series on hard and soft tissue response and aesthetics, *J Clin Periodontol* 38(8):746-753, 2011.

Covani U, Cornelini R, Barone A: Bucco-lingual bone remodeling around implants placed into immediate extraction sockets: a case series, *J Periodontol* 74:268-273, 2003.

Degidi M, Nardi D, Daprile G, Piatelli A: Buccal bone plate in the immediately placed and restored maxillary single implant: a 7-year retrospective study using computed tomography, *Implant Dent* 21(1):62-66, 2012.

Elian N, Bloom M, Dard M, Cho SC, Trushkowsky RD, Tarnow D: Effect of interimplant distance (2 and 3 mm) on the height of interimplant bone crest: a histomorphometric evaluation, *J Periodontol* 82(12):1749-1756, 2011.

Ekfeldt A et al: Clinical evaluation of single-tooth restorations supported by osseointegrated implants: a retrospective study, *Int J Oral Max Impl* 9:179, 1994.

Esposito M, Ekestubbe A, Grondahl K: Radiological evaluation of marginal bone loss at tooth surfaces facing single Branemark implants, *Clin Oral Imp Res* 4(3):151-157, 1993.

Felice P, Soardi E, Piatelli M, Pistilli R, Jacotti M, Esposito M: Immediate non-occlusal loading of immediate post-extractive versus delayed placement of single implants in preserved sockets of the anterior maxilla: 4-month post-loading results from a pragmatic multicentre randomized controlled trial, *Eur J Oral Implantol* 4(4):329-344, 2011.

Gastaldo JF, Cury PR, Sendyk WR: Effect of the vertical and horizontal distances between adjacent implants and between a tooth and an implant on the incidence of interproximal papilla, *J Periodontol* 79(9):1242-1246, 2004.

Gomez-Roman G: Influence of flap design on peri-implant interproximal crestal bone loss around single-tooth implants, *Int J Oral Max Impl* 16:61-67, 2001.

Hoshaw S, Brunski J, Cochran G: Mechanical loading of Branemark implants affects interfacial bone modeling and remodeling, *Int J Oral Max Impl* 9:345, 1994.

Ivanoff CJ, Sennerby L, Lekholm U: Influence of initial implant mobility on the integration of titanium implants. An experimental study in rabbits, *Clin Oral Imp Res* 7:120-127, 1996.

Ivanoff C-J, Sennerby L, Lekholm U: Influence of soft tissue contamination on the integration of titanium implants, *Clin Oral Imp Res* 7:128-132, 1996.

Jemt T: Restoring the gingival contour by means of provisional resin crowns after single-implant treatment, *Int J Periodont Rest Dent* 19:20-29, 1999.

Jemt T, Lekholm U, Grondahl K: Three-year follow-up study of early single-implant restorations ad modum Brånemark, Int J Periodont Rest Dent 10:340-349, 1990.

Kan JYK, Rungcharassaeng K, Lozada J: Immediate placement and provisionalization of maxillary anterior single implants: 1-year prospective study, *Int J Oral Max Impl* 18:31-39, 2003.

Kan JYK, Rungcharassaeng K, Kois JC: Dimensions of peri-implant mucosa: an evaluation of maxillary anterior single implants in humans, *J Periodontol* 74:557-562, 2003.

Kim P, Ivanovski S, Latcham N, Mattheos N: The impact of cantilevers on biological and technical success outcomes of implant-supported fixed partial dentures. A retrospective cohort study, *Clin Oral Impl Res* 25(10):175-184, 2013.

Kuperschmidt I, Levin L, Schwartz-Arad K: Inter-implant bone height changes in anterior immediate and non-immediate adjacent dental implants, *J Periodontol* 78(6):991-996, 2007.

Laney WR et al: Osseointegrated implants for single tooth replacement. Progress report from a multicenter prospective study after 3 years, *Int J Oral Max Impl* 9:49, 1994.

Lazzara RJ: Immediate implant placement into extraction sites: surgical and restorative advantages, *Int J Periodont Rest Dent* 9(5) 333-344, 1989.

Nevins M, Mellonig JT: Enhancement of the damaged edentulous ridge to receive dental implants: a combination of allograft and Gore-Tex membrane, *Int J Periodont Rest Dent* 12(2):97-111, 1992.

Nyman S et al: Bone regeneration adjacent to titanium implants using guided tissue regeneration. A report of two cases, *Int J Oral Max Impl* 5(1):9-14, 1990.

Nyman S: Bone regeneration using the principle of guided tissue regeneration, *J Clin Periodontol* 18:494-498, 1991.

Quirynen M et al: A study of 589 consecutive implants supporting complete fixed prostheses: part 1: periodontal aspects, *J Prosthet Dent* 68:655, 1992.

Roe P, Kan JY, Rungcharassaeng K, Caruso JM, Zimmerman G, Mesquida J: Horizontal and vertical dimensional changes of peri-implant facial bone following immediate placement and provisionalization of maxillary anterior single implants: a 1-year cone beam computed tomography study, *Int J Oral Max Impl* 27(2):393-400, 2012.

Rosenberg ES, Cutler SA: Guided tissue regeneration and GTAM for periodontal regenerative therapy, ridge augmentation and dental implantology, *Alpha Omegan* 85:25, 1992.

Salama H, Salama MA, Garber D, Adar P: The interproximal height of bone: a guidepost to predictable aesthetic strategies and soft tissue contours in the anterior tooth replacement, *Pract Periodontics Aesthet Dent* 10(9):1131-1141, 1998.

Salama H et al: The interproximal height of bone: a guidepost to predictable aesthetic strategies and soft tissue contours in anterior tooth replacement, *Prac Periodontics Aesthet Dent* 10:1131-1141, 1998.

Salama H, Salama M, Kelly J: The orthodontic-periodontal connection in implant site development, *Prac Periodontics Aesthet Dent*, 8(9):923-932, 1996.

Salama H, Salama M: The role of orthodontic extrusive remodeling in the enhancement of soft and hard tissue profiles prior to implant placement: a systematic approach to the management of extraction site defects, *Int J Periodont Rest Dent* 13(4):312-333, 1993.

Schwartz-Arad, Laviv A, Levin L: Survival of immediately provisionalized dental implants placed immediately into fresh extraction sockets, *J Periodontol* 78(2):219-223, 2007.

Siebert J, Nyman S: Localized ridge augmentation in dogs: a pilot study using membranes and hydroxyapatite, *J Periodontol* 61:157-165, 1990.

Small P, Tarnow D: Gingival recession around implants: a 1-year longitudinal prospective study, *Int J Oral Max Impl* 15:527-532, 2000.

Small P, Cho S, Tarnow D: Gingival recession around wide vs standard diameter implants: a 5-year longitudinal prospective study, *Prac Periodontics Aesthet Dent* 15:527-532, 2001.

Tarnow D, Cho S: The effect of inter-implant distance on the height of the inter-implant bone crest, *J Periodontol* 71:546-549, 2000.

Tarnow DP, Magner A, Fletcher P: The effect of the distance from the contact point to the crest of bone on the presence or absence of the interproximal papilla, *J Periodontol* 63:995-996, 1992.

Tarnow, DP, Cho SC, Wallace SS: The effect of inter-implant distance on the height of the inter-implant bone crest, *J Periodontol* 71(4):546-549, 2000.

Tarnow DP, Magner AW, Fletcher P: The effect of the distance from the contact point to the crest of bone on the presence or absence of the interproximal dental papilla, *J Periodontol* 63(12):995-996.

Tarnow D, Elian N, Fletcher P, Froum S, Magner A, Cho SC, et al: Vertical distance from the crest of bone to the height of the interproximal papilla between adjacent implants, *J Periodontol* 74(12):1785-1788, 2003.

Weisgold AS: Contours of full crown restoration, *Alpha Omegan* 10:77, 1977.

Wennstrom JO, Bengazi F, Lekholm U: The influence of the masticatory mucosa on the peri-implant soft tissue condition, *Clin Oral Imp Res* 5:1, 1994.

Zarb GA, Schmitt A: The longitudinal clinical effectiveness of osseointegrated dental implants in anterior partially edentulous patients, *Int J Prosthetics* 6:180, 1993.

Zeren KJ: Minimally invasive extraction and immediate implant placement: the preservation of esthetics, *Int J Periodont Rest Dent* 26(2):171-181, 2006.

CANTILEVER

Aglietta M, Iorio Siciliano V, Blasi A, Sculean A, Brägger U, Lang NP, et al: Clinical and radiographic changes at implants supporting single-unit crowns (SCs) and fixed dental prostheses (FDPs) with one cantilever extension. A retrospective study, *Clin Oral Implants Res* 25(50):550-550, 2012.

Aglietta M, Siciliano VI, Zwahlen M, Brägger U, Pjetursson BE, Lang NP, et al: A systematic review of the survival and complication rates of implant supported fixed dental prostheses with cantilever extensions after an observation period of at least 5 years, *Clin Oral Implants Res* 20(5):441-451, 2009.

Brägger U, Hirt-Steiner S, Schnell N, Schmidlin K, Salvi GE, Pjetursson B, et al: Complication and failure rates of fixed dental prostheses in patients treated for periodontal disease, *Clin Oral Implants Res* 22(1):70-77, 2011.

Hälg GA, Schmid J, Hämmerle CH: Bone level changes at implants supporting crowns or fixed partial dentures with or without cantilevers, *Clin Oral Implants Res* 19(10):983-990, 2008.

Palmer R, Howe L, Palmer P, Wilson R: A prospective clinical trial of single Astra Tech 4.0 or 5.0 diameter implants used to support two-unit cantilever bridges: results after 3 years, *Clin Oral Impl Res* 23(1):35-40, 2012.

Pjetursson B, Lang N: Prosthetic treatment planning on the basis of scientific evidence, *J Oral Rehabil* 35 Suppl 1:72-79, 2008.

Romeo E, Lops D, Margutti E, Ghisolfi M, Chiapasco M, Vogel G: Implant-supported fixed cantilever prostheses in partially edentulous arches. A seven-year prospective study, *Clin Oral Impl Res* 14:303-311, 2003.

Romeo E, Lops D, Margutti E, Ghisolfi M, Chiapasco M, Vogel G: Long-term survival and success of oral implants in the treatment of full and partial arches: a 7-year prospective study with the ITI dental implant system, *Int J Oral Max Impl* 19(2):247-59, 2004.

Romeo E, Tomasi C, Finini I, Casentini P, Lops D: Implant-supported fixed cantilever prosthesis in partially edentulous jaws: a cohort prospective study, *Clin Oral Implants Res* 20(11):1278-1285, 2009.

Salvi G, Bragger U: Mechanical and technical risks in implant therapy, *Int J Oral Max Impl* 24 Suppl:69-85, 2004.

Wennström J, Zurdo J, Karlsson S, Ekestubbe A, Gröndahl K, Lindhe J: Bone level change at implant-supported fixed partial dentures with and without cantilever extension after 5 years in function, *J Clin Periodontol* 31(12):1077-1083, 2004.

Zurdo J, Romão C, Wennström JL: Survival and complication rates of implant-supported fixed partial dentures with cantilevers: a systematic review, *Clin Oral Implants Res* 20 Suppl 4:59-66, 2009.

OVATE PONTICS

Dylina TJ: Contour determination for ovate pontics, *J Prosthet Dent* 82:136-142, 1999.

Garber DA, Rosenberg ES: The edentulous ridge in fixed prosthodontics, *Compend Contin Educ Dent* 2:212-223, 1981.

17

Esthetics and Implant Prosthetics

Yakir A. Arteaga

Long-term success rates for osseointegrated dental implants have been well documented.[1,2] However, achieving true esthetic integration may present additional challenges in implant dentistry.

The original Branëmark protocol required several millimeters of exposed supragingival titanium. However, these early Swedish implants were originally placed into totally edentulous, severely resorbed ridges. The borders of the subsequent restoration were apical to the lip and smile line and did not present an esthetic problem. Acrylic denture flanges and acrylic teeth were used to replace the lost natural teeth and alveolar bone.

There is now an increased demand for esthetic harmony between the peri-implant gingiva and the adjacent dentition. A carefully prepared, interdisciplinary, prosthetically driven treatment plan is indispensable to achieve proper esthetics, function, phonetics, and oral hygiene.

Implant therapy involves six steps (Box 17-1). Step 1 includes establishing a diagnosis and developing a proper treatment plan. Restorative needs, interarch distance and jaw relationships, location of edentulous areas, and the quantity and quality of available bone should be evaluated before implant surgery. Step 2 is the placement of the implant fixture. This step is traditionally divided into two stages. In stage 1 surgery, the implant fixture is placed into the alveolar bone and covered by the soft tissue. This is typically followed by a healing period, during which the process of osseointegration occurs. During stage 2 surgery, the fixture is exposed and a transepithelial abutment is connected. After adequate soft tissue, healing the restorative dentist can fabricate a prosthesis. Step 3 is the placement of a provisional restoration, which aids in the development of the emergence profile of the definitive prosthesis. Step 4 is the fabrication of the definitive restoration. Step 5 is the insertion of the definitive restoration. Step 6 is the re-care of the patient.

TERMINOLOGY

Dental implant technology is continuously evolving with established and new systems undergoing further development. It is beyond the scope of this chapter to provide a detailed description of the different implant systems, but a fundamental discussion will be provided.

An implant restoration consists of three components (Fig. 17-1):
1. The implant fixture, which is placed in the bone and becomes osseointegrated
2. An abutment, which is a prosthetic transmucosal extension
3. A restoration, which is cemented (cement retained) or is part of the abutment and attached directly to the implant fixtures by an internal screw (screw retained)

Implant Fixture

Implant fixtures are designed to integrate with the host's bone and provide stability and retention for the restoration. Fixtures are available in many different lengths, shapes (e.g., tapered), and widths (or platform sizes). Manufacturers produce differing designs, each having unique features. These unique features require clinicians and laboratory technicians to adhere strictly to the individual manufacturer's procedures and guidelines when placing and constructing implant borne prosthetics.

To provide successful osseointegration, the fixture material must be biocompatible. Currently, the most popular material is either commercially pure titanium (typically 99.2% pure) or titanium alloy. Titanium has proved to be biocompatible in long-term evaluations and documentation reporting on the success and longevity of dental implants.[3,4] Titanium is lightweight and noncorrosive (because of its oxide layer); it appears to be the most predictable material for manufacturing implants and implant components. Titanium is graded according to its carbon and iron content. In general tensile and yield strength increases with the grade number.

Titanium 4 is used in most situations because it is stronger than other grades. Recently grade 5 titanium is being used increasingly. This alloy consists of 6% aluminum and 4% vanadium alloy and offers better strength and fracture resistance.

Box 17-1
Steps in Implant Therapy

1. **Diagnosis and Treatment Planning:** Examination and diagnosis consist of an oral examination, full-mouth radiographs, panorex radiographs, or 3-D cone beam CT, diagnostic casts, photographs and diagnostic wax-up.
2. **Placement of the Implant:** A soft diet is recommended during the first 4 to 6 weeks. Osseointegration occurs in 3 to 6 months.
3. **Provisional Restoration:** Implants are uncovered. Implants are checked for osseointegration. Provisional prosthesis is made to develop emergence profile.
4. **Permanent Restoration:** Make impressions for the definitive prosthesis. Permanent restoration: make impressions for the definitive prosthesis.
5. **Insertion of the definitive restoration:** Prosthesis is completed and placed onto the implants. Insertion of the definitive restoration: prosthesis is completed and placed onto the implants
6. **Re-care:** Oral hygiene maintenance is performed at 3 to 6 month intervals following placement of the definitive prosthesis.

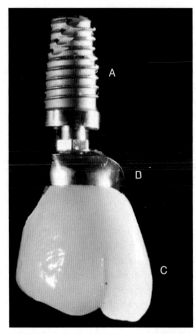

FIGURE 17-1 Implant supported cement retained restoration consists of three parts. **A,** Implant fixture. **B,** Implant abutment with retention screw. **C,** Implant restoration (crown). The components are partially separated to more clearly reveal them.

A more recent development is the use of high strength zirconia ceramics as a material for dental implant fixture. They are considered to be inert in the body and exhibit minimal ion release compared with metallic implants. Yttrium-stabilized tetragonal zirconia polycrystals appear to offer advantages over aluminum oxide for dental implants because of their higher fracture resilience and higher flexural strength.[5] Zirconium appears to offer the same rate of success as titanium in its osseointegration properties,[6] although research in this field is currently limited.

The two most common mating interfaces of the abutment to fixture platform are described as "internal hex" or "external hex" configurations (Fig. 17-2). This configuration prevents rotation of the abutment. Manufacturers have created numerous variations of this basic design. It is beyond the scope of this chapter to discuss every implant design, and esthetic principles may vary because of the limitations and enhancements of any a particular design.

Implant Abutments

The implant abutment links the implant fixture to the restoration. Abutments are available in a variety of different types, each designed to manage a particular clinical situation (Fig. 17-3B,C). The abutment provides an area of retention similar to a prepared tooth for cementation of a crown. Some clinical situations, typically related to angle correction, necessitate the fabrication of a custom cast or CAD/CAM abutment, which is constructed at the implant level (Fig. 17-3A). The definitive prosthesis is placed directly on this custom abutment. The definitive prosthesis or prosthetic superstructure may be cemented to the custom abutment or screw retained. The abutment generally consists of an abutment and an abutment-retaining screw. The abutment retaining screw maintains the abutment's position on the implant.

Prosthetic retaining screws are generally constructed of gold alloy or titanium. They are recessed internally within the occlusal surface of the abutment and hold the definitive restoration in place.

Compressive forces, generated across the implant-abutment interface by tightening the abutment retaining screw to a specific torque help maintain the integrity of the connection and position of the screw, although preload forces slowly decay with time. They are recessed internally within the occlusal surface of the abutment and hold the definitive restoration in place. Preload torque recommendations vary but typically range from 10 to 35 N-cm, depending on screw material and implant/abutment manufacturer. Preload for the abutment screw should ideally be established using a torque wrench and must be sufficient to ensure that lateral forces are distributed to the implant abutment interface rather than to the screw to reduce the likelihood of loosening or fracture.[7]

CLINICAL TIP

Check that your torque wrench is delivering the correct force required. A recent study showed that after repeated use, some devices produce forces far in excess of that needed, and some far less.[8]

The abutment provides an area of retention similar to a prepared tooth for cementation of a crown. Some clinical situations typically related to angle correction necessitate the fabrication of a custom cast or CAD/CAM abutment, which is constructed at the implant level. The definitive prosthesis is placed directly on this custom abutment. The definitive prosthesis is placed directly on this custom abutment. The definitive prosthesis or prosthetic superstructure may be cemented to the custom abutment or screw may be retained.

Implant Restoration

Restorations are cemented or are part of an abutment attached directly to the implant fixtures by internal prosthetic retaining

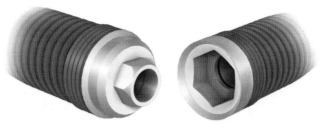

FIGURE 17-2 Implant platforms showing external hex (*left*) and internal hex (*right*).

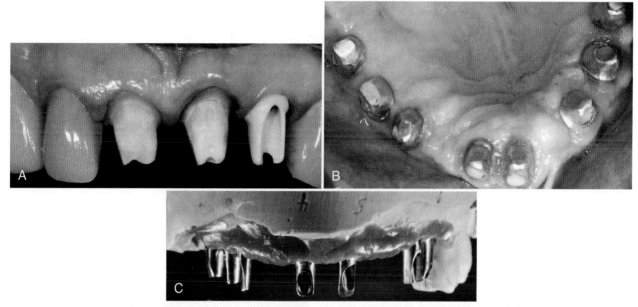

FIGURE 17-3 A, Zirconia abutments are available in multiple shades. **B,** Gold abutments. **C,** Titanium abutments.

screws. Modern porcelain systems provide many options to choose from when planning an implant restoration.

DIAGNOSIS AND TREATMENT PLANNING

To obtain ideal esthetic results it is critical that the restorative dentist, in conjunction with the implant surgeon and laboratory technician, formulate a preoperative plan. Figure 17-4 outlines the potential treatment pathways that can be taken during implant therapy. Treatment planning must address hard and soft tissue deficiencies and combine this with precision in implant placement. This plan culminates in the fabrication of a surgical guide. However, a number of factors must be considered first.

Patient Selection

An appropriate medical history should be obtained and evaluated for systemic conditions to prevent complications during the treatment. The dental examination must consider active infection caries, endodontic lesions, and periodontitis. All the active infections should be treated before implant placement.

Psychological Considerations

The issue of patient expectation must be addressed before implant placement.

> ### CLINICAL TIP
>
> Some patients have unusually high expectations about the esthetics and configurations of the definitive restoration. Be sure to consider this or patients may not be satisfied with the definitive restoration despite biological success.

Patients must be informed that the professionals' ability to satisfy their concerns may be limited. Persistent unrealistic expectations warrant the use of alternate treatment plans.

Oral Examination and Esthetic Factors

To evaluate the implant site in esthetic areas, the following factors should be considered.

Smile Line. The study of the smile line is the most important factor in evaluating the patient's dental esthetics. Lip position relative to the display of teeth and gingiva must be evaluated at rest, while speaking, with a moderately relaxed smile and with a full smile (see Chapter 2).

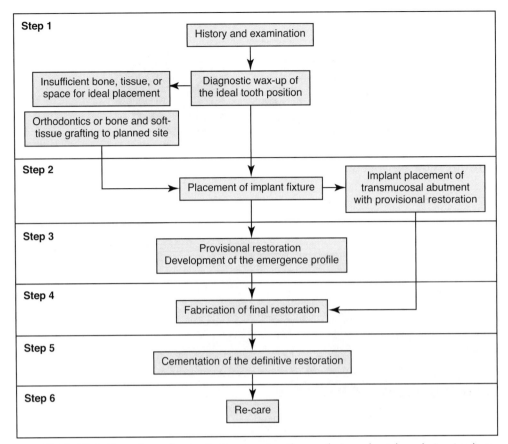

FIGURE 17-4 Flow chart of potential treatment pathways that can be taken during implant therapy.

Tooth Morphology and Periodontal Biotype. The periodontal biotype is an important factor in evaluating the prognosis of implant-supported restorations in the esthetic zone. Two periodontal biotypes related to tooth morphology have been described.[9]

Thin scalloped periodontal biotype. The thin, scalloped biotype (Fig. 17-5A) is associated with less than 15% of clinical situations and is characterized by a delicate soft tissue, a scalloped underlying osseous form, and often has dehiscence and fenestrations and a reduced quantity and quality of keratinized mucosa.

It is associated with a specific dental morphology with anatomically triangular crowns, small interdental contact surfaces in the incisal third, and long thin papillae. It responds to surgical and prosthodontic interventions with recession, apical migration of the periodontal anchorage, and loss of underlying alveolar volume, which results in an empty space known as a *black triangle*.

It is usually is accompanied by thin vestibular cortical bone, with a tendency to form bone defects secondary to bone remodeling and resorption after tooth extraction or implant placement.

Thick flat periodontal biotype. The thick, flat biotype (Fig. 17-5B) exhibits dense, fibrotic soft tissue. The underlying bone is thick and dense. It is associated with dental crowns that are square and convex in the cervical third. The contact points between crowns are long and often extend to the zone of the cervical third. It presents with papillae that are considered short when compared with the thin periodontal biotype. It responds to surgical aggression with scar formation that can jeopardize the aesthetic and functional outcome.

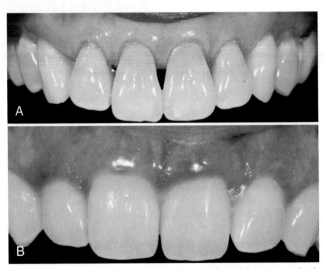

FIGURE 17-5 A, Thin, scalloped periodontal biotype, which can result in the formation of an empty space known as a "black triangle." **B,** Thick, flat periodontal biotype.

MOUNTED DIAGNOSTIC CAST ANALYSIS

Preoperative mounted diagnostic casts can influence decisions concerning the selection of the type of definitive restoration. For example, if the final tooth position will be facial to the residual mandibular ridge, a hybrid-type prosthesis may be considered, as opposed to a conventional crown and fixed partial denture restoration.

In the maxillary arch, an occlusal rim demonstrates the amount of facial positioning required of the replacement tooth to properly support the maxillary lip relative to the residual ridge. This aids in determining whether a conventional crown and fixed partial denture prosthesis, a hybrid prosthesis, or an overdenture should be constructed to best support the lip.

In the fully edentulous patient, it may be necessary to construct a trial tooth setup to precisely determine final tooth position. This is especially true when the location of the teeth is changed both in the arch to be reconstructed with the osseointegrated dental implant and in the opposing arch, which may be restored conventionally. Because tooth position in one arch will affect tooth position in the opposing arch, the location must be determined precisely before constructing the mandibular surgical guide. In those situations, a wax try-in of the maxillary and mandibular teeth should be constructed as part of a diagnostic workup before constructing a surgical guide and placing implants (Fig. 17-6).

The guidelines for selection of a conventional crown and fixed partial denture prosthesis, hybrid prosthesis, or overdenture prosthesis after diagnostic cast analysis are as follows:

- *Patient's desire for a fixed restoration.* For many patients, the avoidance of a removable appliance is paramount.
- *The size of the framework involved.* This may eliminate the possibility of using a conventional crown and fixed partial denture-type prosthesis because of the amount of necessary metal.
- *Amount of interarch distance.* The amount of interarch distance is important because moderate to severe resorption requires a hybrid prosthesis or overdenture to replace missing alveolar bone and soft tissue. If providing adequate lip support is critical, an overdenture is generally necessary, especially in the case of severe resorption.
- *Number and location of implants.* For construction of a conventional crown and fixed partial denture-type prosthesis, implants must be positioned in tooth locations. In addition, the implants must be adequately spaced in the anterior and posterior regions to provide adequate stabilization.

- *Strength and dimension of supporting bone.* When severe resorption has occurred, especially in the mandibular posterior region of totally edentulous patients, placing an overdenture is preferred. An anterior fixed appliance can develop significant functional forces that may overstress the mandible, which thins posteriorly. This may cause fracture of the mandible because of an overload of the anterior region with a fixed restoration.

RADIOGRAPHIC ANALYSIS

Proper radiographic analysis is needed to evaluate the amount of bone available in the area. Computed tomography scans (Fig. 17-7) disclose bone dimension and the contours of the residual ridge and guide proper angling of an implant at a given edentulous site. The sectional portion of the CT scan is especially important because it gives an indication of facial-lingual bone dimension, bone quality, and the location of vital structures.

TYPES OF PROSTHESES

Implant restorations can be attached to the implant fixture with screws (screw-retained) (Fig. 17-8A), or it can be cemented to an abutment, which is attached to the implant fixture with a screw (cement retained) (Fig. 17-8B). Each method has advantages and disadvantages. However, in certain clinical situations, only one method is indicated.

Screw-Retained Prosthesis

Advantages

- *Easy prosthesis retrieval.* Allows for the retrieval of the prosthesis without damage to the restoration or the implant fixture.
- *Reduced interarch dimension.* Used when the interarch dimension is less than 5 mm from the crest of the tissue to the opposing arch.

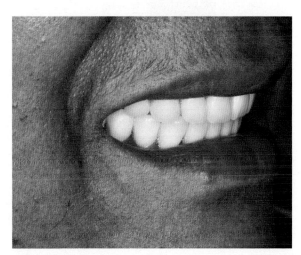

FIGURE 17-6 A wax try-in of the tooth setup is important in the preoperative evaluation of the final tooth position, especially when changing the position of both the maxillary and mandibular teeth.

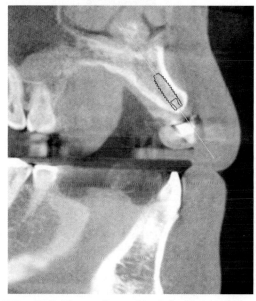

FIGURE 17-7 The radiographic information, along with mounted casts, allows coordination of implant position and angle.

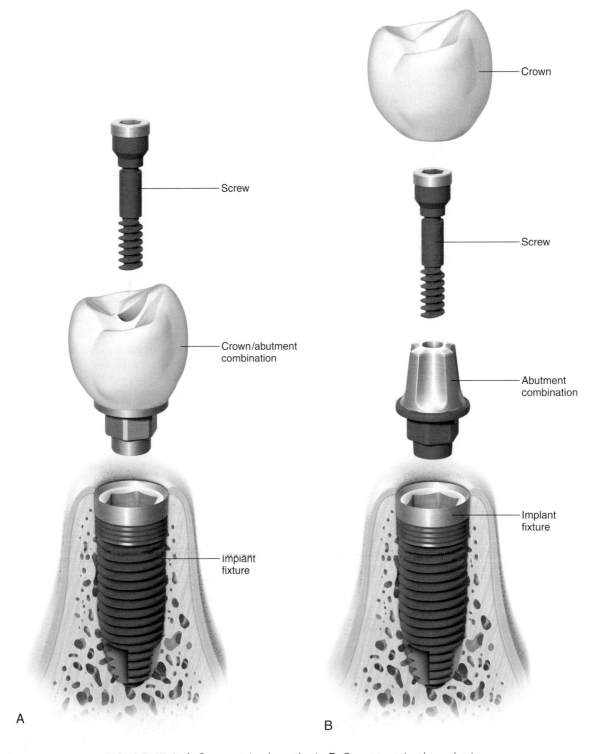

Screw

Crown/abutment
combination

Implant
fixture

A

Crown

Screw

Abutment
combination

Implant
fixture

B

FIGURE 17-8 A, Screw-retained prosthesis. **B,** Cement-retained prosthesis.

+ *Eliminates cement margins.* Absence of cement margins which can result in adverse peri-implant tissue response.

Disadvantages

+ *Occlusal esthetic requirements.* The esthetics of the occlusal surface can be partially compromised when the screw access area is filled with a composite resin, especially when metal-base frameworks are used. The introduction of zirconia-base frameworks has lessened this complication. The white or

shaded substructure facilitates an esthetically pleasing closure of the access opening; however, if the top of the screw is near the occlusal surface it may be difficult to completely mask it.

+ *Requires ideal fixture positioning.* Ideal position and angulations of the fixture in relation to the anticipated definitive restoration are required.

+ *Passive fit considerations.* A passive fit is more difficult to attain for a screw-retained implant restoration with more than one implant. The improving accuracy of CAD/CAM over traditional casting, even when corrective procedures are included, aids in the fabrication of better fitting frameworks.

Cement-Retained Prosthesis

Provisional cements should be used in order to maintain retrievability of the prosthesis. Conventional or CAD/CAM custom abutments or prefabricated (stock) abutments are available.

Advantages

+ *Accessibility.* The cement-retained prosthesis is easier to seat in areas where accessibility with screwdrivers is limited.
+ *Fixture alignment less critical.* The abutment can compensate for misaligned fixtures.
+ *Familiar clinical procedures.* Techniques more closely parallels conventional crown-and-fixed partial denture technique.
+ *Passivity requirements.* Fabrication and seating of passively fitting restorations is easier than screw-retained prostheses.
+ *Cement retained.* The cement layer may act as a shock absorber and enhance the transfer of load throughout the prosthesis-implant-bone system.[10]

Disadvantages

+ *Soft tissue concerns.* There is a potential risk for cement trapping in the peri-implant tissue (Fig. 17-9). Cement extrusion into the sulcular area may result in soft tissue inflammation or even in an exudate.[11]
+ *Cement margins.* Removal of excess cement with plastic and metal scalers may result in scratches and gouges on the implant surfaces.[12,13]
+ *Inadequate interarch distance.* A minimum of 5 mm of abutment is required to provide predictable retention for the definitive restoration.[14] When a reduced amount of interarch distance is available, a screw-retained prosthesis is indicated.
+ *Retrievability concerns.* Despite the use of provisional cements to allow retrievability, removal of the prosthesis should be carried out with great care to avoid damaging the restoration, abutment, or implant fixture.

CLINICAL TIP

Access the cement margins is crucial to providing a successful cement-retained restoration.

ABUTMENT SELECTION

The choice of the implant abutment can be daunting because of different abutment types. Materials such as titanium and various high-strength ceramics (zirconia, lithium di-silicate) are available. Abutments can be categorized as prefabricated abutments (stock abutments), custom abutments (castable abutments or milled), or combined abutment/crown (screw-retained prostheses). Titanium abutments are milled from solid titanium alloy blanks. Zirconia abutments are milled from zirconia blanks and are available in multiple shades. Before selecting an abutment several factors must be considered, including visibility of the region (e.g., high vs. low smile line), the gingival biotype (high scalloped, thin vs. low scalloped, thick), angulation of the implant, inter-arch distance, and peri-implant tissue height (see Chapter 2).

Visibility and Gingival Biotype

In esthetically demanding situations, customized ceramic abutments are indicated to avoid the visible display of metal through the soft tissue, which can occur of when metal abutments are used, particularly in patients with a high smile line and thin biotype. This not only produces the best esthetic results, but also partially compensates for future soft tissue recession (Fig. 17-10A).

CLINICAL TIP

Gingival recession is the most common complication of anterior single-tooth implants.[15]

Angle of the Implant

Precise preplanning and the construction of surgical guides suggest the proper positioning of the implant. However, the clinical acceptability of this predetermined position is determined by the available bone, when bone augmentation is not possible. Sometimes in the maxillary premolar and maxillary anterior regions, implants must be placed with a facial flare to be within the supporting bone. This creates an unesthetic screw access opening in the facial aspect of a screw-retained restoration.

To compensate, a custom abutment can compensate for the angle of the implant so that it emerges from the soft tissue in a favorable position (Fig. 17-10B). A prosthesis can be cemented

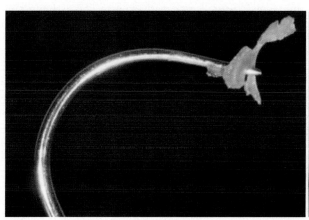
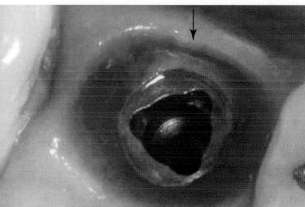

FIGURE 17-9 Cement trapped in the peri-implant tissue.

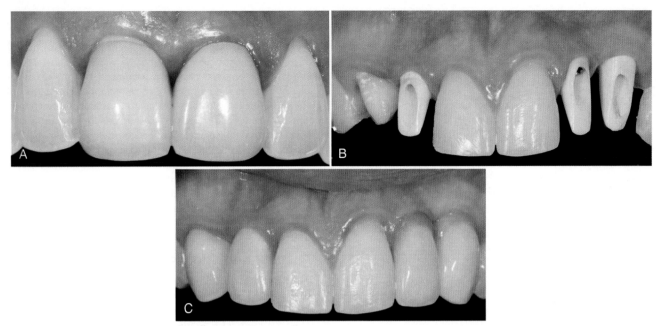

FIGURE 17-10 A, The patient developed recession 4 years after insertion of a zirconia abutment and a ceramic crown. **B,** Custom zirconia abutments were fabricated to compensate for the labially angled implants. **C,** Definitive restorations over the zirconia abutments. Pink-colored porcelain was used to mask a tissue defect in the area of teeth #10 and #11.

over these custom abutments, producing an esthetic result (Fig. 17-10C). Another option is the use of a pre-angled stock abutment.

Interarch Distance

Successfully cemented retained restorations with predictable retention require 5 mm of abutment height. If the vertical distance from the crest of the tissue to the opposing tooth is less than 5 mm, then a screw-retained restoration is indicated.

Peri-implant Tissue Height

If the distance between the platform of the implant and the crest of the tissue is less than 3 mm, a stock abutment (prefabricated) may be chosen, as the margin is sufficiently accessible for cleaning at the time of cementation.[16] If it is greater than 3 mm, a scalloped prefabricated or custom abutment should be used to position the cement in a more accessible, cleansable position relative to the gingival margin.

IMPLANT POSITION AND ALIGNMENT

Osseointegrated implants are ideally positioned in the site previously occupied by the natural tooth, assuming that it was properly located before extraction. Implants placed in an interproximal position can result in considerable restorative difficulties in final crown contour and esthetics when crown and fixed partial denture type restorations are planned.

Considerations with the Peri-implant Papilla

Loss of implant results in a "black triangle" around the implant-supported crown and fixed partial denture type restorations.

Phonetics difficulties and food impactions can also occur. Implant position affects interproximal tissue esthetics between a natural tooth and the implant restoration or between two adjacent implants. Correct three-dimensional placement (mesiodistal, buccolingual, and incisoapical) of the implant in the bone enhances the likelihood of an acceptable result.

Mesiodistal Position. The mesiodistal distance between an implant and a neighboring tooth should be at least 1.5 mm. If this minimum distance is not maintained, the attachment on the tooth side may undergo resorption to the level of that of the implant; this will, in turn cause a loss of interproximal papilla.[17] This also creates restorative problems. Poor embrasure forms and emergence profiles will result in restorations with long contact zones and a compromised clinical outcome.

There should be at least 3 mm between two adjacent implants fixtures.[18,19]

Buccolingual Position. After the implant osteotomy is prepared, the buccal wall should be intact. It should ideally measure at least 2 mm in thickness. This is important to ensure proper soft-tissue support and to avoid the resorption of the facial bone wall following the placement of a restoration.

Apicocoronal Position. The implant platform should be 1 mm apical to the cement-enamel junction of the contralateral tooth in apicocoronal direction.[20] This recommendation, however, is only valid when the contralateral tooth is without periodontal tissue loss.

Considerations with a Congenitally Missing Lateral Incisor

Ideally the definitive restoration will simulate the natural tooth. This can be a challenge if a patient is congenitally missing one or two maxillary incisors. The amount of space required for the restored tooth should be determined by the contralateral incisor.

However, in some patients, the existing lateral incisor may be peg shape and in others, both lateral incisors are congenitally missing. In the latter two situations, the space for the lateral incisor is determined by two factors: esthetics and occlusion clearance. An esthetic relationship exists between the size of the maxillary central and lateral incisor teeth. Ideally the maxillary lateral incisor should be about two thirds the width of the central incisor.[21] One of the most predictable methods to determine the size of the lateral is to fabricate a diagnostic wax-up.

Clinical Case Showing Congenitally Missing Maxillary Lateral Incisor. A 21-year-old female patient presented with an over-retained primary maxillary right canine in need of extraction, and for a consultation on treatment options to replace the congenitally missing maxillary lateral incisor. The patient's medical history was noncontributory. A detailed examination of the teeth and periodontium was performed to assess the esthetic risk for implant dentistry. The patient's gingival biotype was thin

to medium thick and scalloped, presenting a broad band of keratinized mucosa (Fig. 17-11A). The maxillary left lateral incisor was a peg lateral incisor. The maxillary right canine had migrated mesially into the lateral incisor location. The periapical radiograph revealed root resorption on tooth C and distal caries (Fig. 17-11B).

Restorative options included:

1. Extraction of the primary maxillary right canine, placement of a three-unit resin-bonded ("Maryland") fixed partial denture and recontouring of the maxillary right permanent canine so that it would to appear to be a lateral incisor. Also orthodontic creation of the required space for placement of a properly sized restoration on the maxillary left lateral incisor.
2. Extraction of the primary maxillary right canine, placement of a cantilever two-unit fixed partial denture using the canine as the abutment, and recontouring of the maxillary

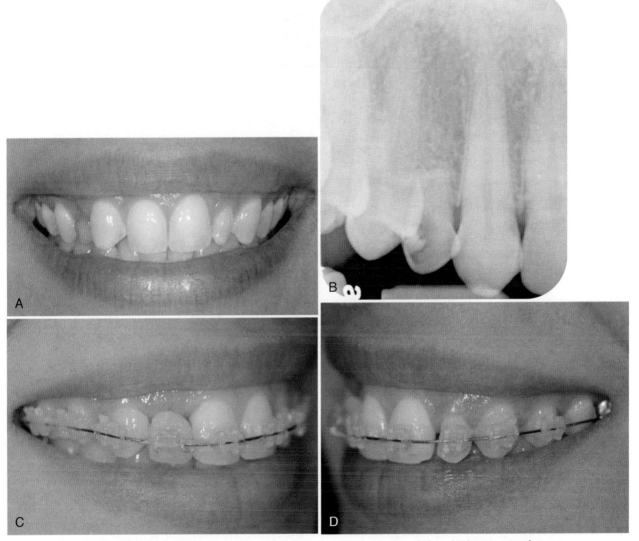

FIGURE 17-11 A, At full smile, the patient presents with a high smile line displaying a significant portion of the gingiva. The thin, scalloped gingival biotype increases the esthetic risk in this patient. **B,** Pretreatment periapical radiograph showing the extent of root resorption of tooth. **C,** Right lateral view of the final orthodontic position, showing sufficient space for the implant restoration of the maxillary right lateral incisor. **D,** Left lateral view of the same patient after orthodontic repositioning, which created sufficient space to restore the maxillary right peg lateral incisor.

Continued

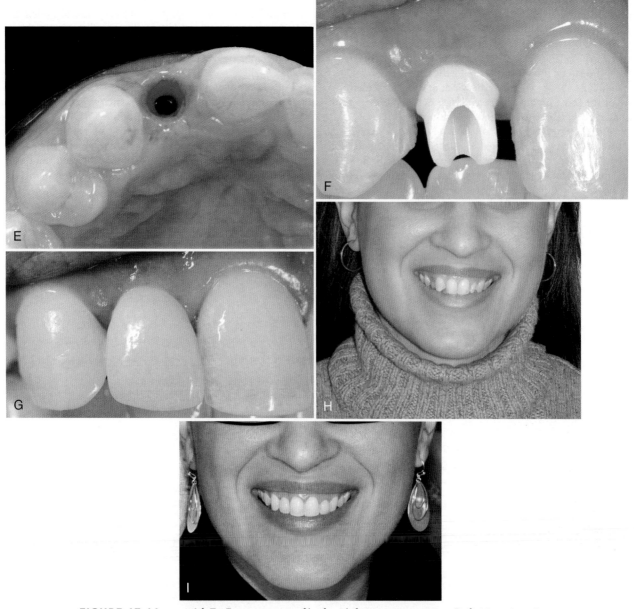

FIGURE 17-11, cont'd E, Emergence profile for definitive restoration. Definitive zirconia abutment (**F**) and definitive restoriation (**G**). Preoperative (**H**) and postoperative (**I**) views.

right canine so that it would to appear to be a lateral incisor. Also, orthodontic creation of the required space for placement of a properly sized restoration on the maxillary left lateral incisor.

3. Extraction of the primary maxillary right canine, placement of a single unit implant, and recontouring of the maxillary right canine so that it would to appear to be a lateral incisor. Also, orthodontic creation of the required space for placement of a properly sized restoration on the maxillary left lateral incisor.

4. Extraction of the primary maxillary right canine, orthodontic distalization of the maxillary right canine to its correct position, and placement of a single unit implant at the proper site the lateral incisor. Also, orthodontic

creation of the required space for placement of a properly sized restoration on the maxillary left lateral incisor.

Option 4 was selected was selected for this patient (Fig. 17-11 C-I).

Considerations with a Small Edentulous Space with Limited Bone

When replacement tooth size or limited bone availability prevents placement of a standard-size implant, an implant of smaller diameter may be indicated. This type of implant can be used for replacing a single mandibular incisor tooth (Fig. 17-12) or a maxillary lateral incisor.

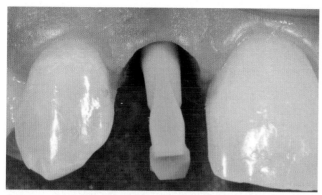

FIGURE 17-12 Zimmer One-Piece Implant, with snap-on impression cap. This implant allows placement in the limited tooth spacing of the maxillary laterals and mandibular lateral areas.

Considerations with Implant-Retained Removable Partial Dentures

Poor removable partial denture (RPD) stability occurs with highly resorbed ridges and an inadequate number of suitable abutment teeth (Fig. 17-13A,B). Removable partial dentures with distal extensions (Kennedy Class I and II) generally have

less stability than those engaging distal abutment teeth.[22,23] Implant-retained removable partial dentures have made treatment options possible to patients who previously may not have been able to benefit from implant dentistry because of limitations in health, anatomy, or finances. This treatment modality provides options for additional treatment in the future and accommodates future changes in the remaining natural dentition.

Implant-retained RPDs can combine the use of natural teeth and implants in one arch when certain requirements are met. Because teeth are considered resilient because of the presence of the periodontal ligament and dental implants are considered rigid because of their osseointegrated state, the use of a "resilient" implant attachment (Locator implant attachment systems) and possibly resilient "clasps" are needed. These attachments to provide the level of resilience needed for an implant-retained, tissue-supported prosthesis, and to allow for normal movement of the teeth[24] (Fig. 17-13B,C). Rigid attachments restrict rotational movement and provide only a limited path of angle insertion, whereas resilient attachments allow varying amounts of rotation and angulation correction. In situations in which implants are even minimally nonparallel, a resilient attachment will consistently show less friction, wear, and breakage.[25]

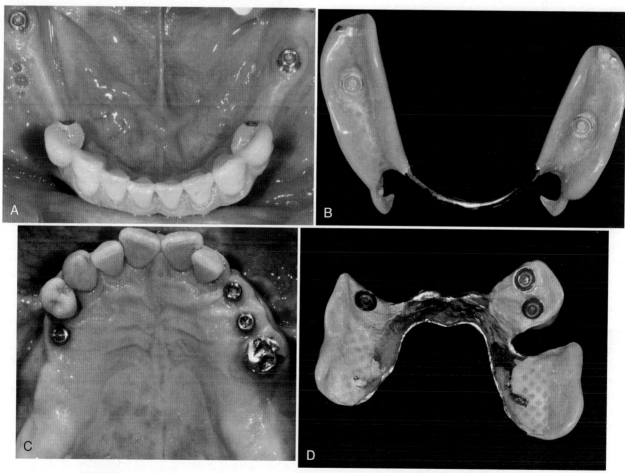

FIGURE 17-13 A, Occlusal view of Zest Locator Abutment. The attachments are picked up and transferred to the denture using autopolymerizing acrylic. **B,** View of the internal aspect of the RPD showing the over-denture attachments. **C,** Occlusal view of Zest Locator Abutment. **D,** View of the internal aspect of the RPD showing the over-denture attachments.

TREATMENT PLANNING*

Radiographic/Surgical Guide

A properly designed surgical guide is particularly essential before implant surgery involving the esthetic display to formulate a comprehensive treatment plan that can address the needs of the treatment team, the desires of the patient, and the requirements of the clinical situation, including:

+ The number of teeth to be replaced
+ The number of fixtures to be placed
+ The preferable fixture sites
+ Whether site development is needed and if so, the types of procedures necessary. (This can be determined from both the clinical examination and the radiographic assessment.)
+ Whether teeth will be removed and whether replacement fixture(s) will be placed immediately or delayed.
+ Whether the restoration will be screw-retained or cemented.

The surgical guide should be anatomically correct and represent the size, shape, and position of the planned restoration. It can be constructed with hard acrylic (e.g., a night guard design with pontics) or with rigid tray material (formed on a diagnostic wax-up), and must rest securely on the adjacent teeth when inserted (Fig. 17-14A). The surgical guide will often serve a dual role both as a radiographic and surgical guide.

CLINICAL TIP

If a single tooth is being replaced, markers are placed on the surgical guide in that location only. If multiple teeth are missing, the markers are placed for each tooth in the restoration regardless of the number of fixtures, thus allowing for identification of the most ideal sites.

A radiopaque material (e.g., barium powder or a piece of lead foil from conventional radiographic film) can be applied to the surface of the teeth on the surgical guide, which will provide an outline of the planned restoration on the scan image. Another method is to prepare a 2- to 3-mm diameter hole in the center of the occlusal table (for posterior teeth) or cingulum (for anterior teeth) in the location of the screw access hole of the fixture (Fig. 17-14B).

The hole in the surgical guide is filled with gutta percha, which will be displayed as a white vertical line over the scanned ridge (Fig. 17-14C). In both instances, the markers will allow both the surgeon and restorative dentist to observe the bone in relation to the planned restoration.

CLINICAL TIP

Lead foil can be placed over the pontic(s) of an existing provisional fixed partial denture for use as a radiographic stent. This can also be done on an acrylic provisional removable partial denture ("flipper") pontic as long as there are no other wires that will interfere with the image.

With this information, the surgeon can relay to the restorative team member the size options for the implant, such as length and diameter ranges, as well as the location the fixture

---

*This section was written by Drs. Edwin S. Rosenberg and James Torosian.

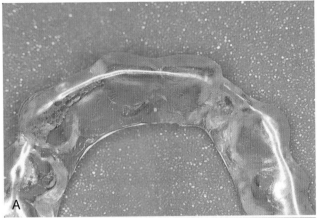

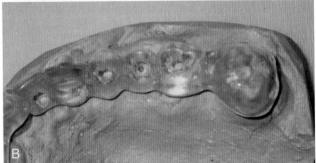

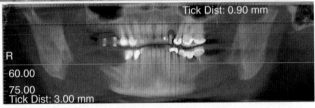

FIGURE 17-14 A, Radiographic/surgical guide for the maxillary left lateral incisor made of a rigid tray material. **B,** Hard acrylic surgical guide with guide holes prepared in the planned implant sites. **C,** The panoramic reconstruction of the CBVT scan displays the gutta percha markers for the planned implants in the maxillary right posterior sextant and the maxillary left canine. (A,B, Courtesy of Edwin S. Rosenberg and James Torosian).

can occupy in the ridge. This allows the restorative dentist to convey his/her preference for fixture placement. For multiple fixture treatment plans, this information can be used to identify the best location for the fixtures supporting the restoration. The radiographic stent can be converted to a surgical guide by repositioning the guide hole.

Gathering as much pertinent information during this diagnostic phase can eliminate most, if not all, potential problems during the course of treatment.

SURGICAL GUIDE CONSTRUCTION

Restoration-driven treatment planning and implant placement requires accurate assessment of the surgical site. The guide ensures proper positioning and angulation of the osseointegrated dental implants, thus coordinating radiographic analysis, clinical analysis, and cast evaluation, leaving most of the decision making at the presurgical stage, diagnostic tooth set up, from a diagnostic wax-up, denture teeth arrangement, or via duplication of the pre-existing dentition or restoration. They may be categorized based on the material used and amount of surgical restriction.

Traditional Surgical Guide

Traditional surgical guides are restoratively driven and are fabricated based on information pertaining to the ideal esthetic and function position of the definitive prosthesis as opposed to the optimal position based on bone morphology. This important information helps the surgeon visualize the restorative requirements and proceed accordingly during the surgical procedure.

Surgical Guide from a Preexisting Removable Complete Denture

When an existing denture tooth position is adequate in the fully edentulous patient, it can be replicated to construct a surgical guide.

Armamentarium
- Basic dental setup
  - Explorer
  - Mouth mirror
  - Periodontal probe
  - High-speed handpiece
  - Low-speed handpiece
- Irreversible hydrocolloid impression material (Jeltrate Dustless Fast Set, Dentsply Caulk)
- Disposable Impression Trays (UltraDent Products, Inc.)
- Denture duplicator (Lang Dental Manufacturing Co., Inc.) (optional)
- Ortho-Jet Power (for clear guide) Jet XR Powder (for radiopaque appliance) (Lang Dental Manufacturing Co., Inc.)
- #10 round Carbide bur
- 2-mm twist drill (DeWalt, Inc.)

Clinical Technique
1. Make an irreversible hydrocolloid impression and pour a diagnostic cast.

2. Mark the desired implant locations on the cast.
3. Duplicate the denture in clear acrylic resin, either in the laboratory or chairside using a denture replication flask (Fig. 17-15*A*).

CLINICAL TIP

Clear acrylic resin permits visualization of the implant location as marked on the diagnostic cast. This expedites precise positioning of the guide holes in the replicated denture stent.

4. Drill openings through the entire thickness of the surgical guide from the desired tooth position to the location marked on the cast (Fig. 17-15*B*). Place the holes with a #10 round bur completely through the surgical guide, followed by a 2-mm twist drill. This provides a location guide and an angulation guide, because the thickness of the replicated denture will guide the angulation of the surgeon's bur.

CLINICAL TIP

Creating a pathway for the surgeon's bur provides a location guide and an angulation guide, because the thickness of the replicated denture will guide the angulation of the surgeon's bur.

Surgical Guide from Inadequate or Nonexistent Removable Complete Denture. If the patient does not have an existing denture or the prosthesis does not have desirable tooth position, an occlusal rim must be fabricated first.

Armamentarium
- Basic dental setup (Refer to the section on Surgical Guides from a Pre-existing Removable Complete Denture earlier in this chapter.)

Clinical Technique
1. Make an irreversible hydrocolloid impression and pour a diagnostic cast.
2. Construct an occlusal rim with a preliminary tooth setup.

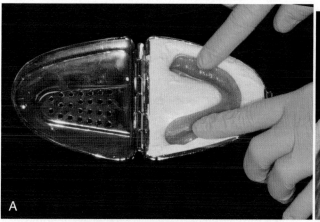
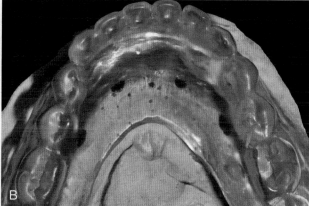

FIGURE 17-15 A, Replication of the patient's existing denture in a denture-replicating flask simplifies construction of a surgical guide. **B,** The replicated denture on the diagnostic cast. Holes will be drilled from the occlusal position of the tooth to the predetermined location of the ridge.

3. After the patient approves the esthetics of the tooth placement, duplicate the wax setup with a denture-replicating flask to construct the surgical guide.
4. Mark the cast and drill holes in the surgical guide in the same manner as for a pre-existing denture. (See the Section on Surgical Guides from a Pre-existing Removable Complete Denture earlier in this chapter.)

Surgical Guide from a Removable Partial Denture. Partial dentures can be replicated in the same manner as pre-existing dentures. (Refer to the section on Surgical Guides from a Pre-existing Removable Complete Denture in this chapter.)

Provisional Fixed Partial Denture. Provisional fixed partial dentures may be used as surgical guides. This requires that teeth adjacent to the implant site are treatment planned for a fixed prosthesis (Fig. 17-16).

Armamentarium
- Basic dental setup (See the section on Surgical Guides from a Pre-existing Removable Complete Denture earlier in this chapter.)

Clinical Technique
1. Prepare the abutment teeth and fabricate a provisional fixed partial denture to span the edentulous area where the implants will be placed.

They can serve as abutments to stabilize the provisional fixed partial denture, which can be used as a surgical guide during implant placement. They can also function as abutments for the provisional restoration during the integration phase of treatment.

CLINICAL TIP

Maintenance of hopeless teeth is acceptable during the osseointegration phase of treatment, if they will not affect implant location and the esthetic success of the definitive prosthesis.

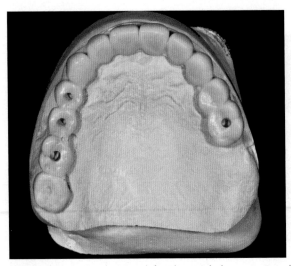

FIGURE 17-16 A provisional fixed partial denture may be used as surgical guides.

2. With a #10 bur, followed by a 2-mm twist drill, place an opening in the pontic areas of the provisional fixed partial denture to act as a surgical guide.
3. After surgery, seal these holes with acrylic resin.

Computer-Assisted Surgical Guide

The combined use of three-dimensional imaging and computers to plan and execute precise implant placement can be used to create a surgical guide (Fig. 17-17). This same technology can also be used to fabricate a provisional prosthesis before the surgical placement of the implant fixture. Precision surgical metallic guides can be fabricated that closely match the diameter of the surgical drills and/or implant fixtures.

Computed Tomography–Derived Tooth-Borne Template
Armamentarium
- Basic dental setup (see the section on Surgical Guides from a Pre-existing Removable Complete Denture earlier in this chapter.)
- Fast set Polyvinyl Siloxane VPS (Aquasil Ultra Smart, Dentsply Caulk)
- Laboratory Putty (Lab-Putty, Coltene/Whaledent)
- bis-Acryl (Luxatemp Automix Plus, DMG America)

Clinical Technique

1. Make an impression with polyvinyl siloxane impression material and pour a stone diagnostic cast.
2. Fabricate a diagnostic wax-up.
3. Make a matrix using laboratory putty and verify complete seating intraorally.
4. Place bis-acryl into the matrix (Luxatemp Automix Plus, DMG America). The tip is placed at the incisal edge and back-filled.
5. Seat the fully loaded matrix intraorally and remove the excess material.
6. After setting remove the matrix and evaluate for fit and position and contour of planned restoration.

Scanning Prosthesis. The scan prosthesis is a radiopaque duplicate of the existing dentition or the diagnostic wax-up. It supplies the clinician with additional information for implant planning. When the patient is scanned with the scan prosthesis, the desired tooth set-up is visible in the CT images. The scan prosthesis is also used to visualize the soft tissue in the planning software. Reference marks are incorporated in the scan prosthesis for the identification of its position in the planning software. The procedure for fabricating the scan prosthesis is dependent on the applied software and chosen template fixation (bone, teeth, or mucosa supported).

Software-Based Planning. Software-based planning allows implants to be virtually designed. In addition, the software company or dental laboratory may be capable of manufacture the surgical guide directly from the software data.

Surgery with Guided Instruments. A surgical guide is helpful when planning the specific surgical instrumentation and location of each implant site. Some systems allow for insertion of the fixture through the surgical guide including a physical depth control.

ESTHETIC MANAGEMENT OF THE PATIENT IN TRANSITIONAL PHASES

The use of provisional restorations during the transitional phase of implant therapy is an important clinical step and should be carefully planned before the surgical phase (Table 17-1). Provisional

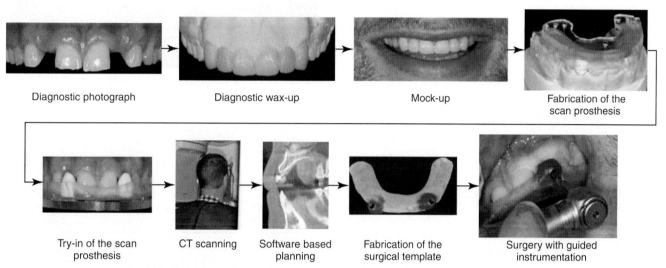

Diagnostic photograph   Diagnostic wax-up   Mock-up   Fabrication of the scan prosthesis

Try-in of the scan prosthesis   CT scanning   Software based planning   Fabrication of the surgical template   Surgery with guided instrumentation

FIGURE 17-17 Steps in computer-assisted surgical guide implant surgery.

Table 17-1 **Selecting Provisional Restorations**

Removable Provisional Restoration				
Types of Provisional	**Advantages**	**Disadvantages**	**Contraindications**	**Recommended Uses**
Using an existing prosthesis	Simplicity; the prosthesis is made at no additional cost to the patient	If the prosthesis is not ideal, it may compromise results	If the prosthesis is ill fitting	If the prosthesis fits well and its comfortable for the patient
Interim removable partial/complete dentures	Easy to fabricate Easy to insert Easy to modify	Initiate soft tissue inflammation Interfere with speech Cause transmucosal loading	Guided bone regeneration Gag reflex	Patients who require multiple procedures
Essix provisional restoration	Quick and inexpensive Free of transmucosal loading	Lack of durability Unesthetic	Long-term provisional	Short-term provisional
Fixed Provisional Restoration				
Types of Provisional	**Advantages**	**Disadvantages**	**Contraindications**	**Recommended Uses**
Adhesive fixed partial dentures	Chairside procedure	Debonding	Long-term provisional	Short-term provisional
Tooth-supported restoration	Esthetics Free of transmucosal loading Contouring of soft tissue	High laboratory cost Adjacent teeth preparation	Adjacent teeth do not need full coverage	Long-term provisional Splinting of periodontally compromised teeth Serial extraction
Transitional implant supported	Esthetics Free of transmucosal loading Contouring of soft tissue	Fracture of implants Prevent definitive fixtures from integrating	Single edentulous sites	Long-term provisional

restorations provide esthetics and adequate function, and can be used to shape the soft tissue and protect the surgical site from occlusal forces during the healing process by preventing micromovement of the implant and grafted site. Controlling micromovement is essential to ensure osseointegration rather than fibrous encapsulation of the implant fixtures. The provisional restoration provides both the prototype and "blueprint" for the definitive prosthesis (Box 17-2).

The most common forms of provisional restorations are fixed prostheses supported by retained natural teeth; and removable interim prostheses ("flipper," existing prosthesis, Essix provisional); and resin bonded fixed partial dentures.

Removable Interim Partial Dentures

Ease of fabrication, cost, and insertion are the most obvious advantages of this provisional restoration. An additional advantage is the ability to modify an acrylic resin interim RPD to accommodate any changes in the anatomy of the ridge for patients who may require multiple procedures of extraction, soft- and hard-tissue augmentation, and implant placement (Fig. 17-18).

> ### CLINICAL TIP
> Denture lining material can dry and become hard over time. Changing the lining material at monthly intervals will keep the lining material of the denture elastic.

In the mandibular arch, a similar procedure can be used, especially for vestibular deepening procedures. Extension of soft reline material in the facial flange area provides a surface guide for tissue healing. However, the lack of stability may compromise function and speech, and encroach upon the surgical site.

For single tooth replacements, a provisional acrylic resin removable denture can be placed. If implant placement is performed at the time of tooth extraction, space over the extraction site must be adequate so as to not load the implant.[26]

Existing Prosthesis. This is beneficial only if the prosthesis is esthetically and functionally acceptable. Wherever possible, hopeless teeth can be maintained to serve as provisional abutments during the integration phase of treatment, allowing the patient to have a fixed restoration during this time (Fig. 17-19).

Although less than ideal because of the undesired pressure, they may apply to the healing surgical site, RPDs and complete dentures replace missing teeth and the flanges; providing necessary lip support.

Essix Provisional Appliance. The Essix provisional is made either in the laboratory or in the dental office from clear

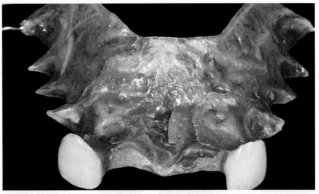

FIGURE 17-18 The provisional is tooth-retained and avoids pressure on the surgical site.

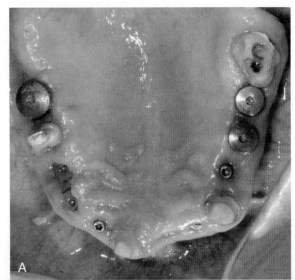

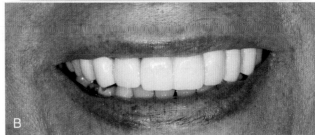

FIGURE 17-19 It is advantageous to maintain strategic nonrestorable teeth (**A**) to support a fixed provisional prosthesis until the restoration can be supported by osseointegrated implants (**B**).

thermoplastic sheets to retain pontics for missing teeth. The pontic is fabricated by applying the vacuum form sheet under high pressure and heat over the denture teeth. Pressure on the surgical sites is avoided because the Essix provisional is tooth retained (Fig. 17-20).[27]

Provisional Fixed Partial Dentures

The most common provisionalization technique is a provisional fixed partial denture using the adjacent teeth as abutments even if they are questionable (stage surgery) (see Fig. 17-19).

Box 17-2		
Functions of a Provisional Prosthesis		
Provide a functional and stable occlusion	Protect the underlying gingival tissues	Restore and enhance esthetics and phonetics
Do not interfere with primary wound closure	Do not exert direct occlusal load on the underlying implants or bone-grafted sites.	Determine the future position, support, and shape the site of the definitive prosthesis

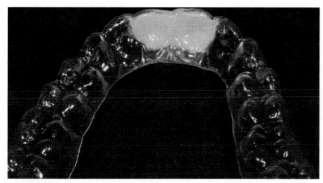

FIGURE 17-20 An interim removable partial denture ("Flipper").

Adhesive Fixed Partial Dentures. A provisional fixed restoration (Fig. 17-21A) can be bonded to the adjacent natural dentition or the replacement tooth may be luted onto orthodontic brackets during the integration phase (Fig. 17-21B). These restorations protect the implant site from occlusal loading, while providing functional occlusion and esthetics.

Tooth-Supported Restoration. If teeth adjacent to surgical sites will ultimately require complete coverage restorations, they can be prepared and used as abutments for tooth supported provisional restorations which can be adjusted to avoid direct contact with the implant site. These teeth are often used even if the long-term prognosis is questionable in staged implant procedures (Fig. 17-22).

Transitional Implants. Mini transitional implants can be use to support fixed and removable provisional restorations.

Provisional Restorations after Osseointegration. A provisional fixed partial denture has many advantages when used after osseointegration. It allows the restorative dentist to evaluate the esthetics, tooth position, lip support, pontic

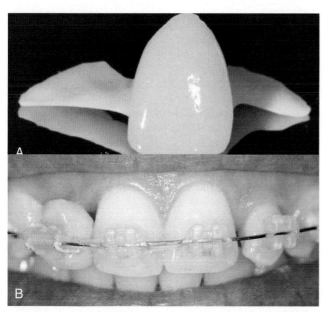

FIGURE 17-21 A, Provisional fixed restoration may be bonded to the adjacent natural dentition. **B,** Provisional replacement of the maxillary right lateral incisor luted onto orthodontic brackets.

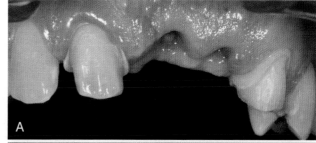

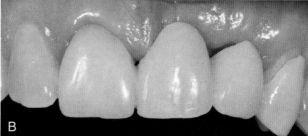

FIGURE 17-22 A, Ridge area of extracted teeth. **B,** If the teeth adjacent to surgical sites will require full coverage restorations they can be used as abutments for a tooth supported provisional restoration. They should be contoured to avoid direct contact with the surgical site.

location, vertical dimension, and control of the gingival margin before constructing the definitive restoration. A provisional fixed partial denture allows full maturation of the gingival tissues without the pressure of a removable appliance during healing. It provides the patient a degree of psychologic confidence by having an esthetically acceptable fixed appliance during soft tissue maturation following stage 2 surgery. In addition, oral hygiene procedures can be reinitiated at an earlier stage.

Provisional fixed partial dentures can be either cement retained using provisional fixed partial denture heads on the standard abutments or screw retained with provisional cylinders. The latter provides long-term stability to the provisional prosthesis.

After Stage 2 Healing. The soft tissue around the abutments in the stage 2 postoperative period can recede considerably. It is therefore recommended that 3 months elapse for the tissue to stabilize before either selecting a definitive abutment or making final impression.[28]

At this point, additional procedures can be performed, such as tissue recontouring or augmentation (see the section on Soft Tissue Management in this chapter), evaluation of vertical dimension, placement of additional implants, or evaluation of tissue maturation after the extraction of hopeless teeth.

SOFT TISSUE MANAGEMENT

Tissue must not be inflamed, bleeding, or hyperplastic. In addition, an adequate zone of healthy attached gingiva is necessary to maintain the level of the marginal tissue around the definitive restoration. Proper tissue type and health also prevents irritation from oral hygiene procedures and decreases the likelihood of marginal recession. Gingival grafting for either tissue augmentation or vestibular extension can be done at the time of stage 2 surgery or after the tissue heals around the provisional healing abutments.

Gingival Papilla

A crucial aspect of successful tissue management in the partially edentulous patient is the maintenance of the interproximal profile of the papilla and the re-creation of normal alveolar contours found in the natural dentition. The shape of the gingival tissues is particularly important in patients with high smile lines because of gingival display in the maxillary anterior and premolar regions.

Gingival Recontouring

The level and contour of the tissue in the implant area can differ from that of adjacent natural dentition (Fig. 17-23). The gingiva can be coronally or apically positioned if surgical correction is indicated.

SOFT TISSUE EMERGENCE PROFILE

Teeth have a natural emergence from the root to the crown of the tooth that provides for smooth transitions well as providing

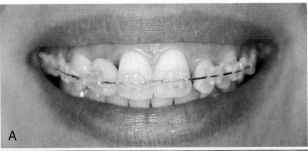

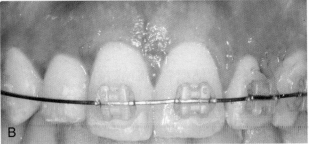

FIGURE 17-23 A, Preoperative facial view showing gingival disharmony. **B,** Gingival re-countering was performed on both maxillary central incisors and the left lateral incisor, creating a gingival architecture, which is more harmonious with the provisional implant restoration of the right lateral incisor.

for soft tissue support. The importance of developing a proper emergence profile is critical to achieving a definitive restoration whose appearance on exiting the soft tissues closely mimics that of adjacent natural teeth tissue as opposed to resting on the soft tissue, as is the situation with ridge-lapped restorations.

Emergence profile of the definitive restoration begins with the dimension of the supporting implant fixture. Wide-diameter implant fixtures and wide implant fixture platforms often allow for the fabrication of crown contours with more gradual transition in dimension from the implant fixture to the crown than do smaller diameter implant fixtures and fixture platforms. A more ideal emergence profile can be obtained when using an implant of similar diameter to the tooth root being replaced. If too large or too small, the resulting emergence angle will be compromised. Additionally, if the implant is not placed properly in a coronal, or apical, facial, or palatal direction, the emergence can also be compromised. It is recommended that the fixture platform be located approximately 3 mm apical to a line drawn between the cementoenamel junctions of the adjacent teeth. This will usually provide enough space for the development of ideal emergence. However, this position needs to be altered if the fixture diameter is significantly different from the diameter of the root it replaces. If a fixture is placed that is significantly smaller than the tooth that it replaces, a more apical placement is necessary. Likewise, if the fixture diameter is larger than the root it is replacing, then a slightly more coronal position is recommended.

The development of an ideal crown emergence also depends on the soft tissue. Healing abutments and provisional abutments can begin the process of recontouring the soft tissues at the time of implant fixture exposure. This can occur immediately following stage 1 or 2 surgery, depending on the clinical situation. The placement of these specially contoured healing abutments allows the soft tissues to heal and mature in a shape that can be incorporated into the provisional restoration and later into the definitive prosthesis.

The use of emergence profile concepts can provide for the fabrication of restorations that more closely resemble the natural dentition. Sculpting of the interproximal papillae and the buccal gingiva is accomplished with sequential fixed provisional restorations. Stepwise addition of provisional composite resin material manipulates tissues and creates proper esthetic contours (Fig. 17-24). Once accomplished, these contours must be accurately and predictably communicated to the laboratory using a custom impression coping.

FABRICATION OF A CUSTOM IMPRESSION POST

Armamentarium
+ Basic dental setup (Refer to the section on Surgical Guides from a Pre-existing Removable Complete Denture in this chapter.)
+ Rubber Dappen dish
+ Fast Set laboratory plaster (Laboratory Plaster–Fast, Kerr Dental Laboratory Products)

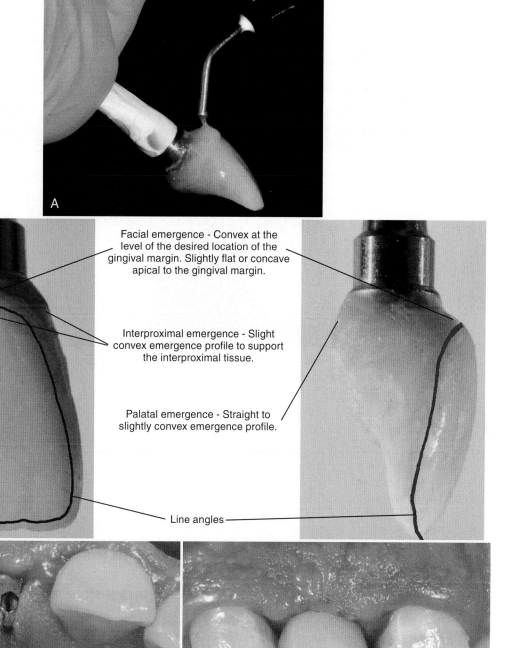

Facial emergence - Convex at the level of the desired location of the gingival margin. Slightly flat or concave apical to the gingival margin.

Interproximal emergence - Slight convex emergence profile to support the interproximal tissue.

Palatal emergence - Straight to slightly convex emergence profile.

Line angles

FIGURE 17-24 A, Step-wise addition of a light polymerized bis-acryl provisional material used to manipulate soft tissue and create proper esthetic contours. **B,** Emergence profiles can be developed with a provisional restoration. **C,** Incisal view of peri-implant tissue before placement of the provisional restoration. **D,** Screw-retained provisional restoration intraorally.

Continued

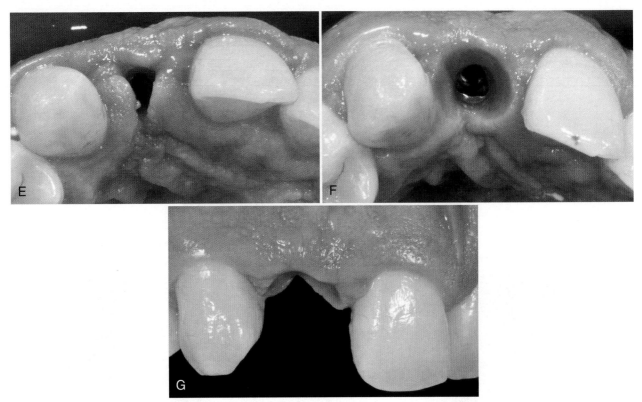

FIGURE 17-24, cont'd E, Incisal view following removal of the healing abutment. **F,** Incisal view of soft tissue developed by the provisional restoration. **G,** Soft tissue levels developed by using the provisional restoration demonstrates a parabolic sulcular form.

+ Implant analog
+ Implant impression coping (manufacture specific)
+ Fast set polyvinylsiloxane (PVS) (Aquasil Ultra Smart, Dentsply Caulk)
+ Auto-polymerizing rapid cure provisional material (Luxatemp Automix Plus, DMG America)

Clinical Technique

1. Fabricate a provisional restoration with the desired emergence profile (see Chapter 10).
2. Place the laboratory analog into the fast set plaster (Fig. 17-25A).
3. Inject a PVS (fast set) around the provisional restoration and once the material is set mark the PVS material to indicate the facial surface of the restoration.

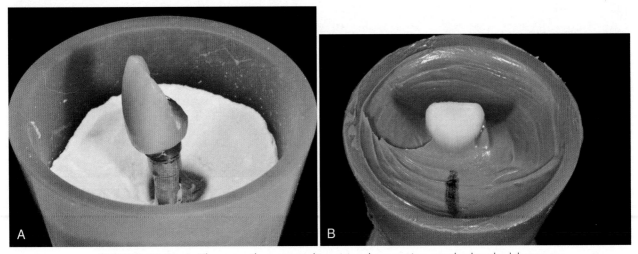

FIGURE 17-25 A, The correctly contoured provisional restoration attached to the laboratory analog is placed into the rubber dappen dish. **B,** Polyether impression material is injected around the provisional and once the material is set the polyether impression material is marked to indicate the facial surface of the restoration.

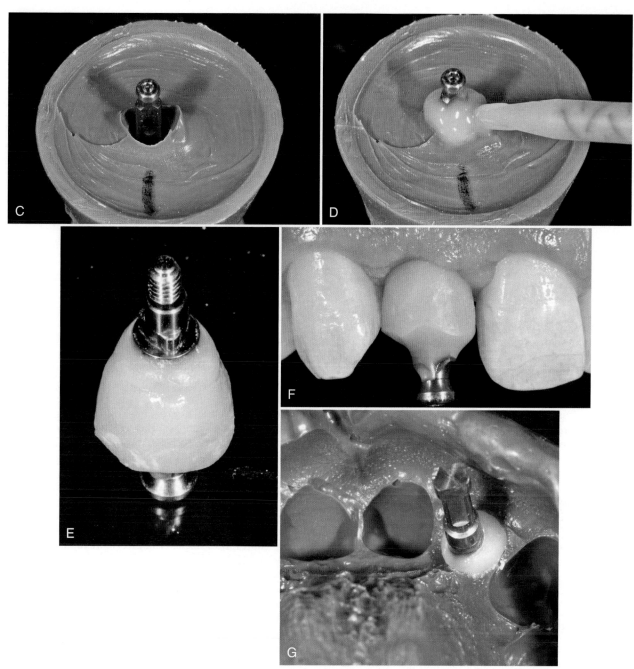

FIGURE 17-25, cont'd C, The provisional restoration is removed and an impression coping is place attached to the embedded lab analog. **D,** The impression post is placed onto the lab analog. Then the impression is filled with cold cure or auto-polymerizing rapid cure provisional material. The material is allowed to set for 2 minutes around the custom impression post. **E,** The custom impression post is unscrewed; trim excess material is trimmed. Any voids are filled, the restoration is polished, and an impression is made. **F,** The custom impression post is screwed into the implant. **G,** An impression is made and the master cast is now ready to be fabricated.

Continued

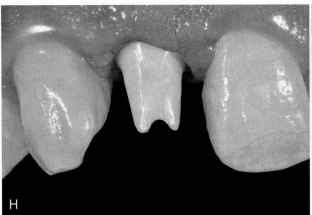
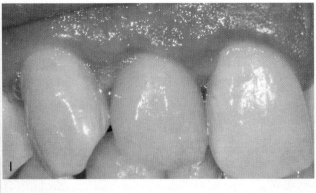

FIGURE 17-25, cont'd H, The definitive abutment in place and proper gingival architecture is observed after maturation of the peri-implant tissues. **I,** The definitive restoration.

4. Remove the provisional restoration and place the impression coping onto the lab analog (Fig. 17-25B).
5. Fill the impression with cold cure or auto-polymerizing rapid cure provisional material and allow the material to set for 2 minutes (Fig. 17-25C).
6. Unscrew provisional post and trim excess material. Fill any voids, polish, and make impression (Fig. 17-25D).
7. Screw the custom impression post into the implant and make an impression (Fig. 17-25E).
8. Once impression material sets the provisional can be removed.
9. The master cast is now ready to be fabricated (Fig. 17-25F-I).

CLINICAL TIP

The custom impression coping captures the transitional zone of the peri-implant mucosa. This tissue is usually greater in depth on the interproximal and palatal positions around the implant.

TYPES OF IMPLANT RESTORATIONS

A variety of treatment designs exist for removable and fixed implant prostheses. They can be classified as removable overdentures, implant-supported removable overdentures, bar overdentures, crown and fixed partial denture types, and crown and fixed partial denture—full arch types.

Removable Overdenture: Full and Partial

Historically, implant-based treatment was focused on fixed prosthetic tooth replacement, however, benefits of implant overdentures is in improving function, emotional stability, physical health, and esthetics is well documented.[30] Removable partial and full overdentures are either implant supported or combined implant retained and soft tissue supported. They generally require fewer implants when compared with the totally implant supported prosthesis design. Fewer implants and a removable prosthesis offer a less complex and less expensive option for an edentulous or partially edentulous patient.

Implant-Supported Removable Overdenture: Bar Overdenture

Indications

1. *Lip support requirements.* A fixed prosthesis may be inadequate to provide sufficient lip support in the anterior regions, especially in the maxillary arch, a because of resorption of the maxillary ridges. The use of an overdenture provides the option of extending the facial flange to provide for additional lip support. This will maximize esthetics and facial contours. Fixed restoration can also contain acrylic flanges or pink porcelain extension, but oral hygiene may be compromised.
2. *Psychologic concerns.* Patients who have worn removable appliances for many years sometimes feel that a removable appliance allows them better access for oral hygiene. They are accustomed to removing their appliance during oral hygiene procedures. These patients may feel more comfortable having a removable prosthesis.
3. *Financial concerns.* The overdenture is usually the least expensive alternative for the restoration of multiple osseointegrated implants in an edentulous arch.
4. *Medical concerns.* The health status of the patient may not allow extensive grafting procedures.
5. *Home care.* Overdentures also allow for easy hygiene maintenance by the patient.

Contraindications

1. *Psychologic concerns.* Many patients have a psychologic aversion to wearing a removable appliance. This aversion can be extremely strong and these patients may desire to avoid a removable prosthesis at all costs.
2. *Hyperactive gag reflexes.* The overdenture requires the extension onto the tuberosity area of the maxillary arch and onto the posterior retromolar area of the mandibular arch. Placement into these areas may activate the patient's gag reflexes.
3. *Unilaterally edentulous areas.* When a patient presents with a unilateral edentulous area, an overdenture is not indicated because it is not possible to adequately stabilize the appliance. Therefore a fixed restoration should be considered in such situations.
4. *Poor supporting bone.* As with any implant, adequate bone type and configuration must be available.

Clinical Case Showing Bar Overdenture with Four Implants. A healthy 67-year-old woman who wore a maxillary complete denture presented with a terminal mandibular dentition, a defective mandibular partial denture, and a severe atrophic posterior mandible. Because of the amount and the pattern of resorption of the edentulous mandible, the only area available for implant placement was the intraforaminal area. The treatment plan was to extract her remaining teeth and replace them with a bar overdenture with four implants.

Teeth # 23, #24, and #25 had a hopeless periodontal/restorative prognosis and were extracted without complications. Straumann NCdental implants were placed in the #21, #23, #25, and #28 positions.

After stage 2 surgery, impression posts were placed and complete seating verified with a periapical radiograph (Fig. 17-26A). An impression was made.

CLINICAL TIP

Open tray impression posts are necessary when the implants have different angulations; a closed tray could lock the impression in the mouth. The open tray may be a more accurate technique because the impression posts remain inside the impression.

The final impression was poured by the dental laboratory producing a cast replicating the position of the implants. An occlusal record/verification jig was fabricated for occlusal records and to confirm the position of the implants (Fig. 17-26B).

A diagnostic tooth set-up was prepared by the dental laboratory (Fig. 17-26C), which was verified intraorally for esthetics and function. The restoration was returned to the laboratory for fabrication of the bar.

The bar can be cast in type 3 or 4 noble alloy or milled from titanium. The most common bar patterns are the Dolder Bar (Preat Corp.), and the Hader Bar (Sterngold Dental, LLC). The bar that was used in this patient was computer designed and milled from a titanium blank using CAD/CAM technology (NobelProcera Implant Bar Overdenture, Nobel Biocare) The bar was designed in NobelProcera software (Fig. 17-26D). The implant bar was milled and the locator attachments were placed.

This milled bar is often more accurate[31,32] than a conventional cast bar. The bar must fit passively on the implants and this is verified by placing only one screw and evaluating radiographically to determine proper fit. If the fit is not passive, the contralateral side will be elevated. Once the fit is verified, the bar is placed back on the cast and returned to the dental laboratory for construction of the overdenture (Fig. 17-26E).

The overdenture was returned, the bar was placed, torqued to the manufacturer's specifications, and checked for fit of denture, balanced contacts, and group function (Fig. 17-26F,G).

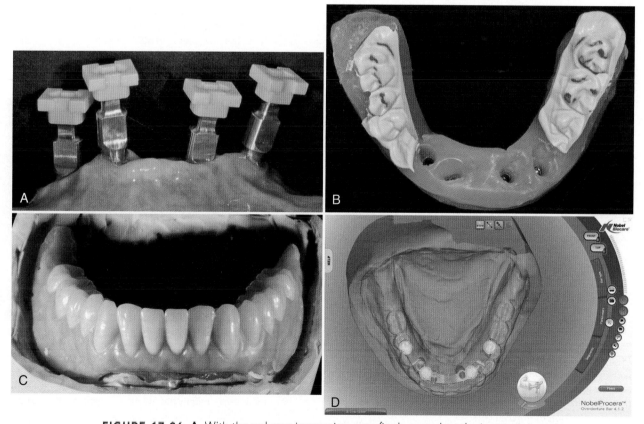

FIGURE 17-26 A, With the polymer impression caps firmly seated on the impression posts, a closed tray impression was made. **B,** Occlusal records/verification jig. **C,** Diagnostic tooth set up. **D,** The bar was computer-designed and milled from a titanium blank using CAD/CAM technology (NobelProcera Implant Bar Overdenture).

Continued

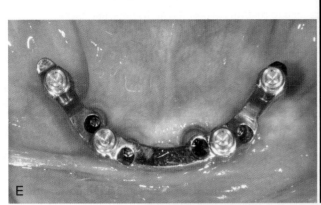

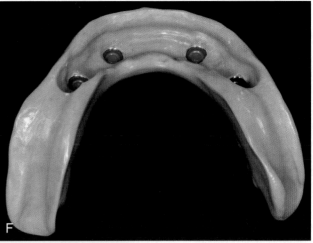

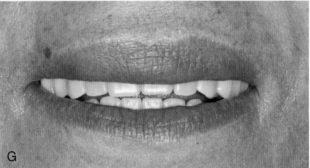

FIGURE 17-26, cont'd E, The milled implant bar with locator attachments. The bar must fit passively on the implants and is verified by placing only one screw and evaluating radiographically for proper fit. Occlusal (**F**) and frontal (**G**) views of the definitive complete mandibular full overdenture with Locator attachments. (ZEST Anchors LLC)

Implant-Retained and Tissue-Supported with Individual, Non-Connected (Non-Bar) Attachments

With implant retained and tissue supported with individual, non-connected (non-bar) attachments abutments screw directly into the implant. They do not require laboratory construction of bars and connections but rather provide immediate connection to the denture. They are usually in the form of an O-ring or ball-and-socket attachment (Dal-RO, BIOMET 3i; Overdenture Kit, Nobel Biocare). The Locator attachment (ZEST Anchors LLC) is a more recent option that provides greater flexibility[33] when restoring overdenture cases (Fig. 17-27). It allows correction between divergent implants angles of up to 40 degrees using identical attachment, eliminating the need for placement and positioning of angled abutments while maintaining a low vertical height of 3.17 mm from the platform to the top of the attachment housing.

Indications

1. *Simplicity requirements.* The overdenture abutments provide a simpler approach to the retention of overdentures, because they do not require impressions or laboratory procedures and construction of gingival bars.
2. *Two to four implants.*

Contraindications

1. *Maintenance requirements.* O-rings or Locator retention males must be changed periodically because they tend to wear during extended use.

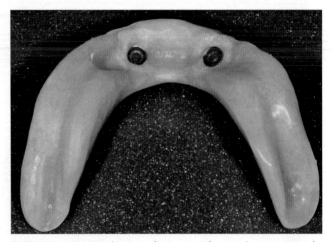

FIGURE 17-27 An overdenture with two Locator attachments. (ZEST Anchors LLC)

2. *Nonparallel implant orientation.* Because these abutments have male posts extending above the implant, they must be relatively parallel to prevent damage to the retaining rings and allow proper seating. The Locator design allows for correction of angles up to 40 degrees between divergent implants using the same abutment.
3. *Immobility requirements.* O-rings and ball-and-socket attachments allow some movement of the overdenture. If the patient

requires absolute immobility to the overdenture, multiple implants and bars should be used to provide a greater area of support for stabilizing the denture.

Treatment Complications with Overdentures

Treatment complications associated with implant overdentures have been discussed in numerous studies.[34,35]

1. Loose, lost, or broken retentive clips accounted for the most common overdenture repairs.
2. Gingival hyperplasia, maxillary denture re-line requirements, and occlusal adjustment.
3. Denture base fracture
4. Overdentures require more adjustment than fixed prostheses, but the adjustments were usually performed within the first year post insertion.

CROWN AND FIXED PARTIAL DENTURE TYPE

Single Tooth

The single tooth replacement is one of the most challenging esthetic restorations.[36] Placement of a dental implant in the esthetic zone is a technique sensitive procedure with little room for error. A subtle mistake in the positioning of the implant or the mishandling of soft or hard tissue can lead to esthetic failure and patient dissatisfaction.

Today, the single-tooth implant has become one of the most common treatment alternatives for the replacement of missing teeth.[37,38] Various studies have shown the successful osseointegration and long-term function of restorations supported by single-tooth implants.[39]

CLINICAL TIP

Dental implants cannot be placed until facial growth is complete.

Indications
1. *Conservation of tooth structure.* The usual alternative to a single tooth replacement is either a conventional or acid-etch composite resin retained fixed partial denture. These require the removal of tooth structure.
2. *Diastema maintenance.* Maintaining adjacent diastemata prevents overcontouring contact areas or placement of a palatal bar.
3. *Existing clinically acceptable adjacent fixed partial dentures.* In some instances a single tooth must be removed and the adjacent multiple unit fixed partial denture is clinically acceptable. Conventionally, this would require replacement of the adjacent fixed partial denture to replace this single tooth. Generally, this also includes extending the fixed partial denture one tooth beyond the edentulous area. Placement of a single implant allows the preservation of the clinically acceptable fixed partial denture, and avoids the preparation of an additional tooth adjacent to the new edentulous area.

Contraindications
1. *Poor supporting bone.* As with any implant, adequate bone type and configuration must be available.

2. *Restoration of adjacent teeth is necessary for other reasons.* If adjacent teeth require extensive rehabilitation, a fixed partial denture should be considered.

Crown and Fixed Partial Denture Type: Full Arch

Full arch crown and fixed partial denture restorations can be constructed on osseo-integrated fixtures, assuming there is adequate supporting structure and that the expected esthetic result can be achieved (Fig. 17-28). Under ideal circumstances, a patient can convert an existing complete denture to a totally fixed restoration.

Indications
1. *Adequate ridge height.* Full arch crown and fixed partial denture restorations can be considered only for totally edentulous patients when adequate ridge height is present to produce a normally sized and shaped definitive restoration. Minimal resorption of the residual ridge permits the definitive restoration to be tooth like in both size and shape. This is the ideal situation for using a conventional crown and fixed partial denture restoration supported by osseo-integrated dental implant fixtures.

Contraindications
1. *Significant ridge resorption.* In the situation of significant bone resorption, a fixed restoration requires replacement of more than just tooth crowns. Root dimension and alveolus height must be replaced. This is difficult to achieve using a conventional crown and fixed partial denture restoration because of framework considerations. In addition, because the ridges generally recede in a lingual or palatal direction, as well as in an apical direction, unusual contours would be required in the definitive restoration or the definitive fixed partial denture.
2. *Inadequate lip support.* The prosthesis may not adequately support the lip in the vestibular area and may produce a soft tissue crease under the nose.

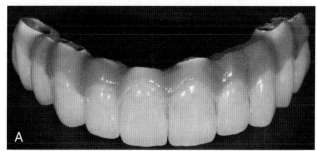

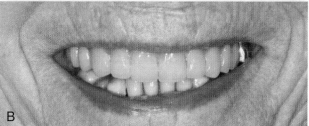

FIGURE 17-28 A, Full arch prosthesis. **B,** Full arch prosthesis in place.

Hybrid Type

The hybrid restoration of osseointegrated dental implants involves components of both the complete removable denture and the traditional fixed restoration. It consists of a metal framework supporting denture teeth. Denture acrylic is processed around the denture teeth, connecting them to the metal framework. This allows replacement of the lost alveolar structures as well as root structures in the edentulous patient with moderate to severe bone resorption. Generally these restorations are associated with extensive cantilevering at the distal aspects of the restoration.

Indications

1. *Totally edentulous arches with moderate to severe resorption.* This hybrid prosthesis is used in moderately to severely resorbed edentulous patients, because it provides maximum flexibility when positioning the teeth despite the location of the implants. The denture teeth can be placed in the proper position to provide lip support and occlusal function. Tooth positions do not need to be directly over the fixtures themselves.
2. *Lip support, speech, and air control requirements.* The hybrid prosthesis provides sufficient bulk to adequately seal areas that otherwise may potentially cause disturbances in air control and speech. The hybrid prosthesis can provide adequate bulk for lip support, especially in severely resorbed areas of the anterior maxilla.

Contraindication

1. *Minimal ridge resorption.* In the situation of minimal ridge resorption, the hybrid prosthesis is contraindicated when the open apical surface of the hybrid prosthesis will be displayed during function.

CONCLUSION

The treatment of patients with dental implants requires knowledge of multiple specialties. Close coordination among the implant surgeon, restorative dentist, and laboratory technician in the preoperative phase will improve the quality of the definitive restoration. An esthetic approach to implant placement and restoration provides patients with stable, predictable restorations that enhance the patient's quality of life both functionally and esthetically.

REFERENCES

1. Branëmark P-I, Hansson BO, Adell R, et al: Osseointegrated implants in the treatment of the edentulous jaw. Experience from a 10-year period, *Scan J Plast Reconstr Surg* 11(suppl 15):1, 1977.
2. Adell R, Lekholm U, Rockler B, et al: A 15-year study of osseointegrated implants in the treatment of the edentulous jaw, *Int J Oral Surg* 10:387, 1981.
3. Branëmark, P-I, Zarb GA, Albrektsson T: *Tissue-integrated prostheses*, Chicago, 1985, Quintessence.
4. Adell R: Clinical results of osseointegrated implants supporting fixed prostheses in edentulous jaws, *J Prosthet Dent* 50:251, 1983.
5. Kohal RJ, Klaus G: A zirconia implant-crown system: a case report, *Int J Periodontics Restorative Dent* 24(2):147-153, 2004.
6. Barter S, Stone P, Brägger U: A pilot study to evaluate the success and survival rate of titanium-zirconium implants in partially edentulous patients: results after 24 months of follow-up, *Clin Oral Implants Res* 23(7):873-881, 2012.
7. Weinberg L: The biomechanics of force distribution in implant-supported prostheses, *Int J Oral Maxillofac Implants* 8:19-31, 1993.
8. McCracken MS, Mitchell L, Hegde R, et al: Variability of mechanical torque-limiting devices in clinical service at a US dental school, *J Prosthodont* 19(1):20-24, 2010. Epub September 17, 2009.
9. Becker W, Ochsenbein C, Tibbetts L, et al: Alveolar bone anatomic profiles as measured from dry skulls. Clinical ramifications, *J Clin Periodontol* 24:727-731, 1997.
10. Bidez MW, Misch CE: Force transfer in implant dentistry: basic concepts and principles, *J Oral Implantol* 18:264-274, 1992.
11. Pauletto N, Lahie BJ, Walton JN: Complications associated with excess cement around crowns on osseointegrated implants: a clinical report, *Int J Oral Maxillofac Implants* 14:865-868, 1999.
12. Agar JR, Cameron SM, Hughbanks JC, et al: Cement removal from restorations luted to titanium abutments with simulated subgingival margins, *J Prosthet Dent* 78(1):43-47, 1997.
13. Razzoog ME, Lang LA, McAndrew KS: AllCeram crowns for single replacement implant abutments, *J Prosthet Dent* 78:486-489, 1997.
14. Shadid R, Sadaqa N: A comparison between screw- and cement-retained implant prostheses. A literature review, *J Oral Implantol* 38(3):298-307, 2012.
15. Kan JY, Rungcharassaeng K, Umezu K, et al: Dimensions of peri-implant mucosa: an evaluation of maxillary anterior single implants in humans, *J Periodontol* 74(4):557-562, 2003.
16. Drago C, Lazzara RJ: Guidelines for implant abutment selection for partially edentulous patients, *Compend Contin Educ Dent* 31(1):14-20, 23-24, 26-27, 2010.
17. Salama H, Salama MA, Garber D, et al: The interproximal height of bone: a guidepost to predictable aesthetic strategies and soft tissue contours in anterior tooth replacement, *Pract Periodontics Aesthet Dent* 10:1131-1141, 1998.
18. Saadoun AP, Le Gall M, Touati B: Current trends in implantology: Part II. Treatment, planning, aesthetic considerations and tissue regeneration, *Pract Proced Aesthet Dent* 16:707-714, 2004.
19. Tarnow DP, Cho SC, Wallace SS: The effect of inter-implant distance on the height of inter-implant bone crest, *J Periodontol* 71:546-549, 2000.
20. Elian N, Ehrlich B, Jalbout ZN, et al: Advanced concepts in implant dentistry: creating the "aesthetic site foundation," *Dent Clin North Am* 51:547-563, 2007.
21. Kokich V: Anterior dental esthetics: An orthodontic perspective III. Mediolateral relationships, *J Esthet Dent* 5:200-207, 1993.
22. Brudvik JS: *Advanced removable partial dentures*, Chicago, 1999, Quintessence.
23. Mitrani R, Brudvik JS, Phillips KM: Posterior implants for distal extension removable prostheses: a retrospective study, *Int J Periodontics Restorative Dent* 23:353-359, 2003.
24. Vogel RC: Expanding the benefits of implant therapy: implant-retained removable partial dentures, *Funct Esthet Restor Dent* 2:2-5, 2008.
25. Vogel RC: Implant overdentures: a new standard of care for edentulous patients—current concepts and techniques, *Funct Esthet Restor Dent* 1(2). http://shop.zestanchors.com/images/articles/article_63_Functional%20Esthetics.pdf. Accessed January 2014.
26. Branëmark, P-I, Zarb GA, Albrektsson T: *Tissue-integrated prostheses*, Chicago, 1985, Quintessence.
27. Moskowitr EM, Sheridan JJ, Celenza F Jr, et al: Essix appliances. Provisional anterior prosthesis for pre and post implant patients, *N Y State Dent J* 63:32-35, 1997.
28. Small ON, Tarnow DP: Gingival recession around implants: a 1-year longitudinal prospective study, *Int J Oral Maxillofac Implants* 15:527-532, 2000.
29. Lazzara R: Immediate implant placement into extraction sites: surgical and restorative advantages, *Int J Periodontics Restorative Dent* 9:333, 1989.
30. Awad MA, Lund JP, Shapiro SH, et al: Oral health status and treatment satisfaction with mandibular implant overdentures and conventional dentures: a randomized clinical trial in a senior population, *Int J Prosthodont* 16:390-396, 2013.
31. Drago C, Saldarriaga RL, Domagala D, et al: Volumetric determination of the amount of misfit in CAD/CAM and cast implant frameworks: a multicenter laboratory study, *Int J Oral Maxillofac Implants* 25(5):920-929, 2010.
32. King AW, Chai J, Lautenschlager E, et al: The mechanical properties of milled and cast titanium for ceramic veneering, *Int J Prosthodont* 7(6):532-537, 1994.
33. Ochiai KT, Williams BH, Hojo S, et al: Photoelastic analysis of the effect of palatal support on various implant-supported overdenture designs, *J Prosthet Dent* 91:421-427, 2004.
34. Engquist B, Bergendal T, Kallus T, et al: A retrospective multicenter evaluation of osseointegrated implants supporting overdentures, *Int J Oral Maxillofac Implants* 3:129-134, 1988.
35. Naert I, Quirynen M, Theuniers G, et al: Prosthetic aspects of osseointegrated fixtures supporting overdentures. A 4-year report, *J Prosthet Dent* 65:671-680, 1991.
36. Belser UC, Schmid B, Higginbottom F, et al: Outcome analysis of implant restorations located in the anterior maxilla: a review of the recent literature, *Int J Oral Maxillofac Implants* 19(Suppl):30-42, 2004.
37. Naert I, Koutsikakis G, Duyck J, et al: Biologic outcome of single-implant restorations as tooth replacements: a long-term follow-up study, *Clin Implant Dent Relat Res* 2:209-218, 2000.
38. Weng D, Jacobson Z, Tarnow D, et al: A prospective multicenter clinical trial of 3i machined-surface implants: results after 6 years of follow-up, *Int J Oral Maxillofac Implants* 18:417-423, 2003.
39. Schmitt A, Zarb GA: The longitudinal clinical effectiveness of osseointegrated dental implants for single-tooth replacement, *Int J Prosthodont* 6:197-202, 1993.

18

Esthetics and Oral and Maxillofacial Surgery

Daniel Buchbinder

The maxillofacial surgeon can dramatically enhance facial esthetics through manipulation of the craniomaxillofacial skeleton, as well as the soft tissue drape. The importance of recognition by the general practitioner of existing skeletal and soft tissue deformities beyond the dental arches and an awareness of the significant impact the correction will have on the patient's overall satisfaction and self-esteem should not be understated. For example, an edentulous patient with an overclosed vertical dimension and deep perioral furrows should not only be restored prosthetically but also should be offered a referral to an oral and maxillofacial surgeon for evaluation for laser-assisted skin resurfacing to enhance the perioral esthetics. Furthermore, the American Dental Association's definition of oral and maxillofacial surgery as "the specialty of dentistry which includes the diagnosis, surgical and adjunctive treatment of diseases, injuries, and defects involving both the functional and esthetic aspects of the hard and soft tissues of the oral and maxillofacial regions"[1] recognizes not only the functional, but also the facial esthetic enhancement procedures that the contemporarily trained oral and maxillofacial surgeon can offer.

This chapter is not meant to cover the complete scope of oral and maxillofacial surgery, but rather to present selected surgical procedures and adjunctive measures that can improve the patient's overall dental and facial esthetic appearance. For a more comprehensive review the reader should refer to a textbook on oral and maxillofacial surgery.

INTRAORAL PROCEDURES TO IMPROVE ESTHETICS

Gingivectomy

Gingival recontouring or laser-assisted sculpting of the gingiva is a relatively simple procedure that can significantly enhance the esthetics of a patient's restored smile. In situations of noninflammatory gingival hyperplasia, laser-assisted gingivectomy can be used to reshape the interdental papilla around an endosteal fixture to improve the emergence profile and enhance esthetics.[2] A more traditional gingivectomy procedure can be done to lengthen the clinical crowns of the anterior maxillary tooth or teeth[3] (see Chapter 14).

Dental Implants

The use of endosteal fixtures to retain implant-supported fixed or removable prostheses has gained wide acceptance over the past decades and has become part of the armamentarium of every practitioner.[4,5] Advances in implant designs and surface treatment have transformed the field of implant dentistry. It is now possible to provide cosmetically acceptable restorations using improved surgical techniques such as computer-assisted planning and judicious selection of appropriate fixtures, restorative components, and materials that can restore natural looking interdental papillae and soft tissue emergence profiles[6] (Fig. 18-1). For a more detailed discussion of hardware and surgical procedures (see Chapters 16 and 17).

Bone Grafting

Minor bone grafts or bone substitutes can be used to augment a regional defect in the alveolus, such as a bony undercut or narrow ridge that may have resulted from buccal plate collapse after tooth extraction (Fig. 18-2A,B) or from traumatic bony avulsion.

After a period of consolidation of the graft, an endosteal titanium fixture can be placed. Particulate bone grafts also can be placed within the maxillary sinus (sinus lift), enabling the dentist to restore implant fixtures distal to the maxillary canine/bicuspid area with a fixed splint[7] (Fig. 18-2C,D). Larger grafts can restore the alveolar height of the complete maxillary or mandibular arches.

Bone grafts are classified as either autologous or homologous (allogenic). Autologous grafts are harvested from the patient

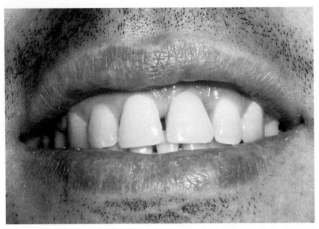

FIGURE 18-1 A single tooth replacement with good gingival contours and tissue emergence profile.

paucity of marrow rich in osteoprogenitor cells and the limited amount of bone available for transplantation.[8]

When the requirement for bone is more significant (e.g., for bilateral sinus augmentations or full-arch onlay grafting), the iliac crest is the preferred site for harvesting the large amounts of corticocancellous bone needed.[9] Up to 100 mL of bone can be harvested from the posterior iliac bone.[10] The tibial plateau is another good source of cancellous bone. Approximately 25 mL of bone can be harvested from this source. Although immediate sequelae, such as pain and gait disturbance, are common, long-term donor site morbidity is very rare. Calvarial bone grafts are mainly cortical in nature and are usually reserved for reconstruction of the midface, nasal, and orbital areas.[11]

Homologous (allogenic) bone is obtained from human cadavers. The material is processed by human tissue banks to remove the antigenic and potentially infectious material (e.g., hepatitis, human immunodeficiency virus) and sterilized with ethylene oxide or gamma irradiation before packaging. Banked bone is available in lamellar strips, corticocancellous blocks, bone chips, and bone powder. The powder form also is available in a demineralized preparation. This process is believed to increase the concentration of an osseoinductive protein, bone morphogenic protein (BMP), which is present in the nonmineralized moiety.[12] In general allogenic bone grafts are used to restore small

and transplanted into the defect. Donor sites can be close to the surgical site (chin and maxillary tuberosity) or distant (calvarium, iliac crest, or tibial plateau). The advantage of the intraoral source, aside from proximity, is the minimal morbidity associated with this type of graft harvest. Disadvantages include the

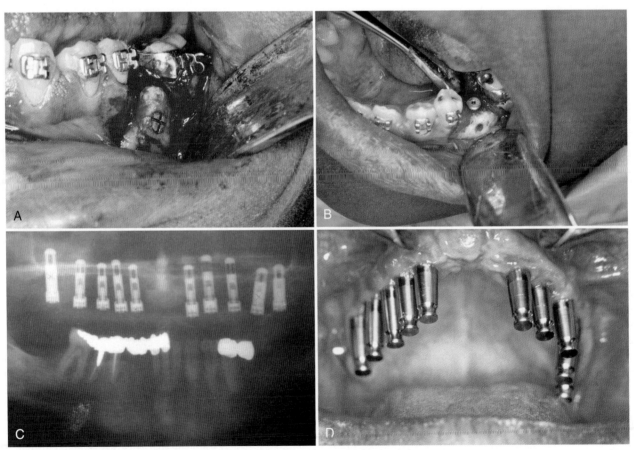

FIGURE 18-2 A, Chin graft to the lateral alveolar ridge to augment the width and allow for implant placement. **B,** The patient after integration of the graft showing removal of the buccal fixation screw and implant placement. **C,** Panoramic radiograph showing implant fixtures placed after bilateral maxillary sinus lifts with cancellous bone graft from the iliac crest. **D,** Frontal view of the patient after bilateral maxillary sinus grafts and implant placement. (Courtesy Alex Montazem, DMD, Smithtown, NY.)

defects or act as graft "expanders" when mixed with autologous bone harvested intraorally. The advantage of this type of grafting material is that it is readily available, thus eliminating the need for a surgical donor site and the associated morbidity. The major disadvantage is the risk of transmission of a disease for which no screening is currently available.

Bone graft substitutes, such as resorbable or nonresorbable hydroxyapatite and other bioactive ceramic granules, can also fill minor contour defects and, to a lesser degree, expand autologous grafts.[13] Although these materials are considered osteophilic, they are not completely replaced by native bone and are not considered to produce good implantation sites. Again the advantage of this material is that it is readily available. The disadvantage is that the material is replaced by bone only on its surface. It generally is not recommended for sinus lifts or significant ridge augmentation in preparation for implant placement.

Alveolar Distraction

Alveolar bone distraction recently was introduced as an alternative to bone grafting for ridge augmentation of traumatically induced, limited alveolar defects (Fig. 18-3A,B). Specially designed expansion devices are used to slowly "distract" an osteotomized bone segment to restore the lost alveolar height.

Once this has been achieved and the regenerate has been allowed to consolidate, the distractors are replaced with endosteal fixtures that will osseointegrate and support a cosmetic prosthesis, which will then have a more acceptable crown to root (fixture) ratio.[14] A similar technique is now used to distract the anterior mandibular alveolus in patients with atrophic mandibles to create a more favorable site for the placement of endosteal fixtures.[15] Changes in the design of alveolar distractors will allow these devices to play a dual role of distractor/implant fixture without having to change the hardware at the completion of the distraction (Fig. 18-3C,D).

Skeletofacial Procedures

Malalignment of the basal and tooth-supporting alveolar structures often result in facial "disharmony" and suboptimal function and appearance. Maxillary and mandibular osteotomies commonly are used to correct dento-skeletofacial deformities.

The first step in the evaluation of a patient suspected of having a dento-skeletofacial deformity is a thorough clinical exam,

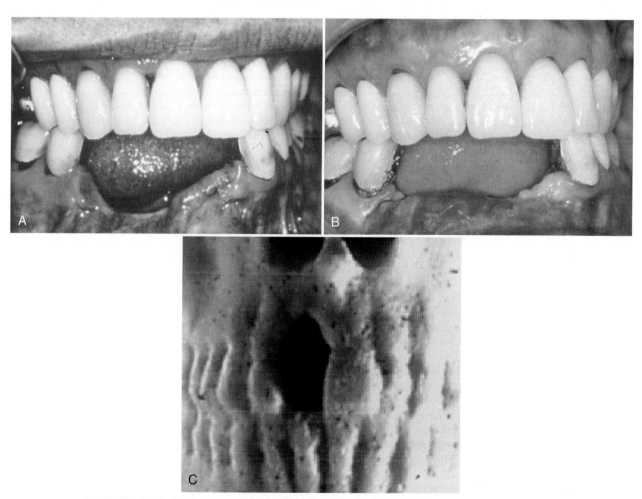

FIGURE 18-3 A, A traumatically induced regional defect of the mandibular alveolus. **B,** Same patient with alveolar height restored using the osteodynamic alveolar distractor. (ACE Surgical Supply Co., Inc.) **C,** Three-dimensional cast of a localized alveolar defect in the region of tooth #8.

Continued

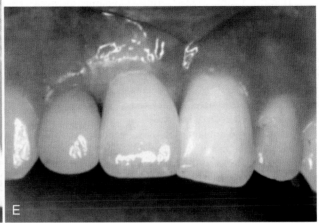

FIGURE 18-3, cont'd D, Intraoperative view of the defect after placement of Implantdistraktor. (SIS Systems.) **E,** Definitive restoration after completion of distraction and consolidation. (Courtesy H. Rainer.) (A,B, Courtesy G. Urbani. D,E, Courtesy H. Rainer.)

good quality extraoral and intraoral photographs, and cephalometric radiographs or a cone beam CT scan (CBCT). The lateral cephalogram can be traced manually or digitized and processed with treatment planning software and a personal computer (Fig. 18-4A,B).

For more complex asymmetries, the Digital Imaging and Communications in Medicine (DICOM) files obtained from the cone beam CT can be used to generate a virtual three-dimensional (3D) cast of the patient's facial skeleton and overlying soft tissue mask (Fig. 18-4C,D). For a more realistic soft tissue representation, a 3D photograph obtained using a special camera can be overlaid on the soft tissue mask (Fig. 18-4E) and used to demonstrate the facial changes that can be expected from the movement of the osteotomized bony segments.

The virtual skeletal cast can then be digitized using conventional cephalometric landmarks and analyzed to generate a problem list. Unlike 2D cephalometry, a number of these landmarks will be subdivided into right and left components to take into account the asymmetry between the two points (ramus height or occlusal cant) (Fig. 18-4F). Once the diagnosis and problem list are generated, a treatment plan is formulated and the proposed osteotomies can then be simulated by creating virtual objects using the planning software's cutting tools. The segments are then repositioned three dimensionally to the desired position (Fig. 18-5A-C). The soft tissue predicted change is calculated using a complicated mathematical algorithm that allows the surgeon and patient to visualize the projected soft tissue changes (Fig. 18-5D).

Computer-assisted design and computer-assisted manufacturing (CAD/CAM)-generated intermediate and definitive splints can also be designed and produced using the planning software and used intraoperatively to help execute the planned procedures (see Fig. 18-1).

Computer-assisted treatment planning is not only a very effective, time-saving technique for the planning of complex maxillomandibular osteotomies, but is also a powerful communication tool. It allows the surgeon to discuss the proposed procedure with the patient using interactive, visual images. It also allows a demonstration of the virtual outcome of the proposed surgery.

However, clinical results that do not reproduce the predicted simulation may lead to patient dissatisfaction, with possible legal implications (for a complete discussion, see Chapter 27). Therefore all discussions with the patient should include a disclaimer that the simulation must be viewed as an aid in visualizing the treatment result, which in no way implies a guarantee of the surgical result.

Most dento-skeletofacial deformities are three dimensional. They must be evaluated and treated in the anteroposterior, vertical, and transverse planes.

Anteroposterior deformities include prognathism, or excessive growth of the jaw in a horizontal plane. Mandibular prognathism (Fig. 18-6A), such as is seen in a Class III skeletal malocclusion, is more common than maxillary or bimaxillary (maxilla and mandible) prognathism.

Retrognathism is an underdevelopment of the jaw in the horizontal plane (Fig. 18-6B). Both the maxilla and mandible may be affected (Fig. 18-6C).

Retrogenia is an underprojected chin, and progenia is an overprojected chin. These deformities are surgically corrected with maxillary or mandibular osteotomies. See the sections on Maxillary Surgery and Mandibular Surgery.

Vertical deformities include vertical maxillary excess (VME), an excessive downward growth of the maxilla that results in a "gummy" smile and a "long face" with a narrow alar base and retrodisplaced mandible, caused by the counterclockwise mandibular rotation prompted by this excessive growth (Fig. 18-7A).

The lip to tooth ratio at rest is excessive (>4 mm) and is accompanied by lip incompetence (the patient is unable to passively oppose the lips without straining the perioral musculature [orbicularis oris and mentalis]). When growth excess is limited to the posterior maxilla, an anterior open occlusion (apertognathia) will result, further accentuating the relative mandibular retrognathia (Fig. 18-7B,C).

Isolated (apertognathia) with occlusal contacts limited to the second molars, anterior maxillary hyperplasia is rare and usually is caused by an overgrowth of the anterior alveolus in a patient with a severe mandibular retrognathia (Class II, division I). Mandibular vertical excess usually is limited to the anterior

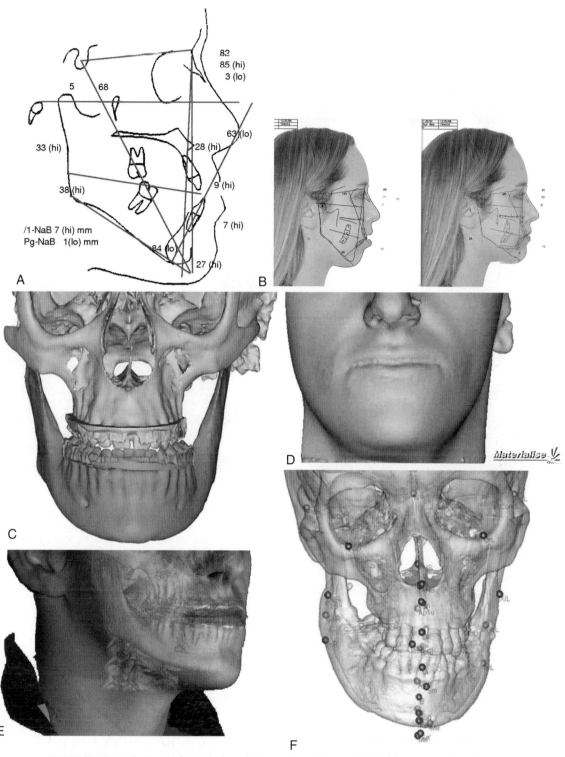

FIGURE 18-4 A, A computerized cephalometric tracing and digital image overlay of patient with dento-skeletetal deformity. **B,** A computerized prediction image. **C,** Virtual cast of the patient's facial skeleton generated from the CBCT data. **D,** Soft tissue mask generated from CBCT data. **E,** 3D photo "fused" to the patient's soft tissue DICOM data from the CBCT. **F,** 3D Cephalometric landmarks. (**B** From Hupp JR, Tucker MR, Ellis E: *Contemporary oral and maxillofacial surgery*, ed 6, St Louis, 2014, Mosby.)

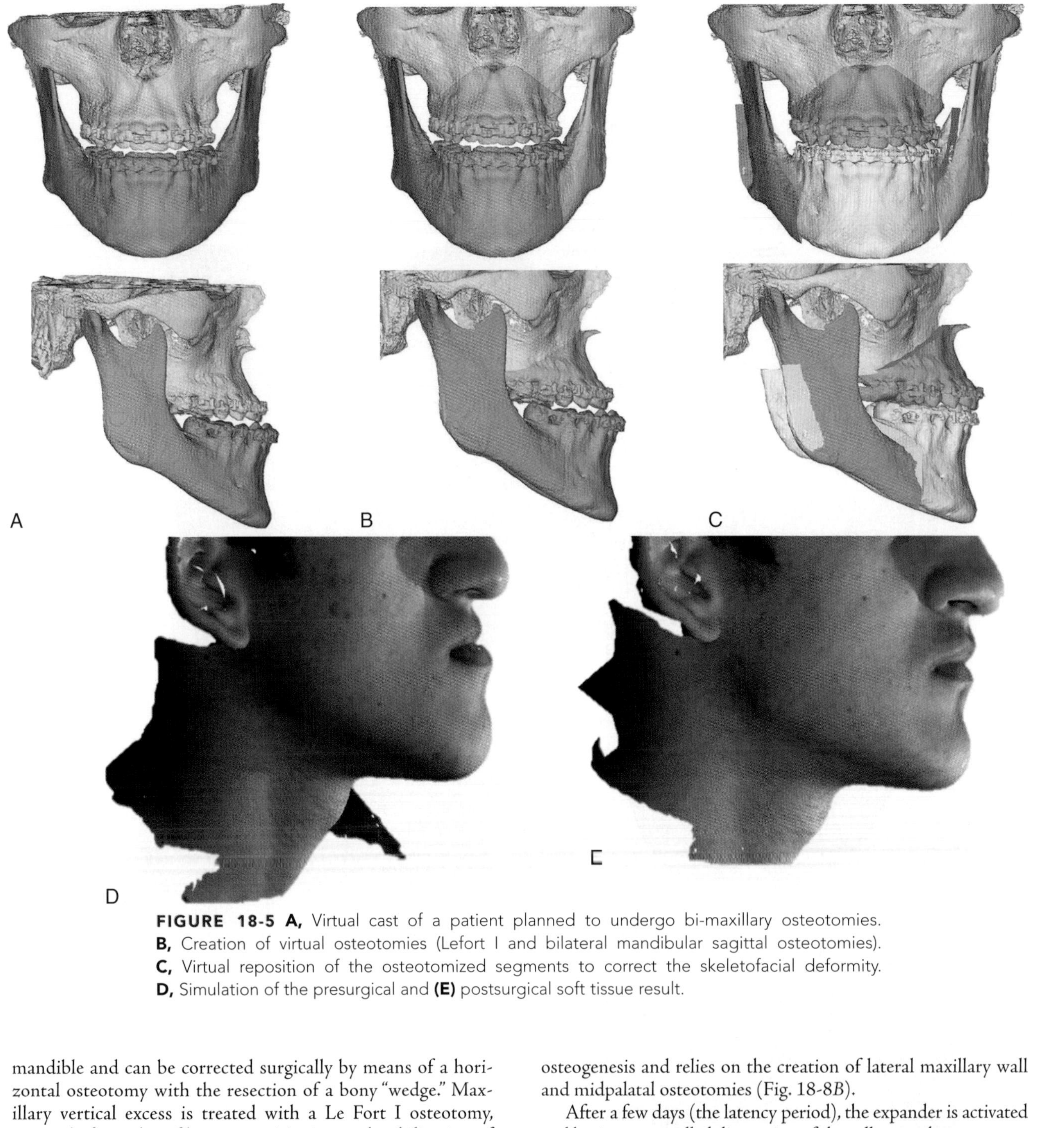

FIGURE 18-5 A, Virtual cast of a patient planned to undergo bi-maxillary osteotomies.
B, Creation of virtual osteotomies (Lefort I and bilateral mandibular sagittal osteotomies).
C, Virtual reposition of the osteotomized segments to correct the skeletofacial deformity.
D, Simulation of the presurgical and **(E)** postsurgical soft tissue result.

mandible and can be corrected surgically by means of a horizontal osteotomy with the resection of a bony "wedge." Maxillary vertical excess is treated with a Le Fort I osteotomy, removal of a wedge of bone, repositioning, and stabilization of the maxilla (Fig. 18-8A).

Maxillary vertical deficiency, another vertical deformity, is also corrected with a Le Fort I osteotomy. In this situation, the placement of a wedge of bone (grafting) between the upper facial skeleton and the repositioned maxilla becomes necessary before stabilization (fixation) (see Fig. 18-8A). Transverse deformities usually result in a constricted arch form with overcrowding and tooth malalignment. The treatment goal is the expansion of the alveolar segment to correct the tooth/arch-length discrepancy. In the maxilla, a palatal expansion device can be used. Surgically assisted palatal expansion is based on the concept of distraction

osteogenesis and relies on the creation of lateral maxillary wall and midpalatal osteotomies (Fig. 18-8B).

After a few days (the latency period), the expander is activated and begins a controlled distraction of the callous at the osteotomy site. Once the expansion is complete, the regenerate bone is allowed to consolidate before the teeth can be moved into the neoalveolar segment. In patients in whom the transverse deformity is not caused by a tooth/alveolar discrepancy and the orthodontist is unable to align the dental units over the alveolar segment, a multiple-segment Le Fort I osteotomy with interpositional bone grafting can be done to correct the transverse problem. A similar procedure can be performed to expand the mandibular arch with an internal bone/tooth-borne distraction device and a midline mandibular osteotomy to expand the mandibular alveolus.[16] This device has now been approved for clinical use.

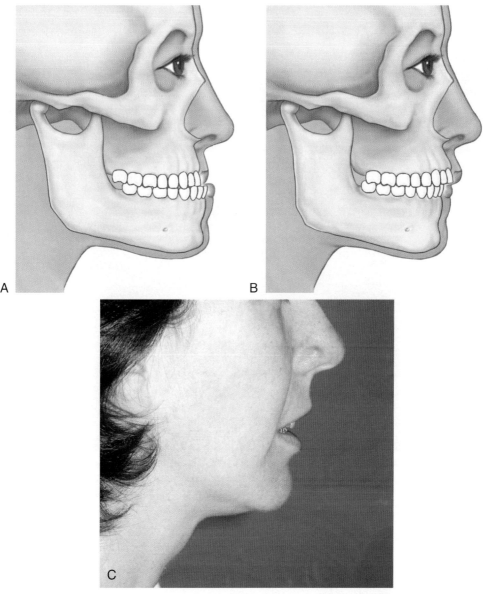

FIGURE 18-6 A, Mandibular prognathism. **B,** Mandibular retrognathism. **C,** Vertical maxillary excess combined with mild mandibular retrognathia. A,B, Adapted from Morcos SS, Patel PK. The vocabulary of dentofacial deformities. Clin Plast Surg 34(3):589-99, 2007.

The deformities described in the preceding can involve both the maxilla and the mandible and may also be associated with facial asymmetries such as laterognathia or facial canting in patients of hemifacial atrophy or hypertrophy (congenital) or condylar hyperplasia (acquired). Temporomandibular joint pain and dysfunction and the resulting masticatory and swallowing difficulties often are associated with dento-skeletofacial deformities and should alert the practitioner to investigate for a malocclusion or jaw malposition. Recognition of the underlying condition and appropriate referral can increase the patient's confidence in the practitioner's ability to provide comprehensive care.

Once the workup has been completed and a problem list has been formulated, the surgeon selects the surgical procedures designed to correct the deformity and discusses the risks and benefits of each procedure with the patient. If the patient agrees with the proposed treatment, the general practitioner and orthodontist optimize the patient's dentition in preparation for the surgical procedure. Dental and periodontal diseases must be either eradicated or controlled before the surgery. The goal of preoperative orthodontics is to level and align the dental units over the alveolus and coordinate the opposing dental arches. The fixed orthodontic appliances will also be used for maxillomandibular fixation at the time of surgery.

SURGICAL PROCEDURES

Mandibular Surgery

Most mandibular deformities are treated by surgery in the ramus or anterior mandible. The two most common ramal osteotomies are the sagittal (bilateral sagittal split ramus osteotomy, or

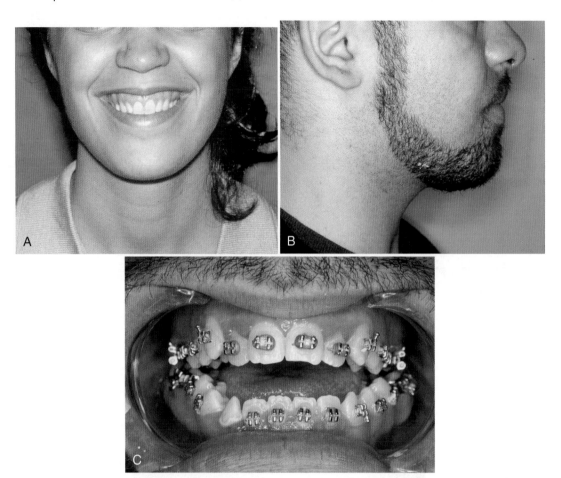

FIGURE 18-7 A, Full face view of a patient with vertical maxillary excess. Note "gummy" smile and narrow alar base. **B,** Lateral view of a patient with apertognathia (the result of posterior maxillary excess) and relative retrognathia. **C,** Frontal view of the patient in part B showing significant open occlusion (apertognathia) with occlusal contacts limited to the second molars.

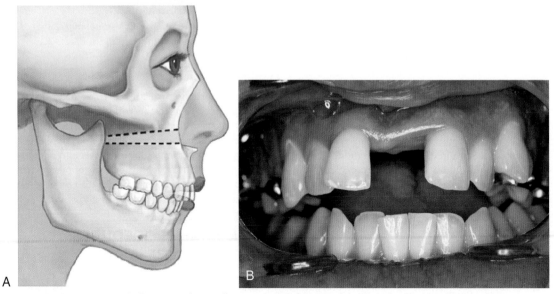

FIGURE 18-8 A, Patient with maxillary vertical deficiency showing a Le Fort I osteotomy at a level immediately below the floor of the nose and placement of a wedge of bone. **B,** A large diastema between the maxillary incisors after surgically assisted maxillary palatal expansion. A, Adapted from Patel PK, Novia MV. The Surgical Tools: The LeFort I, Bilateral Sagittal Split Osteotomy of the Mandible, and the Osseous Genioplasty. Clin Plast Surg 34(3):447-475, 2007.

BSSO), first described by Obwegesser in 1946, and the vertical or subcondylar osteotomy (bilateral vertical ramus osteotomy, or BVRO),[17] originally described as an extraoral procedure, performed from a retromandibular, transfacial approach. Refinement of the instrumentation and introduction of a right-angled oscillating saw now allow an intraoral approach, which eliminates the facial scar. The ramus is sectioned vertically from the sigmoid notch to a point near the angle of the mandible. The cut remains posterior to the lingula to avoid injury to the inferior alveolar neurovascular bundle (Fig. 18-9A).

When performed bilaterally, this procedure allows repositioning of the distal (tooth-bearing) segment while preserving the condyle-fossa relationship of the proximal segments. Once the mandible has been placed in the desired position, as guided by the occlusion or an acrylic surgical guide, maxillomandibular fixation is applied and maintained during the healing phase (4-6 weeks) to allow for bony union at the osteotomy sites (Fig. 18-9B,C).

This procedure is relatively quick, and the risk of injury to the inferior alveolar nerve is minimal. However, the procedure lacks versatility (it can only be used to correct prognathism) and has the obligatory postoperative period of maxillomandibular fixation.[18] During that time the patient's diet is limited to fluids, and oral hygiene care is quite difficult.

The sagittal osteotomy, on the other hand, is perhaps one of the most versatile facial osteotomies. It allows for the correction of prognathism, retrognathia, mandibular rotations, and small anterior open occlusion. This osteotomy is performed entirely intraorally. After dissection of the medial aspect of the ramus in a subperiosteal plane, the neurovascular bundle is identified as it enters the lingula; it is retracted and protected. A horizontal lingual corticotomy is then performed using a bur, a reciprocating saw, or a piezoelectric saw, just above the level of the lingula. The use of the piezoelectric saw reduces the risk of injury to the inferior alveolar nerve. The bone cut extends from the level of the lingula to the anterior border of the ramus, where it is carried vertically just medial to the external oblique ridge. It finally is connected to a vertical corticotomy of the buccal cortex of the mandible in the posterior body usually between the first and second molars (Fig. 18-10A).[18]

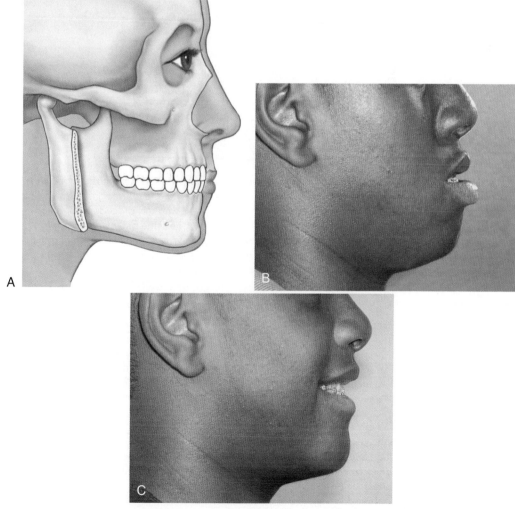

FIGURE 18-9 A, A vertical oblique osteotomy of the ramus allows the mandible to be pushed posteriorly while maintaining the condyles correctly in the articular fossae. **B,** Preoperative lateral view of a patient with mandibular prognathism. **C,** The same patient after undergoing bilateral vertical ramus osteotomies to correct the prognathism. (B,C, Courtesy Alex Montazem, DMD, Smithtown, NY.)

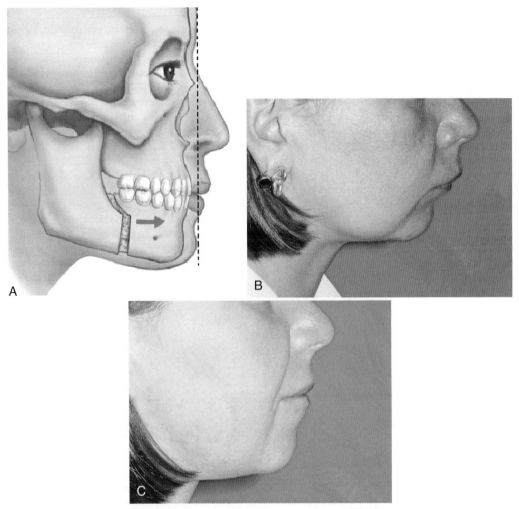

FIGURE 18-10 A, A sagittal split ramus osteotomy allows the surgeon the latitude of moving the mandible forward to correct a retrognathism or posteriorly to correct a prognathism while maintaining condylar position. Often a genioplasty is performed with this procedure. **B,** Preoperative lateral view of a patient with mandibular retrognathia. **C,** The same patient after undergoing mandibular advancement with bilateral sagittal osteotomies to correct the retrognathia. (A, Adapted from Reyneke JP. Basic Guidelines for the Surgical Correction of Mandibular Anteroposterior Deficiency and Excess. Clin Plast Surg 34(3):501-517, 2007.)

Osteotomes

Often a genioplasty is performed with this procedure and chisels are used to complete the osteotomy and separate the proximal ramal segment from the distal tooth-bearing segment. The sagittal nature of this osteotomy allows for a large surface area of bone-to-bone contact when the distal segment is moved to a more anterior position. The proximal segment remains in its preoperative position, maintaining the original condyle-fossa relationship (Fig. 18-10B,C).

During the healing phase the osteotomized segments can be maintained in their new position by maxillomandibular fixation, but this osteotomy design allows for the placement of fixation plates or screws (or both) that can maintain the position during the healing phase, obviating the need for maxillomandibular fixation (Fig. 18-11A).

The internal fixation hardware is made of commercially pure titanium and is generally well tolerated by the body, rarely requiring retrieval once the osteotomies have healed. Occasionally loose hardware may cause a local reaction, necessitating removal. Some patients request that the hardware

be removed after healing. Their concern about the long-term retention of a "foreign body" may not be evidence based, but it is nevertheless understandable. The use of bioresorbable screws and plates made of polylactide stereoisomers obviate concerns about retained internal fixation hardware because these devices are completely resorbed by hydrolysis and, to some extent, phagocytosis (Fig. 18-11B).

Bioresorbable

Plates and screws are used more commonly in craniofacial surgery in very young patients requiring craniosynostosis release or cranial vault reshaping.

The anterior horizontal mandibular osteotomy (AHMO), or genioplasty, can be used to advance, retrude, shorten, or lengthen the patient's chin (Fig. 18-12A,B).

The osteotomy is performed through an intraoral anterior degloving incision. It is important to avoid stripping the muscular attachments to the inferior border to prevent postoperative chin ptosis and the development of the "witch's chin" deformity.

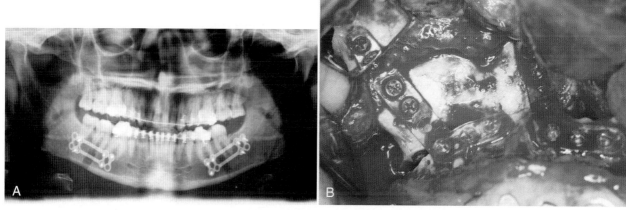

FIGURE 18-11 A, Radiograph showing titanium internal fixation hardware for the sagittal osteotomy. **B,** Intraoperative view of polylactide stereoisomer internal fixation hardware for a Le Fort I osteotomy.

The mental foramina are identified bilaterally, and a bicortical osteotomy is performed below the apices of the incisors, ensuring adequate room for the placement of the fixation plates and extending below the mental foramina as the cut is carried laterally.[18] The distal segment, with its blood supply derived from the lingual attachment of the geniohyoid and genioglossus muscles, is freed from the superior segment and can be repositioned anteriorly, posteriorly, or superiorly after the resection of a wedge from the proximal segment, and inferiorly with the placement of an interpositional graft. The segment is retained with a preformed titanium plate and screws (Fig. 18-12C).

After closure of the mucosal incision, an external elastic dressing is placed to aid in the resuspension of the soft tissue and obliteration of the "dead space" to prevent hematoma formation that

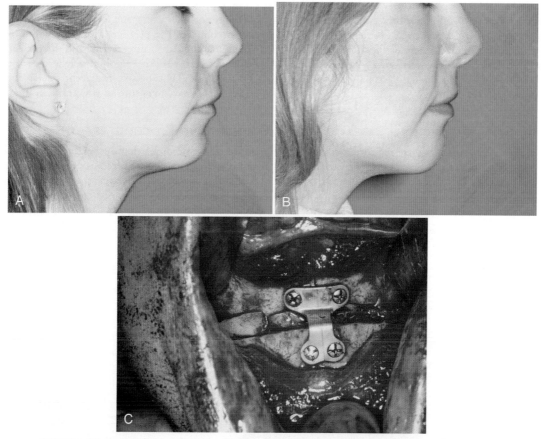

FIGURE 18-12 A, Lateral view of a patient with retrogenia. **B,** The same patient after advancement genioplasty (anterior horizontal mandibular osteotomy). **C,** Intraoperative view of an anterior mandibular osteotomy showing the use of interpositional bone grafting and prebent titanium fixation plate and screws. (Courtesy Alex Montazem, DMD, Smithtown, NY.)

could result in a postoperative infection. As an alternative, an alloplast can be used to augment the patient's chin. See the section on Facial Implants later in this chapter.

Maxillary Surgery

The most common maxillary surgical procedure is the Le Fort I osteotomy. It can be performed as a single piece or the maxilla can be divided into two or more segments to allow for the precise repositioning of each segment. A horizontal osteotomy is performed above the apices of the teeth and through the lateral wall of the maxilla and the lateral nasal walls. The pterygoid plates are then separated from the maxillary tuberosities. Finally the nasal septum and vomer are separated from the maxilla, which is then downfractured.[18] The maxilla can now be repositioned in a more anterior, posterior, superior, or inferior position. Vertical repositioning of the maxilla requires either a resection of a bony wedge for superior positioning or placement of an interpositional bone graft for inferior repositioning (Fig. 18-13).

The osteotomized segments are held in their new position by internal fixation devices made of titanium or a resorbable material[19] as described for the fixation of the sagittal osteotomy. When the maxilla is segmented, an occlusal acrylic splint is wired to the orthodontic appliances and used to unitize and further stabilize the segments during the healing phase. Maxillomandibular fixation is usually not necessary in situations of single jaw, maxillary surgery. Modifications of the standard Le Fort I osteotomy include that in which the lateral osteotomy is carried on to the body of the zygoma before being tapered down in the area of the tuberosity to allow for the advancement of the malar complex. A quadrangular or high Le Fort I osteotomy can be performed where the lateral cut extends superiorly to the infraorbital rim area before tapering anteriorly to the base of the pyriform rim to avoid injury to the nasolacrimal duct and the resulting epiphora (excessive tearing).

Bimaxillary Surgery

The correction of certain dento-skeletofacial deformities requires surgery on both the maxilla and the mandible[18] (Fig. 18-14; see Fig. 18-13B).

Vertical maxillary excess with mandibular retrognathia, maxillary deficiency with mandibular excess, and severe anterior open occlusion secondary to maxillary posterior excess are a few examples of deformities that require two-jaw surgery. The maxilla is osteotomized first and fixed in its definitive position with a prefabricated acrylic intermediate splint based on the "cast surgery" (Fig. 18-13E); the mandibular osteotomies are performed afterward.

CAD/CAM intermediate and definitive splints can be generated from the 3D virtual planning of the surgical procedures. Bimaxillary surgery is more time consuming and may result in additional blood loss. Autologous blood donation before surgery should be encouraged to prevent the need for a homologous (allogenic) transfusion in the rare instance in which the blood loss would require a packed red blood cell transfusion.

Postoperative Care

Most orthognathic surgery, except for genioplasty, is performed as an inpatient hospital procedure with a stay of 1 or 2 days. The patient is discharged when able to tolerate a full fluid or soft diet that provides the proper caloric and nutritional requirements and when the patient can perform activities of daily living. A moderate amount of swelling in the immediate postoperative period is typical; this usually dissipates within the first week. The patient then is followed initially on a weekly basis, then less frequently, until healing is complete (8-10 weeks). During that time the patient's diet is slowly advanced until a regular diet has been established, usually by the end of the seventh week. Physical therapy is instituted at 6 weeks to help the patient regain a good interincisal opening and function and allow the orthodontist to complete the postoperative orthodontic phase. When maxillomandibular fixation is used and the patient is restricted to a liquid diet, a 10- to 15-pound weight loss early in the postoperative phase is expected. Sufficient caloric and nutritional intake is necessary to ensure an uneventful healing phase.

Adjunctive Procedures

Soft tissue procedures that optimize the results of prosthetic and bony reconstructive procedures often are indicated. These procedures can be performed at the time of the orthognathic

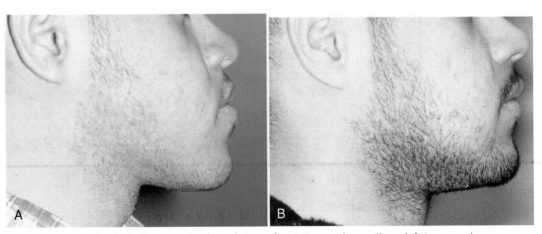

FIGURE 18-13 A, Preoperative lateral view of a patient with maxillary deficiency and mandibular excess. **B,** Postoperative view of the patient after bimaxillary osteotomy.

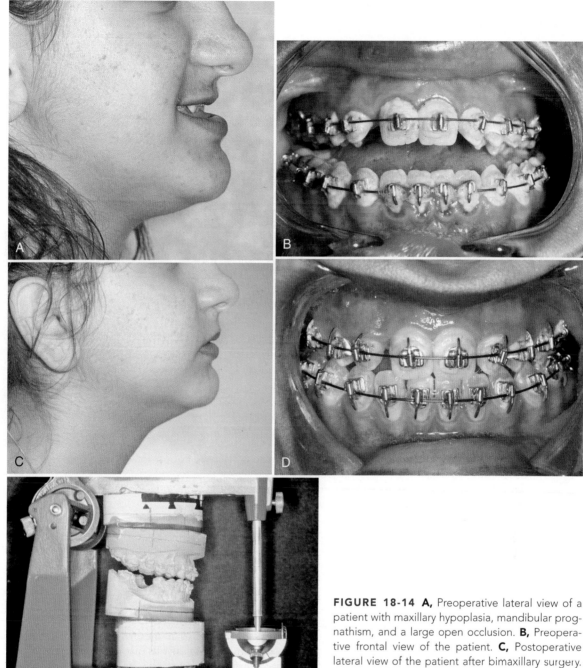

FIGURE 18-14 A, Preoperative lateral view of a patient with maxillary hypoplasia, mandibular prognathism, and a large open occlusion. **B,** Preoperative frontal view of the patient. **C,** Postoperative lateral view of the patient after bimaxillary surgery. **D,** Postoperative frontal view of the patient. **E,** "Cast surgery" for planning bimaxillary surgery.

procedure, or they can be delayed until healing is complete and the surgeon is able to evaluate the effect of the skeletal surgery on the soft tissue drape.

PERIORAL PROCEDURES

Lip Augmentation and Reduction

Reduction of prominent lips is a relatively uncomplicated surgical procedure. A transverse, elliptic segment of mucosa and submucosal tissue is excised down to muscle. The anterior limit of the ellipse is placed behind the free border of the lip so that the scar remains inconspicuous. The excision must be uniform and symmetric to avoid any irregularities in the free border of the lip (Fig. 18-15).

Thin lips usually can be augmented either with submucosal injection of bovine-derived collagen or by placement of a strip of acellular dermis (AlloDerm, LifeCell Corporation) through small incisions and submucosal tunneling.[20,21] The implant is fixed to the overlying tissue with a 5-0 plain gut suture. The results achieved from collagen injection can be expected to last 6 to 8 months; the AlloDerm implant seems to

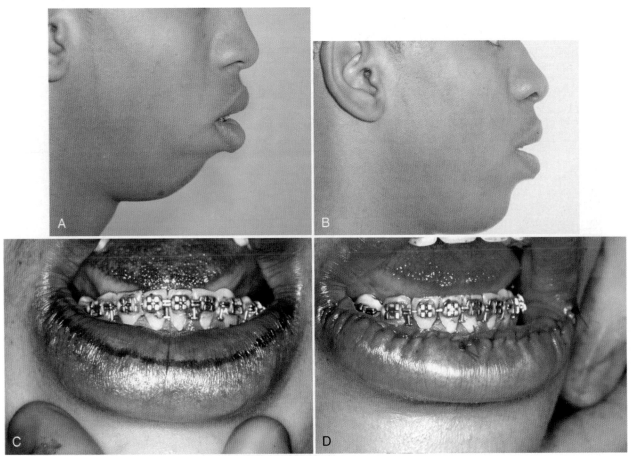

FIGURE 18-15 A, Lateral view of a patient with macrocheilia. **B,** Postoperative view of the patient after reduction cheiloplasty. **C,** Outline of mucosal resection for reduction cheiloplasty for the patient. **D,** The patient after excision of the mucosal wedge and primary closure. Note that the incision line does not extend beyond the free border of the lip.

offer a more "permanent" result, with more than 50% of the volume in place after 1 year (Fig. 18-16).

Skin Resurfacing

The lips and perioral structures are common sites for age-related vertical wrinkles (rhytids) caused by loss of collagen. This condition is accentuated in "sun-damaged" skin. Any treatment that reduces or eliminates these age-related perioral changes effectively enhances the result of the cosmetic dental reconstructive procedure (Fig. 18-17).

Chemical peels, dermabrasion,[22,23] and laser-assisted skin resurfacing[24] are effective techniques for improving perioral wrinkling and hence esthetics. Facelift procedures alone cannot address this problem.[25]

Chemical peeling using agents such as phenol (50%-80%) or trichloroacetic acid (TCA) are applied to the affected skin and covered with an occlusive dressing for 48 hours. The chemical penetrates the epidermis and upper reticular layer of the dermis, resulting in a process very similar to a second-degree burn. The area begins healing in 48 hours, resulting in a consistent formation of a new, stratified collagen layer. This regenerative process is complete in 7 to 10 days, with some erythema lasting up to 6 weeks. A major problem with chemical peeling agents, especially phenol, is that skin bleaching results in sharp lines of demarcation between the treated and untreated areas. Because patients with a dark complexion are more prone to developing hyperpigmentation and discoloration, the patient's skin texture and tone must be carefully assessed before this type of treatment can be offered. Patients must be warned about the possibility of permanent color changes.

Dermabrasion is an inexpensive, safe, and effective method of treating perioral rhytids that does not require highly specialized instrumentation. The epidermis and superficial dermis are abraded in a controlled fashion using abrasive wheels on an electric handpiece. As with the chemical peel, the partial thickness wound heals by the induction of collagen synthesis, upper dermal thickening and contracture, leading to a smoother skin surface.

The success of all skin resurfacing procedures depends on the severity of the rhytids and the pigmentation of the skin. Hypopigmentation and hypertrophic scarring are some of the more common complications associated with skin resurfacing. Proper technique and meticulous postoperative wound care tend to minimize these complications.

Carbon dioxide (CO_2) laser resurfacing has become an increasingly popular method of perioral skin resurfacing.[26] The epidermal cells absorb the laser beam and are heated, leading to vaporization. At the level of the dermis, the conducted heat produces a band of coagulation necrosis. The depth of the injury

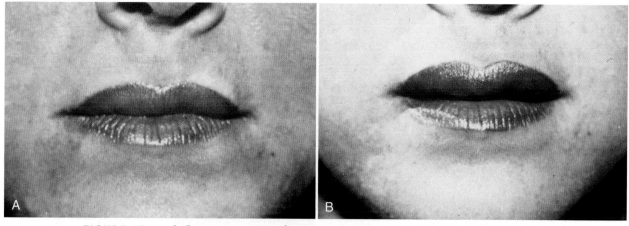

FIGURE 18-16 A, Preoperative view of a patient desiring lip augmentation. **B,** Postoperative view of the patient after lip augmentation with Alloderm strips. (Courtesy B. Schwartz and the Lifecell Corp.)

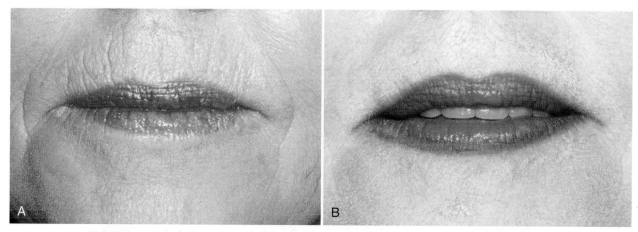

FIGURE 18-17 A, Preoperative view of a patient with deep perioral rhytids. **B,** Postoperative view of the patient after carbon dioxide perioral skin resurfacing. (Courtesy S. Guttenberg.)

depends on the intensity of the beam and the duration of contact with the tissue. The introduction of high-energy, pulsed scanning CO_2 lasers with an ultra-short dwell time has enabled the surgeon to treat superficial wrinkles with minimal thermal injury to the underlying structures. The mechanism of healing is similar to that with other forms of skin resurfacing, with the added advantage that in patients with darker complexions, the CO_2 laser is more sparing of the melanocytes, resulting in a lower incidence of hyperpigmentation or hypopigmentation.

Submental Liposuction

The patient population undergoing orthognathic procedures is becoming older and to a certain degree more discriminating. A desire for not only functional but also cosmetic facial improvement is often expressed. Esthetic neck surgery is by far the most common adjunctive procedure with orthognathic surgery (Fig. 18-18).

Basically, two approaches can be used for cosmetic improvement of the neck line. The first approach involves excision of submental fat with plication of the platysma muscles in the midline when indicated. This lipectomy can be performed with a suction-assisted method. A cannula hooked to a suction machine is introduced into the submental area through a small incision in the skin and used to "extract" the submental fat.[27-29]

As an alternative, a transfacial or transoral "open lipectomy" can be done. When performed in conjunction with a genioplasty, the surgeon can gain direct access to the submental fat through the intraoral mucosal incision by carrying the dissection underneath the anterior border of the mandible.[30] A submental transfacial approach is recommended when the surgeon is planning simultaneous resection of the redundant submental skin. Submental lipectomy can also be performed in conjunction with a rhytidoplasty–neck lift procedure.

After the neck recontouring procedure, the patient must wear a compressive dressing for several days to prevent formation of a seroma or hematoma and ensure good tissue adaptation.

Rhytidectomy (Facelift)

Mandibular skeletal surgery may have either a positive or a negative impact on cervicofacial contours. When the planned mandibular procedure will accentuate a submental fullness, or jowls, elevation of the skin and restoration of the cervicomental contours and a well-defined jaw line will not only correct deformity but also enhance the result of the skeletal surgery (Fig. 18-19).

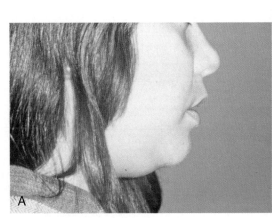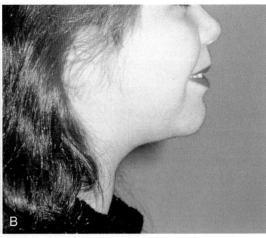

FIGURE 18-18 A, Preoperative view of patient requiring a jaw and neck lift procedure. **B,** Postoperative view.

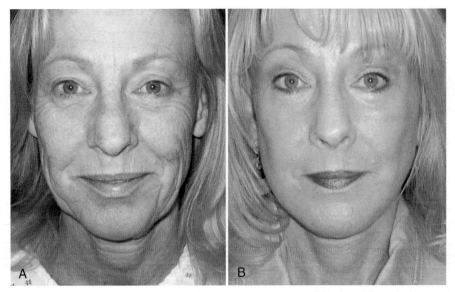

FIGURE 18-19 A, Preoperative view of a patient requiring a "full" face-lift, including endoscopic brow and forehead lifts. **B,** Postoperative view. (From Niamtu J: Cosmetic facial Surgery, St. Louis, Mosby, 2011.)

A skin incision is made in a natural skin crease immediately in front of the ear (preauricular).[31,32] The incision is carried behind the earlobe and into the hair-bearing area behind the ear (postauricular). After the skin flap is undermined, elevation of the preauricular component of the flap allows for the reduction of cheeks and jowls; elevation of the postauricular skin reduces the "sagging" in the neck and submental areas. After the excess skin has been excised, the skin is reapproximated using very fine nylon sutures. A pressure dressing is applied to aid in the adaptation of the tissues and to prevent hematoma formation. (For other indications for the facelift procedure, see Chapter 25.)

Rhinoplasty

Orthognathic surgery of the maxilla often results in minor changes in the width of the alar base or the tip position.[33] For example, impaction of the maxilla in a patient with a wide alar base results in an even greater deformity after surgery unless simultaneous nasal surgery, such as an alar base cinch suture, excision of skin from the alar base (weir), or tip procedures are performed (Fig. 18-20).[34]

Indications for simultaneous maxillary and nasal surgery include functional septal deviations, necessary correction of nasal tip and alar base position, and significant abnormality of the dorsum.[35] Correction of subtle tip position and refined cartilage trimming should be performed as a secondary procedure once the healing from the skeletal surgery is complete. On the other hand, no contraindications exist for performing rhinoplastic procedures when performing isolated mandibular surgery with the use of internal fixation. Furthermore the patient should be informed of the possible need for revision procedures to refine the surgical result.

Cosmetic surgery of the periorbital area, including blepharoplasty, brow lift, and forehead lift, also has a significant impact

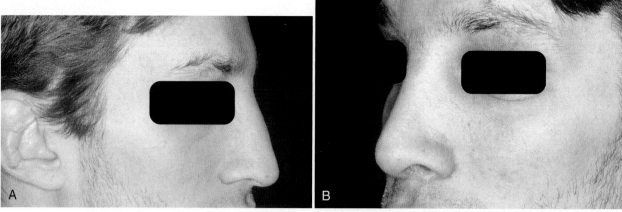

FIGURE 18-20 A, Preoperative view of a patient with a nasal ptotic (drooping) tip and dorsal hump. **B,** Postoperative view of the patient after septorhinoplasty. (Courtesy P. Costantino.)

on the result of skeletal jaw surgery. (These procedures are discussed in Chapter 25.)

Facial Implants

Alloplastic implants have been used to augment the facial skeleton and, more specifically, the malar, mandibular angle, and chin regions (Fig. 18-21 *A,B*).

These solid implants are available in a variety of preshaped sizes. They also are available in blocks that can be carved by the surgeon during surgery in patients of unilateral or asymmetric augmentations. In complex craniofacial situations, the data obtained from a computed tomography (CT) study of the patient can be used to fabricate a custom, patient-specific implant using computer-assisted design (CAD) and a milling machine (Fig. 18-21C).

Alloplastic facial implants are made of Silastic, Proplast, or Medipore. Silastic or silicone implants are made of medical-grade polymer of dimethylpolysiloxane, a noncarcinogenic, biocompatible material that induces very little inflammatory response when implanted subcutaneously. The principal drawback of solid Silastic is the rigidity and memory and nonporous state of this material. The lack of porosity prevents tissue ingrowth into the implant that would fix it to the surrounding tissue. Over time this can lead to migration of the implant, causing resorption of the underlying bone or extrusion of the implant (Fig. 18-21D).[36]

Proplast is a highly porous material made of a Teflon fluorocarbon (PTFE) fiber base and, in the situation of Proplast III, hydroxyapatite.[37,38] Earlier versions of the material contained first carbon (Proplast I) and then aluminum oxide (Proplast II). The advantage of hydroxyapatite is not only its osteoconductive properties and better tissue integration, but also that it eliminates the skin discoloration seen with the earlier material.

Medipore implants, manufactured from a high-density porous polyethylene, are the most popular and widely used implants in facial augmentation. The large pore size (>100 μm) and pore volume ($\approx50\%$) allows good tissue ingrowth. The firm nature of the material allows the surgeon to carve the implant with a scalpel during surgery without collapsing the pore structure. As with all the mentioned materials, the major complication in alloplastic facial augmentation is infection. Inevitable

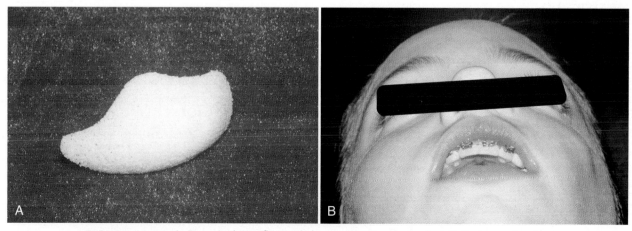

FIGURE 18-21 A, Porex (polytetrafluoroethylene, or PTFE) malar implant. **B,** Postoperative view of a patient with a left Porex malar implant for reconstruction of a defect caused by cancer surgery.
Continued

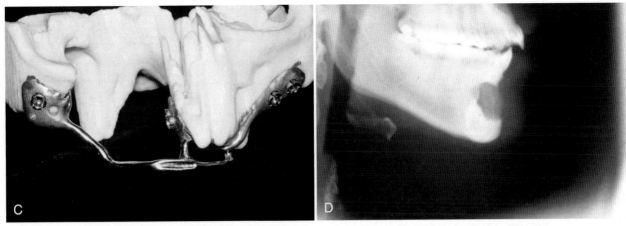

FIGURE 18-21, cont'd C, Stereolithographic cast used in the construction of a custom maxillary subperiosteal implant. **D,** Cephalogram/orthopantomogram showing resorption of the lateral mandibular cortex adjacent to a Silastic chin implant.

contamination of the implants when placed via the intraoral route can lead to colonization of the implant and ultimately an infection that requires its removal. Impregnation of the implant in an antibiotic solution and postoperative administration of an oral antibiotic decrease the chance of infection.

Finally, small soft tissue irregularities can be corrected by subcutaneous placement of sheets of AlloDerm or the injection of dermal fillers (see Chapter 24). This material, made of homologous (allogenic) acellular dermis, is described earlier in the section on Lip Augmentation.

CONCLUSION

Oral and maxillofacial surgery can result in profound facial esthetic improvements. It is vital that the practitioner consider this when assessing and treatment planning dental patient for ssthetic treatment.

REFERENCES

1. Commission on Dental Accreditation: *American Dental Association accreditation standards for advanced specialty education programs in oral and maxillofacial surgery,* Chicago, 1999, American Dental Association.
2. Russo J: Periodontal laser surgery, *Dent Today* 16:80, 1997.
3. Johnson RH: Lengthening clinical crowns, *J Am Dent Assoc* 121:473, 1990.
4. Eckert SE, Wollan PC: Retrospective review of 1170. endosseous implants placed in partially edentulous jaws, *J Prosthet Dent* 79:415, 1998.
5. Keller EE: Reconstruction of the severely atrophic edentulous mandible with endosseous implants: a 10-year longitudinal study, *J Oral Maxillofac Surg* 53:305, 1995.
6. Viassis JM, Lyzak WA, Senn C: Anterior aesthetic considerations for the placement and restoration of nonsubmerged endosseous implants, *Pract Periodontics Aesthet Dent* 5:19, 1993.
7. Tong DC, Rioux K, Drangsholt M, et al: A review of survival rates for implants placed in grafted maxillary sinuses using meta-analysis, *Int J Oral Maxillofac Implants* 13:175, 1998.
8. Montezam A et al: *Chin grafting in maxillofacial surgery: a quantitative analysis.* Presented at the Fourteenth International Meeting of Oral and Maxillofacial Surgeons, Washington, DC, April 28, 1999.
9. Catone GA, Reimer BL, McNeir D, et al: Tibial autogenous cancellous bone as an alternative donor site in maxillofacial surgery: a preliminary report, *J Oral Maxillofac Surg* 50:1258, 1992.
10. Marx RE, Morales MJ: Morbidity from bone harvest in major jaw reconstruction: a randomized trial comparing the lateral anterior and posterior approaches to the ilium, *J Oral Maxillofac Surg* 46:196, 1988.
11. Harsha BC, Tuvey TA, Powers SK: Use of autogenous cranial bone grafts in maxillofacial surgery: a preliminary report, *J Oral Maxillofac Surg* 44:11, 1986.
12. Niederwanger M, Urist MR: Demineralized bone matrix supplied by bone banks for a carrier of recombinant human bone morphogenetic protein (rhBMP-2): a substitute for autogenic bone grafts, *J Oral Implantol* 22:210, 1996.
13. Tomasetti BJ, Munk LK, Zallen R: Treatment of trauma-related bony defects with nonresorbable hydroxyapatite, *Implant Soc* 5:10, 1995.
14. Chin M, Toth BA: Distraction osteogenesis in maxillofacial surgery using internal devices: review of five cases, *J Oral Maxilllofac Surg* 54:45, 1996.
15. Unpublished data or data on file.
16. Guerrero AC, Bell WH, Contasti GI: Mandibular widening by intraoral distraction osteogenesis, *Br J Oral Maxillofac Surg* 35:383, 1997.
17. Steinhauser EW: Historical development of orthognathic surgery, *J Craniomaxillofac Surg* 24:195, 1996.
18. Bell WH, Proffit WR, White RP: *Surgical correction of dentofacial deformities,* Philadelphia, 1980, Saunders.
19. Edwards RC, Kiely KD: Resorbable fixation of Le Fort I osteotomies, *J Craniofac Surg* 9:210, 1998.
20. Tobin HA, Karas ND: Lip augmentation using an AlloDerm graft, *J Oral Maxillofac Surg* 56:722, 1998.
21. Burres S: Lip augmentation, *Dermatol Surg* 24:160, 1998.
22. Branham GH, Thomas JR: Rejuvenation of the skin surface: chemical peel and dermabrasion, *Facial Plast Surg* 12:125, 1996.
23. Baker TM: Dermabrasion as a complement to aesthetic surgery, *Clin Plast Surg* 25:81, 1998.
24. Koch RJ: Laser skin resurfacing: what credentials are necessary? *Dermatol Surg* 24:595, 1998.
25. Fulton JE: Simultaneous face lifting and skin resurfacing, *Plast Reconstr Surg* 102:2480, 1998.
26. Weinstein C: Carbon dioxide laser resurfacing: long-term follow-up in 2123. patients, *Clin Plast Surg* 25:109, 1998.
27. Knize DM: Limited incision submental lipectomy and platysmaplasty, *Plast Reconstr Surg* 101:473, 1998.
28. Kovacs B, Smith RG, Cesteleyn L, et al: Submental liposuction in maxillofacial surgery, *Acta Stomatol Belg* 89:37, 1992.
29. Pinto EB, Rocha RP, Queiroz W Jr, et al: Submental skin: morphohistological study of interest to liposuction, *Aesthetic Plast Surg* 21:388, 1997.
30. Wider TM, Spiro SA, Wolfe SA: Simultaneous osseous genioplasty and meloplasty, *Plast Reconstr Surg* 99:1273, 1997.
31. Becker FF: The preauricular portion of the rhytidectomy incision, *Arch Otolaryngol Head Neck Surg* 120:166, 1994.
32. Stratigos AJ, Arndt KA, Dover JS: Advances in cutaneous aesthetic surgery, *JAMA* 280:1397, 1998.
33. Schendel SA, Carlotti AE Jr: Nasal considerations in orthognathic surgery, *Am J Orthod Dentofacial Orthop* 100:197, 1991.
34. Loh FC: A new technique of alar base cinching following maxillary osteotomy, *Int J Adult Orthodon Orthognath Surg* 8:33, 1993.
35. Cottrell DA, Wolford LM: Factors influencing combined orthognathic and rhinoplastic surgery, *Int J Adult Orthodon Orthognath Surg* 8:265, 1993.
36. Matarasso A, Elias AC, Elias RL: Labial incompetence: a marker for progressive bone resorption in silastic chin augmentation, *Plast Reconstr Surg* 98:1007, 1996.
37. Kent JN, Westfall RL, Carlton DM: Chin and zygomaticomaxillary augmentation with Proplast: long-term follow-up, *J Oral Maxillofac Surg* 39:912, 1981.
38. Robiony M. Costa F, Dimitri V, et al: Simultaneous malaroplasty with porous polyethylene implants and orthognathic surgery for correction of malar deficiency, *J Oral Maxillofac Surg* 56:734, 1998.

19

Esthetics and Pediatric Dentistry

Ali B. Attaie and Nabil Ouatik

The need for pediatric esthetic dental treatment is primarily because of caries and trauma and, less frequently, congenital disorders and disturbances in dental mineralization and development. Although some simple treatments can result in significant esthetic improvement, other treatments are at times very demanding, requiring staged multi-disciplinary approaches that may well extend from early childhood to adolescence.

GENERAL CONSIDERATIONS

The primary maxillary incisors are the most susceptible teeth to sequelae from caries and trauma. Premature loss of primary teeth often delays eruption of the permanent teeth if less than one half the root structure is formed on the primary tooth. Treatment of advanced caries in the maxillary primary incisors with stainless steel crowns or extractions without replacement for a period of 3 to 6 years until the eruption of the permanent dentition may be acceptable options for some dental professionals; however, this will be initially unacceptable to many parents. In addition to the elimination of dental pathology, the practitioner's aim in esthetic dentistry is to follow the concept of biomimesis—the restoration of form, function, and esthetics of affected body structures to their natural state. Parents often seem desirous of preserving esthetically damaged incisors as opposed to the replacement of extracted or missing teeth with an esthetic prosthesis.[1] Hence esthetic restorations of primary teeth are now emerging as an expected standard of care by many parents. Physical appearance and superficial attributes also influence a child's self-esteem and interaction with others. A child who is perceived as attractive is also considered more socially adept than a child who is perceived as unattractive. This assumption is made by both acquainted and unacquainted preschool children[2,3] Children as young as 3 years old are able to distinguish between attractive and unattractive peers and children between the ages of 3½ and 6 display similar judgments to that of adults, preferring attractive children for friends.[4]

CLINICAL CONSIDERATIONS

From a functional perspective, prematurely lost or congenitally missing teeth may affect speech patterns during early childhood, further affecting a child's self-esteem, although most children eventually learn to adapt such speech difficulties.[5] The production of tongue tip sounds (t, d, s, sh, and ch) and labial sounds (f and v), which are most often affected by early loss of maxillary incisors, may be aided by fixed or removable restoration of the missing maxillary anterior teeth.[6,7]

Anatomically, the primary dentition usually has interdental spacing in the anterior portion, which is exaggerated in the primate space mesial and distal to the canine in the maxillary and mandibular arches, respectively. In the posterior teeth, primary molars are larger mesiodistally than the premolars that replace them. This results in provision of additional spacing in the dental arch, which is also known as the leeway space. Leeway space is commonly lost in the posterior dentition through either premature loss of primary teeth or advanced interproximal caries that result in a mesial drifting of the permanent first and the primary second molars. This loss of arch length may result in both anterior crowding and impaction of the permanent premolars. The space in both the anterior and posterior portion of the dental arch may be preserved in children through appropriate treatment planning with space maintenance therapy to ensure that sufficient space is available for alignment of their permanent teeth.[8-10]

The primary teeth are lighter in shade than the permanent teeth and the crowns are smaller but more bulbous than the corresponding permanent teeth. The bell-shaped primary molar crowns have a definite constriction in the cervical region and flat broad interproximal contacts. The sharp constriction at the neck of the primary teeth is associated with occlusally directed enamel rods that necessitate special care when creating the gingival floor during interproximal cavity preparations. Both enamel and dentin are thinner and the pulp is proportionately larger than that of the permanent teeth. The pulpal outline of the primary teeth follows the dentoenamel junction more closely than that of the permanent teeth and the pulpal horns are longer and more pointed than the cusps would indicate.[10]

DIAGNOSIS

Primary maxillary incisors are the teeth in most frequent need of restorative care due to early childhood caries, trauma, and enamel defects or staining. Early childhood caries is an infectious disease, and pathogenic *Streptococcus mutans* are most often the causative agent; diet also plays a critical role in the acquisition and clinical expression of this infection. Primary oral colonization by pathogenic *S. mutans* colonies coupled with caries-promoting behaviors such as frequent bottle feeding at night, and extended and repetitive use of a no-spill training cup with sugary liquids results in accumulation of these organisms and leads to rapid demineralization of tooth structure.[11] Caries Management by Risk Assessment (CAMBRA) is a method of assessing caries risk with age appropriate standards as an aid in making dental treatment and restoration recommendations based on individual caries risk. Using CAMBRA or a similar caries risk management approach should be part of every pediatric dental treatment plan.[12]

Young children are quite prone to accidents, which most often occur between 10 to 24 months of age.[13,14] Children in this age group are gaining mobility and independence while lacking coordination and motor skills. Traumatic injuries may result in concussion, subluxation, intrusion, avulsion, or fractures involving enamel, dentin, and pulpal tissue (Table 19-1). The International Association of Dental Traumatology provides a comprehensive online resource with specific guidelines on diagnosis, treatment planning, and prognosis of traumatic dentoalveolar injuries.[15] Lesions involving enamel defects and staining are perhaps the most difficult to appropriately diagnose and treat, which may explain why no uniform and widely accepted set of guidelines exists for their treatment. These lesions are briefly addressed in the Treatment of Enamel Lesions and Management of Color Changes and Discolorations section in this chapter.

Table 19-1 Classification of Traumatic Injuries

Class	Problem
I	Fracture of the crown into the enamel with little or no dentin involvement
II	Fracture of the crown into the dentin, but not involving the dental pulp
III	Fracture of the crown exposing the dental pulp
IV	Displacement of the tooth without fracture of the crown or root
V	Root fracture without loss of crown structure
VI	Traumatized tooth (vital or nonvital) that may or may not discolor

TREATMENT PLANNING

The primary goals of any treatment of a child's dentition are to atraumatically: (1) restore normal form and function with minimal side effects and disturbance to the overall growth of the dentofacial complex, (2) avoid pain and infection, and (3) protect the forming permanent tooth. Attainment of all of these goals is often not possible, for these goals may not always complement each other. In younger and generally precooperative children under 3 years of age, an attempt to esthetically restore an anterior tooth may prove futile unless the child is moderately sedated or under general anesthesia. If deep sedation or general anesthesia is required, the associated risk, albeit statistically insignificant, may not be accepted by parents and many practitioners for sole purposes of an aesthetic result. For children with initial early childhood caries, medical management of caries may be most appropriate until a child can cooperate for an ideal restorative procedure.[16] In cases of trauma, although it is possible to replant an avulsed primary tooth and restore normal function,[17] this is contraindicated because the long-term success for this procedure is not reliable, the pressure of manipulation may damage the permanent tooth bud, and the child's cooperation is often insufficient to allow the procedure to be properly performed.[18] At about 3 years of age, most children are able to cooperate for dental procedures when approached by clinicians trained and experienced in behavior guidance of the pediatric patient. The appropriate use of the "tell, show, do" technique and effective use of other common nonpharmacological pediatric behavior management approaches are often sufficient in gaining the necessary cooperation for completion of most restorative procedures.[19] In the case of more apprehensive and anxious children in need of more extensive restorative care, the proper use of nitrous oxide and oxygen has been shown to be quite effective in reducing the need for general anesthesia in many cases.[20]

The following checklist is a helpful reminder for documentation, review and obtaining of appropriate records in pediatric and adolescent dental treatment planning and dental treatment:

1. Chief complaint, dental, medical and social history
2. Consent for the exam and proposed treatment including risks, benefits, alternatives, and confirmation of legal guardianship of the adult accompanying the child
3. Diagnostic radiographs of teeth being treated; periapical area in the anterior teeth and at the minimum, the furcation area in the posterior teeth are necessary for any pulp related treatment
4. Determine and document the maximum amount of local anesthesia and plan your behavior management approach (non-pharmacological, nitrous oxide and oxygen, pharmacological sedation, general anesthesia)
5. Always review the clinical and radiographic data and determine, document and communicate the working diagnosis and prognosis for the proposed treatment plan to the legal guardian and adolescent patients prior to initiating treatment; for young children it is imperative that you explain what will happen in age appropriate language as part of the "tell, show, do" approach.
6. Document the amount of local anesthesia and sedative used as well as the child's behavior during the procedure

TYPES OF TREATMENTS

Tooth Fractures

A small enamel fracture of the primary anterior incisors is among the most common esthetic concerns for parents. These lesions are classically of minimal size, rarely extending beyond one millimeter, and are often asymptomatic with no signs or symptoms of pulpal involvement. Conservative treatment of these lesions may range from no treatment to enameloplasty with a polishing disk to smooth any sharp edges and round out the fracture to best complement the tooth anatomy (Fig. 19-1*A,B*). At times it may be necessary to also minimally adjust the enamel of the adjacent unaffected teeth for best esthetic results (Fig. 19-1*C*). Monitoring of the tooth on a more frequent recall schedule to assess pulpal status is advised for cases that are first identified by the provider and are confirmed to be a recent trauma. The treatment of more extensive tooth fractures is discussed later in this chapter.

Treatment of Enamel Lesions and Management of Color Changes and Discolorations

Discolored primary teeth can be yellowish, reddish, brown, grey, green, blue, or black. These discolorations may be due to intrinsic or extrinsic factors. Extrinsic staining can be commonly caused by many agents such as multivitamins, iron supplements, and many food items with high pigment content. Such staining is easily treated by coronal scaling and polishing the teeth with a medium grade prophylaxis paste that removes stubborn stains from tooth enamel in both primary and permanent dentition. In younger pre-cooperative children, such treatment can be achieved by a practitioner experienced in the knee to knee position.[21]

An intrinsically discolored primary incisor most often indicates that the tooth has sustained pulpal injury.[22] Dark discoloration of the primary incisor may be an indication of the release of red blood cells from a ruptured pulpal blood vessel into the dentin. Such discoloration may resolve, persist, or worsen depending on the extent of the pulpal injury. The determination

of the prognoses of these teeth is challenging. Clinical and radiographic evaluation at 4 weeks, 6 to 8 weeks, and 1 year from the time of initial occurrence and diagnosis is advised.[23] An isolated yellow tooth may also be associated with a history of trauma that has resulted in dentinal calcific deposition within the dentin. This calcific degeneration or metamorphosis of the pulp can be confirmed radiographically by the presence of a calcified pulp chamber. Enamel and or dentin dysplasia explain the more generalized irregularities in the surface of the enamel and or underlying dentin causing discoloration in both primary and permanent dentition. These may be caused by a specific etiology such as ingestion of tetracycline during the development of the anterior teeth (generally up to 7 years of age), or they may be multifactorial, ranging from suboptimal or excessive fluoride exposure to other environmental, developmental, and genetic disorders[24-27] Molar-incisor hypomineralization (MIH) is yet another developmental condition resulting in enamel defects in first permanent molars and permanent incisors, with no currently known etiologic mechanism.[28]

Most of the resulting esthetic defects from intrinsic factors and superficial staining resistant to scaling and polishing can be treated with a conservative composite resin veneer technique. Beyond these approaches, bleaching and acid application with mechanical abrasion (microabrasion) and resin infiltration therapy are three other modalities utilized for esthetic treatment of affected anterior teeth (see Chapter 12). These techniques along with a more detailed etiology of the associated lesions are described in Chapter 13. Although bleaching in primary and young permanent teeth may be an option and has been reported in the literature for both selected situations of extrinsic and intrinsic staining, such approaches await long-term studies in children.[29-33] Currently there are no bleaching products in the marketplace that have the ADA's Seal of Acceptance for use in children, and practitioners are encouraged to consider side effects when contemplating dental bleaching for child and adolescent patients.[34,35]

Recently a new remineralizing agent based on Casein Phosphopeptide-Amorphous Calcium Phosphate (CPP-ACP) (MI Paste, GC America Inc.) has been developed. CPP-ACP stabilizes high concentrations of calcium and phosphate ions that bind to pellicle and plaque. When teeth are under acid challenge, this reservoir of ions maintains a supersaturated mineral environment, reduces demineralization, and enhances remineralization of enamel. According to in vitro studies, CPP-ACP supplementation has the potential to be effective in remineralization of the enamel affected by MIH and to result in an aesthetic improvement. This is a therapeutic agent that is particularly promising in the treatment of MIH in conjunction with treatments mentioned thus far and traditional restorative care. The use of CPP-ACP does require a long-term treatment plan that could last months or years, requiring optimal patient cooperation.[36]

Anterior Composite Resin Restorations in Primary Teeth

Dentin/enamel adhesives allow bonding of resin-based composites and compomers to primary and permanent teeth. (See Chapters 3-5 for the treatment of permanent teeth with bonded restorations). Adhesives have been developed with reported dentin bond strengths exceeding that of enamel. In vitro studies have shown that enamel and dentin bond strength is similar for

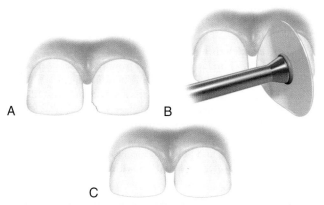

FIGURE 19-1 A, Maxillary left primary central incisor with mesioincisal fracture. **B,** Enameloplasty with a polishing disk. **C,** The maxillary right primary central incisor after enameloplasty. The unaffected maxillary right primary central incisor has also been adjusted to create bilateral symmetry.

primary and permanent teeth. The clinical success of adhesives allows for more conservative preparation when using composite restorative materials. Adhesive systems currently follow either a "total-etch" or a "self-etch" technique. The total etch technique requires 3 steps. It involves use of an etchant to prepare the enamel while opening the dentinal tubules, removing the smear layer, and decalcifying the dentin. After rinsing the etchant, a primer is applied that penetrates the dentin, preparing it for the bonding agent. The enamel can be dried before placing the primer, but the dentin should remain moist. A bonding agent then is applied to the primed dentin. A simplified adhesive system that combines the primer and the adhesive is available. Because the adhesive systems require multiple steps, errors in any step can affect clinical success. Attention to proper technique for the specific adhesive system is critical to success.

Bisphenol A (BPA) is widely used in the manufacturing of many consumer plastic products and can become part of dental sealants and composites in three ways: as a direct ingredient, as a by-product of other ingredients in dental sealants and composites that may have degraded (e.g., bisphenol A glycidyl methacrylate [bis-GMA] and bisphenol A dimethacrylate [bis-DMA]), and as a trace material left over from the manufacturing of other ingredients used in dental sealants and composites. The most significant window of potential exposure to BPA is immediately following the application of resin-based dental sealants and composites. Based on current evidence, the US Food and Drug Administration and the American Dental Association (ADA) do not believe there is a basis for health concerns relative to BPA exposure from any dental material and have concluded that any low-level of BPA exposure that may result from dental sealants and/or composites poses no known health threat.

Measures can be taken to reduce potential BPA exposure from dental materials. A precautionary application technique recommended is removal of residual monomer by rubbing the monomer layer with pumice on a cotton roll or having the patient gargle for 30 seconds and spit immediately after application of the dental sealant or composite. Because rinsing and spitting can be challenging for many children, thorough rinsing with an air-water syringe may be a suitable substitute. As with all dental operative procedures, use of a rubber dam to control the operative field would further limit potential exposures.[37,38]

Isolation Technique

Composite resin is extremely technique sensitive and appropriate isolation technique must be used.[39] Rubber dam isolation has been the traditionally used technique for ideal isolation. The use of ligature ties with dental floss to retract the gingival tissue has been shown to improve rubber dam effectiveness.[40] Gingivectomy with electrosurgery is a less commonly used alternative. Isolite Systems (Fig. 19-2) is a fiber optic and evacuation device with age appropriate sized disposable mouthpieces that is easily administered with no need for anesthesia of the clamped tooth as is the case for rubber dam isolation. This device is well tolerated by most children and serves as bite block and cheek retractor and isolates the maxillary and mandibular arches well beyond the midline of the side of the mouth in which it is placed. It also provides continual evacuation of

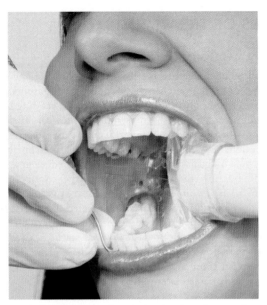

FIGURE 19-2 Isolite device in place intraorally.

fluid and salivary flow, protection of adjacent soft tissues, and assistance in opening the mouth.

Composite Resin Veneer

Armamentarium

- Standard dental setup, basic composite resin restorative tray with nonstick composite resin placement instrument (e.g., Cosmedent, Inc.), high- and low-speed dental handpieces
- Acid-etch gel (see Chapter 3)
- Bonding agent of choice (see Chapter 3)
- Composite resin of choice (see Chapter 5)
- Isolation set up with Rubber dam (e.g., Hygenic Flexi Dam Rubber Dam Coltene/Whaledent. Inc) or other dental isolation system (e.g., Isolite Isolite Systems)
- Diamond flame bur—Medium (862) to Coarse (6862) (Peter Brasseler Series, Brasseler USA)
- Mylar clear strips and Cure-Through Wedge Wands (Garrison Dental Solutions)
- White Store Flame Finishing Bur & CompoSite Polishing Kit (Shofu Dental Corp.)

Clinical Technique
1. Isolate the teeth using a rubber dam or Isolite.
2. Remove a 0.5-mm layer of enamel from the facial portion of the teeth, etch, rinse, dry, and apply bonding agent.
3. Apply a clear Mylar matrix to the teeth being treated and secure with a finger or a palatally placed wedge.
4. Apply a layer of composite resin (microfilled) and a buildup to cover the discolored tooth.
5. Light cure, finish, and polish to ideal esthetics.
6. Thoroughly rinse the restoration with an air-water syringe for 30 seconds.

CLINICAL TIP

The "Pedo Size Isolite" mouthpiece is generally the best size for use with the primary dentition.

For maximal retention, place a 0.5- to 1-mm bevel at the incisal and interproximal areas on the lingual side for extension of the preparation and bonding.

Because of its small size, the S-Max pico high-speed (air-driven) handpiece (NSK Dental) is excellent for pediatric cases and any case in which molar access is difficult.

Composite Resin Restorations (Class III, Class IV, Class V)

The age of a child will not only influence the ability to cooperate with procedures such as rubber dam application and local anesthesia, but the patient's age will also dictate for how long a restoration is required to remain in the mouth. The morphology of the primary anterior dentition is unique in that the actual dimensions of the primary incisors offer little tooth structure for an effective long-term interproximal restoration (Table 19-2). Class III lesions in the primary dentition may best be treated with full coverage crowns, particularly when they are treatment planned in younger children who both are less likely to be fully cooperative and who require a longer period of service from the restoration. Restoration of primary incisors with interproximal caries requires an exacting technique. Prudent evaluation of both the tooth to be restored and the child's ability to cooperate is imperative for successful treatment planning. The lesions should be small compared with the total tooth size. A lock may be placed with generous beveling of the facial or lingual portions of the preparation, rather than in the proximal internal walls where a danger of pulp exposure exists. The small size of the mandibular incisors makes it almost impossible to use this procedure without exposing the pulp, and full coverage composite resin strip crowns (see section on Resin-Bonded Composite Strip Crowns later) are often a more prudent esthetic treatment option. Stripping of interproximal enamel may be used occasionally for minimal caries in the anterior lower primary teeth. Opening of the contact points with a thin diamond bur allows saliva and fluoride to slow and possibly arrest the carious

process, even when the caries involves the dentine. This is often, however, a less esthetic alternative that may be provided until the child is more cooperative and or until pharmacological behavior management options can be used.[41]

Armamentarium
- All materials for composite resin veneers (see section on Composite Resin Veneer earlier in this chapter)
- Round carbide bur 2,4, or 6 depending on lesion size (Brasseler USA)
- #330 high speed carbide bur (Brasseler USA)
- Glass ionomer liner/base material (Vitrebond 3M ESPE)
- Topical and local anesthesia

Clinical Technique
1. Apply topical and local anesthesia.
2. Place a rubber dam or Isolite.
3. Remove interproximal caries with a pear-shaped bur #330 and round bur (Fig. 19-3A). A bevel can be placed if desired.
4. Remove the incisal angle if it is thin and undermined. If both mesial and distal caries exist and/or a mechanical pulp exposure occurs, it is best to prepare the tooth for a full coverage strip crown. In the case of a mechanical pulp exposure, perform a vital pulpotomy. Direct pulp capping in primary teeth is generally contraindicated. (See the section on pulpotomy of vital primary teeth in this chapter.)
5. Place a liner of glass ionomer cement on the dentin. If a pulpotomy or pulpectomy is performed, place glass ionomer cement over the zinc oxide and eugenol, which was placed during the pulpotomy procedure.
6. Acid etch the enamel for 30 to 45 seconds, rinse, and dry.
7. Apply bonding agent (Fig. 19-3B).
8. Depending on the restorative situation
   A. If the dental arch exhibits interdental space between the anterior teeth, place a bonded composite resin (Fig. 19-3C).
   B. If no interdental space exists, place a wedge (if possible) and a mylar strip to aid in shaping the composite resin (Fig. 19-3D).
9. Light cure from the lingual (see Fig. 19-3D) and facial direction. Then, finish and polish the restoration (Fig. 19-3E).
10. Thoroughly rinse the restoration with an air-water syringe for 30 seconds.

Table 19-2 Average Sizes of Primary Teeth

	Maxillary Incisors		Mandibular Incisors	
	Central	Lateral	Central	Lateral
Labial view	1.5 ⊢ 1.5 1.5 ⊢ 1.5 M 2.4 D Enamel: 0.7 (max.)	1.4 ⊢ 1.4 1.4 ⊢ 1.4 M 2.0 D Enamel: 0.6 (max.)	1.7 1.4 ⊢ 1.4 M D Enamel: 0.3 (max.)	1.7 1.4 ⊢ 1.4 M D Enamel: 0.3 (max.)
Proximal view	2.0 ⊢ 2.0 1.5 ⊢ 1.5 Li La	1.9 ⊢ 1.9 1.4 ⊢ 1.4 Li La	1.0 1.4 ⊢ 1.4 La Li	1.0 1.4 ⊢ 1.4 La Li

Modified from McBride WC: *Juvenile dentistry*, ed 4, Philadelphia, 1945, Lea & Febiger.

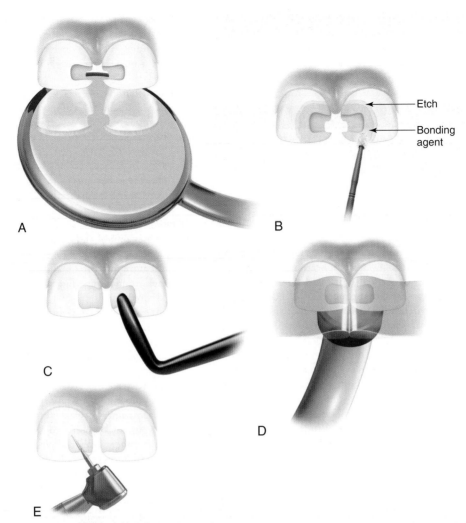

A,

B, Etch
Bonding agent

C,

D,

E,

FIGURE 19-3 A, Class III preparations. A bevel can be placed if desired. **B,** Preparation with bonding agent extended beyond the margins. **C,** Composite resin is placed. **D,** Mylar strips are used to stabilize the resin and the restoration is light cured (wedge not shown). **E,** The resin is finished and will be polished.

INTRACORONAL ESTHETIC RESTORATIONS OF POSTERIOR PRIMARY TEETH

The demand for esthetic restorations in children is no longer limited to the anterior zone. Posterior esthetic options increasingly expected by patients and their parents. A 2009 study in the United States found that esthetics was the main parental concern about dental material.[47,48]

Since the introduction of posterior esthetic options, the restoration of primary teeth with tooth colored materials has been increasing. Studies shows that composite resin is now the most frequently used restorative material for restoration of class I and class II restoration in some regions.[47] The number of esthetic options is now wider than ever. Although amalgam continues to be deemed an acceptable and safe restorative material for children, glass ionomers, resin-modified glass ionomers, and composite resins have allowed for reliable esthetic treatment in the posterior region. Despite the scientific evidence, many areas in the world have experienced a decline in the use of amalgam in children, mostly because of more stringent environmental regulations and

worries about mercury exposure.[42,43] In Scandinavia, Germany, and Japan amalgam is now seldom used in children.

When multisurface carious lesions are present, a full coverage restoration such as a stainless steel crown has been shown to have better long term survival rates[44] and continues to be the most commonly used full coverage restoration for posterior primary teeth. However, these are an unesthetic option and parents often prefer a tooth-colored crown (see full coverage esthetic options in the preceding sections).

Posterior composite resins and compomer restorations (see Chapter 5) allow for almost perfect biomimesis in the posterior primary and permanent dentition for class I, small class II, class V and class VI carious lesions. However, in patients with high caries risk, multi-surface composite resin restorations are not indicated. Typically, a child requiring full-mouth rehabilitation under general anesthesia should receive full coverage restorations[42,45] unless the carious lesions being treated are very small. Multi-surface composite resin restorations can be successful but should be used with caution, especially in patient with higher risk for caries and patients who demonstrate signs of bruxism or erosion. Bonded restorations to primary enamel and dentin present some unique challenges. Because the size of the preparations is smaller than that for permanent teeth, the bonded area is smaller. A lack of cooperation may complicate proper isolation. A conservative slot preparation has been advocated for class II restorations,[46] and this has become the most frequently used design by some pediatric dentists. No studies have shown better survival for a traditional class II preparation (with a dovetail) versus a conservative slot preparation (no dovetail). Clinicians should maintain a good ratio between the occlusal load and the bonded area. A restoration that receives a high occlusal load but has minimal bonded enamel is at a higher risk of dislodging. Because the size of the ideal preparations are rather small, these preparations can be bulk filled.[47] Some clinicians have advocated using a layer of flowable composite resin followed by regular composite resin to achieve better adaptation.

Posterior Glass Ionomer and Resin-Modified Glass Ionomer Restorations

Glass ionomers and resin-modified glass ionomers are unique among dental materials because they release fluoride and physically and chemically bond to tooth structure with no need for etch and prime. However, nonmodified glass ionomers are brittle and have a tendency to wear. They are indicated for class I restorations but not ideal for definitive class II restorations of primary teeth because they have been shown to fail at a higher rate than other restorative materials.[48] Conventional glass ionomers are especially indicated for atraumatic restorative treatment or IRT intermediate restorative treatment wherein partial caries removal is followed by restoration with a fluoride-releasing material in a non-cooperative or pre-cooperative child.

Whereas traditional glass ionomer cements were opaque, newer resin-modified glass ionomers have attained a much better esthetic match to dentin and enamel. In clinical studies, resin-modified glass ionomers have greater longevity than conventional glass ionomers for class II restorations.[49] These restorations do not provide ideal esthetics and are not discussed in this chapter.

Resin-Bonded Composite Strip Crowns

Resin-bonded composite strip crowns are among the most esthetically desirable anterior restorations for primary teeth, but they are also among the most technique sensitive procedures. These are clear celluloid plastic empty crown forms (3M ESPE or Nowak Pediatric Strip Crowns, Nowak Dental Supplies, Inc.) that the clinician sizes appropriately and then fills with resin-bonded composite and bonds to the prepared tooth. With crowding of the anterior teeth, and/or hemorrhage or poor salivary control, it is quite challenging to perform a direct composite resin restoration. These crowns are also more susceptible to loss and fracture when compared with stainless steel crowns. Patients with edge to edge occlusion and moderate to severe bruxism are poor candidates for restorations with these crowns.[50]

There should be sufficient incisal reduction (about 1.5 mm) to avoid incisal fracture. In the preferred design, more reduction on the facial surface is required. On the lingual surface there is often minimal reduction (about 0.5 mm) and a featheredged gingival margin.

Armamentarium
+ All material for composite Class III, IV, and V (see Composite Resin Restorations (Class III, Class IV, Class V earlier in this chapter)
+ Celluloid pediatric strip crown forms (3M ESPE) or (Nowak Pediatric Strip Crowns, Nowak Dental Supplies, Inc)
+ Orthodontic elastomers (Alastiks, 3M Unitek)

Clinical Technique
1. Local anesthesia and rubber dam or Isolite isolation
2. Select the correct celluloid crown form depending on the mesiodistal width of the teeth.

CLINICAL TIP

Always pick the desired crown form size at the beginning of the procedure by holding them against the teeth to be prepared; be sure to account for any additional reduction in cases of crowded incisors and always allow for the minimal 1.5-mm incisal and 0.5-lingual and facial reduction to allow for sufficient composite bulk and to prevent premature fracture.

3. Remove the caries using high-speed #330 carbide and slow-speed round bur.
4. Using a high-speed tapered diamond or tungsten carbide bur, reduce the incisal height by approximately 1.5 to 2 mm and prepare interproximal slices.

CLINICAL TIP

Trim the crown form and, in order to allow for venting of excess composite resin material, make two holes in the incisal corners by piercing with a sharp explorer.

5. Etch the enamel for 15 seconds, and wash and dry.
6. Apply a thin layer of bonding resin and cure for 20 seconds, ensuring all surfaces are covered equally.
7. Fill the crown form with the appropriate shade of packable composite and seat with gentle, even pressure, allowing the excess to exit freely.

CLINICAL TIP

Crown forms may be lined with a thin layer of bond before being filled with composite to reduce the chance of bubble formation and increase ease of removal.

CLINICAL TIP

When treating both or all four central incisors, it is helpful to cure both central filled crown forms simultaneously first to set the guide for the rest of the arch.

CLINICAL TIP

In order to determine the correct shade of composite resin, a tab of composite resin can be placed on the unprepared tooth and light polymerized to account for the shade changes occurring during polymerization.

Although 3M strip crowns are more anatomically esthetic, they do require additional manipulation and fitting time. The Nowak strip crown forms rarely require adjustment and yield excellent esthetic results despite being less anatomically detailed.

Protect the composite filled crown forms from the dental exam light by covering them with an opaque film or cover such as a plastic cup to prevent any premature curing; the dental exam light may be set on lower intensity and pulled away to minimize curing during the positional manipulation of the crowns prior to light curing.

Viewing the pre–light-cured crown forms from the axial view (looking down the incisal edge of the seated crown using a dental exam mirror) is quite helpful in assuring ideal labial positioning of the crown(s) within the arch form.

8. Light cure each aspect (labially, incisally, and palatally) equally.
9. Remove the celluloid crown gently with a spoon excavator, and adjust the form and finish with either composite finishing burs or abrasive discs.
10. Check the occlusion after removing the isolation.
11. Thoroughly rinse the restoration with an air-water syringe for 30 seconds.

For rubber dam isolation, place holes of the smallest size possible for each tooth being treated and an additional tooth each side for retention. Place orthodontic elastomers over each incisor after placement of the rubber dam. This will retract the dam and gingival tissues. Remove the elastomers with the labial floss after completion of the crown. If left in place they can asymptomatically migrate apically along the conically shaped roots, resulting in atraumatic and asymptomatic tooth extraction.[40]

Stainless Steel Crowns with Window Facings

Stainless steel crowns (SSCs) are widely used in pediatric dentistry for restoration of larger multi-surface carious lesions in molars. Although SSCs for anterior teeth exist, they are clearly not esthetic and less commonly used. The facial or buccal aspect of SSCs may be cut out in the anterior or posterior teeth respectively after cementation and a composite facing may be bonded on to improve the esthetics. However, this procedure is time consuming because the composite resin facing cannot be placed until the stainless steel crown cement sets. Also the achieved esthetics are fair to good at best (never excellent) because of the shadowing of the metal color margins surrounding the composite resin resulting in a grayish tinge to the tooth that is further accentuated because of the contrasting white enamel of the approximating or opposing primary teeth. However, SSCs are more retentive and durable on anterior teeth than composite resin strip crowns and

their placement and cementation are not significantly affected by hemorrhage and saliva. Preparing a window on the facial aspect of an SSC and filling it with composite resin material is also an effective method of enhancing the esthetic appearance of a stainless steel crown in posterior teeth especially the first primary molars, which are more visible when a child smiles (Fig. 19-4).

Armamentarium
+ Standard dental set up for composite resin restorations
+ Topical and local anesthesia
+ Isolation set up with Rubber dam (e.g., Hygenic Flexi Dam Rubber Dam Coltene/Whaledent. Inc.) or other dental isolation system (e.g., Isolite Isolite Systems)
+ Pre-crimped stainless steel crowns kit (3M ESPE Crowns, St. Paul, MN or Acero Crowns, Seatle,WA)
+ Carbide burs (#330, #556, #2 and #4 round bur, #169L) (e.g., (SS White Burs, Inc.) or fine tapered diamond bur #6859 (Peter Prasseler Series, Brasseler USA)
+ Heatless stone (Brasseler USA)
+ Polishing rubber point bur (Shofu Dental Corp)
+ Glass ionomer cement (Ketac CEM 3M ESPE or Fuji I, GC America)
+ Composite resin or flowable composite resin (see Chapter 5)
+ SSC crimping pliers (e.g. no. 110 Howe pliers and no. 137 Gordon pliers, Hu-Friedy Inc.)
+ Abrasive discs (Sof-Lex, 3M ESPE)

Clinical Technique
1. Obtain adequate anesthesia
2. Place rubber dam or Isolite isolation.
3. Remove caries using high speed and low speed rotary instrumentation with carbide burs #330, #556, and round burs (Brasseler USA). If pulp therapy is required, it should be completed at this time.
4. Using a carbide 169L bur or a fine tapered diamond bur (#6859 Peter Brasseler Series), reduce the incisal edge by 1.5 mm. Reduce the facial surface by 1 mm and the lingual surface by 0.5 mm. Create a featheredge gingival margin and round all internal line angles.
5. Anterior SSCs are manufactured with a smaller faciolingual dimension and are ovoid shaped. To change the shape and

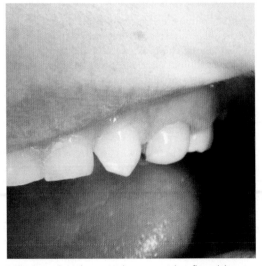

FIGURE 19-4 Stainless steel crown with a flowable composite resin window on the maxillary left primary first molar.

allow the crown to passively fit the tooth, squeeze the crown slightly mesiodistally with a pair of Howe no. 110 pliers in order to increase the faciolingual dimension.

6. The crown should extend 1 mm subgingivally and the fit of the crown should be snug without rocking.

7. Trimming, though rarely necessary, is best done with a heatless stone on a straight slow speed handpiece followed by polishing with a rubber point.

CLINICAL TIP

Contouring and crimping with a crimping plier is often necessary to insure ideal marginal fit, which should be confirmed with an explorer prior to final seating check.

8. Fill the crown with cement and seat it removing the excess cement with wet gauze. The cement must be completely set before preparation and placement of the open-faced veneer.

9. Once the cement is set, cut a labial window in the cemented crown using a # 330 bur and remove the cement until the prepared tooth is reached. Place a continuous circumferential undercut at the level of the margins with a #330 bur.

CLINICAL TIP

When cutting the window on the buccal surface of the stainless steel crown, it is helpful to place a continuous circumferential undercut in order to maximize retention of the composite veneer.

10. Extend the window just short of the incisal edge occlusally, to the height of the gingival crest gingivally, and to the line angles mesially and distally.

11. Place composite resin into the cut window, forcing the material into the undercuts.

CLINICAL TIP

Traditionally, conventional composite resin[51] has been used; however, the use of flowable composite resin provides excellent contour and retention with minimal need to polish or recontour.

CLINICAL TIP

In order to obtain maximal adhesion, it is necessary to remove all cement from the unprepared buccal surface so that bonding can occur on enamel.

12. Finish the restoration with abrasive disks.

CLINICAL TIP

When running the finishing disks from the resin to the metal at the margins, take extra caution not to discolor the resin with metal particles.

Preveneered Stainless Steel Crowns

Preveneered stainless steel crowns are covered on the buccal or facial surface with a tooth-colored coating of polyester/epoxy hybrid composition. They are available with and without resin-covered occlusal surfaces and provide more acceptable and consistent esthetic results compared to SSCs with window facings. However, there are only limited studies regarding their durability.[44] These crowns are relatively inflexible because the resin facing is brittle and tends to fracture when subjected to heavy forces or crimping; therefore only the lingual portion of the crowns can be trimmed or crimped. A significant amount of tooth structure must be removed in order to achieve the required passive fit. Shade choices are limited and the crowns are three to five times more expensive when compared with stainless steel crowns or strip crown forms.

Most manufacturers of anterior preveneered stainless steel crowns also produce posterior preveneered crowns. In general, they are not as successful as anterior crowns[52] because the resin veneer can be subject to high forces that will cause chipping.

Armamentarium
- Preveneered stainless steel crowns (e.g., Nu Smile Crowns (Nu Smile Ltd.), Cheng Crowns (Peter Cheng Orthodontic Laboratory), Kinder Crowns (Mayclin Dental Studio) and Flex Crowns (Space Maintainers Laboratory)
- Standard dental set up for composite resin restorations
- Topical and local anesthesia
- Isolation set up with Rubber dam (e.g., Hygenic Flexi Dam Rubber Dam Coltene/Whaledent. Inc.) or other dental isolation system (e.g., Isolite Isolite Systems)
- Carbide #169L or fine tapered #8650 coarse diamond bur (Brasseler USA)
- Polishing rubber point bur (SuperGreenie, Mini-Point, RA, Shofu Dental Corp.) or finishing disk (Dura-White Stone RE1, Shofu Dental Corp.)
- Glass Ionomer Cement (Ketac CEM 3M ESPE or Fuji I, GC America)
- SSC crimping pliers (e.g., no. 110 Howe pliers and no. 137 Gordon pliers, Hu-Friedy Inc,)

CLINICAL TIP

It is helpful to first size the desired crown for the tooth being treated by placing the incisal edge of the crown against the incisal edge of the tooth. However, when there is any crowding in the dental arch being treated, adjustments must be made to plan for overreduction of the teeth to allow proper fit.

CLINICAL TIP

Too much crimping of the metal substructure may cause fractures in the veneer material.

CLINICAL TIP

The smaller maxillary lateral incisor crowns may be used on mandibular anterior teeth.

CLINICAL TIP

If the veneer fractures, a similar technique to the open-faced crown may be used for repair.

Clinical Technique
1. Anesthetize the area being treated and place isolation.
2. Reduce the tooth a great deal more than would be required for an SSC, particularly if there is crowding in the dental arch. Reduce approximately 2 mm incisally (or occlusally) and reduce the interproximal contacts so that the distance between the contact area of the adjacent tooth and the prepared tooth is 0.75 to 2.0 mm.

3. Create a featheredge margin as far subgingivally as possible. The reduction of the buccal, lingual, mesial and distal may range from 0.75 to 1.5 mm resulting in the tooth being reduced by approximately 25% to 30%. This requires pulp therapy in some cases, (which is addressed later in the chapter which should then be completed at this point.[53] Tapered diamond burs are normally used, proceeding from coarse to fine, when preparing the tooth subgingivally and refining the preparation (Figs. 19-5A,B.

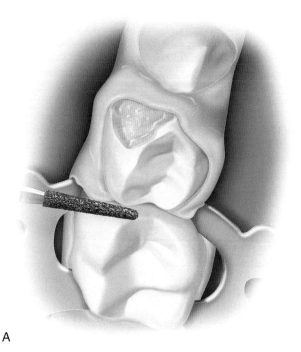

A

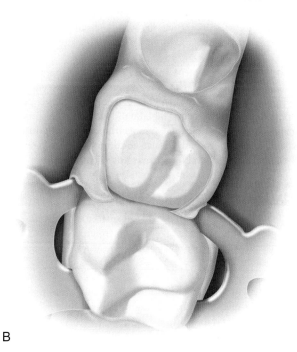

B

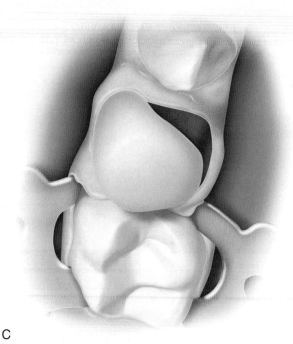

C

FIGURE 19-5 **A,** The maxillary right first primary molar will be prepared for a preveneered stainless steel crown. **B,** Completed preparation for pre-veneered stainless steel crown. **C,** Cemented posterior preveneered stainless steel crown.

4. Try in the crown and refine the preparation for ideal fit as needed.

CLINICAL TIP

Do not force the crown onto the tooth, because this will result in the fracture of the tooth-colored facing. A properly fitted crown should have a passive fit, should not fit past the prepared tooth structure, and should extend 1-mm below the gingival margin.

---

5. Cement the crown with a glass ionomer cement, remove the excess cement, and allow the cement to set (Fig. 19-5C).
6. After cementation and excess cement removal the incisal edges of anterior crowns may be contoured with a finishing point or disk.

CLINICAL TIP

The length of the crown may be altered by trimming the gingival margin with a diamond bur with water spray. For added retention, the lingual aspect of the crown may be crimped slightly with a crimping plier.

Prefabricated Zirconia Crowns

With a continuous decrease in the cost of zirconia manufacturing technology, it is now economically feasible to manufacture prefabricated zirconia crowns (PZCs) for primary teeth. These may be milled directly from a CAD/CAM zirconia block or produced by injection molding. The esthetic outcomes for these crowns are very favorable. PZCs demand a more aggressive preparation when compared with standard SSCs or composite resin strip crowns. Much like other full coverage options, they will be very difficult to adapt in the presence of interproximal space loss due to caries because the crown cannot be crimped. Practitioners and parents should be aware that PZCs are a very recently introduced treatment option that has not been evaluated by long-term clinical studies.

Armamentarium
- Standard dental setup:
  - Topical and local anesthesia
  - Isolation set up with Rubber dam (e.g., Hygenic Flexi Dam Rubber Dam Coltene/Whaledent. Inc.) or other dental isolation system (e.g., Isolite Isolite Systems)
- High-speed handpiece burs (5909 coarse, 5850 coarse, 379 coarse 888 medium (Peter Brasseler Series, Brasseler USA), 369D (Dialite Diamond, Brasseler USA) (Fig. 19-6A)
  - Glass ionomer cement (GC FujiCEM, GC America)
  - Hemostatic agent: (e.g., Hemodent [Premier Dental Products] or ViscoStat Clear [Ultradent Products, Inc.])
  - Cleaning agent for the crown form: 70% ethyl alcohol (American Dental Supply) or Superoxol Dental Bleach (Sultan Healthcare)
- Zirconia crown forms (e.g., all anterior and posterior PZCs are offered by both EZ Pedo [EZ Pedo Inc, Loomis, California, USA], NuSmile [NuSmile Ltd, Houston, Texas, USA], Kinder Krowns [Mayclin Dental Studio, St. Louis Park, Minnesota, USA]; and Zirkiz [Hass Corp, South Korea])

Clinical Technique
1. Administer local anesthesia and place a rubber dam or Isolite.
2. Select crown size (Fig. 19-6B).
3. Reduce the incisal surface of anterior teeth by 1.5 to 2.0 mm and reduce the occlusal surface of posterior teeth by 1 to 1.5 mm (Fig. 19-6C).
4. Reduce the buccal, lingual, mesial, and distal surfaces of both the anterior and posterior teeth by 0.75 to 1.5 mm circumferentially, with posterior teeth and the lingual surfaces of the anterior teeth falling in the higher end of the reduction range (Fig. 19-6D-F).
5. Place an approximately 1- to 2-mm subgingival featheredge margin (Fig. 19-6G).
6. Try-in the crown using no pressure to ensure a passive fit, which will cover the gingival margin.

CLINICAL TIP

PZCs may not be crimped nor trimmed with scissors but it is possible to adjust the gingival margin using a fine diamond in a high-speed handpiece and, to prevent sparks, copious irrigation (Fig. 19-6H).

---

7. Thoroughly clean the interior of the crown with alcohol.
8. Ensure good hemostatic control of the soft tissues using cotton drenched with Hemodent or ViscoStat Clear gel.

CLINICAL TIP

Any manufacturer labeling (which is printed on the surface of the crown) may be scraped off with a spoon or preferably polished off with a coarse prophy paste.

---

9. Cement the crown with a glass ionomer cement using firm stable pressure and do not disturb the seated crown until the cement is set.

CLINICAL TIP

After cementing PZCs, occlusion should be adjusted exclusively on opposing natural teeth.

CLINICAL TIP

It is not always possible to place two zirconia crowns one next to the other in the posterior zone due to existing crowding in the dental arch and/or severe space loss. In some situations it might be preferable to restore the first primary molar with a zirconia crown and the second primary molar with a conventional stainless steel crown (Fig. 19-6I).

SPACE MANAGEMENT AND PEDIATRIC PROSTHODONTICS

Anterior Fixed Space Maintainers

Anterior teeth can be decayed to a point at which infection and resorption of the primary roots precludes endodontic therapy. Trauma and developmental disturbances can also cause early loss of the primary teeth. Anterior fixed space maintainers (also

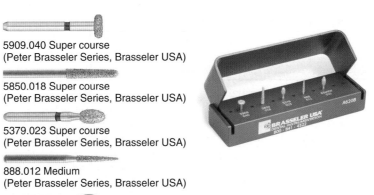

5909.040 Super course
(Peter Brasseler Series, Brasseler USA)

5850.018 Super course
(Peter Brasseler Series, Brasseler USA)

5379.023 Super course
(Peter Brasseler Series, Brasseler USA)

888.012 Medium
(Peter Brasseler Series, Brasseler USA)

8369DF.025 Fine
A   (Dialite Series, Brasseler USA)

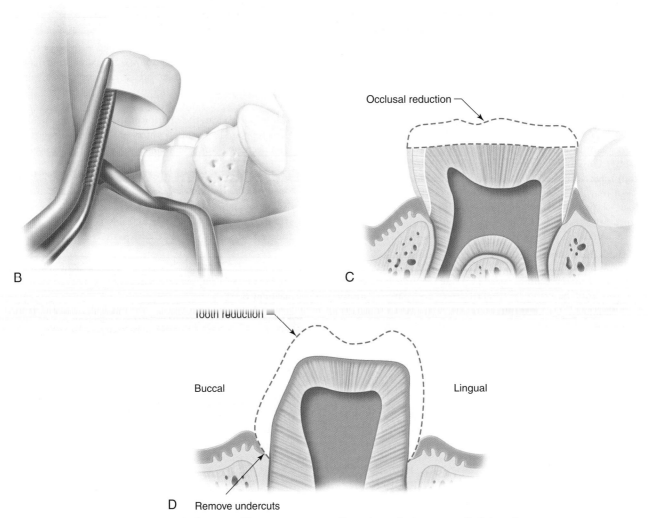

Occlusal reduction

B

C

Tooth reduction

Buccal

Lingual

D   Remove undercuts

FIGURE 19-6 **A,** Suggested bur set to prepare Zirconia pediatric crowns. **B,** Select the proper zirconia crown size. **C,** Occlusal reduction (2.0 mm). **D,** Buccal and lingual reduction (0.75 to 1.5 mm).

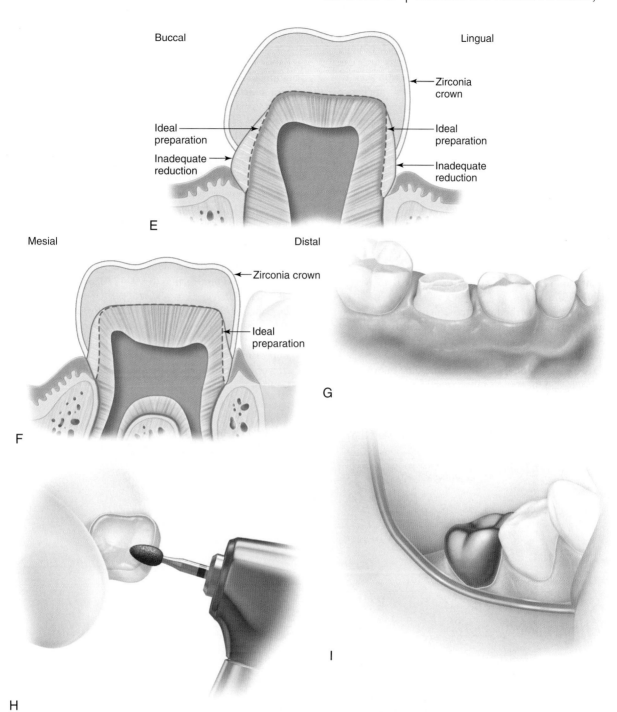

Buccal

Lingual

Zirconia crown

Ideal preparation

Inadequate reduction

Ideal preparation

Inadequate reduction

E

Mesial

Distal

Zirconia crown

Ideal preparation

F

G

H

I

FIGURE 19-6, cont'd E, Insufficient buccal and lingual reduction will result in difficulties when seating the crown. **F,** Mesial and distal reductions must be sufficient to allow for proper seating of the crown. **G,** Mandibular right first primary molar tooth reduction for a zirconia crown, A knife edge finish line should be prepared at the margin. **H,** The margins of the crown can be adjusted using an appropriate diamond bur and a copious amount of water. **I,** Definitive zirconia crown on the mandibular right first primary molar (see clinical tip on page XX).

called Pedipartials, esthetic appliances, or Groper appliances) are an option in this clinical situation (Fig. 19-7A-F). Opinions about their use vary among clinicians. Some make very little use of this type of treatment and discourage parents who seek to replace missing anterior primary teeth, citing low appliance survival rates. Other clinicians find that it is the treatment of choice when a decision is made to treat anterior edentulism in a pediatric patient[54] No clinical study has investigated the survival of these restorations.

The advantages of anterior fixed space maintainers are the following:
1. Good esthetics
2. Restored function
3. Maintenance of posterior space where necessary
4. Prevention of supraeruption of opposing dentition
   Their disadvantages are the following:
1. Cost
2. Decementation of the appliance due to higher than average occlusal forces
3. Possible inadvertent orthodontic movement if not passive.
4. Requires cementation of bands or crowns, which may affect posterior teeth by causing decalcification or caries if the cement washes out.

Before treatment is initiated, parents should be informed of the possibility of decementation and the need for proper follow-up. The level of cooperation of the child should be considered to ensure that treatment will be possible.

Bands are usually placed on caries-free first or second primary molars. They do not require the removal of tooth structure and are sometimes preferable to stainless steel crowns. However, stainless steel crowns are indicated in the following situations:
1. Extensive caries
2. Band retention proves to be insufficient

CLINICAL TIP

Retention can be maximized in children who exert higher masticatory challenge on an appliance, such as bruxers, by using stainless steel crowns instead of bands.

Armamentarium
+ Standard dental setup
+ A high-speed bur, such as #699, #330, or #331 carbide bur (Brasseler USA)
+ Dry angles (Dri-angle, Dental Health Products, Inc.)
+ Stainless steel crowns or orthodontic bands (3M ESPE or Dentsply GAC)
+ Impression compound (Kerr)
+ Irreversible hydrocolloid impression material (Jeltrate, Dentsply Caulk)

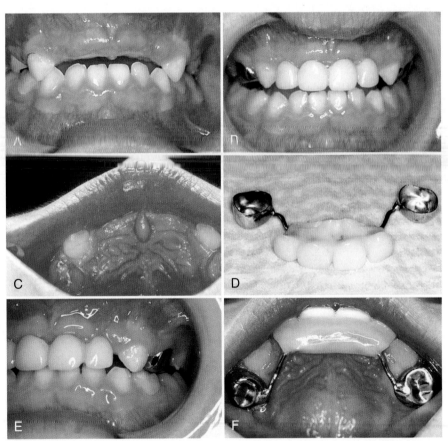

FIGURE 19-7 A, The primary anterior teeth were removed because of early childhood caries. **B,** A fixed space maintainer with acrylic teeth was fabricated to replace the primary central and lateral incisors. **C,** Occlusal view of the edentulous anterior maxilla. **D,** An anterior space maintainer is fabricated on the previously fitted stainless steel crowns. **E,** Three-quarter view of the fixed space maintainer in place. **F,** Occlusal view of the fixed space maintainer in place.

- Stone (Modern Materials Denstone)
- 0.036-in orthodontic wire (Great Lakes Orthodontics, Ltd,)
- Glass Ionomer luting cement (GC FujiCEM Automix, GC America)
  - Wax wafer for occlusal registration (Almore)
  - Sticky wax (Kerr)
  - Prosthetic Acrylic (Lucitone 199, Dentsply Prosthetics)
  - Primary acrylic Bambino Denture Teeth (Major Dental S.p.A., Moncalieri, Italy)

Clinical Technique

1. Fit the stainless steel crowns or bands on the maxillary primary first or second molars.
2. Capture the bands in a compound pick-up impression. Compound creates a firm seat to ensure proper transfer.
3. If possible, obtain a counter irreversible hydrocolloid impression and a wax wafer occlusion registration.
4. Using sticky wax, stabilize the bands or crowns into place in the compound impression.
5. Pour the casts.
6. If the primary teeth were extracted recently, or at the same visit (e.g., when general anesthesia is used), remove a few millimeters of stone from the corresponding portion of the cast. This compensates for the tissue shrinkage that occurs after healing.
7. Adapt a wire to the dental arch.
8. Add acrylic to the wire and position the acrylic teeth.

CLINICAL TIP

Use a dental laboratory that is experienced with the fabrication of anterior fixed space maintainers. It is possible to add pink colored acrylic to complement the soft tissue buccally or as a palatal resting pad.

---

9. Try-in the restoration by seating the crowns or bands into place. Then adjust the wire holding the replacement teeth so the pontics rest passively on the gingiva.
10. Isolate the teeth with a dry angle, dry the teeth with oil-free compressed air, and cement the appliance into place with glass ionomer cement (see Fig. 19-7D-F).

Follow these restorations closely to check for eruption of the anterior teeth. Take maxillary and mandibular radiographs at 6-month intervals. When the mandibular permanent incisors are about to erupt or when evidence of eruption of the maxillary permanent central incisors is noted radiographically, remove the appliance. If the restoration is placed with bands, remove the entire appliance. If crowns are used, cut the wire, leaving the crowns as definitive restorations.

REMOVABLE PROSTHODONTICS

Removable partial and complete dentures are indicated for children when fixed space maintainers are not adequate to replace teeth missing because of trauma and caries (Fig. 19- 8). Hereditary anomalies of tooth number also must be addressed. Anodontia (complete absence of teeth) or oligodontia (partial absence of teeth) is seen in ectodermal dysplasia and Down syndrome. Other diseases cause premature loss of teeth (e.g., histiocytosis X, Papillon-Lefèvre syndrome, and hypophosphatasia). All of these conditions create the need for removable partial or complete dentures. The advantages of removable dentures are the following:

1. Good esthetics
2. Restored function

The disadvantages are the following:

1. Require a mature and compliant patient
2. Easily lost

The concept that the denture must be changed every year is inaccurate. Essentially no interstitial growth occurs in the anterior portion of the mouth from the age of 3 until the permanent anterior teeth erupt. Only vertical growth will occur.

The dentures can remain stable with little adjustment needed in the years before the eruption of the permanent dentition; however, it is necessary to reline the dentures approximately every 12 to 18 months to accommodate vertical growth. With the eruption of the permanent teeth, a proliferation of alveolar bone occurs. It is impractical to cut holes in the denture for these teeth to fit. New dentures must be fabricated at this time.

Armamentarium

- Standard dental setup
- Fast setting Irreversible hydrocolloid impression material (Jeltrate, Dentsply Caulk)
- Thermoplastic Impression compound (Kerr)
- Acrylic custom tray material (SR Ivolen, Ivoclar Vivadent AG)
- Polyvinylsiloxane impression material (Reprosil, Dentsply)
- Primary acrylic Bambino Denture Teeth (Major Dental S.p.A., Moncalieri, Italy)

Clinical Technique

1. Make a preliminary irreversible hydrocolloid impression using stock trays.
2. Pour the impressions.
3. Fabricate custom trays.
4. Make muscle-trimmed impressions, as for adults.
5. Fabricate trays with wax occlusal rims on the master casts.
6. If 1 or 2 teeth are present in the dental arch, it is not difficult to determine jaw relationships. If no teeth are present, use the wax rim as a guide for proper orientation of the teeth. However, it is almost impossible to obtain a correct centric relationship from a child unless he or she is extremely cooperative.
7. With the casts mounted on an articulator, arrange primary acrylic Bambino Denture Teeth (Major Dental S.p.A., Moncalieri, Italy) on the wax rim. Zero-degree plastic denture teeth with a flat occlusal plane can also be used.
8. If any primary teeth are present in the mouth, use them for retention by placing wrought wire clasps.
9. Process and deliver the dentures to the patient.
10. Fit the dentures carefully. Children's vestibules are relatively shallow because they have mostly basal bone and limited alveolar bone.

In addition, follow the patient to determine when (and if) the denture must be replaced.

Overlay complete or partial removable dentures can be fabricated over retained teeth or roots that are not specially prepared to accept copings.[32] These dentures can be used in patients with cleidocranial dysostosis, ectodermal dysplasia, and cleft.

Complete mandibular edentulism in a child is a significant challenge and prosthesis retention is extremely difficult. Implant supported prostheses have been proposed as a possible treatment

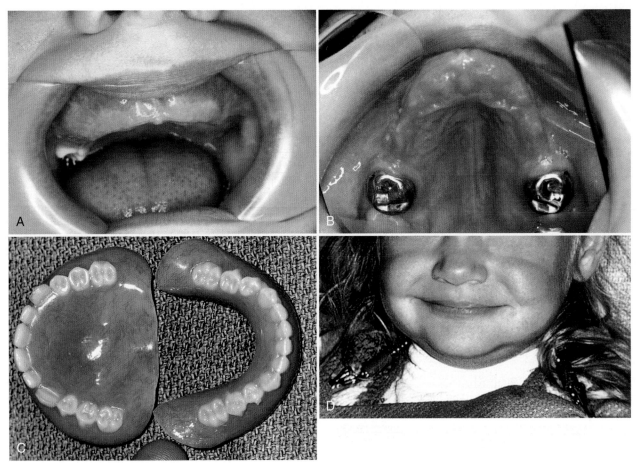

FIGURE 19-8 A, Patient with a loss of primary dentition, except for maxillary second primary molars, because of caries. **B,** Occlusal view of the patient shown in Fig. 19-29, **C,** A complete maxillary and mandibular denture for a patient with Papillon-Lefèvre syndrome. **D,** The patient with the denture in place.

although it is recommended to ideally wait for the completion of dental and skeletal growth before placing dental implants in children and adolescents, except for severe cases of ectodermal dysplasia.[55,56]

CONCLUSION

Esthetic restorations in the primary dentition are proper and necessary. With the many modalities available, children should have their mouths restored to proper form and function.

REFERENCES

1. Holan G, Rahme MA, Ram D: Parents' attitude toward their children's appearance in the case of esthetic defects of the anterior primary teeth, *J Clin Pediatr Dent* 34(2):141-145, 2009.
2. Styczynski LE, Langlois JH: The effects of familiarity on behavioral stereotypes associated with physical attractiveness in young children, *Child Dev* 48:1137, 1977.
3. Shaw WC: The influence of children's dentofacial appearance on their social attractiveness as judged by peers and lay adults, *Am J Orthod* 79(4):399-415, 1981.
4. Dion KK, Berscheid E: Physical attractiveness and peer perception among children, *Sociometry* 1:1, 1974.
5. Gable TO, Kummer AW, Lee L, Creaghead NA, Moore LJ: Premature loss of the maxillary primary incisors: effect on speech production, *ASDC J Dent Child* 62(3):173-179, 1995.
6. Riekman GA, el Badrawy HE: Effects of premature loss of primary maxillary incisors on speech, *Pediatr Dent* 2:119, 1985.
7. Landis P, Fleming J: The interrelationship of speech therapy and prostheses for the handicapped child, *Dent Clin North Am* 3:725, 1974.
8. Baume LJ: Physiological tooth migration and its significance for the development of occlusion: the biogenesis of overbite, *J Dent Res* 29:123, 1950.
9. Macena MC, Tornisiello Katz CR, Heimer MV, de Oliveira e Silva JF, Costa LB: Space changes after premature loss of deciduous molars among Brazilian children, *Am J Orthod Dentofacial Orthop* 140(6):771-778, 2011.
10. Dean JA, Avery DR, McDonald RE: *McDonald and Avery dentistry for the child and adolescent*, ed 9, St Louis, 2010, Mosby.
11. Berkowitz RJ: Causes, treatment and prevention of early childhood caries: a microbiological perspective, *J Can Dent Assoc* 69(5):304-307, 2003.
12. Doméjean S, White JM, Featherstone JD: Validation of the CDA CAMBRA caries risk assessment—a six-year retrospective study, *J Calif Dent Assoc* 39(10):709-715, 2011.
13. Glendor U: Epidemiology of traumatic dental injuries—a 12 year review of the literature, *Dent Traumatol* 24(6):603-611, 2008.
14. Bastone EB, Freer TJ, McNamara JR: Epidemiology of dental trauma: a review of the literature, *Aust Dent J* 45(1):2-9, 2000.
15. The Dental Trauma Guide: Available at: http://www.dentaltraumaguide.org/
16. Ramos-Gomez FJ, Crystal YO, Domejean S, Featherstone JD: Minimal intervention dentistry: part 3. Paediatric dental care—prevention and management protocols using caries risk assessment for infants and young children, *Br Dent J* 213(10):501-508, 2012.
17. Kinoshita S, Mitomi T, Taguchi Y, Noda T: Prognosis of replanted primary incisors after injuries, *Endod Dent Traumatol* 16(4):175-183, 2000.
18. Sakai VT, Moretti AB, Oliveira TM, Silva TC, Abdo RC, Santos CF, et al: Replantation of an avulsed maxillary primary central incisor and management of dilaceration as a sequel on the permanent successor, *Dent Traumatol* 24(5):569-573, 2008.
19. Lekic C: Behaviour management of a pediatric dental patient: audiovisual presentation, *J Can Dent Assoc* 77:b63, 2011.
20. Hennequin M, Collado V, Faulks D, Koscielny S, Onody P, Nicolas E: A clinical trial of efficacy and safety of inhalation sedation with a 50% nitrous oxide/oxygen premix (Kalinox) in general practice, *Clin Oral Investig* 16(2):633-642, 2012.
21. Access to Baby and Child Dentistry: *Dental techniques protect teeth and put kids at ease*. Available at: http://abcd-dental.org/for-dentists/techniques. Accessed March 10, 2014.

22. Holan G, Fuks AB: The diagnostic value of coronal dark-gray discoloration in primary teeth following traumatic injuries, *Pediatr Dent* 18(3):224-227, 1996.

23. Andreasen JO, Andreasen FM, Bakland LK, Flores MT: *Concussion. Traumatic dental injuries. A manual,* Oxford, 2003, Blackwell/Munksgaard Publishing Company, pp 38-39.

24. Cruvinel VR, Gravina DB, Azevedo TD, Rezende CS, Bezerra AC, Toledo OA: Prevalence of enamel defects and associated risk factors in both dentitions in preterm and full term born children, *J Appl Oral Sci* 20(3):310-317, 2012.

25. Seow WK: Clinical diagnosis of enamel defects: pitfalls and practical guidelines, *Int Dent J* 47(3):173-182, 1997. Review.

26. Azevedo TD, Feij√≥ GC, Bezerra AC: Presence of developmental defects of enamel in cystic fibrosis patients, *J Dent Child (Chic)* 73(3):159-163, 2006.

27. Stevenson RE, Hall JG, editors: *Human malformations and related anomalies,* Oxford, 2005, University Press, pp 452-454.

28. Balmer R, Toumba J, Godson J, Duggal M: The prevalence of molar incisor hypomineralisation in northern England and its relationship to socioeconomic status and water fluoridation, *Int J Paediatr Dent* 22(4):250-257, 2012.

29. Croll TP: Esthetic correction for teeth with fluorosis and fluorosis-like enamel dysmineralization, *J Esthet Dent* 10(1):21-29, 1998.

30. Croll TP, Sasa IS: Carbamide peroxide bleaching of teeth with dentinogenesis imperfecta discoloration: report of a case, *Quintessence Int* 26(10):683-686, 1995.

31. Croll TP, Segura A: Tooth color improvement for children and teens: enamel microabrasion and dental bleaching, *ASDC J Dent Child* 63(1):17-22, 1996.

32. Arikan V, Sari S, Sonmez H: Bleaching a devital primary tooth using sodium perborate with walking bleach technique: a case report, *Oral Surg Oral Med Oral Pathol Oral Radiol Endod* 107(5):e80-84, 2009.

33. Sharma DS, Barjatya K, Agrawal A: Intra-coronal bleaching in young permanent and primary tooth with biologic perspectives, *J Clin Pediatr Dent* 35(4):349-352, 2011.

34. American Dental Association: *Statement on the safety and effectiveness of tooth whitening products;* June 2002. http://www.ada.org/1902.aspx http://www.ada.org/5266.aspx?attributes=Whitening http://www.ada.org/5266.aspx?category=Whitening+Products%2c+Dentist+Dispensed%2fHome-Use. Accessed April 7, 2013.

35. American Academy of Pediatric Dentistry: *Policy on the use of dental bleaching for child and adolescent patients,* 2009. Available at: http://www.aapd.org/media/Policies_Guidelines/P_Bleaching.pdf. Accessed April 5, 2013.

36. Mastroberardino S, Campus G, Strohmenger L, Villa A, Cagetti MG: An Innovative approach to treat incisors hypomineralization (MIH): a combined use of casein phosphopeptide-amorphous calcium phosphate and hydrogen peroxide-a case report, *Case Rep Dent* 3795. 3, 2012.

37. Fleisch AF, Sheffield PE, Chinn C, Edelstein BL, Landrigan PJ: Bisphenol A and related compounds in dental materials, *Pediatrics* 126(4):760-768, 2010.

38. American Academy of Pediatric Dentistry: *Guideline on pediatric restorative dentistry,* 2012. Available at: http://www.aapd.org/media/Policies_Guidelines/G_Restorative.pdf. Accessed March 10, 2014.

39. Kameyama A, Asami M, Noro A, Abo H, Hirai Y, Tsunoda M: The effects of three dry-field techniques on intraoral temperature and relative humidity, *J Am Dent Assoc* 142(3):274-280, 2011.

40. Psaltis GL, Kupietzky A: A simplified isolation technique for preparation and placement of resin composite strip crowns, *Pediatr Dent* 30(5):436-438, 2008.

41. Cameron AC, Nowak AJ, Widmer RP, Hall RK: *Handbook of pediatric dentistry,* ed 3, St Louis, 2009, Elsevier.

42. DeRouen TA, Martin MD, Leroux BG, Townes BD, Woods JS, Leitão J, et al: Neurobehavioral effects of dental amalgam in children: a randomized clinical trial, *JAMA* 295(15):1784-1792, 2006.

43. Bellinger DC, Trachtenberg F, Barregard L, Tavares M, Cernichiari E, Daniel D, et al: Neuropsychological and renal effects of dental amalgam in children: a randomized clinical trial, *JAMA* 295(15):1775-1783, 2006.

44. Randall RC, Vrijhoef MM, Wilson NH: Efficacy of preformed metal crowns vs. amalgam restorations in primary molars: systematic review, *J Am Dent Assoc* 131(3):337-343, 2000.

45. Seale NS: The use of stainless steel crowns, *Pediatr Dent* 24(5):501-505, 2002.

46. Guelmann M, Mjör IA, Jerrell GR: The teaching of Class I and II restorations in primary molars: a survey of North American dental schools, *Pediatr Dent* 23(5):410-414, 2001.

47. Sarrett DC, Brooks CN, Rose JT: Clinical performance evaluation of a packable posterior composite in bulk-cured restorations, *J Am Dent Assoc* 137(1):71-80, 2006.

48. Qvist V, Poulsen A, Teglers PT, Mjör IA: Clinical performance of resin-modified glass ionomer cement restorations in primary teeth: a retrospective evaluation, *JADA* 132(8):1110-1116, 2001.

49. Croll TP, Bar-Zion Y, Segura A, Donly KJ: Clinical performance of resin-modified glass ionomer cement restorations in primary teeth. A retrospective evaluation, *J Am Dent Assoc* 132(8):1110-1116, 2001.

50. Ram D, Fuks AB. Clinical performance of resin-bonded composite strip crowns in primary incisors: a retrospective study, *Int J Paediatr Dent* 16(1):49-54, 2006.

51. Hartmann CR: the open-face stainless steel crown: an esthetic technique, *ASDC J Dent Child* 50(1):31-33, 1983.

52. Leith R, O'Connell AC: A clinical study evaluating success of 2 commercially available preveneered primary molar stainless steel crowns, *Pediatr Dent* 33(4):300-306, 2011.

53. Coll JA: Indirect pulp capping and primary teeth: is the primary tooth pulpotomy out of date? *Pediatr Dent* 30(3):230-236, 2008. Review.

54. McMillan AS, Nunn JH, Postlethwaite KR: Implant-supported prosthesis in a child with hereditary mandibular anodontia: the use of ball attachments, *Int J Paediatr Dent* 8(1):65-69, 1998.

55. Waggoner WF, Kupietzky A: Anterior esthetic fixed appliances for the preschooler: considerations and a technique for placement, *Pediatr Dent* 23(2):147-150, 2001.

56. Mankani N, Chowdhary DR, Patil DB, E DN, Madalli DP: Dental implants in children and adolescents: a literature review, *J Oral Implantol* 2012. Jan 3. Epub ahead of print.

20

Esthetic Dentistry and Occlusion

Dewitt C. Wilkerson, III

In 1896, American architect Louis Sullivan stated that form followed function, a principle that has been become an integral part of modern architecture and engineering design. Sullivan believed that the shape of a building or object should be primarily based on its intended function or purpose. This rule is evident in the dynamics of the masticatory system. Clinicians must understand the multiple relationships involved with occlusion to achieve results that are both esthetically pleasing and functionally stable. Restored smiles remain stable only when dental occlusion is established in precise functional harmony with the temporomandibular joints and the neuromuscular system (Fig. 20-1).

CONCEPTS OF OCCLUSION

A comprehensive discussion of occlusion is beyond the scope of this textbook. However, some fundamental concepts applicable to most dental treatments are, therefore, appropriate for esthetic dental procedures. The dental literature contains numerous definitions of specific occlusion terminology that can result in conceptual misinterpretations. Therefore this chapter uses the definitions provided in the *Glossary of Prosthodontic Terms* published in the 2005 *Journal of Prosthetic Dentistry*.[1]

Centric occlusion. The occlusion of opposing teeth when the mandible is in centric relation. This may or may not coincide with the maximal intercuspal position.

Maximal intercuspal position (also called maximal intercuspation). The complete intercuspation of the opposing teeth independent of condylar position sometimes referred to as the best fit of the teeth regardless of the condylar position.

Centric relation. The maxillomandibular relationship in which the condyles articulate with the thinnest avascular portion of their respective disks with the complex in the anterior-superior position against the shapes of the articular eminencies. This position is independent of tooth contact. (This is a partial definition. The entire definition can be found in the *Glossary of Prosthodontic Terms* published in the 2005 *Journal of Prosthetic Dentistry*.)[1]

Temporomandibular Joints and Surrounding Structures

Predictably, stable occlusion depends on proper joint mechanics and masticatory muscle activity. The joints must be evaluated for stability before any occlusal therapy. A screening evaluation should include a review of the patient's joint history. Questions should be asked to identify any known signs or symptoms related to pain, joint noise, joint locking, limited range of movement, or trauma to either jaw joint. Further clinical testing may include joint palpation, orthopedic load testing[2] (Fig. 20-2), Doppler auscultation, and joint vibration analysis.

If joints are identified with apparent intracapsular disorders, further testing through imaging may be indicated. Such joints often require stabilization therapy before initiating dental treatment. Therapy for damaged joints may include occlusal splint therapy, physical therapy, and in severe cases, joint surgery.

In complex restorative cases, centric relation may be the only reference point available to the clinician. Centric relation is precise, repeatable, and stable, in healthy joints with properly aligned condyle-disk assemblies.[3] Dawson's bilateral manipulation is one of numerous methods method of reproducing mandibular centricity.

Uniform Tooth Contacts

Proper occlusion refers to the simultaneous contact of both posterior and anterior teeth. This provides the following benefits:
1. It protects the joints and surrounding structures by reducing the percentage of absorbed force.[4] The positioner muscles of mastication, especially the lateral pterygoids, can fully release

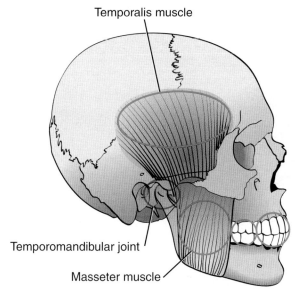

FIGURE 20-1 A healthy masticatory system is the result of harmonious function of the joints, muscles, and posterior and anterior teeth. (From Newman MG, Takei HH, Klokkevold PR, et al. (eds): Carranza's clinical periodontology, ed 10, St. Louis, 2006, Saunders.)

Temporalis muscle

Temporomandibular joint

Masseter muscle

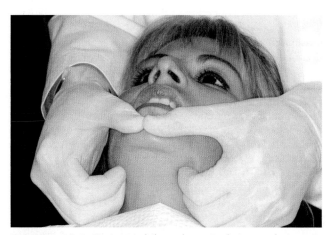

FIGURE 20-2 Dawson's bilateral manipulation technique is one method used to guide the joints into centric relation when this positioning is desired.

their contraction, as the elevator muscles guide the end closure. This release of the positioner muscles protects the muscles.[5]
2. It protects the teeth by reducing the percentage of force through each tooth.[6]

Noninterfering Teeth

The goal of all occlusal therapy is to position teeth so that none interfere with normal jaw function from border to border when the teeth are in occlusion. Ideally, all teeth should touch simultaneously on first contact. New restoration should not cause a shift off the arc of closure (anterior slide), the line of closure (left or right),[7] or vertical hyperocclusion.

It is critical that these interferences be meticulously eliminated. Articulating ribbon is a helpful aid in identifying gross

interferences, but an inconsistent quantifier of small occlusal interferences.[8] Patient feedback can help to identify occlusal prematurities at the 50-μm level, half the thickness of a human hair. In certain cases the T-scan II computerized occlusal analysis (Tekscan, Boston) is helpful (Fig. 20-3). It uses a thin Mylar film containing sensors to record occlusal contacts at the micron level. This information is relayed to a computer monitor for immediate interpretation. This is the most sophisticated means of evaluating occlusal forces presently available.[9]

Coupled Anterior Teeth (Mutually Protected Occlusion)

Anterior coupling is a term used to designate the approximation of the maxillary and mandibular anterior teeth when the posterior teeth are at maximal intercuspation.[10] It is desirable for both anterior and posterior teeth to simultaneously touch in maximal intercuspation (Fig. 20-4). This creates a sharing of occlusal forces over the maximum number of teeth on closure. It also is critical to fulfill the goal of excursive occlusal contacts, namely, immediate anterior teeth guidance and immediate posterior teeth disclusion.

"Several authors believe that mutually protected occlusion (disocclusion through anterior teeth) is ideal, since the canine teeth present higher proprioception, are ideally located (thus promoting immediate disocclusion of posterior teeth),

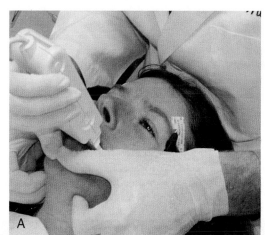

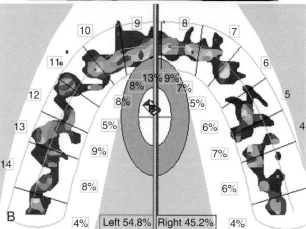

FIGURE 20-3 **A,** Patient undergoes T-scan II occlusal analysis. **B,** Data are relayed to a computer monitor for immediate interpretation.

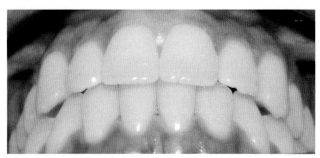

FIGURE 20-4 Ideally anterior teeth should uniformly couple and guide all excursive contacts.

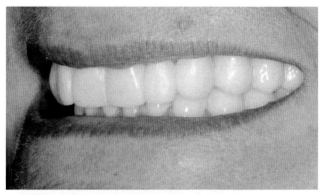

FIGURE 20-5 Phonetics must be tested in the provisional restoration stage to verify correct occlusal relationships.

have considerable volume and bone support and present lower electromyographic activity, i.e. they promote higher muscular relaxation, besides presenting better conditions to distribute and afford occlusal loads without harmful consequences to posterior teeth and supporting structures."[11]

It is necessary for anterior teeth to couple, that is, simultaneously contact, with the posterior teeth so as to maximize physiologic health of the masticatory system.

By harmoniously sharing contact exclusively on the six anterior teeth, in all excursive movements several beneficial effects are realized:

1. The posterior teeth are protected from tooth-to-tooth-abrasive wear, harmful lateral stresses, cervical abfraction, and the damaging effects of parafunctional habits, because they are disoccluded.
2. The EMG activity of elevator muscles is significantly reduced by the disocclusiondistoclusion of the posterior teeth.[12-18]

    Anterior teeth have a mechanical advantage over posterior teeth because they are farther from the fulcrum. This positioning gives them better leverage to offset the closing muscles of mastication. The mechanical advantage is apparent when one tries to "bite hard" with the front teeth as compared to biting hard with the back teeth. This has been shown to significantly reduce chronic myofascial pain in some patients.[26]
3. The reduction of elevator muscle force reduces the loading forces applied at the joint level.

T, D, S, F, V Phonetics

When maxillary and mandibular anterior teeth are properly positioned, they will function in harmony with normal speech. T, D, S, F, and V are the strategic sounds that relate to tooth position affecting proper phonetics (Fig. 20-5).

"T" and "D" sounds are affected by the position of the lingual cingulum of the maxillary anterior teeth, from the maximal intercuspation contact to the gingival margin.[27]

Overcontouring or undercontouring this area can adversely affect clear phonetics. Sharp angles should be avoided.

"S" sounds are used as a critical guideline in removable and fixed prosthetics. "The vertical dimension of speech should be used as the primary guide for establishing the vertical dimension of occlusion. When "s" sounds are being enunciated at conversational speed, the mandible moves to the most forward and upward (closed) position it ever assumes during speech. Because the posterior teeth must never contact during speech, the greatest vertical dimension of occlusion for any person must be 1 mm less than the vertical dimension of speech. Otherwise speech contacts will occur.

Therefore the vertical dimension of speech should be located first and can be used as a protective guide to determine what the vertical dimension of occlusion should be.[28]

The relationship of the lower incisal edges to the maxillary incisors when pronouncing crisp "S" sounds should occur with a clearance of 1 to 1.5 mm. This can occur in a near edge-to-edge position, the "Classic S Position," or in some Class I and II cases, sharp enunciation may occur in an "Atypical S Position," as far apical as the gingival tissues.

Using the "S" sound to assist in determining the ideal relationship between the maxillary incisors lingual contours and the mandibular incisors horizontal and vertical position is described as the "closest speaking space." This can occur in a near edge-to-edge position, the "Classic S Position," or in some Class I and II patients, sharp enunciation may occur in an "Atypical S Position," as far apical as the gingival tissues. "F" and "V" sounds relate directly to the position of the incisal edges of the maxillary incisor teeth. The positions in which these sounds are made are also strategic markers for the ideal length and horizontal position of the maxillary central incisors. The maxillary incisor teeth should contact the inner vermillion border of the lower lip as air is sealed to form a clear F and V sound. This should occur with repetitive unstrained effort of the facial muscles, when the incisal edges are in harmony with the lower lip and speech.

INCISOR-CANINE GUIDANCE

In all mandibular excursions only the incisor and canine teeth should be in contact and the posterior teeth should immediately disocclude.

Two primary factors determine the guiding angles of the maxillary anterior teeth. The first factor relates to the eruption of the teeth, into what is described as the *neutral zone*.

A popular term in denture prosthetics, the neutral zone is an area between the oral musculature, where forces generated by the tongue are neutralized by the forces generated by the lips and cheeks. Denture teeth and flanges placed into this zone of equal and opposite muscle forces, are stable.[29,30] Natural teeth erupt into the neutral zone. Muscle forces the position of each tooth. Strong forces from the lips will result in maxillary incisors that are steep and even potentially lingually inclined. Conversely, strong tongue forces pushing outward, may create maxillary incisors with a very shallow inclination. There are no norms or averages to create standardized anterior guidances for comfortable and stable restorative/cosmetic dentistry outcomes. The neutral zone creates the second factor that determines the guiding angles of the maxillary anterior teeth, the envelope of function.[31] In natural dentition the movement of the mandibular incisor teeth when masticating, swallowing, and speaking is dictated by the position of the maxillary incisors. Neuromusculature harmony occurs when muscle memory engrams coordinate jaw movement within the available parameters, set by the maxillary incisors and canines. The steepness or shallowness of the lingual contours of the maxillary teeth dictates how vertically or horizontally the mandibular teeth function. The exquisite sensitivity of this system, through tooth mechanoreceptors, creates a very refined relationship for the protection of the teeth. The maxillary anterior teeth create a neuromusculature "electrified fence" that the mandibular teeth must function within for long-term stability. Functioning outside of these parameters results in damage to the teeth and supporting structures, as is observed with parafunctional habits. The position of the maxillary incisors and canines, as dictated by the neutral zone, creating the envelope of function, have important clinical significance in many cases. For example, when a "tight neutral zone" is observed, with steep tooth inclinations (Fig. 20-6), it is very important that new restorations not extend facially from the original position. In this case, if teeth leave the neutral zone of balanced muscle forces, they will be unstable (i.e., if maxillary anterior veneers are placed, the patient returns later complaining that "the front teeth are hitting too hard." This occurs because the restored teeth were in violation of the positional parameters determined by the musculature. Another notable example

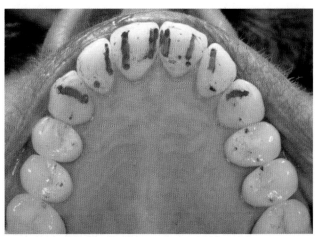

FIGURE 20-7 Maxillary anterior teeth must be positioned in harmony with the patient's neutral zone and envelope of function.

occurs when the lingual contours of maxillary anterior teeth are restored to a steeper angle than the natural teeth. This frequently creates an apparent parafunctional erasure mechanism to regain lost freedom of function, resulting in mobile maxillary anterior teeth, excessive wear of the mandibular incisal edges, and discomfort. Shallowing anterior guidance creates greater functional freedom, but steepening the guidance can create dysfunction in many cases. The patient should be instructed to be very cognizant and communicative about the comfort, phonetics, function, and esthetics of the provisional restorations before the clinician communicates to the laboratory through "approved provisional restorations." This is absolutely vital to achieving predictable and successful outcomes (Fig. 20-7).

CLINICAL TIP

A restored anterior guidance that is stable long-term, involves not only separating posterior teeth, but also verification of functional harmony with the muscles.

OCCLUSAL VERTICAL DIMENSION

Clinical experience has demonstrated that the masticatory system is very amenable to reasonable changes in occlusal vertical dimension (OVD), if the functional guidelines previously discussed are meticulously followed. In general, OVD is determined by muscle. Similar to the neutral zone concept, whereby muscles determine the horizontal position of teeth, the repetitive contraction of the elevator muscles upon swallowing will dictate the eruptive position of opposing teeth.[27] When a full complement of teeth is present, even with significant tooth wear, the concept of "lost vertical" may be a misnomer. It appears that although tooth structure may be lost, alveolar bone is added as compensation, and muscle contraction length remains relatively the same. Nevertheless, the clinician is faced with a restorative challenge. There is decreased tooth structure, and lack of room to restore, at the present OVD. It is typically acceptable to open the OVD enough to restore lost tooth structure back to its original form within reason. If the OVD must be altered, it is

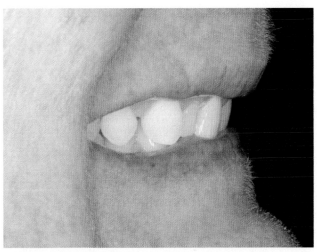

FIGURE 20-6 A "tight neutral zone" with steeply inclined maxillary incisors and strong lower lip pressure must be carefully managed restoratively to avoid a neutral zone violation.

prudent to make the most conservative changes possible to achieve an optimal esthetic and functional result.

Research has shown that alterations of OVD, accompanied in the optimum condylar position, are well tolerated by the TMJ. When altering OVD, problems are often encountered when bilateral tooth contacts are uneven or anterior guidance is adversely managed.[33]

For every 1 mm, the condyles are seated superiorly; from their position in maximal intercuspation (an average of 1 mm down/forward from centric relation)[34] the anterior teeth can open 2 mm without changing the contracted muscle length of the masseter muscles. Therefore when the occlusion is restored in centric relation, it is possible to gain restorative room anteriorly, without changing muscle-contracted length.[35] Increasing OVD changes anterior facial height primarily by rotational condylar movement without the accompanied changes in posterior facial height or muscle length.[35] An adaptive muscle response with concurrent long-term stability is anticipated as long as vertical support and anterior guidance are present.

Occlusal Evaluation for Restoring a Worn Anterior Dentition[36]

Armamentarium
- Semiadjustable articulator
- Patient study models
- Appropriate occlusal relation record

Clinical Technique. This technique is used to establish centric occlusion (condyles in centric relation) with the teeth in maximal intercuspation.

1. Mount the casts on a semiadjustable articulator to establish centric relation.
2. Evaluate tooth-by-tooth conditions and treatment requirements.
3. Evaluate the maxillary and mandibular occlusal planes and determine any treatment requirements.
4. Determine the optimal vertical and horizontal position of the mandibular anterior incisal edges determine the optimal vertical and horizontal position of the maxillary anterior incisal edges.
5. Select the occlusal vertical dimension.
6. Wax to provide ideal centric occlusion contacts on all teeth.
7. Eliminate balancing and working posterior interferences.
8. Harmonize the anterior guidance.
9. Reevaluate the overall functional and esthetic results.

Changes in OVD must be evaluated with provisional restorations for acceptable comfort, phonetics, function, and esthetics, before communicating to the laboratory through "approved provisional restorations" (Fig. 20-8).

CLINICAL TIP

Occlusal vertical dimension can be conservatively altered to accommodate a worn dentition, as long as all other factors of an ideal occlusion are meticulously fulfilled. The results must be evaluated and approved by the patient using provisional restorations.

Nonfunctional Factors

Before restoring a damaged dentition the cause of the damage and whether or not restoring the dentition will eliminate the

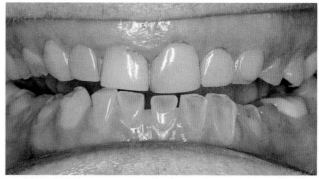

FIGURE 20-8 Severe wear cases may require some increase in OVD, which should evaluated by the placement of provisional restorations, with an idealized occlusion.

cause of the damage should be determined. Occlusal disharmony can be a cause of structural destruction, discomfort and dysfunction.[37]

Another destabilizing factor is parafunction activity unrelated to mastication or speech that can be injurious to the teeth and supporting structures. It appears to have multiple causes, including malocclusion. Studies have shown that sleep bruxism, in many instances, is related to sleep arousal, with a change in cardiac and brain activity preceding jaw motor activity. Peripheral microarousals can affect sleep-wake mechanisms.[38] Systemic disease, such as Parkinson's bruxism, will naturally persist after restorative therapy is complete.

Sleep apnea is a condition of airway obstruction and cessation of breathing for periods of 10 seconds or greater during sleep.[39] Studies are being conducted to analyze the relationship between apnea, reduced oxygen saturation, "fight or flight" responses, increased cortisol release, accelerated heart rate, and bruxism.[40] Gastric reflux caused by negative airway pressure and positive gastric pressure is also associated with sleep apnea.[41] Nonfunctional factors of occlusal/dental instability are also associated with eating disorders, low pH beverages, toothpaste abrasion, and fruit mulling (Figs. 20-9 and 20-10).[42]

When parafunctional factors persist, after ideal occlusal therapy is completed, an oral appliance is indicated to control the parafunction and its deleterious effects.

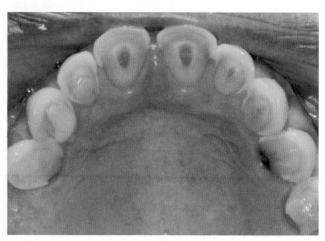

FIGURE 20-9 Classic signs of nonfunctional bulimic disorder, destroying maxillary anterior tooth structure.

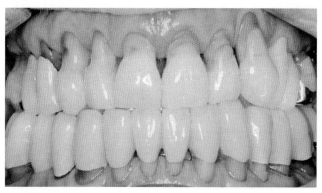

FIGURE 20-10 Nonfunctional factor of severe root damage caused by coarse "natural dentifrice" 15 years after dentition has been restored.

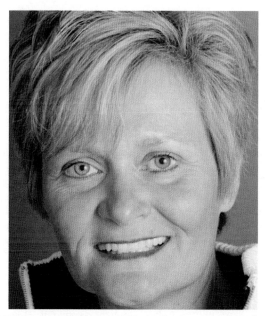

FIGURE 20-11 Understanding the basic principles of occlusion enables clinical results that will endure the test of time.

Dietary discussions are important for patients with a low pH intake. The reduction of low pH beverages and acidic fruits is sometimes critical for long-term restorative integrity.

Patients with eating disorders such as bulimia and anorexia live in a life-threatening situation physically and psychologically. Dentists are often the first health professionals to recognize the problem. It is often uncomfortable but necessary to address the issue with the patient, the family, and the physician (see Chapter 29). Patients who damage their teeth and/or gingiva by excessive toothbrushing and/or overly abrasive dentifrices should be properly advised.

Functional esthetics brings a beauty to the outcome of smile enhancement that extends far beyond a youthful appearance. When beauty includes relaxed comfort, confident stability, clear phonetics, effortless function, and natural esthetics, a service has been provided that is life altering, in the most positive way (Fig. 20-11).

CONCLUSION

It is critical that clinicians understand the multiple relationships involved with occlusion in order to achieve results that are both esthetically pleasing and functionally stable. Restored smiles remain predictably stable only when dental occlusion is established in precise functional harmony with the temporomandibular joints and the neuromuscular system.

REFERENCES

1. The glossary of prosthodontic terms, *J Prosthet Dent* 94(1):10-92, 2005.
2. Dawson PE: *Functional occlusion: from TMJ to smile design*, St Louis, 2006, Mosby.
3. Smith DM, McLachlan KR, McCall WD Jr: A numerical model of temporomandibular joint loading, *J Dent Res* 65(8):1046-1052, 1986.
4. Mahan PE, Wilkinson TM, Gibbs CH, Mauderli A, Brannon LS: Superior and inferior bellies of the lateral pterygoid muscle EMG activity at basic jaw positions, *J Prosthet Dent* 50(5):710-718, 1983.
5. Kerstein R: Combining technologies: a computerized occlusal analysis system synchronized with a computerized electromyography system, *Cranio* 22(2):96-109, 2004.
6. Maness WL: Computerized occlusal analysis: a new technology, *Quint Intl* 18:287-292, 1987.
7. International Academy of Gnathology: *Glossary of occlusal terms*, ed 2. http://www.gnathologyusa.org/got_a-q.html. Accessed November 1, 2013.
8. Matos DA, Teixeira ML, Pinto JH, Lopes JF, Dalben Gda S: Pattern of disocclusion in patients with complete cleft lip and palate, *J Appl Oral Sci* 14(3):157-161, 2006.
9. Lee R: Anterior guidance. In: Lunden JC, Gibbs CH, editors: *Advances in occlusion*, Boston, 1982, John Wright, pp 51-79. http://www.panadent.com/1ADVANCES_IN_OCCLUSION.pdf. Accessed November, 2013.
10. Grubwieser G, Flatz A, Grunert I, et al: Quantitative analysis of masseter and temporalis EMGs: a comparison of anterior guided versus balanced occlusal concepts in patients wearing complete dentures, *J Oral Rehabil* 26(9):731-736, 1999.
11. Fitins D, Sheikholeslam A: Effect of canine guidance of maxillary occlusal splint on level of activation of masticatory muscles, *Swed Dent J* 17(6):235-241, 1993.
12. Williamson EH, Lundquist DO: Anterior guidance: its effect on electromyographic activity of the temporal and masseter muscles, *J Prosthet Dent* 49(6):816-823, 1983.
13. Manns A, Chan C, Miralles R: Influence of group function and canine guidance on electromyographic activity of elevator muscles, *J Prosthet Dent* 57(4):494-501, 1987.
14. Miralles R, Bull R, Manns A, et al: Influence of balanced occlusion and canine guidance on electromyographic activity of elevator muscles in complete denture wearers, *J Prosthet Dent* 61(4):494-498, 1989.
15. Okano N, Baba K, Akishige S, et al: The influence of altered occlusal guidance on condylar displacement, *J Oral Rehabil* 29(11):1091-1098, 2002.
16. Kerstein RB, Wright NR: Electromyographic and computer analyses of patients suffering from chronic myofascial pain-dysfunction syndrome: before and after treatment with immediate complete anterior guidance development, *J Prosthet Dent* 66(5):677-686, 1991.
17. Pound E: The vertical dimension of speech: the pilot of occlusion, *J Calif Dent Assoc* 6(2):42-47, 1978.
18. Beresin VE, Schiesser FJ: The neutral zone in complete dentures, *J Prosthet Dent* 36(4):356-367, 1976.
19. Kois JC, Phillips KM. Occlusal vertical dimension: alteration concerns, *Compend Contin Educ Dent* 18(12):1169-1177, 1997.
20. Lundeen HC, Gibbs CH: *The function of teeth: the physiology of mandibular function related to occlusal form and esthetics*, Gainesville, FL, 2005, L and G Publishers.
21. Kois JC, Phillips KM: Occlusal vertical dimension: alteration concerns, *Compend Contin Educ Dent* 18(12):1169-1174, 1176. 1177, 1997.
22. The Dawson Academy: *Manual*, St. Petersburg, FL, 2012, The Dawson Academy.
23. Kato T, Thie NM, Huynh N, Miyawaki S, Lavigne GJ: Topical review: sleep bruxism and the role of peripheral sensory influences, *J Orofac Pain* 17(3):191-213, 2003.
24. The Free Dictionary: *Sleep apnea.* http://medical-dictionary.thefreedictionary.com/sleep+apnea. Accessed November 1, 2013.
25. Simmons JH: Neurology of sleep and sleep-related breathing disorders and their relationships to sleep bruxism, *J Calif Dent Assoc* 40(2):159-167, 2012.
26. Rosario IC: Obstructive sleep apnea: a review and update, *Minn Med* 94(11):44-48, 2011.
27. Abrahamsen TC: The worn dentition—pathognomonic patterns of abrasion and erosion, *Int Dent J* 55(4 Suppl 1):268-276, 2005.

21

Esthetics and Laser Surgery

Robert A. Strauss and Kenneth S. Magid

The use of lasers in dentistry has burgeoned at an astonishing rate over the past few years. Once relegated to use on soft tissue, now even hard tissue esthetic surgery can be done with lasers. Because of their many advantages, lasers are indicated for a wide variety of intraoral and extraoral esthetic procedures. To use them safely and successfully, however, a thorough understanding of their indications, contraindications, and safety parameters is imperative.

HISTORY

The word *laser* is an acronym for light amplification by stimulated emission of radiation. The theory has its roots in several basic principles of physics first described by Einstein in 1917.[1] Amazingly it was almost another 50 years before these principles were sufficiently understood and the technology could be converted into practical reality. The first laser to use visible light was developed by a physicist, Dr. Theodore Maiman, in 1960. Maiman used a ruby gemstone as the lasing medium, producing the red beam of intense light typically associated with lasers.[2] This was followed in 1961 by another crystal laser using a neodymium-doped crystal of yttrium, aluminum, and garnet (Nd:YAG). In 1964, physicists at Bell Laboratories produced a gaseous laser using carbon dioxide (CO_2) as the lasing medium. That same year another gaseous laser that would prove important in dentistry, the argon laser, was invented.

Dental scientists investigating the effects of Maiman's ruby laser on the enamel of teeth found that it caused cracking and fissuring of enamel.[3,4] The studies concluded that lasers had no place in dentistry, and few other studies were undertaken. In medicine, however, research and clinical use of lasers proliferated. In 1968, the CO_2 laser was used for the first time to perform soft tissue surgery. An increasing variety of laser wavelengths, as well as general and oral surgical indications, evolved. In the mid-1980s, the expanded availability of different wavelengths and the improved understanding of laser physics and tissue interaction created a resurgence of interest in the use of lasers in dentistry for hard tissues such as enamel.[5-8]

Although a few wavelengths, such as that of the Nd:YAG laser, can be artificially manipulated for hard tissue use, their danger potential and lack of specificity for dental tissues make them less than ideal. Other lasers, such as the excited dimer (excimer) laser, which was studied extensively in the late 1980s and early 1990s, were shown to cause little damage to teeth. However, they were plagued by problems of cost, size, and efficiency.[9] Not until 1997 did the US Food and Drug Administration (FDA) finally approve a well-known laser, the Erbium:YAG (Er:YAG) laser and later the Er, Cr:YSGG laser (henceforth collectively referred to as "erbium" because of their similarities), for hard tissue use.[10,11]

BASIC CONCEPTS

Laser energy is unique in that laser light is coherent. This means that laser light has three distinct properties that distinguish it from regular light. Ideal laser light is monochromatic (composed of a single wavelength of light), collimated (the light waves run parallel to each other instead of diverging), and uniphasic (the peaks and valleys of the waves are synchronous (Fig. 21-1).

Monochromatic Property

Because lasers are monochromatic, each has a single frequency and wavelength and therefore a single "color." Thus, lasers often are defined by their visible color (e.g., red light or green light lasers), their position in the electromagnetic spectrum (e.g., infrared, ultraviolet or radiograph lasers), or the chemicals that create the light (e.g., CO_2, argon, or Nd: YAG lasers).

Collimated Property

All laser beams are parallel, or collimated, unlike regular light. Because the laser beam does not diverge significantly over distance, the source can be positioned at great length from the target tissue or can be very efficiently focused down to a small spot with a convex focusing lens.

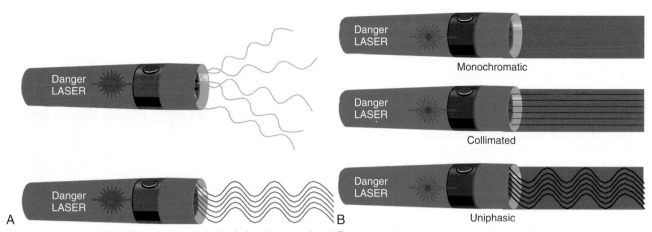

FIGURE 21-1 A, Regular light showing the different wavelengths present and the random spread of the beam. Laser demonstrating uniform, coherent light. **B,** Laser light showing monochromatic wavelength, collimation, and uniformity of phase, which constitute coherent light.

Uniphasic Property

The peaks and troughs of a laser light wave are directly in line (synchronous) with one another, making them uniphasic. All the peaks and troughs of the energy beam are stacked on top of each other.

Intensity Property

Collimation, monochromaticity, and uniphasicity together produce a very intense and powerful flash or beam of light. The ability to efficiently focus the beam down to a small spot size (an effect of the collimation on a convex lens) produces an extremely powerful, condensed energy source.

Laser beams may reflect off, transmit through, scatter (break up) within, or be absorbed by organic target tissue. The first three conditions elicit no effect within the tissue, but when absorbed, a laser beam may produce several different results. The most important is the photothermal effect, or tremendous heat generation that occurs almost instantaneously within the tissue. In soft tissue, this causes the intracellular water to boil or vaporize and literally explodes and disintegrates the cell. In hard tissues, similar effects may be seen in hydroxyapatite. Unlike other heat sources, however, the laser can be applied with incredible precision and with such speed that only microns of tissue can be removed at a time with very controlled and minimal damage to adjacent tissues and structures. Conversely it sometimes is advantageous to have a lateral heat effect in tissue that results in thermal coagulation of adjacent blood vessels and a bloodless field. Lasers can be controlled to provide this as well.

The many lasers now available for medical and dental use differ in several aspects. The primary difference is the active medium (i.e., the material that undergoes stimulated emission). The specific material used determines the wavelength of energy produced and therefore the clinical indications. Few materials in nature can undergo this process because the material must be capable of sustaining population inversion, an unnatural condition in which most atoms are in a highly excited state.

The ideal system uses fiberoptic delivery of the laser beam to the target tissue. These systems are flexible and precise, they allow for both contact and noncontact surgery, and they are capable of endoscopic delivery. Unfortunately, not all wavelengths (e.g., CO_2) can be transmitted through the currently used quartz fiberoptic fibers. These other types of lasers use articulated arm delivery in which a series of hollow metal tubes connected by mirrored flexible joints or "knuckles" allow the beam to be passed from the laser to the tissues. Although this is functional for superficial tissues, it is less than ideal for deeper tissues or areas of difficult access, such as the oral cavity. Some newer lasers use a hollow wave guide, a variation of the articulated arm. The hollow wave guide is a flexible metal tube internally lined with a mirrored surface or foil, which allows the beam to reflect down the guide to the tissues. Although not as flexible as a fiberoptic fiber and incapable of endoscopic delivery, this system has dramatically improved the dentist's ability to provide convenient, precise delivery within the oral cavity.

Some lasers produce a continuous beam of laser light as long as the machine is energized, whereas others can be pulsed. These very high power, short duration pulses of laser light minimize the time available for lateral tissue heating and damage.[12] Other lasers can be electronically enhanced to produce extremely fast, high-powered laser bursts ("superpulsed" or "ultrapulsed") for situations such as dermatologic skin surgery in which lateral thermal damage produces scarring.

Selecting the appropriate laser for a given procedure usually is a simple matter of determining which laser wavelength is best absorbed by the target tissue while producing the least reflection, scatter, and transmission. Laser wavelengths that are absorbed by water (e.g., CO_2, erbium) are appropriate for soft tissue surgery. Those well absorbed by hemoglobin are better suited for vascular tissues or lesions (e.g., argon, KTP: YAG, tunable dye, copper vapor lasers). Argon laser wavelengths are well absorbed by composite resin, and the erbium laser wavelength, which is absorbed by both hydroxyapatite and water, allows for hard tissue use. Some lasers with wavelengths that are absorbed by a number of different tissues (i.e., chromophores) may be useful for a variety of tissue effects. In addition, some transmission may actually be desirable in certain situations to allow deeper penetration of tissues (e.g., when deep hemostasis is desired in vascular lesions). To allow for precise tissue effects and clinical uses, some devices can produce more than one wavelength (i.e., CO_2 and Er: YAG, KTP: YAG and Nd: YAG, and tunable dye), which allows the operator to select the desired tissue effect by varying the wavelength used. The choice of an appropriate wavelength involves a combination of known tissue effect and the operator's clinical experience.[13]

Currently the most commonly used laser in general dentistry is the diode laser. Used primarily for soft tissue incisional procedures, it has the advantage of being small, relatively inexpensive, and comparatively easy to use. However, its mechanism of action is widely misunderstood. Some lasers function by the direct effect of laser energy on soft tissue, whereas diode lasers used in dentistry do not have sufficient power to cut tissue.[13] Therefore the laser tip needs to be activated (initiated) by touching the tip to a light absorbing material such as articulating paper, cork, or other dark substance, which produces a "charring" of the tip. The tip is now capable of absorbing laser light and when activated by the laser will heat up and vaporize the underlying tissue (Fig. 21-2).

Laser Tip Consideration

Laser tip activation deposits carbon on the tip of the laser fiber, which becomes the target of the diode laser energy.

CLINICAL TIP

Initiate the tip and a portion of the side of the laser fiber with light absorbing material.

CLINICAL TIP

The light-absorbing material used for initiating the laser fiber is not consumed by the laser energy. However, with some lasers it may be wiped or broken off during use. In that situation it must be reinitiated.

It is also the cause of more extensive collateral thermal damage as the power of the unconverted laser energy penetrates deeper into the tissues (Fig. 21-3)[5]

Because the diode laser functions tip cutting with a hot tip, the specific wavelength of the diode laser is of less significance than in other lasers. The remaining parameters of power, time, and spot size are, however, still critical. Sufficient power is necessary to maintain the hot tip once it is in contact with the cooler tissue. If the tip cools beyond the temperature required to efficiently incise the tissue the resulting increase in contact time will

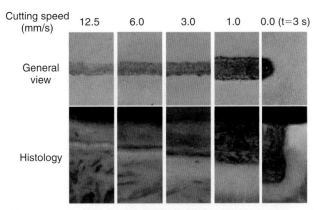

FIGURE 21-3 Effects of cutting speed on collateral thermal damage.

increase the collateral thermal damage as in other lasers. Spot size (or in the situation of diode laser, fiber size) is significant because the heat of the laser tip is concentrated in a smaller area that increases the heat energy per unit area.

ADVANTAGES AND DISADVANTAGES

Many laser wavelengths either are absorbed by hemoglobin or constrict vascular wall collagen, allowing for bloodless surgery.[14] This allows the dentist to work in a clean, dry environment unobstructed by bleeding. When used correctly, lasers also can remove precise and minimal amounts of tissue with minimal effect on adjacent tissues. They are ideal for detailed, exact tissue manipulation.[15] Lasers have an effect on neural tissue that generally results in less pain after surgery compared with other types of treatment.[16] In fact, because of their great speed, some pulsed lasers may even be used for soft or hard tissue surgery without the need for anesthesia.[17] Minimal postoperative pain and absence of bleeding usually precludes the need for suturing, tissue closure, or coverage with splints or dressings except when cosmetic requirements dictate otherwise.

The elimination of lateral tissue damage is especially important in dentistry because of the proximity of such chemically diverse yet clinically vital structures as dental pulp, bone, tooth structure, and oral soft tissue. Lasers also make possible procedures such as perioral cosmetic skin resurfacing, in which even minimal adjacent dermal tissue damage would translate

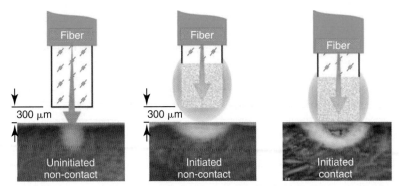

FIGURE 21-2 The experiment shows the inability of the diode laser to cut with either an uninitiated or initiated tip in non-contact. Only an initiated tip in contact is capable of cutting tissue at power levels found in dental diode lasers.

into inevitable and devastating scarring. Sealing of the lymphatic system during laser surgery and the minimal tissue trauma result in little or no postoperative edema in most patients.[18] Finally because of the minimal tissue damage and the decrease in the number of myofibroblasts in laser-treated wounds compared with wounds made by scalpel or electrosurgical instruments, postoperative scarring and contracture are minimized, allowing dramatic surgery without the fear of significant postoperative cosmetic deformity or functional deficits.[19]

Disadvantages are few but important. The preeminent concern with lasers in dentistry is safety. Lasers require tremendous diligence to maintain a safe operative environment for both the patient and the dental team (see the section on Laser Safety later in this chapter). Other disadvantages include the generally high cost of purchasing and maintaining the laser, the loss of tactile sensation with noncontact lasers, the learning curve necessary to obtain uniform results, and the specificity of some laser wavelengths, necessitating the occasional need for more than one laser for a particular procedure. Finally although healing after laser surgery generally is excellent, usually much better than with other instruments such as a scalpel or electrosurgical instrument, it also generally is slower because of the vascular sealing.[20]

CLINICAL INDICATIONS

Restorative and intraoral esthetic modification can be divided into soft tissue or combined soft and hard tissue.

> ### CLINICAL TIP
>
> To determine which procedures are required, and therefore what types of lasers will be used, measurements and planning must be performed to determine if the changes will violate the biologic width of the teeth involved.

Soft tissue procedures include excision of excess tissue, either normal or pathologic, and recontouring of tissue. There are few soft tissue surgeries in which the laser cannot be used and used advantageously. Teeth or bone intimately involved with the target tissue or lesion must be protected from the laser beam, which increases the difficulty of the procedure, but with reasonable precaution and care, this usually is not a problem. For example, a standard mucoperiosteal flap around the dentition can be created with a laser, but it is more easily and safely accomplished with a scalpel. Once the incision has been made, the rest of the surgery may well be enhanced by the use of lasers.

Despite the many different types of lasers available, the techniques for their use do not vary significantly. The three basic techniques are incision, vaporization, and hemostasis.[12] The clinician should evaluate the lesion before surgery and determine which of these is most appropriate.

Incision is accomplished by placing the laser at its focal length (i.e., the smallest possible spot size) near the tissue or touching the tissue if a contact tip laser is used. This increases the density of the power and condenses the effect into a small area. This laser-target distance varies according to the delivery system and ranges from contact with a contact laser to 0.5 mm for a hollow wave guide to more than 1 cm for an articulated arm laser (Fig. 21-4).

Vaporization, also called ablation, allows the removal of large areas of very superficial tissue (e.g., removal of the surface mucosal epithelium) without affecting deeper structures. This is accomplished by defocusing or backing the laser away from the target to increase the spot size. Defocusing effectively lowers the density of the laser energy per unit area and causes the laser to act more superficially over a larger surface area. The target distance may vary dramatically depending on the type of delivery system, the available power, and the desired depth of penetration.

Most lasers are intrinsically hemostatic to a degree, depending on the laser's depth of penetration and whether hemoglobin

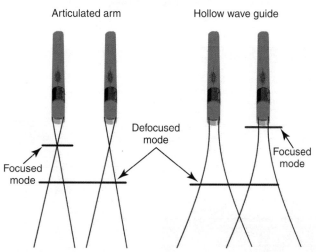

FIGURE 21-4 Focused mode technique (for incision) and defocused mode technique (for vaporization). Note the different distances from target to laser for the hollow wave guide and the articulated arm.

or vascular collagen is the chromophore for a particular laser wavelength. The CO_2 laser generally seals vessels 500 μm or less in diameter, whereas the more hemoglobin-specific KTP:YAG, Nd:YAG, and argon lasers may provide deeper hemostasis. Even when another modality is used, the laser may be used to control hemorrhage. This is done by passing the laser over the surgical site somewhere between the focusing and defocusing distances to produce a hemostatic effect without causing significant tissue cutting or ablation.

The indications for the use of lasers in cosmetic dentistry are presented in Box 21-1. More than one wavelength may be suitable for a specific clinical situation; therefore proper wavelength selection is important. Because of the variety of manufacturers, wavelengths, machines, and clinical variations, there is no "cookbook" for laser surgery. Any clinician using lasers should receive appropriate instruction in that particular wavelength and device and should use known protocols along with individual clinical judgment.

The following sections give some examples of laser cosmetic dental procedures and the lasers most commonly used for that purpose, although other lasers may be used.

SOFT TISSUE

Gingivoplasty/Gingivectomy

Soft tissue procedures can be can be useful in correcting an unesthetic "gummy smile" of delayed passive eruption or medication

Box 21-1
Soft Tissue Clinical Indications for Esthetic Dental Laser Surgery
Frenectomy
Gingivoplasty
Tissue and papilla resculpting
Gingivectomy
Access gingivectomy
Lesion removal
Pigment and tattoo removal

induced hyperplasia (Fig. 21-5). A gingivectomy is also frequently required to expose subgingival root surface carious lesions (Fig. 21-6). This procedure is becoming more common in the aging population using many of the medications that result in decreased salivation. The ability of the laser to remove the soft tissue while leaving a bloodless field permits immediate restoration or impressioning.

Gingivectomy or gingivoplasty may be accomplished with a CO_2, erbium, diode, or Nd:YAG laser. Each of these has its own advantages and disadvantages. For hyperplastic tissue, the CO_2 laser is very effective at altering the location of the gingival margin by incision and then reducing the extensive hyperplastic tissue by ablations. It is, however, necessary to protect the teeth using a thin nonreflecting instrument as a barrier between the tooth and the laser energy, and the noncontact

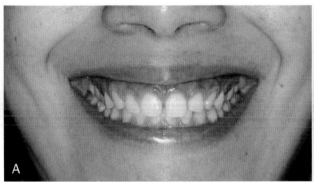
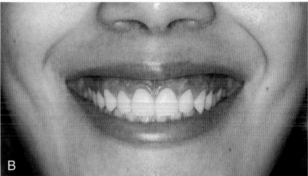

FIGURE 21-5 A, Preoperative view. **B,** Four-week postoperative view showing excellent healing.

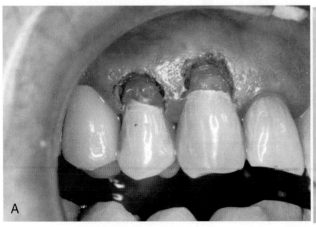
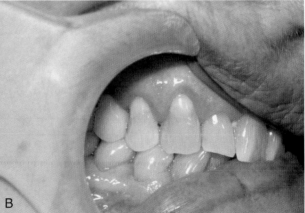

FIGURE 21-6 A, CO_2 laser-assisted access gingivoplasty and recontouring to allow immediate placement of restorations in a bloodless field. **B,** Postoperative view of same patient 2 weeks after restoration. (Courtesy Alan Winner, DDS, New York, NY.)

nature of the CO_2 laser[21] makes learning its use and control more demanding.

Although the erbium laser may be used for gingivoplasty, the pulsed nature of this laser often results in an uneven, ragged cut. Hemostasis and tissue fluid control with the erbium laser can also be problematic even when used without water spray because tissue heating is required for cauterization and the erbium laser's ablation removes tissue but does not create sufficient collateral heat to cauterize any but the smallest vessels. There has been some improvement in these characteristics with newer Er, Cr:YSGG lasers that use high pulse rate and longer pulse width to smooth the cut and increase the heat transfer to the tissue for hemostasis. Potential damage to tooth structure is possible the erbium laser wavelength if excessive power density is used.

The diode laser's hot tip is used in contact mode, which permits easier control for these procedures than the CO_2 or erbium. The dry field left by these devices does not require the removal of soft tissue considerably beyond the desired margin as with erbium lasers and permits immediate restoration.

Although lasers are generally said to be "end cutting," the diode laser hot tip can be used on the side of the tip to the extent the initiation can be maintained. This permits moderate tissue sculpting, which is a benefit in these procedures. Although it is frequently shown that the hydroxyapatite of tooth structure is mostly unaffected by diode laser wavelengths, the hot tip actually used is relatively safe around enamel if contact time is limited but can leave a burned area on root structure or dentin, which is more susceptible to heat damage than enamel.

Frenectomy

Almost any dental laser (CO_2, diode, erbium, Nd:YAG) can easily and quickly remove either a lingual or facial frenum. The frenum can either be excised in continuous, focused mode (or with a contact tip) or ablated in continuous or pulsed, defocused mode. In any situation, no closure is necessary, and healing generally is excellent. The lack of bleeding and elimination of sutures makes this an ideal technique for children. Some lasers may also permit this procedure to be accomplished without anesthesia, although most generally require an anesthetic unless

the frenum is small, in which situation a topical anesthetic may suffice (Fig. 21-7).

Removal of Benign Lesions

The laser (CO_2, diode, erbium,) is an ideal tool for removal of cosmetically undesirable benign neoplastic or hamartomatous lesions. If a benign diagnosis has been confirmed, the laser may be used to excise the lesion in focused mode or to ablate it in defocused mode. Fibromas, mucoceles, granulomas, amalgam tattoos, and small lip, gingival, and tongue hemangiomas, and lymphangiomas can be managed in this manner (Fig. 21-8).[22]

Gingival Troughing

The CO_2 and diode lasers are useful in bloodless gingival troughing before impressioning. This eliminates the need for retraction cords and vasoconstrictors. The laser tip is placed below the height of the gingival crevice, and the tissue is "ledged" to expose the margin of the preparation. This procedure is technique sensitive and must be done carefully to prevent inadvertent damage to the tooth (Fig. 21-9).

HARD TISSUE

Osseous Crown Lengthening

Cosmetic and restorative surgery may involve osseous tissue. The erbium laser has been shown to be safe and effective at removing

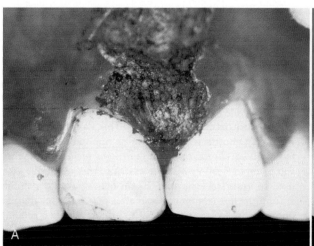 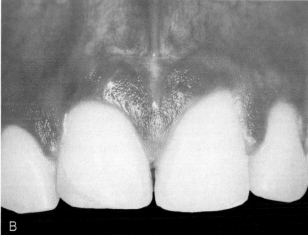

FIGURE 21-7 A, Immediate postoperative view. **B,** Two-week postoperative view showing removal of a maxillary frenum. (Courtesy Alan Winner, DDS, New York, NY.)

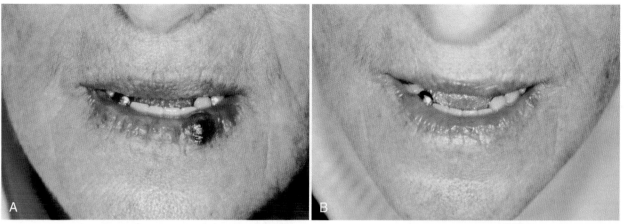

FIGURE 21-8 A, Venous lake of mandibular lip. **B,** Lip after ablation of lesion with argon laser. (Courtesy John Sexton, DMD, Boston, MA.)

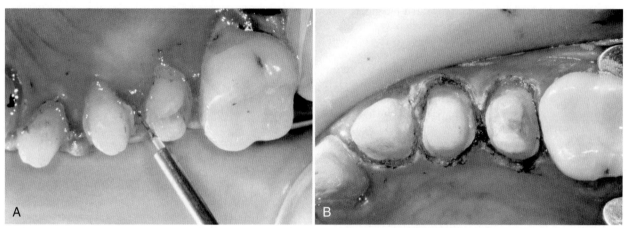

FIGURE 21-9 A, Intraoperative view of gingiva surrounding crown preparations. **B,** Gingival troughing before impression making using a diode laser and fiberoptic delivery.

osseous tissue.[23] Because all lasers are "end cutting" and "side safe," they may be used in a novel approach to osseous crown lengthening. The small fiber diameter and the ability of the erbium laser to affect both soft and hard tissue in the gingival sulcus permit this "flapless" osseous crown lengthening procedure to be used to apically reposition the osseous crest and alter the soft tissue morphology so that proper contours are achieved (Fig. 21-10).

Although the healing rate following bone removal with an Er:YAG laser "bone drilling" has been reported to be equivalent or even quicker than that following bone removal with a bur the healing rate observed following "flapless" crown lengthening made possible by using an erbium laser has been seen to be extremely fast relative to standard osseous surgery, usually with no evidence of the surgery after 2 weeks.[24] It would be expected that the Er, Cr:YSGG would have similar results (Fig. 21-11).[17]

Tooth Preparation. The Er:YAG, Er, Cr:YSGG, and excimer lasers can efficiently remove tooth structure without damage to adjacent structures or the dental pulp.[i] Advantages of laser use include the elimination of anesthesia in some situations[26] and the quiet function of the laser compared with the sound of the dental handpiece. Disadvantages include the

lack of long-term clinical studies, the difficulty in performing complex restorative procedures, and the irregular surface produced by the laser, which makes it unsuitable for indirect restorations such as inlay or crown preparations.[27] With time and new technological modifications, these disadvantages may become less problematic.[27]

Cosmetic Skin Resurfacing

The Er:YAG laser and the CO_2 laser (using a high power, short pulse configuration such as "superpulsing") can selectively remove the surface epidermis and the papillary dermis of the skin while leaving the underlying reticular dermis and adnexal (epithelial-based) structures. This allows internal wound vertical migration of epithelium as opposed to the adjacent basal cell horizontal migration normally seen. Because the result is rapid healing without scarring, this technique can be used to "resurface" the skin. It can help remove the wrinkles around the lips commonly seen after prosthetic rehabilitation of an overclosed stoma and with chronic smoking, prolonged sun exposure, and aging skin. The procedure is performed by oral and maxillofacial surgeons and can be extended to include the entire perioral region or even the entire face.[23,28]

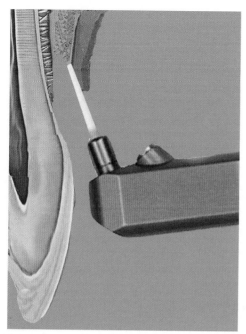

FIGURE 21-10 A cross-section of the dental architecture after soft-tissue gingivoplasty and access to the crestal bone. (From Magid KS, Strauss RA: Laser use for esthetic soft tissue modification. *Dent Clin North Am* 51:525-545, 2007).

LASER SAFETY

Despite being outstanding surgical tools, lasers are inherently dangerous.[29] However, with proper caution and case selection, laser surgery should be as safe as any other modality.

Safety parameters vary to some extent based on differing absorption patterns. Each particular wavelength requires a different set of safety glasses to absorb that particular wavelength. One constant, however, is that all persons in the operatory, especially the patient, must wear appropriate eye protection with side shields.

Flammable items should be eliminated from the surgical field or thoroughly saturated with water to prevent them from igniting. Such items as gauze, cotton rolls, and cotton pellets are especially likely to be a problem if dry and touched by the laser beam. Flammable liquids or gases used for anesthesia or in the operatory should also be considered a danger and avoided. Cleaning agents and alcohol are common flammables. Although oxygen and nitrous oxide are not flammable, they do support combustion and if present in the surgical field could lead to a catastrophic event should something within the field catch fire. The current scientific literature should be consulted before these agents are used in conjunction with lasers.

Wet gauze should be placed in the mouth to protect adjacent tissues and teeth. A CO_2 laser needs only 1 watt-second (i.e., one watt of power in contact with the tooth for 1 second) to cause enamel damage.

A common byproduct of the photothermal laser effect is steam mixed with cellular and tissue debris. This smokelike material, the *laser plume*, contains intact biologic material, including some particles. It is vital for the surgical team to avoid surface contact or inhalation of the plume to prevent disease transmission. This can be avoided by using high-power smoke evacuators fitted with biologic filters and special laser masks that filter out smaller than usual particulate matter.

Because the laser can work at great distances from the target, it is important to take appropriate steps to prevent accidental lasing of unintended targets. This can be prevented by placing the laser in standby mode before removing the handpiece from the mouth using a covered foot pedal and having an assistant engage and disengage the laser for the dentist (in place of the dentist reaching over to put the machine in standby while it is still active).

Other safety rules exist, and it is important to consult the current scientific literature before using a laser.

CONCLUSION

Laser use in cosmetic dentistry has many advantages. A thorough understanding of related physics, control parameters, indications and contraindications, and safety is essential. As more wavelengths become available, laser use for both hard and soft tissue cosmetic procedures will inevitably increase.

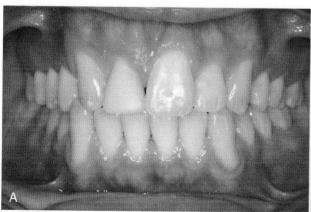
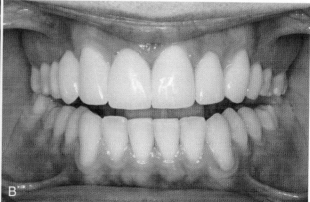

FIGURE 21-11 A, Patient with asymmetric gingival architecture between the two maxillary central incisors. **B,** The same patient after laser "flapless" surgery and placement of esthetic restorations.

REFERENCES

1. Einstein A: Zur Quanten Theorie der Stralung, *Phys Zeit* 18:121, 1917.
2. Maiman TH: Stimulated optical radiation in ruby, *Nature* 187:493-494, 1960.
3. Stern RH, Sognnaes RF: Laser beam effect on dental hard tissues, *J Dent Res* 43:873, 1964.
4. Goldman L et al: Effect of laser beam impact on teeth, *J Am Dent Assoc* 70:601-606, 1965.
5. Myers TD, Myers WD: In vivo caries removal utilizing the Nd:YAG laser, *J Mich Dent Assoc* 67:66, 1985.
6. Keller V, Hibst R: Experimental studies of the application of the Er:YAG on dental hard substances. I, *Lasers Surg Med* 9:338, 1989.
7. Keller V, Hibst R: Experimental studies of the application of the Er:YAG on dental hard substances. II, *Lasers Surg Med* 9:345, 1989.
8. Featherstone JDB, Nelson DGA: Laser effects on dental hard tissues, *Adv Dent Res* 1(1):22, 1987.
9. Neev J et al: Scanning electron microscopy and thermal characteristics of dentin ablated by a short-pulse XeCl excimer laser, *Lasers Surg Med* 13:353-362, 1993.
10. Cozean C et al: Dentistry for the 21st century: Erbium:YAG laser for teeth, *J Am Dent Assoc* 128:1080, 1997.
11. Keller U, Hibst R: Effects of Er:YAG laser in caries treatment: a clinical pilot study, *Lasers Surg Med* 20(1):32, 1997.
12. Strauss RA: Laser management of discrete lesions. In Catone G, Alling C, editors: *Laser applications in oral and maxillofacial surgery*, Philadelphia, 1997, Saunders.
13. Bornstein E: Near-infrared dental diode lasers: scientific and photobiologic principles and applications, *Dent Today* (3):102-108, 2004.
14. Gaspar L, Szabo G: Removal of benign oral tumors and tumor-like lesions by CO_2 laser application. *J Clin Laser Med Surg* 7(5):33-36, 1989.
15. Pogrel MA, McCracken KJ, Daniels TE: Histologic evaluation of width of soft tissue necrosis adjacent to carbon dioxide laser incisions, *Oral Surg Med Oral Pathol* 70:564-568, 1990.
16. Basu MF, Frame JW, Rhys-Evans PH: Wound healing following partial glossectomy using the CO2 laser, diathermy, and scalpel: a histologic study in rats, *J Laryngol Otol* 102:322, 1988.
17. White JM, Goodis HE, Rose CL: Use of the pulsed Nd:YAG laser for intraoral soft tissue surgery, *Lasers Surg Med* 11:455, 1991.
18. Aranoff BL: CO2 laser in surgical oncology. In Kaplan J, editor: *Laser surgery*, Proceedings of the First and Second International Symposiums on Laser Surgery, 1978, Tel Aviv, OTPAZ, pp 191-216.
19. Fisher SE, Frame JW: The effects of the carbon dioxide surgical laser on oral tissues, *Br J Oral Maxillofac Surg* 22:414, 1984.
20. Rhys Evans PH, Frame JW, Branddrick J: A review of carbon dioxide laser surgery in the oral cavity and pharynx, *J Laryngol Otol* 100:69, 1986.
21. Wlodawsky RN, Strauss RA: Intraoral laser surgery, *Oral Maxillofac Surg Clin North Am* 16: 149, 2004.
22. Strauss, RA Coleman M: Lasers in major oral and maxillofacial surgery. In Convissar RA, editor: *Principles and practice of laser dentistry*. St Louis, 2011, Mosby.
23. Lewandrowski KU, Lorente C, Schomacker TJ, et al: Use of the Er:AYAG laser for improved plating in maxillofacial surgery: comparison of bone healing in laser and drill osteotomies, *Lasers Surg Med* 19(1):40-45, 1996.
24. McGuire MK, Scheyer ET: Laser-assisted flapless crown lengthening: a case series, *Int J Periodont Restor Dent* 31(4):357-364, 2011.
25. Dostálová T, Jelínková H, et al. Dentin and pulp response to Erbium:YAG laser ablation: a preliminary evaluation of human teeth, *J Clin Laser Med Surg* 15(3):117-121, 1997.
26. Zanin F et al: Er:YAG Laser: Clinical experience based upon scientific evidence, *SPIE* 2(6), 2001.
27. Visuri SR, Walsh JT, Wigdor HA: Erbium laser ablation of dental hard tissue: effect of water cooling, *Lasers Surg Med* 18:294, 1996.

22

Esthetics and Oral Photography

Kenneth W. Aschheim and Franklin D. Wright

DIGITAL DENTAL PHOTOGRAPHY

Dental photography has become an important adjunct to dental records, informed patient treatment planning, and communications with dental laboratories and dental insurance companies. But perhaps its most important use is in the field of esthetic dentistry. Technologic advances involving computers, large format interoperatory video monitors, and high quality digital photography have ushered in an exciting new era in dental esthetic management.

Because intraoral and extraoral digital dental photography has become an essential tool in documenting esthetic outcomes, proficiency in digital photography is necessary. It is important to understand how to incorporate photography into the esthetic practice, to master the appropriate photographic techniques, and to possess the suitable armamentarium.

The evolution of digital photography from a fledgling, inferior-quality, emerging technology to one that produces precise, detailed images has occurred very rapidly. Historically, film-based photography, which had not evolved significantly from its peak in the 1970s, remained the standard form of photography for dental use. The cumbersome process of exposing an image on film, removing the film from the camera, and transporting it to a laboratory for development and printing was time consuming and fraught with potential errors. The time delay between "clicking the shutter" and viewing the photograph resulted in the use of photographs being a "luxury" rather than a routine part of dental practice, particularly when esthetics was involved.

The current dental digital camera system is composed of a high quality 35-mm format digital single lens reflex (DSLR) camera body with a minimum image size of 12 megapixels and through-the-lens (TTL) exposure metering. The system will also require a compound zoom lens for taking orientation images, a macro (close-up) setting for highly detailed macro images, and a ring flash or an outboard point flash that attaches to the barrel of the lens (either single or dual). All flashes should have a power source (battery) that is independent of the camera's power source.

A new class of cameras, mirrorless interchangeable lens cameras (MILCs), offers some of the advantages of a DSLR camera (e.g., interchangeable lenses) but is smaller and less expensive because they do not have mirror-based optical systems. However, sensors size (see later), lens quality, and choices of flash accessories can vary greatly in MILCs, making a direct comparison with DSLR cameras difficult.

Additional armamentarium includes cheek retractors and mirrors. Digital camera technology continues to evolve with minimal cost differences between newer generations of equipment.

USES OF DENTAL PHOTOGRAPHY

Quality Control

Dental photography can be an effective quality control measure. An image resolution of twelve megapixels or larger will allow sufficient magnification of the dental image to highlight imperfections that the clinician may be unable to see without magnification.

Patient Records

Digital photographs are an effective treatment-planning adjunct. With a thorough medical history, intraoral charting, study casts, radiographs and intra- and extraoral photographs, treatment planning may be accomplished almost as if the patient were present. In addition, attaching a photographic image to the patient's chart or digital record facilitates instant recall of that patient by all staff members.

The authors and publisher wish to acknowledge Dr. Mark King for his contribution on this topic to previous editions.

Case Presentation

Digital photographs of the patient's preoperative clinical situation enhance the patient's understanding and acceptance[1-3] of a proposed treatment plan, especially when accompanied by a portfolio of "before" and "after" images of similar successfully treated patient. Digital photographs combined with computer imaging software can be used to predict clinical results.

CLINICAL TIP

Although the computer simulation may yield mutually agreeable results between the dentist and the patient, only the dentist can determine if a treatment plan exists that can produce these results. Because most of the techniques used by computer software to "rehabilitate" an arch are different from those used by a dentist to fabricate a prosthesis, a less desirable clinical result may occur. Computer imaging systems (CISs) can be extremely valuable in these patients because the dentist can simulate these limitations. This prevents unrealistic patient expectations and documents the possibility of less-than-optimal results.

Treatment Documentation

Before and after digital photographs provide accurate and instant visual documentation of treatment.

Laboratory Communication

A color image of the restorative case facilitates communication with the dental laboratory. Sending digital images to the dental laboratory is simple and instantaneous. Images of the shade tab positioned over the prepared tooth to show the shades of the adjacent teeth increases the chance of esthetic success. In addition, a shade tab can be placed adjacent to the prepared tooth if the underlying shade (stump shade) is required (e.g. when a porcelain laminate veneer is to be fabricated). A high-quality image may not capture the subtle differences between shades with complete accuracy, but the important parameter is the shade of the tab relative to the shade of the tooth. When the laboratory technician compares the actual tab with the image, appropriate adjustments can be made.

CLINICAL TIP

Careful metering of the flash is necessary to prevent "flash burn," which is an overexposed (white) area in a digital photograph created when too much light is emitted from the flash. A flash-burned image prevents the laboratory from compensating for the color discrepancy of the tooth/shade tab in the image when compared with the shade tab they will use to make the restoration. Flash burn can be prevented by raising the ISO or increasing the distance of the flash from the lens by using a point flash with a longer bracket.

Dental Specialist Communication

High-quality digital images can be sent to other clinicians, thus facilitating the "team" approach to comprehensive dental care. Images of oral or perioral pathology can be captured and forwarded to an oral pathologist or oral surgeon for macroscopic review.

Insurance

Submitting color images as part of dental insurance claims may increase the chances of treatment plan acceptance. Often the condition in question is not radiographically evident and a color image may be more helpful. A claim can be made for possible reimbursement for digital photographs using the American Dental Association code 00471.

Education

Digital photographs can be used when lecturing at dental meetings, study clubs, or in table clinics. Images can also be used in publications or, as mentioned above, in patient consultation. Again, a release signed by the patient is necessary before any such use of images.

Community Service

Presentations to local organizations raise the dental health consciousness of the community, improve the image of the profession and expand the dentist's future patient base by creating a greater awareness of advances and available services.

Marketing

The effective use of digital photographs can be a tremendous asset to a dental practice wishing to market its services. The photographs can be used for both internal and external marketing.[1-3] Patients may feel more welcome and important when images of their teeth are created, and on completion of treatment pre- and postoperative images can be sent to them. Additionally, before and after images of different treatments can be incorporated into a patient newsletter (see Chapter 26). Representative esthetic cases can be illustrated in a three-panel brochure format, printed, and made available in the dental office reception area. Digital photographs significantly enhance the effectiveness of a practice's website (see the section on the Internet in Chapter 26). If the dentist involves the staff in this area of the practice, the collective creative capacity of the group can be tapped.

CLINICAL TIP

The dentist should obtain a signed release from the patient to display his or her images (especially full-face photographs) on a website or in other marketing or educational materials (see Chapter 27).

Medicolegal Concerns

Any and every form of record keeping is vital for the historical preservation of patient consultation and treatment, particularly if needed for defense litigation. Color preoperative and postoperative images can be critical in esthetic treatments because the quality of the result is subjective.

BASIC PRINCIPLES OF PHOTGRAPHY

Terminology[4-7]

It is possible to use equipment that is so automated the operator needs no particular knowledge to achieve the desired results.

However, knowledge of the workings of the digital camera is advantageous (Fig. 22-1).

Shutter. The shutter is a device inside the digital camera body that controls the flow of light into the camera, allowing it to strike the digital sensor (where the digital image is created) for a defined period of time (the shutter speed). Each shutter speed setting is exactly one-half the speed of the next highest setting. When a flash unit is attached to the camera, the digital camera's programming will usually calculate the precise amount of additional light required, and time the flash with the shutter speed to create an optimum image. A flash is usually needed to produce additional light. Macro images, which are a significant component of dental photography, require precise flash timing and proper shutter speed. DSLR cameras will automatically calculate the correct aperture setting (see the following section on Aperture.) when the user selects a specific shutter speed if the camera is set in shutter priority mode. Macro flashes typically require a 1/125th second shutter speed.

Aperture. The aperture is the opening inside the lens that controls the amount of light that strikes the digital sensor. The terms "aperture setting," "aperture size," and "f-stop" are synonymous. The terms refer to the size of the opening of the aperture selected by the operator (or the camera when it is in a fully automatic setting) (Fig. 22-2).

The various aperture settings are indicated on a dial of the lens, in the viewfinder, or both. The aperture is set before the image is captured and indicates the amount of opening of the lens. Each successive increase in aperture size allows exactly one-half the amount of light to reach the sensor. However, the larger the aperture, the smaller the corresponding f-stop number. If the camera is set in aperture priority mode, DSLR cameras will automatically calculate the correct shutter speed setting (see earlier) when the user selects a specific aperture setting. The smaller the aperture, the greater the depth of field.

Dentistry uses two significantly different aperture settings. Portrait style images showing the full-face and smile usually require an f-11 setting. For intraoral images, more depth of field is necessary, which is compensated for by changing to an f-16 or f-22 setting.

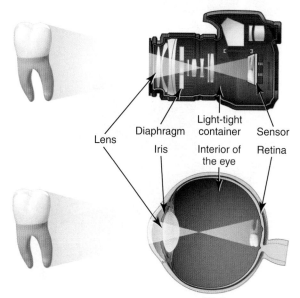

Lens   Diaphragm   Light-tight container   Sensor

Iris   Interior of the eye   Retina

FIGURE 22-1 An DSLR camera mechanism "sees" in a manner similar to the human eye.

CLINICAL TIP

When using an automatic setting for image capture, the camera's focus programming may not produce an adequate depth of field.

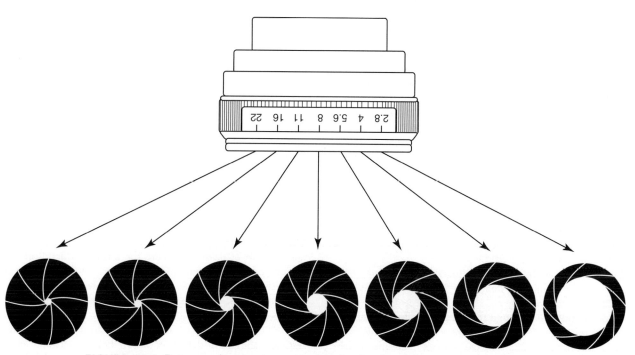

FIGURE 22-2 F-stop numbers are inversely related to the size of the aperture; that is, a lower number means a larger opening. Above, from left to right, F-22 to F5.6.

If not, it may be necessary to switch the camera to either an aperture priority mode or manual mode (both the aperture and shutter speed are set by the user) and manually change the aperture to f-22. A ring flash attached to the front of the lens and synchronized automatically with the digital camera may be necessary to provide enough light to properly expose intraoral images.

Focus. Focusing refers to the degree of clarity of the image. This clarity is controlled by viewing the object being photographed in the view finder or LCD screen and either moving the entire camera toward or away from the object until it becomes focused. The lens controls the magnification of the object being photographed in addition to the f-stop. The lens barrel can be moved to change the magnification by rotating the focusing ring of the lens toward the object to increase the magnification or away to decrease magnification. Often, changing the magnification will require refocusing.

If the dentist desires to create before and after images of an esthetic case, the lens should be focused at a fixed distance. This is done by setting the focal length of the lens at 3 feet and then moving the camera toward and away from the object until it is properly focused. By maintaining the same focal length for a series of images, their magnification will be identical and the resulting images will be the same size. These images serve as effective and attractive marketing materials.

In aperture priority setting, f 5.6 is usually a good starting point for full-face images and f 22 for intraoral images. In aperture priority, setting the camera will automatically synchronize the flash so that the correct amount of flash filled lighting is added to optimize the image. Because of the depth of field issues in taking intraoral images, it may be necessary to manually increase the flash exposure time one setting for proper expose, especially when taking images of molars. Because of the depth of field issues in taking intraoral images, it may be necessary to manually increase the flash exposure time one setting for proper exposure, especially when taking images of molars.

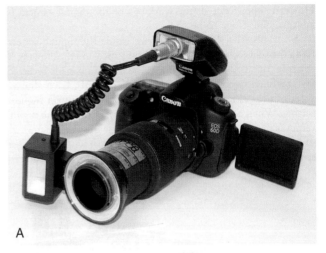

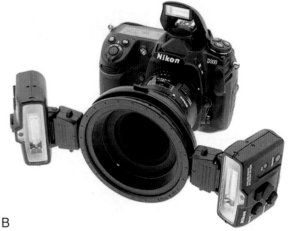

FIGURE 22-3 A, Lester Dine Canon 60D body with a Tamron 90mm Macro Lens with both a point source flash and a ring flash. **B,** Nikon D300 with a macro lens and wireless dual point source flash.

Image Capture Speed (ISO/ASA) Setting

In film photography, ISO/ASA was a measurement of how sensitive the film was to light. Film with lower light sensitivity had a lower ISO/ASA number but produced images with less graininess; therefore the quality of the image was not decreased when it was greatly enlarged. The principal is identical in digital photography wherein the ISO/ASA controls the sensitivity of the image sensor. Higher ISO/ASA settings increase light sensitivity but also increase digital "noise." Modern digital cameras have been automatically programmed to set the ISO/ASA. If the dentist chooses to override the automatic setting of this parameter, a setting similar to the normal daylight setting of ISO/ASA 100 is recommended. Because dental macro photography is always performed with a macro flash, the lack of optimal lighting conditions is rarely an issue. However, the ISO/ASA may need to be increased if the aperture cannot be set to F16 to allow for adequate depth of field.

Light Source. In macro photography, the usual light source is either a single or dual point flash or ring light flash (Fig. 22-3).

By connecting the flash unit to the camera, either by cable or wirelessly, the camera's settings for the exposure will be transmitted to the flash unit and the exact amount of additional light necessary from the flash to properly create the image will be produced.

Depth of Field. The depth of field is the range of distance from the lens within which objects appear in focus (Fig. 22-4).

In dental photography, the more depth of field achieved, the sharper the image in front of and behind the specific object being focused on. In flash photography, the two variables that control depth of field are the aperture size and the distance from the focused image. A smaller aperture (i.e., a larger f-stop) and a larger distance from the image will increase the available depth of field. Therefore macro photography requires more light because smaller aperture openings are used in order to maximize the depth of field. As the camera is moved farther away from the subject for full-face images, the lighting requirements demand a larger aperture size. This greater distance from the object helps compensate for the larger aperture opening, thus maintaining good depth of field. To achieve the maximum depth of field, the photographer should focus one-third the distance into the desired depth of field (see clinical tips following).

Magnification. Magnification indicates the relationship between the size of the object captured by the sensor and the size of the actual object. These relationships are expressed as ratios. If the size of the object captured on the sensor is exactly the same size as the actual object, the magnification is 1:1. A magnification of 1:2 means the object captured on the sensor

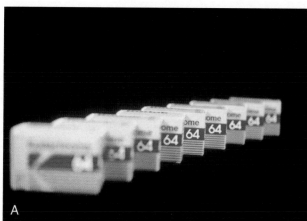

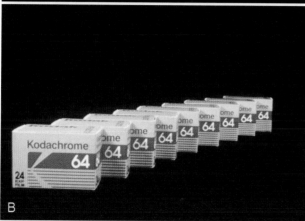

FIGURE 22-4 A, Small depth of field, large aperture size (f/2.8). **B,** Large depth of field, small aperture size (f/32).

is one-half the actual size of the object. Most macro photographs are taken at approximately 1:1.2 or 1: 1.5. Full-face views are usually taken in the 1:8 or 1:10 range. Uniform magnification should be used when documenting various stages of a dental case because this produces images of identical sizes. In dental esthetic cases, with uniform magnification, the before, during, and after images will all be the same size and thus be easier to compare when viewing.

Composition. The term *composition* simply refers to the content of the photograph. The image should contain only those items intended for viewing. Often magnification is the only variable that needs to be changed to achieve proper composition. Superfluous objects in images are very distracting.

Bracketing. Bracketing is the process of creating a series of images from slightly underexposed to slightly overexposed. The photographer can then select the preferred image. Many DSLR cameras (and some more advanced compact cameras) have a feature called automatic exposure bracketing that can automatically create these images.

CLINICAL TIP

Ideally the dentist should take a series of test pictures when the camera is initially purchased in order to determine the optimal settings for different types on intraoral and extraoral photographs as well as becoming familiar with the camera operation.

DIGITAL CAMERAS FUNDAMENTALS

Camera Sensor

Sensor Type. The two main digital image sensors used today, the charged coupled device (CCD) and complementary metal oxide semiconductor (CMOS), were invented in the late 1960s and early 1970s. CCDs are based on analog capacitive technology, which converts incoming light into electron charges that are then converted to a digital signal.[8,9] The CMOS image capture devices are composed of arrays of tiny sensors that capture the light energy and transfer it to a voltage converter as an analog signal that the image sensor's algorithm converts to a digital image. CMOS sensors consume less power and are less expensive to manufacture than CCD sensors.[10]

Because all the energy of the photodiodes on the CCD chip is dedicated to image capture, CCD image quality is more uniform (better) than CMOS. One tradeoff is that CCD image processing takes more energy to create the image than CMOS, which slows the image capture (images per second). This difference in burst rate can be a problem when taking images in a continuous image capture camera mode.

Some modified CCD cameras use three separate CCDs, one each for red, blue, and green light, to capture the light energy that composes the image. "Light coming into the camera lens is split by a trichroic prism assembly, which directs the appropriate wavelength ranges of light to their respective CCDs."[11] Because these cameras use a separate CCD for red, blue, and green light, there is no Bayer filter and they achieve much better precision than single CCD cameras.[12] These cameras are referred to as three-CCD or 3CCD cameras and are more expensive than single CCD cameras.

CMOS sensors capture light in the same manner as CCD sensors with one major difference. Each pixel on the CMOS chip "... has its own charge-to-voltage conversion, and the sensor often also includes amplifiers, noise-correction, and digitization circuits, so that the chip outputs digital bits ... With each pixel doing its own conversion, uniformity is lower"[13] when all the pixels are assembled to create the image. Therefore, compared with CCD images, CMOS image quality is not as good. Generally CMOS-based cameras use less energy and are usually less expensive than comparable CCD cameras. Most manufacturers produce CCD-based cameras because of their superior image quality, although the CMOS cameras are improving. Either sensor type is perfectly acceptable for dental digital photography.

Sensor Resolution. Resolution is measure of the number of pixels (the smallest resolvable area) of an image. Sensors are also available in different sizes; the larger the size, the greater the number of pixels. Both sensor size and resolution have a direct bearing on the quality of the image produced. Traditionally, resolution was used as the single metric to define image quality, although this is no longer the case. The number of pixels was approximated by multiplying the number of horizontal pixels by the number of vertical pixels (typically measured in megapixels, or million, pixels). As sensor size increased the number of pixels became less significant, with low-end cameras capable of resolving the same number of pixels as more expensive DSLR cameras. For dental photography, a resolution of 12 megapixels is considered acceptable.

Sensor Size. A more important sensor metric is its actual size. Sensor sizes are often measured by aspect ratio (width: height), typically 4:3, as well as the diameter measured in mm. The sensor size was typically considered the usable area of this as approximately two thirds of the designated size (Fig. 22-5).

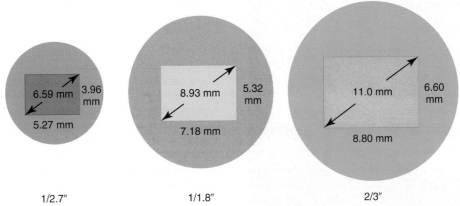

1/2.7"   1/1.8"   2/3"

FIGURE 22-5 Image quality is related to sensor size, with larger sensors yielding higher quality pictures.

Point-and-shoot cameras and mobile phones have very small sensors, whereas DSLR cameras and MILCs have larger sensors. Sensor size is also measured by name such as, Full Frame, APS-C, Micro Four Thirds, and Four Thirds (Box 22-1).

Pixel Density

Pixel density is simply the measurement of the number of individual photoreceptors (pixels) or dots per inch (dpi). The more dpi a sensor has the higher the pixel density. Cameras often have the same resolution but one camera may have a smaller sensor and thus a higher pixel density. Higher pixel densities increase the amount of random digital noise (random distortion in brightness and/or color) as well as decrease the dynamic range (the range of tones from black to white). In addition, higher densities decrease the maximum number of f-stops the camera sensor can capture and thus limit the depth of field capabilities of the camera. Unfortunately, manufactures rarely report a camera's pixel density and it must be calculated based on image resolution and sensor size.

DSLR Sensors Size

DSLR sensors are much larger those found in compact cameras and have lower pixel densities. Therefore DSLR cameras are preferred for dental photographs because they are better able to produce quality photographs in lower light clinical situations, with less noise. Low light sensitivity also allows smaller aperture openings to be used, producing greater depth of field.

Higher-end DSLR cameras use full frame sensors that are the size of traditional 35-mm film (1.7 inches measured diagonally or 864 mm2). Less expensive DSLR cameras use APS size sensors and half the surface area of a full sensor (1.18 inches measured diagonally or 329 mm^2). Another common type is Four-Thirds (0.85 inches diagonal or 225 mm2), which has an even smaller surface area.

Digital Image Capture

When an image is captured by a digital camera, the light energy that the camera's sensor (either CCD or CMOS) captures is then converted to digital electric energy. This directed digital energy is then collected and processed so that the image is created and can be viewed. Because manufacturers produce their own unique processing algorithm, uniform standard digital image file formats have been created. Most digital camera systems produce final images using one of two (or sometimes both) of the most widely recognized standard file formats: raw image files and Joint Photographic Experts Group (JPEG)

Image File Types

Raw Image Files. Raw image files are usually proprietary to the individual camera manufacturer. Only the computer program supplied by the camera manufacturer (and a few stand-alone programs such as Adobe Photoshop) can read, open, and view the files. Raw data files for digital photographs are uncompressed and contain all the information for that particular image file. Consequently, these files are usually large.

Box 22-1			
Approximate Sensor Size of Common Sensor Formats			
Name	Width × Height	Area	≈Aspect Ratio
Full Frame	36 × 24 mm	864 mm^2	3:2
APS-H	28.7 × 19 mm	548 mm^2	3:2
APS-C	22.2 × 14.8 mm	329 mm^2	3:2
Foveon	20.7 × 13.8 mm	286 mm^2	3:2
Four Thirds System	17.3 × 13 mm	225 mm^2	4:3
Point and Shoot 1/1.7"	7.6 × 5.7 mm	43 mm^2	4:3
Point and Shoot 1/1.8"	7.18 × 5.32 mm	38 mm^2	4:3
Point and Shoot 1/2.5"	5.76 × 4.29 mm	25 mm^2	4:3

Raw image files format digital photographs are "read only" and the files cannot be changed or altered in any way unless saved as a separate new file using a different name. This protects the integrity of the original image, which always remains exactly as it was created. This is particularly important from a legal perspective, because the raw image files can be authenticated as being original and unaltered.

A disadvantage of raw image files is that they require a stand-alone program to be viewed. This may require the photographer to purchase an addition computer program, which can be costly and difficult to learn to use.

In addition, transferring raw image files over the internet can be time consuming and cumbersome because of their large size. If a dentist wishes to send several raw images to share with a specialist or dental laboratory, the images may have to be compressed using an additional program (for example a "zip" file) before they can be sent electronically. The recipient must then have the ability to uncompress (reopen or "unzip") the files before the individual images can be viewed. It is also possible to share large files using web hosting and "cloud" technology such as www.DropBox.com or www.DropSend.com.

JPEG Files. JPEG files have built in compression, usually at a ratio of 10:1, with very little perceptible loss of image quality. Because JPEG files are smaller than raw image files, they require less storage space and can be easily emailed. JPEG files are the most commonly used file format for digital images and can be used by virtually any digital imaging software, including many free packages in the public domain.

JPEG files can be altered and resaved with the original file name. Therefore it is impossible to verify and authenticate if a photograph is the original image captured by the camera or if it has been altered.

If digital photographs will be used in a legal proceeding, the courts demand that the original file is authenticated as being unaltered or manipulated. Without this authentication, the courts can choose to disallow the images as evidence.

Whenever any file is altered and saved with the original name, the already compressed file is recompressed, which can affect the image quality. Digital image specialists recommend only opening the original JPEG file but not re-saving it with the same name if any changes are made. If the file with changes (enhancements) is saved, the "save as" choice in the computer drop down box should be used and the files should be renamed. The original JPEG file should remain unaltered.

Some higher quality digital cameras allow for the creation of both raw and JPEG files, simultaneously, when the images are created. This feature allows the ease of opening and electronically sharing the JPEG files while the security and image details of the digital file are preserved with the raw file format.

Memory Cards

Memory cards, removable storage cards, or flash drives are different names for an electronic data storage device used by digital cameras to store the recorded images on a temporary basis. They are capable of retaining images without the need for power and can be used multiple times.

The type and size of the removable storage card must be matched with the system designed for each specific digital camera.

Memory cards vary in storage capacity and speed. Before use these cards must be prepared (formatted) in order to receive and store the data. The amount of information a memory card can hold (capacity) varies with the resolution setting of the camera, the quality of the image being stored, and the file type (i.e., raw or JPEG) of the image.

Bundled Software

Manufacturers supply an installation and setup program disk with a digital camera to facilitate the use of an individual digital camera and the digital image files it creates. The camera is connected to the computer with a physical cable or wirelessly after the program disk installation is completed as part of the camera setup process. This final setup step verifies the camera is recognized by the computer so the images created by the camera can be uploaded (sent) to the computer.

Digital Image Storage

Digital imaging requires devices to store the captured images. Many DSLR cameras have extremely limited or no built-in memory to store the digital photographs, therefore another means to store the captured images is required. This storage is managed with two different methods: direct image storage and indirect image storage.

Direct Storage. The direct method of image storage allows the camera to send images electronically to a computer or stand-alone storage device, either wirelessly using Bluetooth or with Wi-Fi technology.

Most wireless technology requires that the receiving device be within a specified distance or within the same network group of the storage device to function

Indirect Storage. A DSLR camera stores images on a media storage card that can be removed from the camera and placed in a computer's digital card reader. The camera can also be physically connected to the computer via a Universal Series Bus (USB) or Firewire cable, and the images can be copied to a specified folder on the computer.

Storage and Archiving Digital Images

After the digital photographs are transferred, the images must be protected from inadvertent, unexpected, catastrophic, and unrecoverable loss from computer or hard drive "crashes" (when a computer or hard drive permanently fails to operate), computer virus or malware infections, flooding, fire, or computer theft, to name a few. Storing and preserving the digital images requires a standardized technique to ensure that the digital image files are redundantly and repeatedly backed up.

Most digital photographers create files on their computer that collect and store all the digital photographs associated with that particular event. Once these files are uploaded (copied) to the computer, they are erased from the camera's digital storage card and the only copy that exists is the single copy on the host computer. To protect against a corruption or loss of the file, the files stored on the host computer must then be backed up so they are protected. There are many ways to create identical digital copies of these files.

The first line of a protection against data loss is an automated, stand-alone, routine backup program. Alternatively, the dentist should manually copy all digital image data to a dedicated stand-alone onsite storage device, such as a computer, on a weekly basis. Additionally, weekly, or more frequent, data backup to a removable hard drive, which is then stored off site (out of the office) to protect it from an electrical surge, fire, or other disaster that could destroy the onsite backup, is also prudent.

The host computer can also suffer from computer or hard disk drive failure. In a dental office the host computer is often a server (a computer that manages software and storage for a group of networked computers). The server can be configured with an automatic redundancy file replication and storage system known as a Redundant Array of Independent Disks (RAID) array. The dental photographer should consult with an information technologist for more information about using a RAID array to protect against data loss.

With the expansion of the uses for the Internet, the use of cloud data transfer and storage can be automatically done via the Internet. Companies that operate cloud data storage systems can be contracted by the dental photographer to automatically copy all the digital image data (and any other data stored on the office computers) every night at a specified time. This method of data backup and storage can be quite cost effective and simple to implement and use. Although most cloud data backup involves some form of data encryption (a protection against the unauthorized viewing of that data), there have been instances of data from cloud storage systems having been accessed illegally and altered, copied, or destroyed. Once the data is uploaded to the cloud of a given vendor, the photographer is no longer in complete control of who can actually ever see access or otherwise use the stored data.

The best solution for the storage and archival preservation of digital photographs is a combination of on-site, off-site, and cloud data storage. This combined approach should provide adequate backup protection. The protocol would include nightly automatic cloud and on-site backups and at least weekly data backup on a removable hard drive that is stored off site.

BASIC ARMAMENTARIUM

The basic equipment required for proper dental photography is a digital camera, a macro lens, a flash unit, accessories such as mirrors and lip retractors, and the memory card.

Digital Camera Body

A DSLR camera with a minimum image resolution of 12 megapixels should be used. High quality need not be expensive. The most common manufacturers of quality camera bodies are Nikon, Fuji, Cannon, and Sony. A DSLR camera body is a minimum requirement for high-quality esthetic images. A mirror and prisms displays an image through the viewfinder (or on the LCD display), which precisely duplicates the image that the camera will produce. This is referred to as "through the lens" (TTL) viewing (Fig. 22-6A). The mirror is repositioned when the "picture" is "taken" to allow the image to be exposed on the sensor (Fig. 22-6B).

Most DSLR camera bodies allow for automatic exposure settings; the programming in the camera automatically adjusts the f-stop, exposure time, and supplemental flash-delivered light for a host of manual settings selected by the photographer. However, using automatic settings will, more often than not, result in an inferior image, especially in macro photography. It is preferable to select a manual setting and bracket image exposures by altering either the exposure time and/or the aperture setting to compensate for issues such as depth of field, focal length, and the amount of light.

Higher quality digital cameras will record date and time information as a permanent part of the image. This data can be important and useful in documenting "before" and "after" images of an esthetic case as well as authenticating the image in a legal proceeding.

Macro Lens

Macro refers to the close-up focusing capability of the lenses. Several reliable macro lenses are on the market that perform well in dentistry. High quality glass lenses allow sharp focus in the entire range of magnification as well as nearly perfect transmission of the light to the digital sensor of the camera, rendering an extremely high-quality image.

With a higher quality DSLR camera, lenses will often be interchangeable (one can be removed and another lens can then be attached to the same camera body). The lens magnifies, focuses, and projects the images onto the camera's sensor.

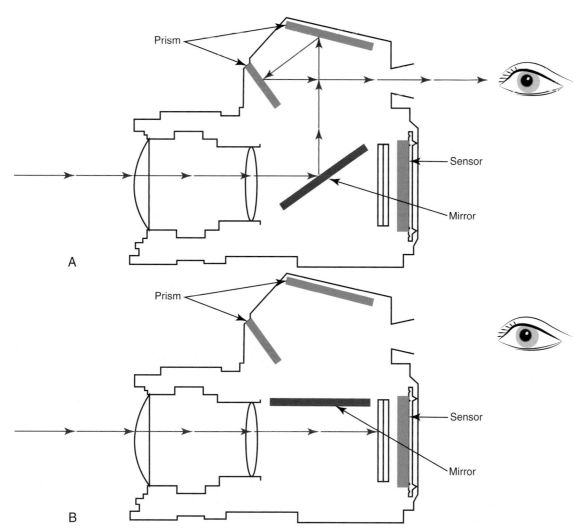

FIGURE 22-6 A, Single lens reflex (SLR) camera with the mirror in the view-finding position. The mirror and prism mechanism allows the viewer to see the exact same image as the camera lens (known as "through the lens" (TTL) viewing). **B,** An SLR camera with the mirror in the "exposing" position. The mirror is lifted out to allow light to expose the sensor.

It is perhaps the most important part of the esthetic image capture process. Better lenses are constructed with high quality glass, which provide sharper optics, better light conduction to the camera's capture device, and magnification that is more precise. This should be seriously considered when purchasing camera components. One crucial feature of the lens is the ability to change its optical properties from a standard exposure setting to a macro setting. Macro images are a critical part of esthetic dentistry because they capture discriminate details that would be overlooked when using lenses that do not have a macro setting. Some macro lenses actually create images greater than life-sized when working at their maximum magnification.

Digital lens size recommendation partially depends on sensor size (see the section on DSLR Sensors Size). Recommendations based on 35-mm film cameras still hold true for DSLR cameras that use 35-mm CCD or CMOS sensors. If the camera's sensor is smaller than the same size lens, it will produce a more magnified image. There is a direct correlation between lens recommendation and sensor size. If a 100-mm lens is recommend for a 35-mm CCD or CMOS sensor, a 60- to 70-mm lens would be recommended for a ⅔ size.

With full-size sensors, full-face views can be easily captured with a 55-mm lens. The best focal length for the macro lens is typically 105 mm, which will allow the dentist to create a 1:1 image without creating a working distance that is too uncomfortably close to the front of the patient's face. Older 105-mm lenses required additional converters or extenders to create an acceptable magnification range and should be avoided.

Flash

To obtain proper lighting effects in intraoral photographs, the light source must be mounted on the end of the lens barrel; otherwise the lips and cheeks will create harsh and unwanted shadows. The choices for proper lighting are a single point, a ring flash, or a ring flash combined with a single point flash or a dual point flash (Figs. 22-4 and 22-5) depending on the photographer's needs and preferences.

A single-point source is mounted on a rotating bracket on the front end of the lens. It can be rotated around the lens to achieve the most advantageous lighting for the image. Generally this type of flash creates a visual environment that is similar to natural light, producing an image with more shadows and with greater depth, contrast and texture (see Chapter 2). The operator must be completely familiar with the proper position of the point light or an entire series of images may not be correctly created. Experimentation by the photographer is necessary to properly coordinate the position of the point flash in dental photography.

Another type of flash used in macro photography is the ring light that completely encircles the end of the lens barrel and provides more even lighting than a point flash, resulting in a flatter surface with less depth, less contrast, and less texture. The major advantage of the ring light is that its position remains unchanged, resulting in one less variable for the operator to control. It is also better suited for the posterior dentition, where it has less of a tendency to wash out some of the color, shadows, and details of the dentition.

The dual-point flash directs light from both sides. Because illumination is bilateral, rather than circumferential as in the ring flash, shadowing and depth for anterior teeth are maintained. The ability of some units to position the flashes closer to the lens produces more optimal posterior photography then when using a single-point flash. However, the dual-point flash is the largest and most expensive of the flash unit configurations.

There is no consensus regarding the optimal light source. Many photographers prefer the more even disbursement of light produced by a ring flash, whereas others favor the depth of field provided by a point flash. Some believe that the dual-point flash is the most ideally suited for dental photography despite its larger size and greater cost. The photographer should be familiar with all types of flashes and the indications for each.

Retractors and Mirrors

Lip and cheek retractors are made of clear or opaque plastic or metal (Fig. 22-7). Clear plastic retractors allow the tissue to be seen through the retractor and the different size double end allows versatility. Plastic retractors can also be reshaped with an acrylic bur to any size the photographer finds useful. Sometimes metal retractors can be used in combination with facial

mirrors (long slender mirrors that reflect facial views and fit between the zygomatic arch and the lower border of the mandible). Front surface glass mirrors perform best because they produce a clearer image when compared with the double (shadowed) view of back surface mirrors. Chrome-plated mirrors also perform well, but due to lower reflectivity may require a larger aperture setting for proper exposure. Two differently shaped mirrors are required, one for full occlusal views and one for facial and lingual views (Fig. 22-8). The clinician with a practice composed of all age groups probably needs at least two sizes of each.

CLINICAL TIP

To determine the type of mirror, place an explorer directly onto the mirror's surface. On a front surface mirror, the "tips" will meet. On a back surface mirror, a space will be seen between the tips. This space represents the distance between the glass and the reflecting surface on the back.

CLINICAL TIP

A commonly encountered problem is mirror fogging caused by the patient's breath. This can be eliminated either by soaking the mirrors in warm water or by having the assistant gently blow air from the syringe onto the mirror while it is in use.

CLINICAL TIP

If saliva comes in contact with the mirror's surface, the mirror must be removed and cleaned to avoid a significant distraction on the finished photograph.

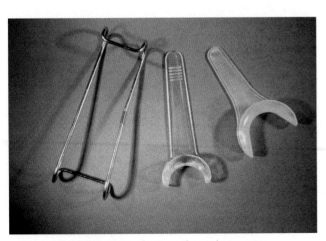

FIGURE 22-7 Plastic and metal retractors.

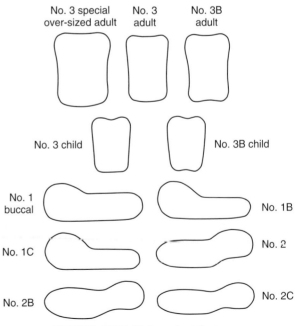

FIGURE 22-8 Various dental mirrors.

CHOOSING A DENTAL PHOTOGRAPHY SYSTEM

Many prepackaged dental photography systems are available. These systems have been created to facilitate the ease of acquiring a "turnkey" system but may limit the specific features the photographer may wish to include. Most large dental supply companies either supply a complete system or can recommend a system available from another vender. The components of the system and how well they work individually and together are more important than cost alone. The camera body, lens, and flash must meet minimum requirements. Treatments involving esthetic makeovers are the most demanding for the dental photographer. Compromises in the selection of components of a digital photography system can result in the creation of poor quality "before and after" images.

CLINICAL TIP

Products are continually updated and revised. Before purchasing a system, confirm with the manufacturer which options are still available, the changes that have been made, and if limitations still exist. New products may have been introduced that result in current products becoming obsolete. Reputable camera shops and specialized online retailers can provide some direction and expertise when assembling a system.

DIGITAL PHOTOGRAPHIC TECHNIQUES

After perseverance and practice, the ability to create high-quality images will become routine. The dental photographer should develop a standard routine for each series of images that are created. For example, the dental office may adopt a practice of taking a series of digital photographs of all new patients. This would include a full-face view, an anterior view with the teeth in occlusion, an anterior view with the incisal edges of the anterior teeth separated, lateral views with the teeth in occlusion, mandibular and maxillary occlusal views, and macro images of the maxillary and mandibular anterior teeth. All images should be created using retractors to separate the lips and cheeks from the teeth. The use of mirrors will facilitate creating images where access with the lens and mounted ring flash would otherwise be impossible.

A specific standard routine should be developed for all esthetic cases, which could include a baseline full-face view and macro images of the maxillary and mandibular anterior teeth, canines and premolars in occlusion, and with the teeth slightly separated. This series of images would then be repeated when the esthetic treatment is completed.

Additional routines can be developed for documentation of dental problems such as fractured cusps, cracked tooth syndrome, caries around large old leaking restorations, or other hard or soft tissue abnormalities.

If a tooth fracture or the size of a defective direct restoration is not sufficiently evident radiographically, a high-quality digital image either attached to a dental insurance claim form or uploaded digitally to third-party payers may facilitate the granting of benefits as well as a significant decrease in the time involved to have the claim processed and paid.

Digital photographs can document treatment complications such as pulpal exposure after caries removal, fractures in teeth after crown preparations, or any other anomaly in the routine delivery of dental care. Despite proper communication to patients at the time of the occurrence, they often do not recall the circumstances at a later date. An image documenting the issue can be quite advantageous.

INTRAORAL TECHNIQUE

A good image is the product of proper equipment, organization, a procedural checklist, and good photographic technique. It is important that the procedure be organized and simplified to reduce the learning curve for new dental team members.

CLINICAL TIP

Care should be taken that the preoperative photograph captures all of the necessary details. The posttreatment image can be repeated at any time but, obviously, the pretreatment image can never be reproduced once treatment has started.

CLINICAL TIP

The dental camera should be readily available near the work area, stored at room temperature in a wall-mounted bracket, a drawer, or on a counter. If the camera is not conveniently accessible, it will be less likely to be used. Similarly, the camera should always remain in the designated area and should not be used for recreational purposes.

Patient Position

Although there are many opinions regarding optimum patient position when creating the images, the least desirable is a supine position. When a patient is lying back, it is very difficult to position the camera so that the front of the lens is parallel with the teeth being photographed. This results in very poor image angles, creating either elongated or foreshortened images. The ability to create the identical camera to object angle in the subsequent posttreatment image is also nearly impossible. Additional problems include shadowing from ambient room lighting, the overhead dental lamp casing shadows from behind the photographer, and flash burn (the flash burst overwhelms the object of the image and only a bright white "cloud" is captured).

Ideally, the patient should sit upright and face the photographer so that both the camera height and teeth being imaged are in the same horizontal plane. The dental chair can be raised or lowered to achieve the proper height. This simple positioning technique will help eliminate the previously described angulation problems. The magnification on the lens should be established and recorded, positioned approximately three feet from the object. Using this magnification for all the photographs in a series will ensure that the before and after treatment photographs are the same size, in the same plane, have the same object to lens distance, and have similar lighting and focus.

Retractors and Mirrors

Once the magnification is set, the retractors and mirrors are placed. The photographer will need to physically move forward or backward and/or slightly laterally until ideal focus at the set magnification is achieved and the plane of the front of the camera lens and the teeth being imaged are parallel.

CLINICAL TIP

Position the retractors so that there is not only a lateral spread of the perioral tissues but also a slight anterior pull. In this position the lips and cheeks are repositioned both laterally and anteriorly away from the teeth and intraoral tissues, providing sufficient access for the flash unit to properly expose the image.

Mouth mirrors are required for a maxillary or mandibular full arch occlusal or lateral facial views.

CLINICAL TIP

To prevent mirror fogging, they can be warmed under running water or the dental assistant can gently blow on with the air syringe.

Camera Mode. Although the camera can be set in automatic mode, manual adjustment is often required.

CLINICAL TIP

When the camera is first purchased, the dentist should experiment to determine which settings produce optimal results.

The camera will most likely need to be set to aperture priority mode with the appropriate f-stop setting—f-5.6 to f-8 for distant anterior views (minimal depth of field) and f-16 to f-22 for macro anterior occlusal or facial views (more depth of field). The flash unit mounted on the front of the lens should be automatically synchronized with the camera setting (or for wired models, the flash cable should be attached to the camera body) so that all that needs to be done is to turn the flash on.

An ideal set of images would include a face view, an anterior dentition view with the lips and cheeks retracted and the teeth in occlusion, a macro image of both the maxillary and mandibular teeth with lip and cheek retraction, a maxillary and mandibular occlusal view, bilateral canine views, and bilateral facial posterior teeth views. Ideally a full set of images should be performed for new patients undergoing extensive treatment as well as all esthetic cases.

A simplified checklist will prevent error:

Armamentarium
+ Appropriate digital camera
+ Appropriate macro lens
+ Appropriate retractors

Clinical Technique
1. Turn on the power unit.
2. Check that the memory card is in place and that there is sufficient free memory on the card.
3. Set the camera in the appropriate mode and f-stop for macro photography.
4. Position the subject, flash, retractors, and mirrors.
5. Choose the desired magnification.
6. Focus while correcting the magnification.

CLINICAL TIP

The single most common beginner's error is incorrect choice of magnification. A typical magnification error involves including the nose and chin in a frontal view of the oral cavity. This extraneous information is distracting for the viewer. The photographer must decide what the photograph should contain and choose the magnification that eliminates everything else.

7. Release the shutter.

CLINICAL TIP

Good intraoral photographs should appear as if the camera were aimed directly at the desired subject regardless of whether mirrors were used. The photographs should be devoid of mirror edges, fingers or thumbs, fog, saliva, lip retractors, or any elements other than the desired aspect of the oral cavity.

CLINICAL TIP

Lip retractors are not always easily eliminated, but clear retractors are an excellent compromise. Some photographs may require only the patient's assistance, whereas others require assistance from the patient, the photographer, and one or even two staff members.

Anterior (Frontal) View

The anterior or frontal view is the most common view used in dental photography (Fig. 22-9*A*). It ranges from a single tooth to a full-face view and may be obtained with or without retractors (Fig. 22-9*B,C*).

Armamentarium
+ Appropriate digital camera
+ Appropriate macro lens
+ Appropriate retractors
(See the section on the Basic Armamentarium earlier in this chapter.)

Clinical Technique
1. Seat the patient semi-upright with the head turned toward the photographer.
2. Place retractors at the corners of the mouth and pull gently outward and forward so that the facial tissue is away from the teeth.
3. If a point light is used, it should be at the 3 o'clock or 9 o'clock position to create a sense of depth with shadows.
4. Set the camera in the appropriate mode and f-stop for macro photography.
5. Hold the camera so that the occlusal plane is perpendicular and centered horizontally to the plane of the digital sensor.
6. Align the patient's midline with the center of the frame. Adjust the magnification (usually 1:2). Compose the photograph to include all relevant teeth and soft tissue.
7. Focus the camera while correcting the magnification.

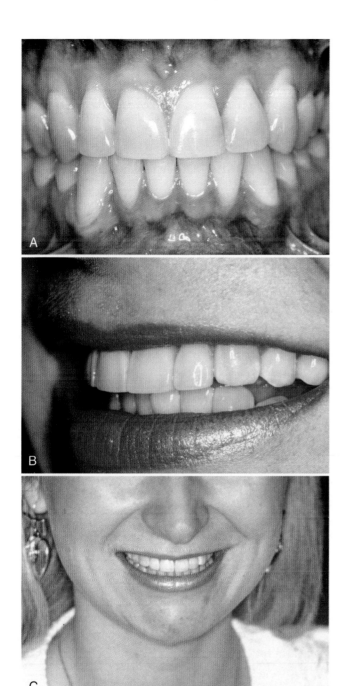

FIGURE 22-9 A, Anterior (frontal) view (1:2 magnifications) with lip retractors (not visible in image). **B,** Relaxed, casual three-quarter view without lip retractors. **C,** Relaxed, casual frontal view without lip retractors.

CLINICAL TIP

To achieve maximum sharpness of the image, focus the camera on the canines, not the central incisors.

Maxillary Occlusal View

The maxillary occlusal view is the most difficult view to obtain and requires patience (Fig. 22-10A). This photograph usually requires assistance from two staff members.

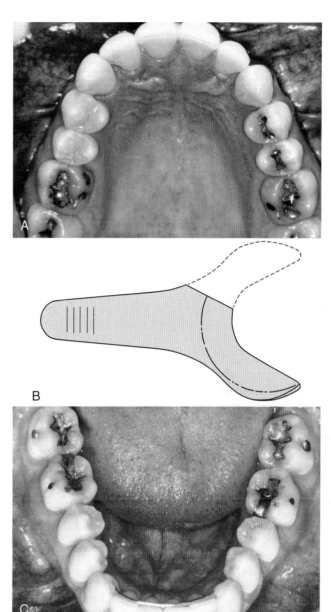

FIGURE 22-10 A, Maxillary occlusal view (1:2 magnification). **B,** A standard cheek retractor can be modified by removing a flange from one of its sides. This provides more working space and allows for better visualization of the dental arch. **C,** Mandibular occlusal view (1:2 magnification).

Armamentarium
+ Appropriate digital camera
+ Appropriate macro lens
+ Appropriate retractors
+ Appropriate mirrors (see earlier)

(See the section on the Basic Armamentarium earlier in this chapter.)

Clinical Technique
1. Seat the patient in a semi-upright position with the head turned toward the photographer.
2. Instruct one of the assistants to gently rotate the retractors upward and outward.

3. Instruct the other assistant to rest a full-arch mirror on the maxillary tuberosity, not on the teeth. The mirror should diverge from the occlusal plane as much as possible so that the camera can be held 90 degrees to the plane of the mirror.
4. If a point light is used, it should be at the 9 o'clock or 3 o'clock position.
5. Set the camera in the appropriate mode and f-stop for macro photography (see earlier).
6. Hold the camera so that the plane of the digital sensor is parallel to the full arch in view.
7. Align the midline of the palate with the center of the frame and adjust the magnification (usually 1:2). Compose the photograph to include all relevant teeth and soft tissue.
8. Focus on the premolar area while correcting the magnification.

Mandibular Occlusal View

The mandibular occlusal view is the reverse of the maxillary occlusal view (Fig. 22-10C).

Armamentarium
+ Appropriate digital camera
+ Appropriate macro lens
+ Appropriate retractors
(See the section on the Basic Armamentarium earlier in this chapter.)

Clinical Technique
1. Seat the patient in the supine position, parallel to the floor.
2. Tip the patient's head back slightly and turn it toward the photographer so that the occlusal plane is parallel to the floor.
3. Rotate the retractors gently downward toward the mandible and outward.

4. Rest a full-arch mirror on the retromolar pad not on the teeth.
5. The mirror should diverge from the occlusal plane as much as possible so that the camera can be held 90 degrees off the plane of the mirror.
6. If a point light is used, it should be at the 9 o'clock or 3 o'clock position.
7. Set the camera in the appropriate mode and f-stop for macro photography.
8. Hold the camera so that the plane of the film is parallel to the full arch in view.

9. Align the midline of the tongue with the center of the frame and adjust the magnification (usually 1:2). Compose the photograph to include all relevant teeth and soft tissues.
10. Focus on the premolar area while correcting the magnification.

Buccal View

Buccal views are ideal for photographing the patient's centric occlusion (Fig. 22-11).

Armamentarium
+ Appropriate digital camera
+ Appropriate macro lens
+ Appropriate retractors
(See the section on the Basic Armamentarium earlier in this chapter.)

Clinical Technique
1. Seat the patient in a semi-upright position with the head facing straight for left buccal views and toward the photographer for right buccal views (reverse for left-handed dental units).
2. Place a buccal mirror distal to the last tooth in the arch. Move it as laterally as possible while at the same time retracting the lip. The mirror also serves as a retractor.

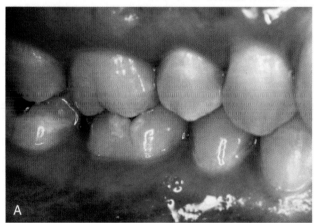
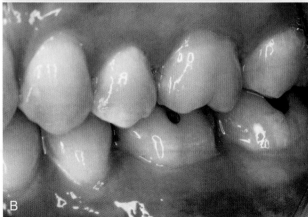

FIGURE 22-11 A, Right buccal view (1:1.2 to 1:1.5 magnification). **B,** Left buccal view (1:1.2 to 1:1.5 magnification).

CLINICAL TIP

Buccal views can be taken without mirrors if a view of the distal end of the terminal molar is not required.

3. If a mirror is used, passively hold a single retractor on the side opposite the mirror.
4. If no mirror is used, pull the retractor on the side being photographed as distally as comfortably possible for the patient. Passively hold the retractor on the side that is not being photographed.
5. If a point source light is used, place it on the same side of the camera as the mirror.
6. Set the camera in the appropriate mode and f-stop for macro photography.
7. Hold the camera so that the plane of the digital sensor is as perpendicular to the mirror as possible.
8. Set the magnification (usually 1:1.2 to 1:1.5 depending on the size and number of teeth in the photograph). Compose the photograph to include from the distal area of the canine to the most posterior tooth, with the plane of occlusion parallel to the film plane and in the middle of the frame.
9. Focus the camera on the premolar area while correcting the magnification.

Lingual View

Lingual views of the maxilla (Fig. 22-12*A,B*) or the mandible (Figs. 22-12*C,D*) are obtained similarly.
+ Appropriate DSLR camera
+ Appropriate macro lens
+ Appropriate film
+ Appropriate retractors
(See the section on the Basic Armamentarium earlier in this chapter.)

Clinical Technique
1. Position the patient semi-upright with the head facing straight for right views and toward the photographer for left views (reverse for left-handed dental units).
2. Place retractors at the corners of the mouth, rotated toward the photographed arch and passive on the opposite side.
3. For a mandibular photograph, place a mirror between the tongue and the quadrant being photographed, distal to the terminal tooth, parallel to the long axis of the teeth, and angled as much as possible so the face of the mirror faces the camera lens. For a maxillary photograph, place the mirror against the palate in the midline, distal to the terminal tooth, parallel to the long axis of the teeth, and angled medially as much as possible so the face of the mirror faces the camera lens.
4. If a point source light is used, place it on the same side of the camera as the mirror.
5. Set the camera in the appropriate mode and f-stop for macro photography.
6. Hold the camera so that the plane of the film is as perpendicular to the mirror as possible.
7. Set the magnification (usually 1:1.5 to 1:1.2). Compose the photograph to include from the distal area of the canine to the most posterior tooth, with the plane of occlusion parallel with the sensor plane and in the middle of the frame.
8. Focus the camera on the distal side of the canine while correcting the magnification.

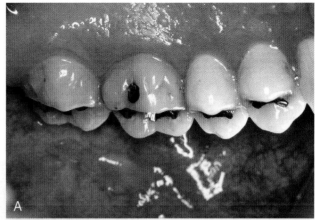
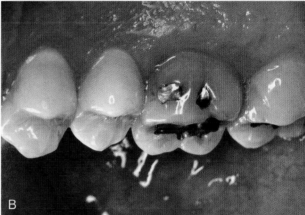
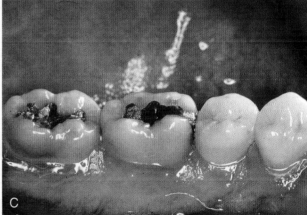
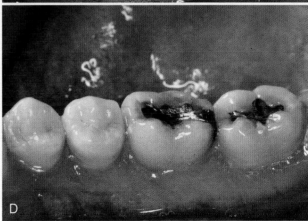

FIGURE 22-12 A, Maxillary left lingual view (1:1.2 to 1:1.5 magnification). **B,** Maxillary right lingual view (1:1.2 to 1:1.5 magnification). **C,** Mandibular left lingual view (1:1.2 to 1:1.5 magnification). **D,** Mandibular right lingual view (1:1.2 to 1:1.5 magnification).

Other Views

Any of the above views can be modified to meet the needs of the user. Usually only changes in magnification and composition are necessary to suit specific needs. For example, if only an occlusal view of a quadrant is necessary, the facial or lingual mirror can be used in a similar manner as that described for the full-arch occlusal view, along with a modification in the magnification. For a view of only the premaxilla, only the necessary portion of a full-arch mirror is used and the magnification is adjusted (1:1.2). The creativity of the photographer can allow for any other specific views that are needed (Fig. 22-13).

EXTRAORAL TECHNIQUE

High quality full-face, and profile photographs require a pleasant colored background (Fig. 22-14). An art store can furnish art paper in a number of suitable colors. The best usually is a

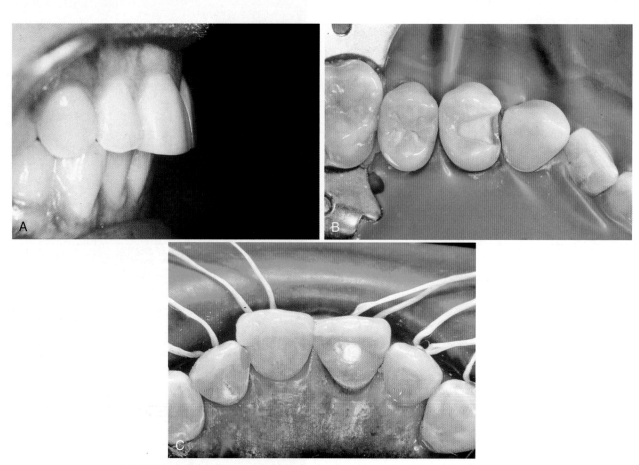

FIGURE 22-13 A, Lateral view. **B,** Occlusal quadrant view. **C,** Premaxilla view.

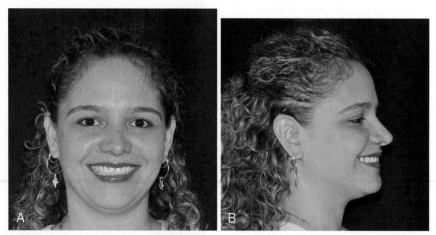

FIGURE 22-14 A, Full-face view (1:10 magnification). **B,** Profile view (1:10 magnification). (From Proffit WR, Fields HW, Sarver DM: *Contemporary orthodontics*, ed 5, St. Louis, 2013, Mosby.)

pastel color that contrasts with normal hair color and skin tones. A soft blue is the best overall. This paper can be taped to the wall in the operatory and removed as needed.

Full-Face View

Armamentarium
* Appropriate DSLR camera
* Appropriate lens
* Appropriate background (optional)
  (See the section on the Basic Armamentarium earlier in this chapter.)

Clinical Technique
1. Position the patient approximately 18 to 24 inches in front of the background to help minimize shadows.
2. Position the head such that a line from the ala of the nose to the tragus of the ear is parallel to the floor.
3. If a point source light is used, place it at the 12 o'clock position.
4. Set the camera in the appropriate mode and f-stop for extra-oral photography.
5. Position the camera vertically at the level of the patient's eyes.

CLINICAL TIP

Many cameras feature a "red eye" reduction flash. Pulsating the flash before taking the photograph causes the subject's iris to contract, thus eliminating the reflection of light off the retina and minimizing the "red eye" effect seen in some photographs.

6. Set the magnification (usually 1:10). Compose the photograph to include from the inferior border of the hyoid to above the top of the head.
7. Focus the camera on the patient's eyes while correcting the magnification.
8. Take a photograph with the teeth in occlusion.
9. Take a second photograph with the patient smiling.

Profile View

Armamentarium
* Appropriate DSLR camera
* Appropriate lens
* Appropriate background (optional)
  (See the section on the Basic Armamentarium earlier in this chapter.)

Clinical Technique
1. Position the patient approximately 18 to 24 inches in front of the background to help minimize shadows.
2. Position the head such that a line from the ala of the nose to the tragus of the ear is parallel to the floor. The teeth should be in occlusion.

CLINICAL TIP

The head should be turned slightly toward the photographer so that the off-side eyelash is just visible. This avoids the appearance of the patient looking away from the camera.

3. If a point source light is used, place it on the side of the camera that the patient is facing. The camera should be in a vertical position at the level of the patient's eyes.
4. Set the camera in the appropriate mode and f-stop for extra-oral photography.
5. Set the magnification (usually 1:10). Compose the photograph so that the profile dominates the center of the frame, with the area just behind the ear visible.
6. Focus the camera on the patient's eyes while correcting the magnification.

CLINICAL TIP

A more relaxed or casual view without lip retractors is useful and appropriate for esthetic dentistry, especially when designed for patient viewing (see Figs. 22-9*B,C*). Never show patients with lips retracted when illustrating esthetic dentistry for patient viewing.

TECHNICAL ERRORS

Some of the problems commonly encountered in the finished photograph can be caused by technical errors. Table 22-1 presents some of the major mistakes made in using the camera and lens system; however, this is not meant to be an exhaustive list.

INTRAORAL IMAGING SYSTEMS

Intraoral imaging systems (IISs) were among the first electronic imaging devices to be used in dentistry. Original IISs were modified gastroenterology endoscopes; however, newer models were designed exclusively for dental use. They are primarily used to enhance clinical visualization by displaying intraoral images on a monitor. These systems can store, retrieve, and reproduce the images. As a category, IISs are slowly becoming integrated with CISs. Digital technology and the integration of image storage and manipulation into dental management programs will change IIS from an independent category to an "acquisition device" for CISs. In addition, many dentists use extraoral digital cameras to capture intraoral images. Newer systems that use smaller, higher resolution

Table 22-1 Common Photographic Problems and Possible Causes

Problem	Possible Causes
Black image	Improperly connected flash Broken flash Improperly positioned point flash Extraneous overhead lighting reflected into mirrors, disrupting the flash Weak flash batteries
Shadows	Weak flash batteries Improperly set flash Incorrect f-stop
Improper exposure	Improperly focused Fog on the mirror
Out of focus image	Camera movement Patient movement

CCD or CMOS sensors combined with light emitting diode (LED) technology have reduced the cost and size of these systems. Some of these systems have been combined with alternative lighting for use as caries detection systems.

Advantages

Intraoral imaging systems have the same advantages as digital photography plus the following.

Greater Intraoral Visibility. They provide an unparalleled view of the oral cavity, allowing the clinician to view areas that are otherwise difficult to see. Systems equipped with special macro lenses allow visualization within endodontic canal systems and periodontal pockets.

Disadvantages

Intraoral imaging systems have the same disadvantages as digital photography plus the following.

Complexity. These systems have a considerable learning curve, although newer models have simplified user interfaces.

Limited Extraoral Imaging. All IISs have been optimized for intraoral viewing. Early models produced a distorted "fish-eyed" appearance when used extraorally. The image quality of a moderately priced digital camera is still superior to that of an IIS when used for extraoral imaging.

Components

Although hardware varies from system to system, all have certain common elements.

1. *Input device.* Input is through a small camera mounted in a hand-held device shaped like a dental handpiece (Fig. 22-15). The image is acquired through a front or side mounted lens coupled with a high-resolution sensor. An LED light source is integrated into the handpiece.
2. *Transmission cable.* A transmission cable is the "wire" that transmits the image from the handpiece to the central processing unit. Current systems typically use a USB cable, although a few wireless models are available.

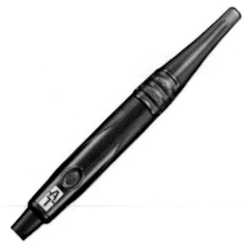

FIGURE 22-15 The optics and broad focal range of the Polaris intraoral camera deliver high quality images which help to improve diagnosis and case presentation. (Courtesy Air Techniques, Inc., Melville, NY.)

3. *Light source.* Early IIS units required a xenon or quartz light source to produce the extremely bright light required by early CCDs. These lights were expensive and required pulsing (repeated switching on and off at a set rate) to function. This produced a stroboscopic flashing accompanied by an audible clicking. Current IIS technology uses continuously illuminating LED light sources similar to those found in light-curing units.
4. *Display/Central processing unit.* Most units communicate directly with an operatory computer.
6. *Video storage unit.* Most units use the computer's hard drive for storage.
7. *Video output device.* Video output devices provide a hard copy (printout) of the displayed image. An office ink jet or color laser printer using photographic quality paper can produce excellent results

---

CLINICAL TIP

Products are continually updated and revised. Before purchasing a system, confirm with the manufacturer which options are still available, the changes that have been made, and if limitations still exist. New products may have been introduced that result in current products becoming obsolete. It is also import to know if a system is upgradable when future enhancements become available.

CLINICAL TIP

A great deal of time and effort is required to master the complexities of intraoral imaging systems. A dealer who provides ample instruction and maintenance support is important. If a "bargain system" does not include servicing, the full capabilities of the system may never be realized.

Clinical Procedure

Although the individual controls of different systems vary greatly, certain elements are common.

Armamentarium
+ Intraoral imaging system

Clinical Technique
1. Adjust the operatory lights for optimum viewing according to the manufacturer's recommendation.
2. Install a new infection control sheath on the handpiece.
3. Aim the camera at the desired image (Fig. 22-16*A*).
   Freeze the image on the screen by activating the appropriate switch or foot pedal.
4. Store the image (Fig. 22-16*B*).
   Print the image (optional).

CLINICAL TIP

A specialized intraoral camera that uses a fluorescence LED/sensor combination can detect incipient caries and cracks in teeth that are not captured may not be captured in normal radiographs for example, the Spectra Caries Detection aid [Air Techniques, Inc.]). The camera detects porphyrins in bacterial populations, which glow red when stimulated with 405 nm light; noncarious enamel glows green (Fig. 22-17).

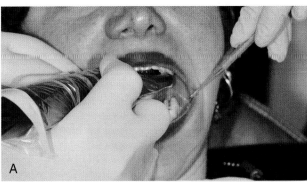

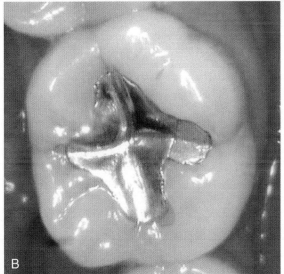

FIGURE 22-16 A, The camera (Polaris) is aimed at the desired image. **B,** The image is stored.

COMPUTER IMAGING SYSTEMS

The computer imaging system (CIS) has revolutionized diagnosis, treatment planning, and case presentation. Intraoral and extraoral images can be accessed, stored, and manipulated. Patients can be shown their current dental condition and the possible results of various treatment plans.

Most CISs perform the following tasks:

1. *Magnify or shrink an image.* CISs can alter the size of the entire image or an individual section of the image.
2. *Crop an image.* CISs can crop (isolate) sections of the image and remove extraneous information, thus focusing on problem areas.
3. *Move an image.* CISs can move a section of an image from one area to another demonstrating, for example, the possible results of proposed orthodontic treatment.
4. *Copy an image.* CISs can duplicate images of individual teeth and move the duplicated image to edentulous areas, enabling the patient to see the possible results of tooth replacement.
5. *Change shading.* The shade of any section of an image can be altered, allowing patients to see the possible results of bleaching, restorations or other shade altering treatments.
6. *Change the shape of an image.* The shape of any section of an image can be altered to allow patients to see the possible results of restorations, esthetic recontouring, or other procedures.

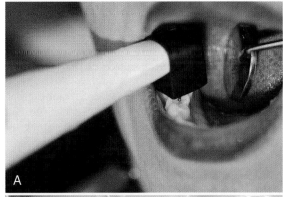

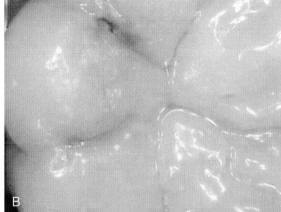

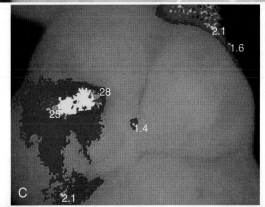

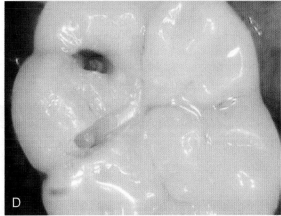

FIGURE 22-17 A, The Spectra caries detection aid uses an interchangeable cable with the intraoral camera to detect incipient caries. **B,** Possible occlusal carious lesion. **C,** The presence of caries is found, see the red areas. **D,** Excavation of the lesion confirms the presence of caries.

7. *Store and retrieve image cutouts.* CISs can save small sections of an image, retrieve them instantly and add them to the appropriate position on the display screen. This creates a "library" of prosthetic parts. The dentist can, for example, instantly show a patient the effects of placing a pontic or wrought wire clasp.

8. *Create a print of the altered image.* Once a treatment goal has been established, a print of the image can be conveyed to the laboratory to aid in the fabrication of the definitive prosthesis.

9. *Take measurements directly from the screen.* Most systems can take measurements of the image on the viewing screen. The measurements can be used when fabricating the restoration.

10. *Manipulate entire facial features.* Some systems were first developed for plastic and cosmetic surgery and can predict the possible results of orthognathic and other maxillofacial surgical procedures.

Advantages

CISs have the same advantages as IISs plus the following:

1. *Create "what-if" scenarios.* Treatment alternatives can be explored by manipulating of images.

2. *Decrease the chance of patient misunderstanding.* Because the patient sees predicted treatment results, less chance of miscommunication exists (however, see the first item listed under "Disadvantages"). However, the patient needs to understand that the computer simulation of the expected treatment results may appear slightly differently than the actual completed treatment (see Chapter 27).

3. *Convey the desired treatment goals to the dental laboratory.* After the dentist and patient produce an acceptable treatment plan, the information can be conveyed to the dental laboratory.

4. *Contain a large capacity storage system.* CISs have large capacity hard disks that can store thousands of images. This increases the ease and efficiency of information retrieval.

5. *Accept images from multiple sources.* All units can accept images obtained from an IIS.

Disadvantages

CISs have the same disadvantages as IISs plus the following:

1. May inaccurately predict results. The major drawback of these systems is that the optimal results predicted on a preoperative computer simulation will not be achieved clinically.

CLINICAL TIP

The method by which images are manipulated is different from the way teeth are clinically treated. Emphasize to the patient that a predictive simulation may not be realized.

CLINICAL TIP

It is uncertain at this time if an inadequate clinical result after a favorable prediction by a computer simulation is a valid basis for litigation. (See the section on Medicolegal Considerations later in this chapter.)

Hardware Components

Initial CISs were sold as proprietary dedicated computers or standard computers preloaded with the CIS software. Current CISs are either hardware- or software based (usually combined with an IIS) or just software based and accept images from any digital imaging device. They share common components.

1. *Input device.* Early CISs used bulky extraoral *RGB* video cameras. Current systems use a digital camera, an IIS, or a digital scanned image from a photograph.

2. *Light source.* Early CISs used extraoral RGB video cameras and they required large photographic studio lights to obtain proper color balance. Current systems use the light source of the input device.

3. *Video display.* CISs are always attached to a computer and use a standard computer flatscreen display.

4. *Video board.* CISs use the standard high-resolution computer graphics adaptor built into computers. Many have additional NTSC/HDMI inputs for analog IISs and video inputs.

5. *Alternate input devices.* All systems manipulate the image with a mouse, trackball, light pen, or other similar device.

6. *Video storage unit.* All systems use standard hard drives or other similar computer-based storage devices

7. *Video output device.* These devices are identical to those discussed for IISs.

Software Components

The major difference between the different computer imaging systems is the software. Software is the most critical part of a CIS system and evolves rapidly. It is important to evaluate the most current version of the software before purchasing a system. Most software programs have certain common elements.

CLINICAL TIP

Because most software allows the importation of an image from almost any source, a user is not limited to a particular hardware/software combination.

1. *Graphical interface.* All programs use a graphical interface, usually under the Microsoft Windows operating system.

2. *Multiple windows.* This allows the simultaneous viewing of multiple images.

3. *Menu driven.* All programs use a cascading menu system, usually under the Microsoft Windows operating system.

4. *Drawing tools.* All use computer "tools" that allow the user to manipulate an image. They include the following:

   A. *Selection/highlighting tool.* This tool aids in selecting the parts of the teeth upon which the dentist wishes to perform a function. The ease in which areas can be selected, usually the most frequent function performed, often determines the general ease of use of the entire *software* package.

   B. *Cut/copy/paste tools.* These allow the removal, duplication, or placement of "teeth."

   C. *Move/flip/rotate tools.* These allow the movement and manipulation of highlighted "teeth."

   D. *Color tools.* These allow color manipulation of teeth.

   E. *Other tools.* These specialized tools perform numerous preprogrammed functions, such as "bleaching."

5. *Annotation.* This allows the insertion of text into the image.
6. *Stock image libraries.* Manufacturers include libraries of "ideal teeth" to simplify "pasting" an ideal smile (see the section on Medicolegal Considerations later in this chapter).
7. *Specialized functions.* Software developers are continually adding specialized functions that simplify image manipulation.

CLINICAL TIP

Products are continually updated and revised. Before purchasing a system, confirm with the manufacturer which options are still available, the changes that have been made, and if limitations still exist. New products may have been introduced that result in current products becoming obsolete.

CLINICAL TIP

Mastering the complexities of computer imaging systems requires a great deal of time and effort. A dealer who can provide ample instruction and maintenance support is important. If a "bargain system" does not include servicing, the full capability of the system may never be realized.

CLINICAL PROCEDURE

Esthetic Dental Workup

Although system operation techniques vary greatly, the following are common to all.

Armamentarium
+ Extraoral camera and computer imaging software (e.g., SNAP Instant Dental Imaging simulation software [SNAP Instant Imaging Systems, Inc.] and Nikon D900 with dual point flash [Nikon Corp.]).
  Clinical Technique. Because of the flexible nature of the software, many methods exist for achieving the same result. Personal experience with a system is required to understand which method will have the greatest predictive value of the outcome of treatment.
1. Obtain an extraoral image of the dentition using a digital camera (Fig. 24-15).

CLINICAL TIP

If a digital camera is not available, a patient-supplied photograph can be digitized using a flatbed scanner.

---

2. After consulting with the patient, determine a proposed result.
3. Highlight the teeth using the highlighting tool (Fig. 24-16).
4. Select the correct amount of whitening of the highlighted image (Fig. 24-17).

CLINICAL TIP

If an individual tooth requires additional whitening, it can be highlighted separately and individually whitened (Fig. 24-18).

---

5. Use the pull brush and the clean brush to reshape and whiten individual teeth (Fig. 24-19).
6 The results in steps 3 to 5 can also be accomplished by selecting an ideal tooth and pasting it over the tooth to be corrected (Fig. 24-20).

CLINICAL TIP

Bookmark (temporarily store an image change) and save work often to prevent accidental loss.

---

7. After an acceptable result is obtained, save the image.

CLINICAL TIP

Comparing the predicted postoperative image with the true postoperative image is instructive. Repeatedly performing this procedure enables practitioners to improve the predicative accuracy of their computer manipulations (Fig. 24-21).

Repair of Missing Teeth

Armamentarium
+ Extraoral camera and computer imaging software (e.g., SNAP Instant Dental Imaging simulation software [SNAP Instant Imaging Systems, Inc.] and Nikon D900 with dual point flash [Nikon Corp.]).

Clinical Technique
1. Obtain a macro image of the dentition using a digital camera (Fig. 22-18*A*).
2. After consulting with the patient, determine a proposed result.
3. Load the image into the computer imaging software (Fig. 22-18*B*).
4. Highlight the segment of the image which will be duplicated (Fig. 22-18*C*).
5. Duplicate the highlighted segment (Fig. 22-18*D*).
6. Select the correct orientation of the highlighted image (Fig. 22-18*E*).
7. Move and paste the image to the proper position (Fig. 22-18*F*).

CLINICAL TIP

Any necessary resizing of the tooth should be performed at this time

---

9. Repeat pasting and reorienting teeth as necessary (Figs. 22-18*G,H*).
10. Complete the process as necessary (Fig. 22-18*I*).
11. Save the images (Fig. 22-18*J*).

Medicolegal Considerations

Often the technique used to create the simulation is designed for simplicity and is not related to the technique that will be used to restore the teeth. The simulations may not take into account the relative position of any of the remaining teeth, root locations, alveolar bone, and other vital structures. Whenever possible the manner in which the images are manipulated should be identical to the way the teeth are clinically treated. Failure to attempt to simulate clinical technique as closely as possible could create simulated results that cannot be achieved clinically.

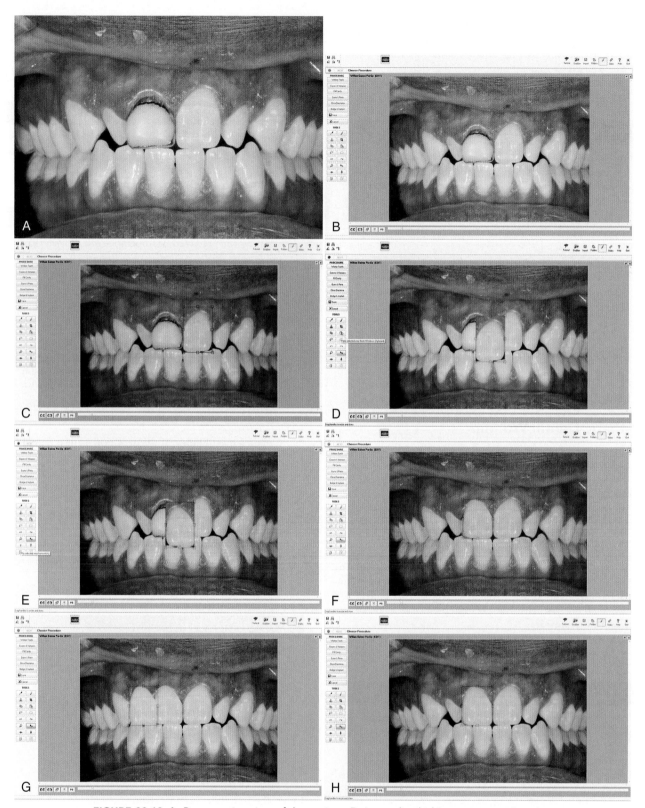

FIGURE 22-18 A, Preoperative view of the patient. **B,** Image loaded into computer imaging software. **C,** The segment which will be duplicated is highlighted. **D,** The highlighted segment is duplicated. **E,** The highlighted image orientation is corrected. **F,** The highlighted image is moved to the proper position. **G,** A second tooth is pasted in order to mimic restoring the lateral incisor. **H,** The lateral incisor is resized to the proper dimensions.

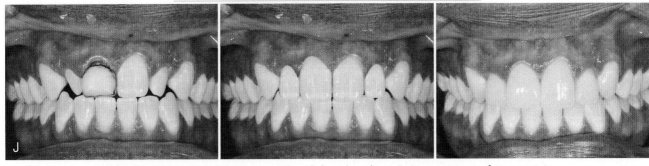

FIGURE 22-18, cont'd I, The completed digital workup. **J,** A comparison of preoperative (*left*), predicted (*middle*) and postoperative (*right*) work-ups (Case courtesy of Yakir A. Arteaga, DDS, New York, NY.)

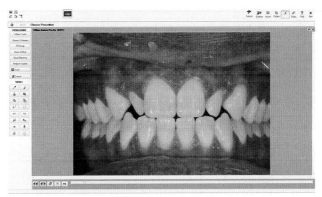

FIGURE 22-19 Simulation showing a single tooth replacement which will produce an oversized maxillary right central incisor.

CLINICAL TIP

Although the computer simulation may display mutually agreeable results, only the dentist can determine if a treatment plan exists that can clinically reproduce the simulated results. Because most of the techniques used by the computer to "rehabilitate" an arch are different from those used by a dentist to fabricate a prosthesis, a less desirable final result sometimes must be accepted. CIS can be extremely valuable in these cases because the dentist can also simulate these limitations (Fig. 22-19). This prevents unrealistic patient expectations and documents the possibility of less-than-optimal results.

CLINICAL TIP

Because various proposed final results may be contemplated, mark clearly and save each result before manipulating a new image.

CLINICAL TIP

It is vital that all images are clearly annotated with a disclaimer stated that they are a computer simulation and results cannot be guaranteed (see Chapter 27).

CONCLUSION

The use of photography in the practice of dentistry can be highly rewarding. It is extremely gratifying to share a "before" and "after" image with a patient and observe the elated facial expression as the images are opened beside each other. The ability to repeatedly create high quality digital photographs develops as the skill of the dental photographer increases and repetition perfects techniques. Once that level of skilled digital photographic image creation is achieved, the images will add to the degree of patient satisfaction, provide a means to document case histories indefinitely, and more likely than not prove to be a significant practice builder.

REFERENCES

1. Agarwal T: Using digital photography to increase case acceptance in hygiene, *Dent Today* 26(5):62-63, 2007.
2. Helvey GA: How to increase patient acceptance for cosmetic dentistry: cosmetic imaging with Adobe Photoshop Elements 4.0, *Dent Today*. 26(2):148-153, 2007.
3. Almog DM, Meitner SW, Even-Hen N, Grant JP, Soltys JL: Use of interdisciplinary team approach in establishing esthetic restorative dentistry, *N Y State Dent J* 71(5): 44-47, 2005.
4. Digital Dictionary: *A glossary of photographic terms*. Available at: http://www.all-things-photography.com/digital-dictionary.html. Accessed Nov, 2012.
5. *Digital Cameras Made Easy*. Available at: http://www.digicamguides.com/. Accessed Nov, 2012.
6. Glossary of Photography Terms: *Photography terms & their definitions*. Available at: http://www.photographytips.com/page.cfm/1587. Accessed Nov, 2012.
7. A Glossary of Photographic Terms: Available at: http://store.kodak.com/store/ekconsus/en_US/html/pbPage.termsA/ThemeID.16765600. Accessed Nov, 2012.
8. Terry DA, Snow SR, McLaren EA: Contemporary dental photography: selection and application, *Compend Contin Educ Dent* 29(8):432-436, 2008.
9. Image Sensors for Professional Photography: Available at: http://www.teledynedalsa.com/sensors/applications/dsc.aspx. Accessed Nov, 2012.
10. Camera Image Sensor: Available at: http://cameraimagesensor.com/. Accessed Nov, 2012.
11. Three-CCD camera: Available at: http://en.wikipedia.org/wiki/Three-CCD_camera. Accessed Nov, 2012.
12. Dorion RBJ: *Bitemark evidence: A color atlas and text*, ed 2, Boca Raton, FL, 2011, CRC Press.
13. Background Information on CCD and CMOS Technology: http://www.tedpella.com/cameras_html/ccd_cmos.htm. Accessed Nov, 2012.

Esthetics and Computer-Aided Design and Computer-Aided Manufacturing (CAD/CAM) Systems

Masly Harsono and Gerard Kugel

. . . .

In the mid-1980s, the earliest generation of computer-aided design/computer-aided manufacturing (CAD/CAM) technology was designed to fabricate immediate chairside inlay and onlay ceramic restorations.[1] This initial technology required an excessive amount of fabrication time. The first generation of computer software and hardware that accompanied this technology offered only a limited, two-dimensional view of the scanned images because the system's hard drive was incapable of storing the volume of data required for a three-dimensional view. CAD/CAM technology has evolved to become a practical and useful resource for dental professionals to perform chairside restorations.[2]

In CAD/CAM technology, a digital impression is substituted for the traditional elastomeric impression using an intraoral digital scanner.[3] Alternatively a digital scan of a cast made from a traditional elastomeric impression also can be performed. An intraoral digital impression that "captures" the data of the teeth and their supporting soft-tissue structures is recorded by a scanning wand using an optic laser, digital imaging, and/or video technology. A specialized three-dimensional (3D) rendering program allows the images of the intraorally scanned impressions to be actualized in three dimensions and in real time on a computer monitor. The software allows the dental professional to mark margins, digitally design wax-up proposals of the restoration, place accurate occlusal contacts, and refine the proximal contact areas with adjacent teeth. The clinician can perform any or all of these procedures at the chairside "design center" before sending the definitive data to the computer-controlled milling unit. The workflow is summarized by the following steps:

1. Tooth preparation
2. Intraoral scan
3. Restoration design
4. Milling of the restoration
5. Finishing of the restoration (coloring, glaze, polish) and adhesive luting

Advantages

The CAD/CAM system eliminates the need for traditional impression making because systems can make direct impressions. By enhancing tooth preparations the new technologies allow dentists to make better observations and assessments of the tooth preparation based on the enlarged 3D images. Most modern CAD system software can also check for undercuts. Other advantages of the CAD/CAM system include the following:

1. **Manufacturing of the restoration (not all systems).** An in-office portable milling is capable of immediate milling of the restoration, generally in less than an hour, eliminating the use of an off-site dental laboratory.
2. **Alternative materials.** All CAD/CAM systems use milling technology meaning that the dentist is not limited to restorations fabricated from by casting and pressing procedures.
3. **Open architecture system (not all systems).** Digital impressions made with devices that feature an open architecture system are compatible with any milling machine, as opposed to a closed architecture system in which the digital impression and the restoration milling machine must be from the same manufacturer. An open system, therefore, provides more freedom of choice when it comes to the selection of materials and a restoration fabrication partner (either a dental laboratory of the manufacturer of the CAD/CAM

system. Once the restoration is digitally designed by the dentist or technician, it is electronically sent to the facility with the milling machine center for fabrication.

Disadvantages

Following are some of the disadvantages of using CAD/CAM technologies:

1. **Expense.** CAD/CAM technologies are expensive. Most are leased and the cost of the actual restorations sometimes rival laboratory fees.
2. **Learning curve.** To use this new technology properly, the dentist or technician must be well-acquainted with computer design, implying an inherent learning curve for the system.
3. **Multiple unit limitations.** Currently only some systems are able to manufacture multiple-unit restoration.
4. **Inability to image in a wet environment.** Optically based imaging systems are incapable of obtaining accurate images in the presence of excess fluids. Impression-based systems have similar limitations. Nevertheless hydrophilic impression material is better equipped to overcome this limitation.
5. **Incompatibility with other imaging and CAD/CAM systems.** Because of the 3D file format used by CAD/CAM systems, they are not compatible with the 2-D IIS (intraoral imaging) system. Although stereolithography (STL) is a standard file format employed by 3D CAD software, some CAD/CAM systems use their own 3D file formats.
6. **Bulky scanning wand.** Current commercial CAD systems use a bulky, corded scanning wand. The slightly inconvenient design of this wand may prove to be an awkward limitation in some intraoral situations.

CLINICAL PRODUCTS

CLINICAL TIP

Proper tissue management and cord retraction must be performed during the digital impression the scanning procedure. Hardware systems and software versions are regularly updated by the manufacturer, making it crucial to verify the current status with the manufacturer before making a purchase.

The Cerec 4.0

The Cerec system (made by Sirona Germany and distributed by Paterson Dental Co., St Paul, MN) was first introduced in the United States in 1996.[4-6] It requires the use of a white, glare-free powder containing titanium oxide to enhance the contrast of the tooth. A CCD sensor wand makes a 3D infrared scan of the preparation in roughly 0.1 seconds at a resolution of 25 μm.[5,7] The digital image is displayed on the self-contained microprocessor display where the dentist designs the restoration. The Cerec is capable of fabricating porcelain inlays, onlays, crowns, and veneers, and allows immediate, single visit esthetic restorations. Version 4 can mill a single-unit definitive or provisional restoration and a provisional three-unit fixed partial denture from an acrylic block. The system also contains a block that functions as a wax casting (burnout block) for a cast metal crown. The system also contains a portable, six-axis micromilling machine that can be used in the dental office. The clinician can electronically send a design and the digital impression with Cerec Connect to the off-site laboratory for fabrication of casts,

multiple units, fixed partial dentures, implant abutments, and zirconium or metal crowns. Cerec can also be integrated with the Galileos System to construct surgical guides for implant placement. The Cerec's Biogeneric software can analyze individual patient occlusion and the anatomy of adjacent teeth so that the restoration is patient-specific. Preparation evaluation software (prepCheck) is included. This is a learning tool that provides an analysis of either a computer-simulated tooth preparation or a scan of an actual tooth preparation.

Cerec AC Bluecam CAD System was released in 2009 and used a short wavelength blue-diode LED laser light that the manufacturer claimed produces increased illumination to aid in scanning difficult access areas. It acquired single quadrant high-resolution 3D images in less than a minute and occlusion registrations in a few seconds and has electronic image stabilization. The 3D data obtained from the system could be exported into a standard STL (stereolithography) file format for use with any industry standard 3D software. In 2013, CEREC Omnicam system was introduced which the manufacture claims does not require titanium oxide application for scanning. However, the company still offers the CEREC Optispray to cover the reflective tooth surface for more precise imaging in difficult scanning situations.

The E4D Dentist

Unlike the earlier models of the Cerec system, the E4D system (made by D4D Technologies, Richardson, TX, and distributed by Henry Schein, Melville, NY) does not require the use of titanium oxide. The system wand contains a digital micromirror device and uses red diode laser to acquire a grayscale 3D image. The E4D system contains a chairside portable milling unit. E4D's Compass software allows the pairing of the E4D CAD/CAM technology with i-CAT (Gendex Dental Systems, Hatfield, PA) cone beam Technology for the coordination surgical implant planning. Like the Cerec, E4D Version 2.0 software allows the E4D to export digital files in an open-architecture stereolithography CAD data format widely used by other 3D software packages. This will allow rapid prototyping and CAM on a wide array of devices. The E4D software product named Compare serves as an evaluation tool for tooth preparation.[8]

The Lava COS

The Lava COS system, originally developed by Brontes Technologies (Cambridge, MA) and now made by 3M ESPE, is a scanner-only system (it does not contain a portable milling machine). It uses Brontes' 3D-in-motion technology to capture continuous 3D video images for digital impressioning. The scanner/software combination is capable of capturing approximately 20 3D datasets per second, each with more than 10,000 data points. At its highest capture rate, more than 2400 3D datasets and more than 24 million data points per arch can be acquired within 2 minutes. The scanner is claimed to have an accuracy of between 6 and 11 μm.[9] Similar to early model Cerec CAD/CAM systems, Lava COS requires the use of a powder for scanning. The scan data are electronically sent to the dental laboratory, which in turn electronically sends the information to a centralized cast manufacturing facility where the cast is fabricated from an epoxy resin using stereolithography. The cast is then returned to the dental laboratory for conventional restoration fabrication.

iTero

The iTero System (Align Technology, Inc.) uses parallel/confocal technology to capture the digital images and generate a 3D model. The scanner wand is capable of capturing a digital impression of 100,000 data points with a resolution of 0.5 μm. A powder coating of the teeth is not required. The preparation is scanned and the dentist sends the data to iTero for conversion into a file format that is compatible with an in-office milling system. The data are then returned to the dentist for in-office milling. Alternatively the data can be sent to iTero for refinement of the digital impression and delineation of margins and then sent to a local dental laboratory for a quality check. The dental laboratory can then mill the restoration using an in-laboratory milling machine or fabricate a conventional cast on a 3D printer and create the restoration using traditional methods. A final alternative is to send the data to iTero for data refinement, have the local dental laboratory perform the definitive quality check and then returned the data to iTero for fabrication of a polyurethane milled cast. The cast is then shipped to the local dental laboratory for creation of a restoration using traditional methods.

TRIOS

Like the iTero, the TRIOS system (3Shape A/S) is a scanner-only system that does not require the use of titanium oxide powder and the wand does not need to be held at any specific distance or angle. The scanning wand is capable of capturing more than 3000 2D images per second and the autoclavable tip can be rotated for alternation between the maxillary and mandibular jaws. The system uses a touch screen monitor to display live 3D images and its motion-sensor interface and hand-held scanner allows the dentist to virtually rotate and turn the 3D digital impression without touching the screen. The TRIOS software contains tools for instant clinical validation of the impression and tooth preparation at chairside such as the *Occlusal Clearance* tool ensures adequate tooth reduction and the *Insertion Direction* tool verifies convergence/divergence issues. Scanning information is sent to the dental laboratory that accepts STL file format using 3 Shape's Communicate solution software system

NobelProcera

The NobelProcera system (Noble Biocare) was originally designed to fabricate a titanium substructure core beneath a low-fusing ceramic for use as a fixed partial denture.[10] It has since been modified to include a sintered high-purity alumina coping combined with compatible veneering porcelain to create all-ceramic crown restorations.[11-14]

Unlike office-based CAD/CAM CAM systems, the NobelProcera system is designed for dental laboratory use only. The laboratory scans the stone cast poured from a conventional impression sent by the dentist. After the stone replicated cast is properly ditched, it is placed into the cast holder platform of the scanner. The optical impression scanner uses conoscopic holography technology, which the manufacturer claims offers more accuracy and shorter scanning time compared with stylus scanner technology.

> ### CLINICAL TIP
>
> The outcome of the CAD/CAM restoration is dependent upon the experience of the dentist or operator. There is a learning curve involved with operation of the scanner and/or software.

CAD/CAM RESTORATION MATERIALS

Advances in CAD/CAM CAM technology occurred simultaneously with innovations in esthetic restorative materials. Modern monoblock ceramic materials have been engineered to resist masticatory stress and milling induced damage. Feldspathic ceramic materials have been mostly replaced by reinforced ceramic with silica (feldspar, leucite, and lithium disilicate), nonsilica (alumina and zirconia), and a combination of resin-ceramic based materials, resulting in a three- to 11-fold increase in flexural strength.[15,16] Computer modeling simulation shows that a single, thick, monolithic all-ceramic crown materials performed better under stress when compared with ceramic core material with veneering porcelain.[17,18] Furthermore the coefficient of thermal expansion mismatch between core and veneer materials may initiate the internal stress that causes delaminating or internal cracking of porcelain.

Advantages

1. **Immediate crown fabrication.** The crowns are able to be immediately fabricated eliminating traditional laboratory fabrication procedures.
2. **Monolithic crowns.** Single layer ceramic materials exhibit better strength than dual layer core and veneer porcelain.
3. **Marginal integrity.** CAD/CAM milling crowns exhibit the same marginal integrity as those made with conventional laboratory-made crown restorations.[19-21]

Disadvantages

1. **Limited color shades.** The blocks are only available in a few selected shades and frequently require staining before glazing.
2. **Monochromatic color/appearance.** The monochromatic appearance can only be overcome by staining or by using a polychromatic block.

The monoblock ceramic can be rectangular, tubular, or in the shape of the dental arch depending on the type of milling machine used. Most frequently in-office/portable milling machines use the rectangular or tubular shapes. Porcelain restoration materials can be categorized into the following categories: reinforced ceramic with nonsilica (alumina and zirconia), silica (feldspar, leucite, and lithium disilicate), and a combination of resin-ceramic based materials. Only some of these materials are currently used in office based CAD/CAM milling systems

NON–SILICA-BASED CERAMICS

Zirconia

Millable zirconia is generally the strongest ceramic material. Zirconia is difficult to mill; therefore the blocks are usually presintered and less dense. The material will only be fully sintering after the milling procedure is completed. Fabrication of zirconia restorations require a higher degree of skill than that required for other ceramic materials because of its density and hardness.

The restorations are, therefore, usually fabricated by laboratory technicians. Glass particles are included in the composition of this material to enhance esthetics.

Alumina

Alumina-based systems typically use an alumina substrate over which a conventional layer of feldspathic porcelain is placed. Currently there are only limited alumina blocks available for office based CAD/CAM systems such as VITA In-Ceram Alumina block (Vident) and inCoris Al (Sirona Dental Inc. USA).

SILICA

Feldspathic Porcelains

Feldspathic porcelains are typically available in sintered, pressed and milled block form. Examples are fine particle ceramic blocks: Vitablocs Triluxe Forte and Vitablocs RealLife (Vident). Both have a graded variation in chroma. The incisal/occlusal third exhibits a low, less intense chroma with high translucency, the body layer exhibits regular chroma and the cervical layer exhibits the highest chroma and the lowest translucency (Fig. 23-1*A,B*).

The Vitablocs RealLife (Fig. 23-1*C*) blocks better mimic the enamel-layered-over-dentin design of the natural tooth and reproduce translucency, chroma, and value by positioning the restoration to be milled within a spherical dome of dentin that is surrounded by more translucent enamel.

Leucite-Reinforced Ceramics

Leucite-reinforced ceramics are available in sintered pressed and milled block CAD/CAM forms. Examples are IPS Empress and IPS Empress CAD (Ivoclar Vivadent). Early chairside ceramic milling blocks were available in limited shades and therefore required external staining. Recently a greater selection of incrementally chroma and value gradated polychromatic ceramic blocks (IPS Empress CAD) for both the PlanScan CAD/CAM Restoration System (E4D Technologies) and CEREC CAD/CAM System (Sirona Dental Inc. USA) have become available. These tri-shaded blocks contain different cervical, body, and incisal segments in an attempt to mimic the polychromaticity of natural teeth. Blocks are also available with high and low translucency.

Lithium Disilicate

Glass ceramics are characterized based on their crystalline structure and/or application with lithium disilicate ranking among the best known and most widely used types of glass ceramics. Lithium disilicate is an esthetic, high-strength material that can be conventionally cemented or adhesively bonded. For example, IPS e.max (Ivoclar Vivadent) composed of lithium dioxide, quartz, phosphor dioxide, alumina, potassium oxide, and other components is a composition that yields a highly thermal shock-resistant glass ceramic because of its low thermal expansion during processing. It can be processed using either well-known, lost-wax hot pressing techniques or state-of-the-art CAD/CAM milling procedures.

The pressable lithium disilicate (IPS e.max Press, Ivoclar Vivadent) is produced according to a unique bulk casting production process in order to create the ingots. This process involves a continuous manufacturing process based on glass technology (melting, cooling, simultaneous nucleation of two different crystals, and growth of crystals) that is constantly optimized in order to prevent the formation of defects. The microstructure of the pressable lithium disilicate material consists of approximately 70% lithium disilicate crystals, which are needle-shaped and measure 3 to 6 μm in length, embedded in a glassy matrix.

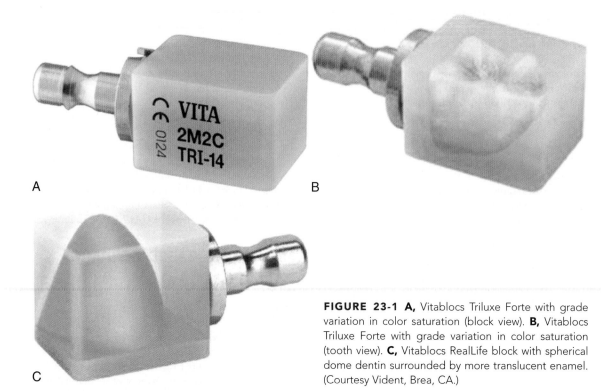

FIGURE 23-1 A, Vitablocs Triluxe Forte with grade variation in color saturation (block view). **B,** Vitablocs Triluxe Forte with grade variation in color saturation (tooth view). **C,** Vitablocs RealLife block with spherical dome dentin surrounded by more translucent enamel. (Courtesy Vident, Brea, CA.)

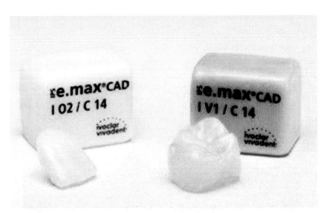

FIGURE 23-2 IPS e.max CAD impulse blocks in different brightness and shades. (Courtesy Ivoclar Vivadent, Amherst, NY.)

The machinable lithium disilicate blocks (IPS e.max CAD blocks) (Fig. 23-2) are produced by bulk casting but are only formed to a softer intermediate blue translucent state, to ensure that the blocks can be milled efficiently. The intermediate crystallization process yields lithium metasilicate crystals that have properties that include ease of machinability and good edge stability. After milling, the restorations are fired to their definitive higher strength crystallized state. The microstructure of the intermediate crystallized lithium disilicate consists of 40% platelet-shaped lithium metasilicate crystals embedded in a glassy phase. These crystals range in length from 0.2 to 1.0 μm. Post-crystallization microstructure of IPS e.max CAD lithium disilicate material consists of 70% fine-grain lithium disilicate crystals embedded in a glassy matrix.[22-25]

Ivoclar Impulse lithium disilicate blocks are available in different brightness values and opalescence shades. The opalescence blocks are mainly designed to create thin veneers and other partial coverage restorations and single crowns (see Fig. 23-2).

REINFORCED RESIN-CERAMIC

A reinforced resin-ceramic block (Lava Ultimate CAD/CAM, 3M ESPE). is a unique resin nano-ceramic material. The manufacturer claims long-lasting esthetics and performance, however,

data on material wear properties are not yet available and currently, there is only limited clinical data in the literature. The most significant advantage of this product is that post-milling oven firing is unnecessary.

CLINICAL TIP

It is essential for clinicians to have knowledge of what type of ceramic are needed in every situation.

CLINICAL TECHNIQUE

Case Study

A healthy 85-year-old woman presented to the dental office on an emergency basis with a coronal fracture of the maxillary right lateral incisor. The medical history was noncontributory. It was determined that the tooth required endodontic therapy, a post and core and a crown. The tooth was endodontically treated followed by the placement of a prefabricated post (RelyX fiber post, 3M ESPE) and a core build-up of composite resin (Filtek Z250, 3M ESPE) (Fig. 23-3*A,B*).

A shade was selected with Vita shade guide and a digital photograph (Canon D50 with macro lens, Canon Inc.) was made to aid the laboratory technician in fabricating proper tooth color and morphology. A digitally designed virtual wax-up of the tooth was constructed following margin marking (Fig. 23-3*C*).

After the sprue location was determined digitally, the data for the designed crown were sent to the computer-controlled milling machine. A provisional crown was made with bis-acrylic material (Tuff-Temp, Pulpdent Corp.) and delivered to the patient due to the lengthy procedure in the initial unscheduled emergency visit and scheduling requirements that precluded completing the restoration during the initial visit. The final restoration was completed using a D3-V1 Impulse mono-ceramic block (Ivoclar Vivadent). Following milling, the crown was customized using laboratory burs (Fig. 23-3*D*).

The crown was then stained and glazed using the IPS e.max ceram shade kit (Ivoclar Vivadent) on a white dental stone working model (Fig. 23-3*E*).

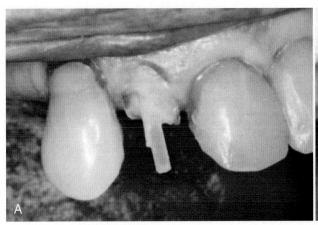
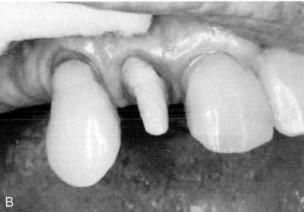

FIGURE 23-3 A, Endodontically treated teeth with fiber post placement. **B,** Composite resin core build-up.

Continued

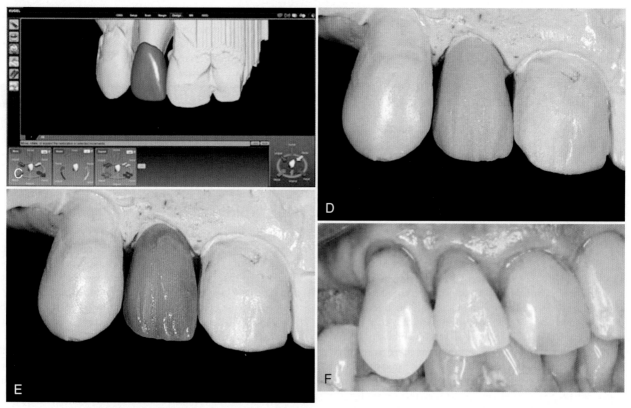

FIGURE 23-3, cont'd C, Virtual digital wax up (E4D Technologies) on the maxillary right lateral incisor. **D,** IPS e.max CAD impulse blocks after milling and customization with laboratory burs. **E,** IPS e.max CAD impulse esthetic stain and glaze on stone die. **F,** Postoperative images following crown cementation.

The crown was tried in and adjusted and, after the patient approved the esthetics, the restoration was cemented using a definitive composite resin luting cement (Multilink Automix, Ivoclar Vivadent) (Fig. 23-3F).

CONCLUSION

The success of CAD/CAM technology depends on the clinical skills of the dentist and the ability to properly employ technology. This begins with proper diagnosis and tooth preparation followed by proper use of the CAD/CAM technology. Many of the procedures involved with the fabrication CAD/CAM restorations are major departures from traditional techniques. A distinct learning curve is involved with attaining the skills necessary to become clinically facile with this technology.

REFERENCES

1. Mörmann WH: The origin of the Cerec method: a personal review of the first 5 years, *Int J Comput Dent* 7(1):11-24, 2004.
2. Miyazaki T, Hotta Y, Kunii J, Kuriyama S, Tamaki Y: A review of dental CAD/CAM: current status and future perspectives from 20 years of experience, *Dent Mater J* 28(1):44-56, 2009.
3. Mörmann WH: The evolution of the CEREC system, *J Am Dent Assoc* 137(Suppl) 7S-13S, 2006.
4. Brandestini M et al: Computer machined ceramic inlays: in vitro marginal adaptation, *J Dent Res* 64:208, 1985.
5. Mormann WH, Brandestini M, Lutz F, Barbakow F, Gotsch T: CAD-CAM ceramic inlays and onlays: a case report after 3 years in place, *J Am Dent Assoc* 120(5):517-520, 1990.
6. Mormann J et al: Marginal adaptation von adhasiven Porzellaninlays in vitro, *Schwizerische Monatsshrift fur Zahnmedizin* 85:1118-1129, 1985.
7. Mormann J: Method for the manufacture of dental reconstructions and blank for carrying out this method.
8. Renne WG, McGill ST, Mennito AS, Wolf BJ, Marlow NM, Shaftman S, et al: E4D compare software: an alternative to faculty grading in dental education, *J Dent Educ* 77(2):168-175, 2013.
9. Balakrishnama S, Wenzell K, Bergeron J, Ruest C, Reusch B, Kugel G: *Dimensional repeatability from the LAVA COS 3D Intra-oral Scanning System*, Boston, 2009, Boston Center For Oral Health.
10. Smedberg JI, Ekenbäck J, Lothigius E, Arvidson K: Two-year follow-up study of Procera-ceramic fixed partial dentures, *Int J Prosthodont* 11(2):145-149, 1998.
11. Awliya W, Odén A, Yaman P, Dennison JB, Razzoog ME: Shear bond strength of a resin cement to densely sintered high-purity alumina with various surface conditions, *Acta Odontol Scand* 56(1):9-13, 1998.
12. Andersson M, Razzoog ME, Odén A, Hegenbarth EA, Lang BR: Procera: a new way to achieve an all-ceramic crown, *Quintessence Int* 29(5):285-296, 1998.
13. Wagner WC, Chu TM: Biaxial flexural strength and indentation fracture toughness of three new dental core ceramics, *J Prosthet Dent* 76(2):140-144, 1996.
14. Persson M, Andersson M, Bergman B: The accuracy of a high-precision digitizer for CAD/CAM of crowns, *J Prosthet Dent* 74(3):223-229, 1995.
15. Seghi RR, Sorensen JA: Relative flexural strength of six new ceramic materials, *Int J Prosthodont* 8(3):239-246, 1995.
16. McLaren EA, Giordano RA: Zirconia-based ceramics: material properties, esthetics, and layering techniques of a new veneering porcelain, VM9, *Quintessence Dent Technol* 28:99-111, 2005.
17. Rekow ED, Harsono M, Janal M, Thompson VP, Zhang G: Factorial analysis of variables influencing stress in all-ceramic crowns, *Dent Mater* 22(2):125-132, 2006. Epub 2005. Jul 5.
18. Rekow ED, Zhang G, Thompson V, Kim JW, Coehlo P, Zhang Y: Effects of geometry on fracture initiation and propagation in all-ceramic crowns, *J Biomed Mater Res B Appl Biomater* 88(2):436-446, 2009.
19. Reich S, Wichmann M, Nkenke E, Proeschel P: Clinical fit of all-ceramic three-unit fixed partial dentures, generated with three different CAD/CAM systems, *Eur J Oral Sci* 113(2):174-179, 2005.
20. Tinschert J, Natt G, Mautsch W, Spiekermann H, Anusavice KJ: Marginal fit of alumina and zirconia-based fixed partial dentures produced by a CAD/CAM system, *Oper Dent* 26(4):367-374, 2001.

21. Bindl A, Mormann WH: Marginal and internal fit of all-ceramic CAD/CAM crown copings on chamfer preparations, *J Oral Rehabil* 32(6):441-447, 2005.
22. Deany IL: Recent advances in ceramics for dentistry, *Crit Rev Oral Biol Med* 7(2): 134-143, 1996.
23. Sorensen JA, Cruz M, Mito WT, Raffeiner O, Meredith HR, Foser HP: A clinical investigation on three-unit fixed partial dentures fabricated with a lithium disilicate glass-ceramic, *Pract Periodontics Aesthet Dent* 11(1):95-106, 1999. quiz 108.
24. Höland W, Schweiger M, Frank M, Rheinberger V: A comparison of the microstructure and properties of the IPS Empress 2 and the IPS Empress glass-ceramics, *J Biomed Mater Res* 53(4):297-303, 2000.
25. Kheradmandan S, Koutayas SO, Bernhard M, Strub JR: Fracture strength of four different types of anterior 3-unit bridges after thermo-mechanical fatigue in the dual-axis chewing simulator, *J Oral Rehabil* 28(4):361-369, 2001.

24

Esthetics and Dermatologic Pharmaceuticals

Zev Schulhof

Minimally invasive cosmetic facial procedures are quickly becoming the most exciting and controversial topic in esthetic dentistry. Over the past decade these procedures have experienced tremendous growth because of their increasing popularity and virtually painless, office-based administration.

DENTAL USE OF DERMATOLOGIC PHARMACEUTICALS

The use of dermatologic pharmaceuticals by dentists has become common in a number of states. Dental practice laws place various restrictions on their use, so the practitioner must verify the legality of performing these procedures.

Municipalities that explicitly allow dentists to use dermatologic pharmaceuticals may follow the ADA's definition of dentistry as "the evaluation, diagnosis, prevention, and/or treatment (non-surgical, surgical, or related procedures) of diseases, disorders, and/or conditions of the oral cavity, maxillofacial area, and/or the adjacent and associated structures and their impact on the human body."[1]

There are many instances in which the dentoalveolar complex influences the drape of the facial tissues. For example, because the lips frame the dentoalveolar complex, it is important to consider them when performing any esthetic procedure. The practitioner must evaluate lip support, in both relaxed and animated positions, because it may be affected by the placement of anterior restorations. This must be considered if lip augmentation is planned, to achieve an ideal esthetic result.

THE AGING FACE

It is important to understand the underlying processes that cause facial aging before attempting to correct any age-related changes in the face. Facial aging occurs at every level of the soft tissue envelope. Changes occur in the skin, subcutaneous fat,

superficial muscular aponeurotic system (SMAS), deep fat, and muscles of facial expression[2] (Fig. 24-1).

There is an ongoing loss of collagen and elasticity in the skin, resulting in the skin becoming lax.[3] Collagen loss causes tissue atrophy and thinning of the skin, with increased rhytid (wrinkle) formation (Fig. 24-2). Loss of the underlying fat causes descent of the overlying structures Fig. 24-3A).[4,5]

These changes lead to loss of the volume and curves of the cheeks, resulting in bony contours. Tissue descent also causes increased nasolabial and labiomandibular folds and increased "jowling" (Fig. 24-3B).

There are two types of wrinkles: dynamic wrinkles and static wrinkles. The dynamic wrinkle is caused by animation or muscle function (Fig. 24-4A).

Use of botulinum toxin is appropriate for treating dynamic wrinkles because it weakens the underlying muscle and causes a "chemical denervation." This prevents wrinkling of the overlying skin.

A static wrinkle occurs in the absence of facial movement when the musculature is completely relaxed (Fig. 24-4B).

Botulinum toxin cannot be used alone to treat static wrinkles because it has little effect on wrinkles that appear when the facial muscles are completely at rest. In these cases, filler or combination therapy (with the Botulinum toxin correcting against dynamic wrinkles that can occur in conjunction with static wrinkles) would be preferable.

BOTULINUM TOXIN

Botulinum toxin is a clear fluid medication in a lyophilized (freeze-dried) form. It contains a pure neurotoxin that is surrounded by non-toxin proteins, which are used to stabilize and protect the neurotoxin (Fig. 24-5).

The practitioner mixes the toxin with saline and injects the medication subcutaneously or intramuscularly, with

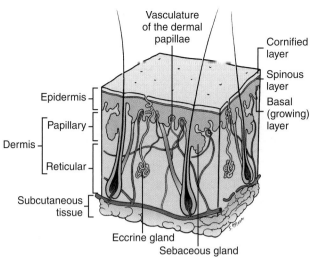

FIGURE 24-1 Anatomy of the skin layers. (From Hupp JR, Ellis E, Tucker MR: *Contemporary oral and maxillofacial surgery, ed 6*, St Louis, 2014, Mosby.)

the intention of weakening the target muscle. Contrary to popular belief, it does not "fill" lines, nor does it "smooth" wrinkles.

History

Botulinum toxin is derived from *Clostridium botulinum*, a gram-positive, spore-producing bacteria first identified by Emile Van Ermengen in 1897[6] when he was investigating fatal cases of food poisoning associated with sausage meat. (*Botulus* is Latin for sausage.) Serotypes A, B, and E cause the classic food-borne disease, which can cause flaccid paralysis of motor and autonomic nerves.

During World War II, scientists investigated botulinum toxin as a means of chemical warfare and isolated serotype A. This research was going on simultaneously in the United States, the United Kingdom, and Russia.[7] Research products first created in the United States and the United Kingdom eventually became the products Botox and Dysport, respectively.

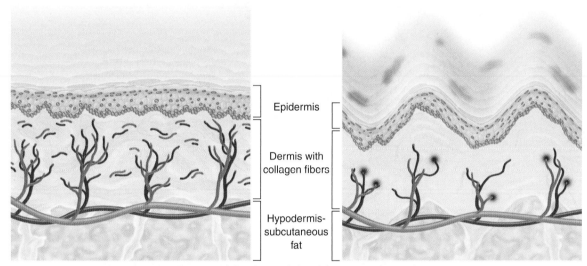

FIGURE 24-2 Thinning of the skin and rhytid formation during the aging process.

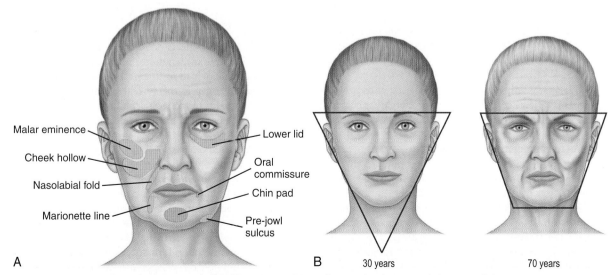

FIGURE 24-3 A, Areas of the face that will be influenced with age and descent of the tissues. **B,** Descent of the facial tissues causing facial folds and "jowling." (From Cantisano-Zilkha M, Haddad A: *Aesthetic oculofacial rejuvenation*, St Louis, 2010, Saunders.)

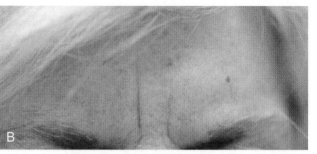

FIGURE 24-4 A, Dynamic wrinkles occur with movement. **B,** Static wrinkles visible at rest.

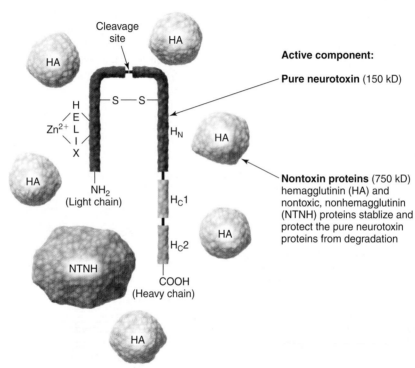

FIGURE 24-5 Structure of botulinum toxin type A.

In 1978, botulinum toxin was tested in clinical trials for strabismus.[8-10] Throughout the 1980s it was used extensively to treat blepharospasm,[11,12] hemifacial spasm,[13,14] and cervical dystonia.[15-17]

In 1987, Jean Carruthers, an ophthalmologist, was treating her blepharospasm patients with botulinum toxin, while her husband, Alastair Carruthers, a dermatologist, noticed that the patient's wrinkles were "disappearing" in the treated areas.[18] In 2002, the FDA approved botulinum toxin type A (Botox) for cosmetic use.

Currently, three types of commercial botulinum toxin Type A are available for cosmetic use in the United States: Botox (Allergan, Inc.), Dysport (Medicis Aesthetic), and Xeomin (Merz Aesthetics, Inc.). One type of commercially available botulinum toxin Type B, Myobloc (Elan Pharmaceuticals), is licensed for the treatment of cervical dystonia. Type B toxin differs from Type A toxin by serotype and is not approved for cosmetic use.

Mechanism of Action

Botulinum toxin's effects occur at the motor end plate. Muscle contraction occurs when motor nerve terminal impulse reaches a nerve ending, which in turn releases acetylcholine across the neuromuscular gap to the muscle signaling muscle contraction. Botulinum toxin blocks acetylcholine release. This blocking of acetylcholine occurs as a four-step process (Fig. 24-6).

1. *Binding.* The free end of the neurotoxin molecule binds to the cholinergic receptors located on the presynaptic neuron of the neuromuscular junction.
2. *Internalization.* The botulinum toxin passes through the cell membrane and cytoplasm via endocytosis.
3. *Release.* Botulinum toxin is released into the cytoplasm.
4. *Block acetylcholine release.* Botulinum toxin blocks acetylcholine release by cleaving SNAP25. SNAP25 is an integral protein required for successful docking and release of acetylcholine from vesicles situated in the nerve endings.

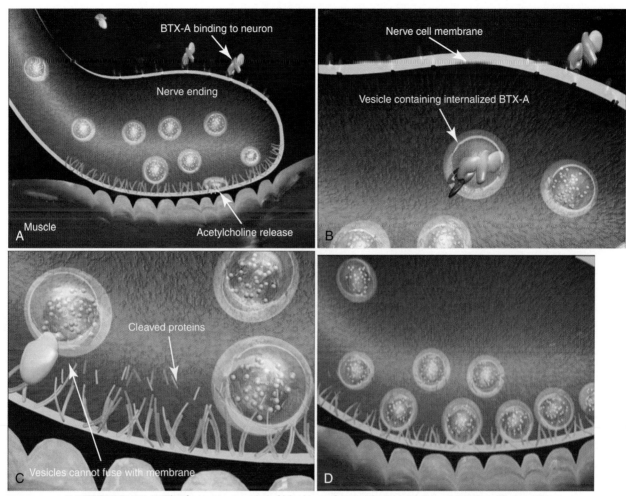

FIGURE 24-6 The four-step process of blocking of acetylcholine. **A,** Step 1: Binding. **B,** Step 2: Internalization. **C,** Step 3: Toxin released into cytoplasm. **D,** Step 4: Release and blocking of acetylcholine release. (Copyright Allergan Inc., Irvine, CA.)

The toxin therefore causes a "chemical denervation" of the muscle. If acetylcholine cannot be released from the nerve ending, the muscle cannot contract. If the muscle cannot contract, then the overlying skin cannot wrinkle.

Wrinkle formation of the overlying skin can be compared to "Roman shades" (Fig. 24-7).

When the shade is raised, it folds over upon itself. Similarly, muscle contraction causes the overlying skin to shorten or fold over upon itself. This wrinkle is perpendicular to the direction of the muscle fibers. For example, horizontal wrinkles are caused by vertical fibers of the frontalis muscle, whereas radial wrinkles run perpendicular to the fibers of the orbicularis oculi.

Onset of Action and Duration

The onset of action of botulinum toxin varies, depending on the type of formulation, ranging from 24 hours to 5 days. Final results may take 2 weeks. Results should last for 3 to 4 months. Toward the end of this period, most patients will feel a gradual return of muscle function, and repeat therapy can be initiated. The repetitive use of botulinum toxin has not resulted in muscle degeneration or atrophy.[19]

Safety and Contraindications

Examination of nearly 20 years of research reveals a high degree of safety and efficacy.[20] A review of 36 randomized trials with 1425 patients revealed no serious adverse events.[21]

Most adverse events are reported to be transient in nature. They include lack of intended cosmetic effect, injection site reaction, ptosis (drooping of the eyelid), muscle weakness, and headache.[22]

There are relatively few contraindications for botulinum toxin therapy. These include muscle movement disorders (e.g., amyotrophic sclerosis [ALS], myasthenia gravis and Lambert-Eaton syndrome) and known allergy to botulinum toxin, which is extremely rare.[23] Botulinum toxin is a pregnancy category C drug and therefore is not recommended during pregnancy or nursing. Caution is advised in the presence of pre-existing skin infections or rashes at the intended injection site.

Storage, Preparation, and Injection Technique

Most types of botulinum toxin require refrigeration. The toxin is packaged in lyophilized (freeze-dried) form, in a multidose vial (Fig. 24-8A).

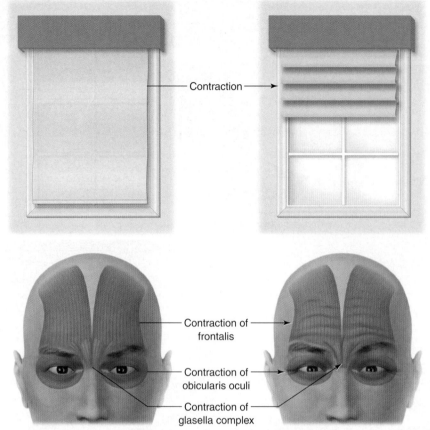

FIGURE 24-7 Wrinkle formation of the overlying skin compared with "Roman shades." Muscle contraction causes the overlying skin to fold over on itself, and this wrinkle is perpendicular to the direction of the muscle fibers. Horizontal wrinkles caused by vertical fibers of the frontalis muscle; radial wrinkles run perpendicular to the fibers of the orbicularis oculi.

The toxin is constituted with saline before use by drawing the desired amount of saline from another vial and transferring it into the vial containing the toxin. According to the manufacturers, the toxin should be drawn up through the rubber stopper on top of the vial, and then a needle tip should be left behind to draw up future doses.

Many practitioners choose to open the multidose vial by removing the rubber stopper, aseptically drawing up the desired toxin into an insulin syringe (Fig. 24-8C), and then recapping the vial for future use.

The insulin syringe has a very fine needle, which can make receiving the injection much more comfortable for the patient than if a larger-diameter needle were to be used. Once constituted, all neurotoxin should be stored in the refrigerator. Sterile techniques must be used as with any multidose vial and the constituted, unused neurotoxin must be used within a given time frame.

> **CLINICAL TIP**
>
> When using an insulin syringe to withdraw the toxin, tilt the bottle 45 degrees and try to avoid touching the glass with the needle tip. This will dull the needle and cause the injections to be more painful for the patient.

> **CLINICAL TIP**
>
> Before injection, most practitioners will mark the areas on the face to be injected (Fig. 24-8D).

The desired units are drawn up in a syringe using a fine-gauge needle (30 or 31 gauge), and injected into the pre-marked areas. For most areas, either a subcutaneous or intramuscular injection is acceptable. However, some areas require deeper injections, to ensure that the neurotoxin will infiltrate the target muscle. No local anesthetic is required. However, for added comfort, some patients prefer to place an ice-pack on the area before injection for about 30 seconds.

Areas of Treatment

Classically, botulinum toxin was used in the muscles of the upper face. The FDA approval for Botox Cosmetic reads, "indicated for the temporary improvement in the appearance of moderate to severe glabellar lines associated with corrugator and/or procerus muscle activity in adult patients ≤65 years of age."[24] Since FDA approval for cosmetic use, it has been used in all areas of the face and neck. For example, an injection can be given intraorally for a gummy smile or into the temporalis tendon muscle for TMJ pain; however, these are off-label uses.

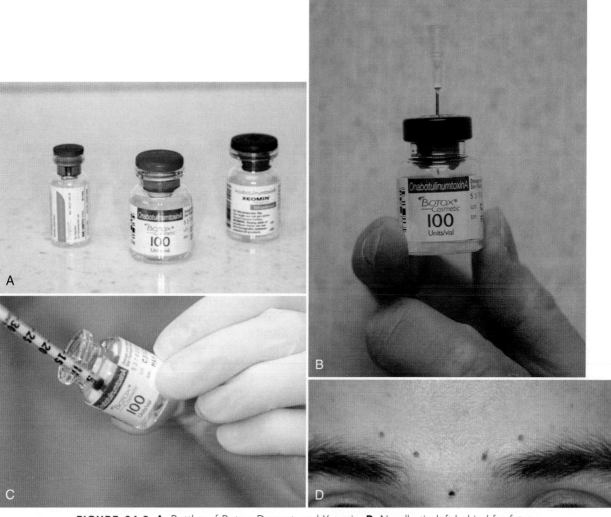

FIGURE 24-8 A, Bottles of Botox, Dysport, and Xeomin. **B,** Needle tip left behind for future withdrawals. **C,** Opening the bottle to withdraw desired toxin using an insulin syringe. **D,** Marking the areas before injection.

Upper Face. In the upper face, botulinum toxin is generally used in three major areas, the forehead, glabella, and peri-orbital areas.

Forehead. Horizontal forehead wrinkles are caused by contraction of the frontalis muscles.

The frontalis muscles are two large fanlike muscles that extend from the eyebrow region to the top of the forehead (Fig. 24-9). Using multiple low dose injections, the practitioner can relax the frontalis muscles. The key to achieving an aesthetically pleasing result is to maintain or enhance eyebrow position and movement. By relaxing the forehead wrinkles without paralyzing brow movement, the patient receives a very natural result.

CLINICAL TIP

Injecting too close to certain anatomic structures surrounding the eyebrows can cause brow ptosis, lid ptosis, or an uneven "brow lifting" effect.

Glabellar Complex. The glabellar complex is made up of two muscles, the corrugator and procerus (Fig. 24-10).

The corrugator muscle is a longitudinal muscle that goes from the medial of the orbits to the mid eyebrow, running approximately 30 degrees above horizontal. The procerus in a flat vertical muscle extending from the bridge of the nose and interdigitates with the corrugator, frontalis, and orbicularis oculi. These two muscles, working in concert, move the eyebrows downward and medial. This causes a perpendicular wrinkling of the overlying skin, that can appear as vertical fan lines (sometimes referred to as "frown lines" or "eleven lines") over the medial eyebrows. Injecting botulinum toxin in a V pattern in this area usually relieves these wrinkles.

In many patients, the deepest of the vertical lines in the glabella complex become static lines. (After treatment with botulinum toxin, these lines remain despite the musculature being at rest.) Therefore combination therapy of botulinum toxin and filler material is required. The filler should be threaded directly into the deep wrinkles to correct them.

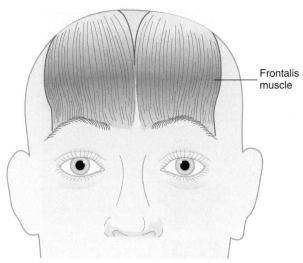

FIGURE 24-9 Frontalis muscle. (From Kaminer MS, Arndt KA, Dover JS: *Atlas of cosmetic surgery,* ed 2, Philadelphia, 2009, Saunders.)

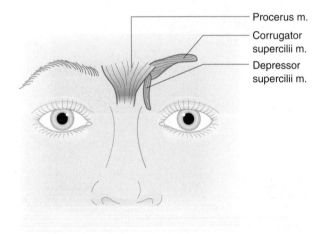

FIGURE 24-10 Glabellar complex made up of the corrugator and procerus muscles. (From Kaminer MS, Arndt KA, Dover JS: *Atlas of cosmetic surgery,* ed 2, Philadelphia, 2009, Saunders.)

Periorbital Area. The lateral canthus area is a common area for wrinkles that form lateral to the eye with aging. These wrinkles form in a radial fashion ("crow's feet") because the underlying orbicularis oculi muscle is round (Fig. 24-11). Following the curve of the lateral orbital rim, three to five low-dose injections of botulinum toxin can greatly reduce or eliminate these wrinkles.

There are other areas around the eye that can benefit from botulinum toxin therapy. However, these areas are usually reserved for the advanced injector (e.g., "chemical brow lift") and lower eyelid injections.

Midface and Lower Face. Although very exciting and inherently intuitive for the dental practitioner, the mid and lower face have traditionally been reserved for the advanced practitioner. The intricacy and anatomy of these areas require an advanced knowledge of anatomy, as well as an artistic eye, to achieve a subtle, yet aesthetically pleasing result. Many times, therapy is accomplished by combining facial fillers and botulinum toxin to "sculpt" the face to the desired result.

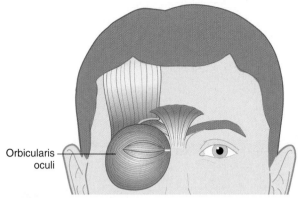

FIGURE 24-11 Orbicularis oculi. (From Kaminer MS, Arndt KA, Dover JS: *Atlas of cosmetic surgery,* ed 2, Philadelphia, 2009, Saunders.)

Some examples of cosmetic augmentation of the mid and lower face using botulinum toxin include:

1. *Vertical maxillary excess* ("*gummy smile*"). When a LeFort I osteotomy is to be avoided, this may be treated by injecting one of the muscles that are raising the lip to such a high level. A small amount of botulinum toxin in the levator labii superioris alaeque nasi (LLSAN) can decrease the pull of the upper lip in the superior direction. This in turn will decrease excessive gingival exposure during smiling (Fig. 24-12*A,B*). Paralyzing all of the muscle movement must be avoided.

2. *The depressor anguli oris* (DAO muscle extends from the corner of the lips to the inferior border of the mandible). With aging, patients may complain of a "down-turned mouth" (Fig. 24-12*C*) in which the corners of the lips seem to turn down in a frown at rest. This area that can be supported with facial fillers, and/or can be injected with botulinum toxin. Injection of the toxin at the base of the DAO relaxes the muscular pull at the corner of the mouth and causes the commissure to "lift up" to relieve the frown.

3. Small doses of botulinum toxin can also be used to relieve "smoker's lines" or "lipstick lines" around the mouth (lines perpendicular to the orbicularis oris, similar to the manner in which "crow's feet" form around the orbicularis oculi) by injecting the orbicular oris.

4. A "pebbly chin" is treated by injecting the mentalis muscle.

5. The lower face can be "narrowed" by injecting a hypertrophic masseter muscle.

6. Some of the nasal muscles can be "sculpted" (with botulinum toxin and/or filler material).

7. Neck wrinkles can be treated with botulinum toxin.

Temporomandibular Disorders and Myofascial Pain. Botulinum toxin has been used with great success in the treatment of temporomandibular disorders, myofascial pain, and migraine headaches. It is important to understand that treating these disorders is a multimodal approach and not every patient will benefit from botulinum toxin. However, with its proper place in the treatment protocol (e.g., if other conservative therapy such as soft foods, appliances, and NSAIDs are ineffective), botulinum toxin has become an important part of therapy for these patients. Botulinum toxin can be injected into various head and neck muscles, both via

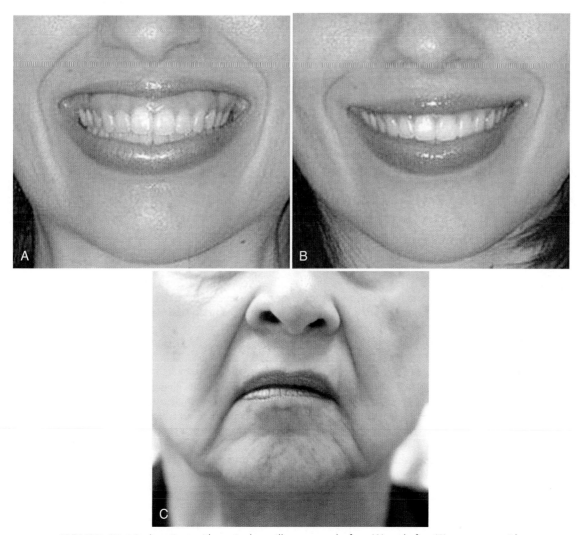

FIGURE 24-12 A patient with vertical maxillary excess before (**A**) and after (**B**) treatment with botulinum toxin. **C,** Patient exhibiting a "down-turned mouth."

an extraoral or even intraoral route, to relax muscle function and/or spasm. A typical example would be a patient with severe bruxism who cannot find relief with appliance therapy. By placing botulinum toxin into strategic points in the masseter muscle, a significant decrease in force of contraction of the masseter muscle can be achieved, thereby providing months of relief for the patient.

FACIAL FILLERS

Facial fillers are injected into the skin to fill in wrinkles or depressions. They are gel-like in consistency, clear, and are packaged in prefilled syringes (Fig. 24-13A).

During the aging process the face loses fat and volume, whereas the skin loses collagen and elasticity (see Fig. 24-1). Facial fillers can add volume or contour to the face, and in some cases can actually stimulate new collagen production. Facial fillers differ from botulinum toxin in that they are injected into one of the layers of the skin and cause an immediate physical "plumping" of the overlying wrinkle. They have no effect on the underlying muscle.

History

For more than 100 years, clinicians have been attempting to find an ideal filler material that could be injected under the skin to replace lost volume and smooth wrinkles and folds.

During the 1890's, clinicians injected fat collected from patients' arms into their faces. This technique, still in use today, and is called autologous fat transfer. During the 1900s clinicians began using paraffin as a filler in the skin until it was discovered that that paraffin would cause foreign body granulomas.[25]

In the 1940s, silicone emerged as the exciting new dermal implant, however there were problematic adverse effects including irregularities in contour, chronic inflammation, migration, granuloma, pulmonary embolism, and silicone pneumonitis. These can lead to organ failure and death.[26] Because silicone was a permanent filler material, these adverse effects could not be changed. Therefore silicone has since been banned as a cosmetic filler material in the United States.

In the early 1980s bovine collagen was FDA approved for use as an injectable filler material (Zyderm 1 and 2 and Zyplast, Inamed Aesthetics, a division of Allergan Inc.). This became the first easy-to-use and readily available filler

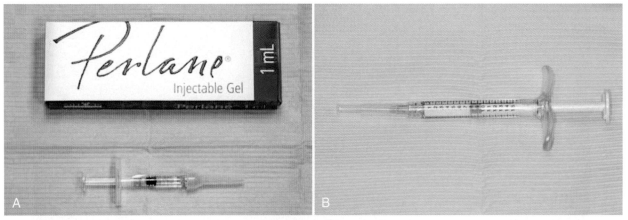

FIGURE 24-13 A, Hyaluronic acid in its prefilled syringe. **B,** Radiesse is white in color.

material that was cost effective and achieved natural results. However, because these were bovine derived products, skin testing for allergic reactions to the material was required.[27] Two skin tests were administered 2 weeks apart, followed by a waiting period of 4 weeks after the second skin test. Thus, performing the procedure on the day of consultation was not possible. Three percent of patients with a normal skin test still developed a sensitivity reaction.[28]

Soon thereafter, human collagen became available (Cosmo-Derm and CosmoPlast, Inamed Aesthetics, a division of Allergan Inc). FDA approval in the United States was granted in 2003. This immediately became more popular than bovine collagen because no testing was required. The collagen is derived from a highly purified human cadaveric collagen, which is cultured from a single cell line and undergoes extensive testing for viruses etc.[27] It requires refrigeration.

Later in 2003, the FDA approved Restylane (Medicis Pharmaceutical Corporation), which became the first non-animal stabilized hyaluronic acid (NASHA) available in the United States. It is a synthetic product that lasts longer than previous materials, has virtually no risk of allergy, and requires no refrigeration. Soon thereafter, Perlane was created with slightly larger gel particles, to increase longevity.

To become competitive in the facial filler market, Allergan, Inc. (the makers of Botox) created its own NASHA product (Juviderm Ultra and Ultra Plus). These two products compete with Restylane and Perlane.

In 2006, another filler material, Radiesse (Merz Aesthetics, Inc.), was FDA approved. Radiesse is composed of calcium hydroxylapatite (CaHA) microspheres suspended in a water-based gel carrier. This is similar to the hydroxylapatite found in teeth and bones. It is thicker than hyaluronic acids and has a greater longevity. However, it is white in color, thus limiting its use to deeper applications (Fig. 24-13B). It is usually not recommended for use in the lip or any area with thin skin because of the risk of the white color being visible through the skin.

Current Filler Materials

The most common types of filler materials currently used in the United States are the hyaluronic acids (Restylane, Perlane, and Juviderm), and CaHA (Radiesse). Although there are many other materials currently or soon to be available emerging on the market, these two are currently the most commonly used.

Non-Animal Stabilized Hyaluronic Acid (NASHA). Hyaluronic acid (HA) is a polysaccharide complex found in the normal connective tissue of all living species.[29] The risk of allergic reaction is extremely low because it is not a protein. Therefore no allergy patch testing is required.

As skin ages, the content of HA decreases, causing wrinkling and decreased moisture of the skin.[30] After injection of HA, the skin changes are maintained by absorption of the body's own moisture.[31] One gram of HA can hold one thousand times its weight in water.[32] It also contains flexible dextran beads, which are thought to stimulate the skin's own collagen production. Hyaluronic acid provides immediate volume to the skin and continues to attract water from the body as it degrades, thus continuing to maintain its shape and form. Results tend to last from 6 to 12 months, depending on the product chosen.

Calcium Hydroxylapatite. CaHA is a naturally occurring substance found in bone and teeth.[33] Radiesse is composed of CaHA microspheres (30%) embedded in a methylcellulose carrier (70%). The methylcellulose carrier dissipates relatively quickly, leaving behind the CaHA microspheres to act as a scaffolding that promotes collagen ingrowth.[34] Although there was an initial discussion about possible bone formation in the area, after many years of clinical use this has shown not to be the case.[31,35] Results tend to last 12 to 18 months.

Safety and Contraindications

There are very few contraindications to facial injectables. The contraindications are usually site-specific (i.e., using the right filler for the right location, not injecting into a rash or infected site, avoiding blood vessels).

Complications of filler material injection usually include bruising, swelling, pain, granuloma formation, and rare cases of tissue necrosis.[36,37] An enzyme, hyaluronidase, can dissolve HA and help in areas of overfilling or nodules.[38-40]

Storage, Preparation, and Injection Technique

Unlike botulinum toxin, there are no special storage or preparation requirements for filler materials. They usually are packaged in prefilled, disposable syringes, with an enclosed needle tip (see Fig. 24-13A). They do not require refrigeration.

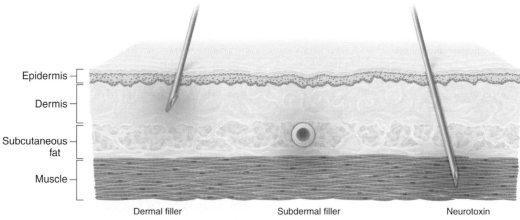

Epidermis
Dermis
Subcutaneous fat
Muscle

Dermal filler   Subdermal filler   Neurotoxin

FIGURE 24-14 Layers of the skin for injectable pharmaceuticals.

Recently, local anesthetic has been premixed into the Hyaluronic acid fillers for patient comfort. Radiesse does not have local anesthesia mixed into the material, but is packaged with a mixing kit, so the clinician can add anesthetic. Because filler material is a particle/gel mix, the needle must be a larger diameter than the needle tip that is used for botulinum toxin. Therefore even with local anesthetic incorporated into the filler material, many patients prefer a local anesthetic be used before filler injection.

CLINICAL TIP

If injecting local anesthesia before the treatment, do not inject copious amounts of anesthetic directly into the area being corrected; this will distort the area, making the deficiency appear to be better than it actually is. Either inject away from the area or use regional blocks.

Patients should be seated upright during evaluation and treatment planning and during the administration of facial fillers so that the shadows of the depressions in the face can be properly evaluated and treated. If a patient is reclining, gravity will cause an immediate "facelift" and many depressions and folds will disappear. It is best to avoid shining the dental light directly into the patient's face, because this will cause the shadows of the face to disappear. Overhead ceiling lights provide a true representation of the effects of aging on the patient's face.

When introducing the filler material into the skin, the needle should be placed subcutaneously, at the mid-dermis level, or at the reticular dermis level (Fig. 24-14). This depends both on the area to be corrected and the type of filler selected. Fillers can be "layered" by placing a heavier body filler deeper in the skin to give support to the area and then placing a lighter body filler above to achieve a natural "smoothing" of the finer wrinkles in the area.

There are many different injection techniques (Fig. 24-15), which vary widely among practitioners and often are a matter of personal preference. These techniques are briefly described as follows.

Serial Puncture. The needle is inserted to the appropriate level in the skin and a deposit of material is expressed. The needle is then removed and the procedure is repeated immediately adjacent to the first deposit. This procedure is continued so that all the deposits connect along the line of the desired correction.

Linear threading   Serial puncture

Fanning   Cross-hatching

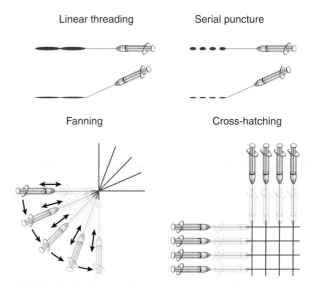

FIGURE 24-15 Various injection techniques. (From Cantisano-Zilkha M, Haddad A: *Aesthetic oculofacial rejuvenation*, St Louis, 2010, Saunders.)

Threading. The needle is inserted to the appropriate level in the skin. The product is then injected as the needle is being withdrawn (retrograde). This technique is ideal for the beginner.

Fanning. Fanning is a threading technique, but after the retrograde injection and before removing the needle from the skin, it is redirected through the skin multiple times in a fanlike manner in the area. This is a popular second step after learning the threading technique. It allows for fewer puncture sites.

Cross-Hatching. Cross-hatching is a series of parallel "threads" followed by another series of parallel threads placed perpendicular above or below the first series of threads. This technique is ideal when large volumes of filler are needed or heavy support is required for a deep fold of skin.

After injection, some practitioners prefer to massage the area to smooth any irregularities ("lumpiness"). A viscous material, such as ultrasound gel, can be placed on the skin to increase tactile sensation of the "lumps and bumps" during the massaging process. It is not advisable to overfill the area in hopes that it will "settle-in." It is preferable to achieve a full correction followed by a 2-week re-evaluation, at which time more filler material can be added if necessary.

Areas of Treatment

As with botulinum toxin, the beginner usually begins with three main areas. Once confidence is attained, other areas can be attempted. Facial fillers are more versatile than botulinum toxin. Filler material has the potential to lift, sculpt, smooth, and contour almost any area on the face.

Nasolabial Folds. One of the most prominent signs of facial aging is descent of the midfacial soft tissues inferiorly and medially.[30] This causes a fold of skin that extends from the ala of the nose toward the corners of the mouth (Fig. 24-16A). Filler material can easily be injected along this fold to fill in the depression, thus making the fold less noticeable. The type of filler material chosen should depend on the depth of the fold, among other considerations. The deeper the fold, the heavier the body of material should be, to lend support to the area (Fig. 24-16B).

When a practitioner has achieved a certain level of experience, the malar area should be evaluated at the same time as the nasolabial folds. If the patient will benefit from correction of the malar area (i.e., "liquid cheek lift"), this should be performed before correction of the nasolabial folds.

> ### CLINICAL TIP
>
> Many times, by correcting the malar area, the cheek will be lifted and the nasolabial fold will receive a tremendous correction without placing any material in the area itself (Fig. 24-17). If still needed, the nasolabial fold can be corrected afterward.

Labio-mandibular Folds (Marionette Lines). The descent of the midfacial soft tissues causes an extension of the nasolabial folds called the labiomandibular fold (see Fig. 24-17A). These are commonly referred to as "marionette lines" because of its similarity to lines of the movable mouth on marionette dolls. These lines are usually corrected at the same time as the nasolabial folds in patients requiring such a correction.

Before correction of this area, the practitioner should evaluate the oral commissures. With age, the commissures will appear to invert causing patients to appear as if they are frowning. With some support from facial fillers, this area can be corrected as well (see Fig. 24-17B).

Malar Area. As described, when the naso-labial and labio-mandibular folds are significant, the advanced practitioner can augment the malar area by placing filler over the malar bone. This will stretch the overlying tissue and "lift the midface" (Fig. 24-18).

There are a group of patients that may complain of "hollowness" of the cheek area. This can be caused by both normal aging and extreme weight loss. Using filler material, these areas can be corrected.

> ### CLINICAL TIP
>
> The skilled practitioner can administer many of the facial fillers through intraoral injections. The patient in Figure 24-18 was treated solely with intraoral injections. By using intraoral injections, facial bruising and injection marks can be avoided.

Lips. No other area on the face is as important to the esthetic dentist as the lips, which are the "frame" for the dentition. During the aging process, the lips can experience changes, including atrophy of the tissue, flattening of the lip architecture, inversion of the vermilion border, loss of distinct vermilion line, loss of philtrum ridges, and perioral rhytids (lipstick/smoker's lines) (see Fig. 24-19A). The goal is to correct as many of these deficiencies as possible, yet retain a natural appearance (see Fig. 24-19B). Although the upper lip tends to lose the most volume during the aging process, thus requiring the greatest amount of correction, the lower lip should always remain larger (as it is during youth). The lower lip should form a proper base for the upper lip to rest upon. Keeping this natural proportion usually necessitates some injection of filler in the lower lip after correction of the upper lip.

Techniques to correct the aging lips include outlining the vermilion border, adding volume to the lips, creating a natural "pout," re-creating philtrum ridges, and correcting perioral rhytids. These corrections can be completed by linear threading, fanning, or serial puncture generally requiring a combination of

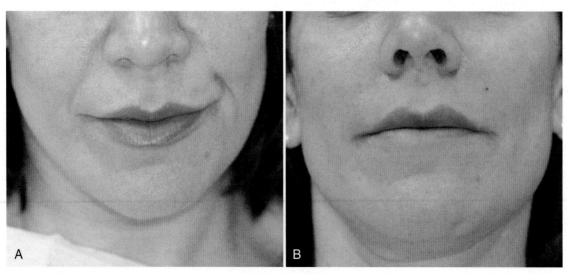

FIGURE 24-16 A, Preoperative view of patient requiring nasolabial fold correction. **B,** Postoperative view of same patient after treatment with Radiesse.

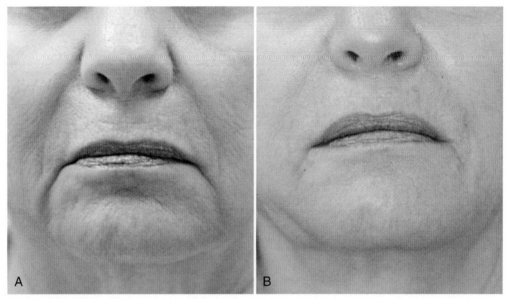

FIGURE 24-17 A, Patient with prominent nasolabial and labio-mandibular folds ("marionette lines"). **B,** Postoperative view of same patient shows correction of naso-labial and labio-mandibular folds and the malar area.

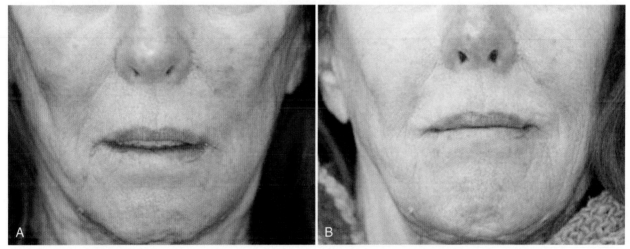

FIGURE 24-18 A, A patient with deficient malar areas showing "hollowness of the cheeks." **B,** The same patient in the rest position after correction of the malar area with Radiesse.

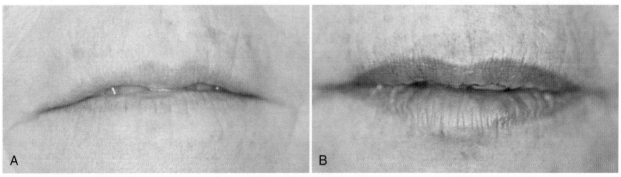

FIGURE 24-19 A, A patient requiring dermal fillers to correct lip volume. **B,** Postoperative view of the same patient after correction with Restylane.

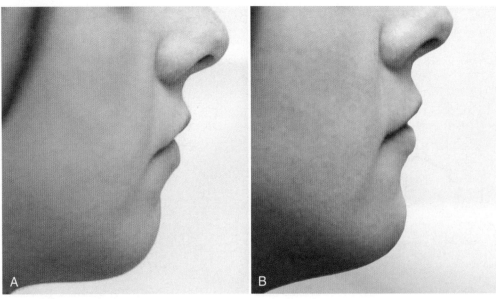

FIGURE 24-20 A, Preoperative "chin advancement" with Radiesse. **B,** Postoperative view of the same patient after "chin advancement" with Radiesse.

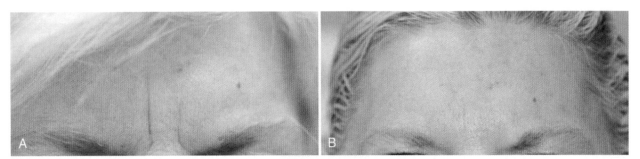

FIGURE 24-21 A, A patient with (both dynamic wrinkling and) static lines, that would be more exaggerated with dynamic animation. **B,** Postoperative view of the same patient after treatment with a combination botulinum toxin and hyaluronic acid filler to correct static lines.

these techniques. Because of the great variation of lip anatomy as well as consideration of lip support and tooth/gingival display, both during rest and animation, the lips can be one of the most challenging, yet rewarding, areas for filler correction.

Advanced Areas and Techniques

The experienced practitioner can perform cheek lifts, brow lifts, nasal correction, earlobe correction, chin augmentation (Fig. 24-20), mandibular contouring, and tear trough correction. Currently there are no set parameters regarding the exact procedures allowed under various state dental practice acts, but this is likely to change in the near future.

COMBINATION THERAPY

Many patients require a combination of botulinum toxin and facial fillers to achieve an ideal aesthetic result.

It is important to educate patients about the different products available and their mechanisms of action so that they will understand the rationale behind treatment recommendations.

For example, if a patient complains of "frown lines" in the glabella complex, the clinician might also observe that both dynamic wrinkling, and distinct vertical static lines (eleven lines) at complete rest (Fig. 24-21A). In this case botulinum toxin would prevent the underlying muscles from causing wrinkling during animation, but a facial filler will be required to correct the lines at rest (Fig. 24-21B).

In addition, many studies demonstrate that combination therapy will extend the time for return to preinjection furrow compared with one modality alone.[41-43]

CONCLUSION

Adequate didactic and hands-on training is required before facial injection treatment is attempted. In addition, individual state laws vary regarding facial injectable treatment requirements. Regardless of who provides the therapy, dermatologic pharmaceuticals should be considered an important adjunct to esthetic dental procedures.

REFERENCES

1. ADA definition of dentistry, Adopted, American Dental Association House of Delegates, 1997.
2. Greco TM, Antunes MB, Yellin SA: Injectable fillers for volume replacement in the aging face, *Facial Plast Surg* 28(1):8-20, 2012. Epub March 14, 2012.
3. Gilchrest BA: Cellular and molecular changes in aging skin, *J Geriatr Dermatol* 2:3, 1994.
4. Rohrich RJ, Pessa JE: The fat compartments of the face: anatomy and clinical implications for cosmetic surgery, *Plast Reconstr Surg* 119(7):2219-2227, 2007 discussion 2228-2231.
5. Rohrich RJ, Pessa JE: The retaining system of the face: histologic evaluation of the septal boundaries of the subcutaneous fat compartments, *Plast Reconstr Surg* 121(5):1804-1809, 2008.
6. Gunn RA: Botulism: from van Ermengen to the present, a comment, *Clin Infect Dis* 1(4):720-721, 1979.
7. Lowe NJ: Overview of botulinum neurotoxins, *J Cosmetic Laser Ther* 9(suppl 1):11-16, 2009.
8. Scott AB, Rosenbaum A, Collins CC: Pharmacologic weakening of extraocular muscles, *Invest Opthamol* 12:924-927, 1973.
9. Scott AB: Development of botulinum toxin therapy, *Dermatol Clin* 22:131-133, 2004.
10. Scott AB: Botulinum toxin injection into extraocular muscles as an alternative to strabismus surgery, *Ophthalmology* 87:1044-1049, 1980.
11. Helveston EM: Botulinum injections for strabismus, *J Pediatr Ophthalmol Strabismus* 21(5):202-204, 1984.
12. Frueh BR, Felt DP, Wojno TH, Musch DC: Treatment of blepharospasm with botulinum toxin. A preliminary report, *Arch Ophthalmol* 102(10):1464-1468, 1984.
13. Wabbels B, Roggenkämper P: Botulinum toxin in hemifacial spasm: the challenge to assess the effect of treatment, *J Neural Transm* 119(8):963-980, 2012.
14. Tsoy EA, Buckley EG, Dutton JJ: Treatment of blepharospasm with botulinum toxin, *Am J Ophthalmol* 99(2):176-179, 1985.
15. Tsui JK, Eisen A, Mak E, Carruthers J, Scott A, Calne DB: A pilot study on the use of botulinum toxin in spasmodic torticollis, *Can J Neurol Sci* 12(4):314-316, 1985.
16. Brin MF, Fahn S, Moskowitz C, Friedman A, Shale HM, Greene PE, et al: Localized injections of botulinum toxin for the treatment of focal dystonia and hemifacial spasm, *Mov Disord* 2(4):237-254, 1987.
17. Jankovic J, Orman J: Botulinum A toxin for cranial-cervical dystonia: a double-blind, placebo-controlled study, *Neurology* 37(4):616-623, 1987.
18. Carruthers JD, Carruthers JA: Treatment of glabellar frown lines with C. Botulinum A exotoxin, *J Dermatol Surg Oncol* 18:17-21, 1992.
19. Dutton JJ, Buckley EG: Long-term results and complications of botulinum A toxin in the treatment of blepharospasm, *Ophthalmology* 95(11):1529-1534, 1988.
20. Carruthers JD, Carruthers JA: Botulinum toxin in facial rejuvenation: an update, *Obstet Gynecol Clin North Am* 37:571-582, 2010.
21. Naumann M, Jankovic J: Safety of botulinum toxin type A: a systematic review and meta-analysis, *Curr Med Res Opin* 20:981-990, 2004.
22. Cote TR, Mohan AK, Polder JA, et al: Botulinum toxin type A injections: adverse events reported to the US Food and Drug Administration in therapeutic and cosmetic cases, *J Am Acad Dermatol* 53:407-415, 2005.
23. LeWitt PA, Trosh RM: Idiosyncratic adverse reactions to intramuscular botulinum toxin type A injection, *Mov Disord* 12:1064-1067, 1997.
24. Botox cosmetic (onabotulinumtoxinA) package insert, Allergan Inc., 2012.
25. Kontis TC, Rivkin A: The history of injectable facial fillers, *Facial Plast Surg* 25(2):67-72, 2009. Epub 2009 May.
26. Narins RS, Beer K: Liquid injectable silicone: a review of its history, immunology, technical considerations, complications and potential, *Plast Reconstr Surg* 118(3S):77S-84S, 2006.
27. Eppley BL, Dadvand B: Injectable soft-tissue fillers: clinical overview, *Plast Reconstr Surg* 118(4):98e-106e, 2006.
28. Narins RS, Bowman PH: Injectable skin fillers, *Clin Plast Surg* 32:151-162, 2005.
29. Laurent TC: Biochemistry of hyaluronan, *Acta Otolaryngol Suppl* 442:7-24, 1987.
30. Longas MO, Russell CS, He XY: Evidence for structural changes in dermatan sulfate and hyaluronic acid with aging, *Carbohydr Res* 159:127-136, 1987.
31. Dayan SH, Bassichis BA: Facial dermal fillers: selection of appropriate products and techniques, *Aesthet Surg J* 28(3):335-347, 2008.
32. John HE, Price RD: Perspectives in the selection of hyaluronic fillers for facial wrinkles and aging skin, *Patient Prefer Adherence* 3:225-230, 2009.
33. Greco TM, Antunes MB, Yellin SA: Injectable fillers for volume replacement in the aging face, *Facial Plast Surg* 28(1):8-20, 2012. Epub 2012 March 14.
34. Shumaker PR, England LJ, Dover JS, et al: Effect of monopolar radiofrequency treatment over soft-tissue fillers in an animal model: part 2, *Lasers Surg Med* 38:211-217, 2006.
35. Jacovella PF, Peiretti CB, Cunille D, Salzamendi M, Schechtel SA: Long lasting results with hydroxylapatite (Radiesse) facial filler, *Plast Reconstr Surg* 118(3 Suppl):15s-21s, 2006.
36. Friedman PM, Mafong EA, Kauvar AN, Geronemus RG: Safety data of injectable nonanimal stabilized hyaluronic acid gel for soft tissue augmentation, *Dermatol Surg* 28:491, 2002.
37. Park TH, Seo SW, Kim JK, Chang CH: Clinical experience with hyaluronic acid-filler complications, *J Plast Reconstr Aesthet Surg* 64(7):892-896, 2011. Epub February 9, 2011.
38. Rzany B, Becker-Wegerich P, Bachmann F, Erdmann R, Wollina U: Hyaluronidase in the correction of hyaluronic acid-based fillers: a review and a recommendation for use, *J Cosmet Dermatol* 8(4):317-323, 2009.
39. Narins RS, Coleman WP 3rd, Glogau RG: Recommendations and treatment options for nodules and other filler complications, *Dermatol Surg* 35(suppl 2):1667-1671, 2009.
40. Grunebaum LD, Bogdan Allemann I, Dayan S, Mandy S, Baumann L: The risk of alar necrosis associated with dermal filler injection, *Dermatol Surg* 35(suppl 2):1635-1640, 2009.
41. Carruthers JD, Glogau RG, Blitzer A; Facial Aesthetics Consensus Group Faculty: Advances in facial rejuvenation: botulinum toxin type a, hyaluronic acid dermal fillers, and combination therapies-consensus recommendations, *Plast Reconstr Surg* 121(5 Suppl):5S-30S, 2008; quiz 31S-36S.
42. Coleman KR, Carruthers J: Combination therapy with BOTOX and fillers: the new rejuvenation paradigm, *Dermatol Ther* 19(3):177-188, 2006.
43. de Maio M: Botulinum toxin in association with other rejuvenation methods, *J Cosmet Laser Ther* 5(3-4):210-212, 2003.

25

Esthetics and Plastic Surgery

Gregory E. Rauscher

The use of cosmetic plastic surgery to enhance self-image, once accessible to only a small and privileged segment of society, has now spread to mainstream America. Today's patients want their outward appearance to reflect their healthy lifestyles. The benefits of exercise, proper diet, and skin care combined with plastic surgery can improve the overall quality of one's life.

The American Society of Plastic Surgeons has defined cosmetic surgery as "that surgery which is done to revise or change the texture, or relationship with contiguous structures of any feature of the human body judged by competent medical opinion to be without jeopardy to physical or mental health."[1] The American Medical Association accepted this definition.[2]

The following sections briefly discuss various techniques for enhancing facial appearance. They techniques vary from superficial adjustment of skin tone to facial skeletal alteration with implants.

RHINOPLASTY

Rhinoplasty, or nose surgery, is one of the most commonly performed procedures in plastic surgery. Depending on the patient's needs, the nose can be reduced in size (Fig. 25-1), or the shape and size of the nasal tip, bridge, or nostrils can be altered (Fig. 25-2) All of the preceding procedures can be done simultaneously. At the time of the nasal surgical operation, the relationship of the nose to the upper lip can be changed. Breathing problems can be relieved concurrently.

The best candidates for rhinoplasty are patients seeking reasonable improvement in their appearance. Several factors can prevent perfection, including individual healing properties, facial asymmetry, and unrealistic expectations. In most circumstances psychologically stable, healthy patients seeking natural results are good candidates. One in 10 patients who choose rhinoplasty requires a touch-up or revision. Nasal surgery is usually performed in less than 2 hours. A nasal splint is necessary for 1 week after surgery. After the first week a night splint is required for at least 2 weeks. Most nasal surgery is performed on an outpatient basis. Surgical incisions are necessary, but are usually undetectable and are placed internally in the nasal sill or the base of the nose. In corrective nasal surgery, the underlying cartilage and bone are sculpted. In some traumatic cases, septal or ear cartilage may be needed to support the tip or nasal bridge.

RHYTIDECTOMY

A rhytidectomy or face lift is the removal of loose skin on the face and neck. Each patient has a unique characteristic of skin texture, plasticity, in addition to facial wrinkles and facial folds. Some patients have mid face bone resorption which produces a deep line or fold that runs from corner (ala) of the nose to the angle of the mouth.

Some patients develop jowls, which is a condition with loss of a well-defined jaw line. Jowls may require removal of fat, facial muscle tightening, or a combination of both techniques. Some candidates have loose skin, wrinkles, as well as excessive fat in the neck. Surgical treatment may require lifting of the neck, cheek, and forehead. In certain cases just a neck or cheek lift can achieve a fresh youthful face without a full face lift (Fig. 25-3).

The best candidates for facial surgery are patients whose cheek and neckline have begun to sag but have skin that has some remaining elements of elasticity and also have good bone structure. The initial consultation may be uncomfortable for the patient, but honest discussion and communication are essential for the plastic surgeon to determine if the patient's expectations are realistic and what the patient hopes to achieve. Prior medical history is important and includes previous operations and medications taken. Smoking should be discontinued well in advance of surgery. Certain antiinflammatory drugs, aspirin, herbs, and alcohol are to be avoided to reduce bruising and bleeding. Poor general health, excessive sun exposure, and use of tobacco and alcohol negatively influence healing and accelerate aging. All cosmetic procedures can turn back the clock; however, aging cannot be stopped. Results of facelift surgery usually last 5 to 10 years, and face and neck surgery can be improved with effective alternate treatments such as laser resurfacing, chemical peel, liposuction, or augmentation of cheek and chin. All these treatments have some degree of risk.

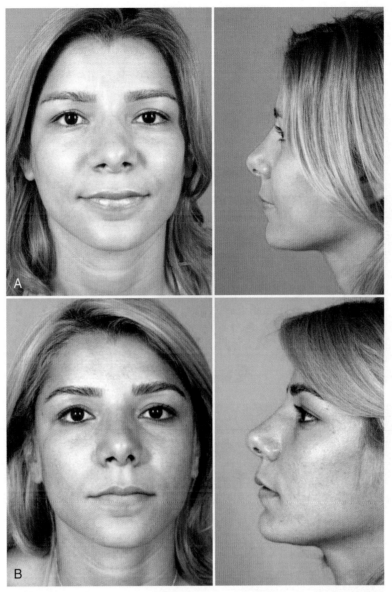

FIGURE 25-1 A, Preoperative view of a female patient who was unhappy with her nose. **B,** Postoperative view of the patient after conservative reduction of all nasal elements.

Minor unexpected complications such as bleeding and unfavorable scarring can affect the final result, but dire complications such as facial paralysis are relatively rare.

BLEPHAROPLASTY

Blepharoplasty (eyelid lift) is a procedure in which excess skin and fat from the upper and lower eyelids is removed. Blepharoplasty can be done through the normal upper eyelid crease and lower eyelid lining producing minimal to no visible scars (Fig. 25-4). Recovery requires 1 week and the results can last several years. In certain cases the patient believes the results are permanent even though the aging process continues.

FACIAL IMPLANTS

Facial implants can change the basic shape of the face by carefully building up the receding jaw, chin, or cheekbones. Implants may be composed of natural or artificial materials. Results with

facial implants are generally permanent and the procedure is performed in less than 1 hour on an outpatient basis. The insertion of facial implants is usually combined with other plastic surgery procedures as seen in the previous case (Fig. 25-5).

OTOPLASTY

Otoplasty (ear surgery) is a procedure to reposition prominent ears closer to the head (Fig. 25-6). Lobe reduction may be necessary to create a harmonious outcome. Results are permanent. The patient generally is back to school or work in 1 week.

BROW LIFT

Forehead or brow lifting can minimize eyebrow drooping, reduce forehead wrinkles, and restore a youthful appearance to the upper third of the face. Depending on the degree of eyebrow ptosis or forehead elevation desired, correction can be performed endoscopically (Fig. 25-7) through small incisions on

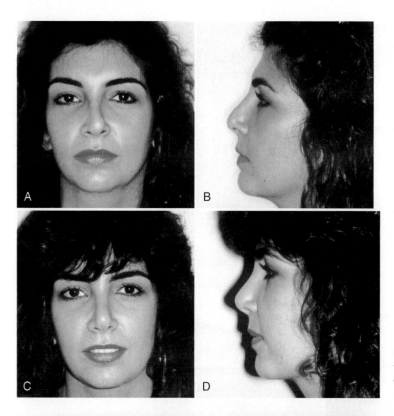

FIGURE 25-2 **A** and **B,** Preoperative view of a 29-year-old female patient with a post-rhinoplasty nasal deformity. **C** and **D,** Postoperative frontal view of the patient after augmentation of the nose with cartilage and bone.

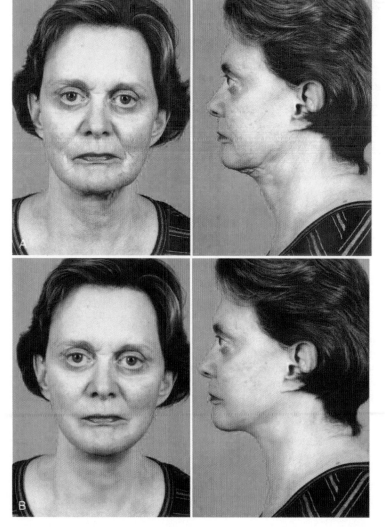

FIGURE 25-3 **A,** Preoperative views of a patient before standard fat grafting to the cheeks and a neck lift. **B,** Two year postoperative views of a patient after fat grafting to the cheeks and necklift

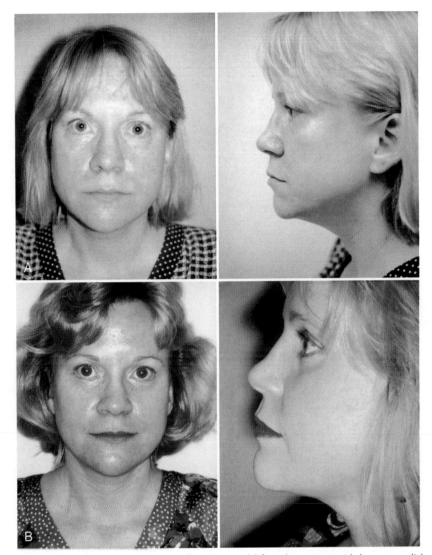

FIGURE 25-4 A, Preoperative views of a 45-year-old female patient with baggy eyelids and underdeveloped cheek bones who complained of looking tired. **B,** Postoperative views of the patient after lower eyelid blepharoplasty and cheek augmentation.

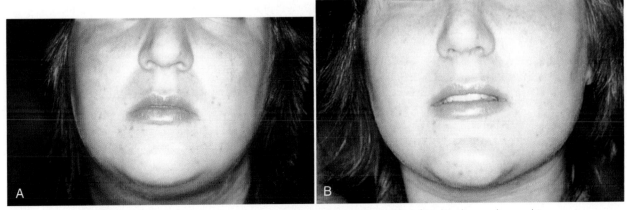

FIGURE 25-5 A, An 18-year-old female patient with an obtuse, ill-defined jawline and poor chin definition. **B,** Postoperative view of the patient after combined chin augmentation, rhinoplasty, and liposuction of the neck.

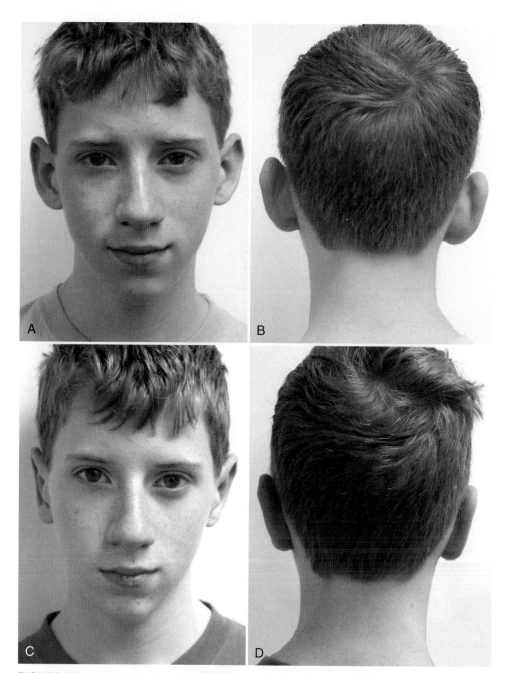

FIGURE 25-6 A, Preoperative views of a patient with prominent ears. **B,** Postoperative views of the patient after surgery to correct the prominent ears. (*From Niamtu J:* Cosmetic Facial Surgery, *St. Louis, Mosby, 2011.*)

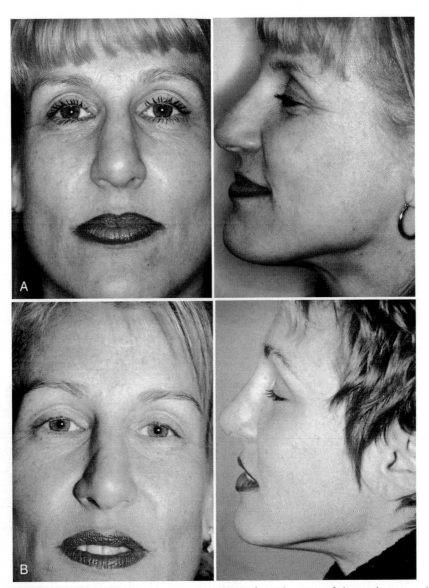

FIGURE 25-7 A, Preoperative views of a patient before elevation of the eyebrows and tip rhinoplasty. **B,** Postoperative views of the patient after endoscopic elevation of the eyebrows and nasal tip reduction.

the scalp or through a more extensive scalp incision. Recovery takes one week. Results generally last 5 to 10 years.

SKIN RESURFACING: CHEMICAL PEEL, DERMABRASION, AND LASER ABRASION

Skin resurfacing and rejuvenation are procedures that can be accomplished through chemical peeling, dermabrasion, or ablative laser resurfacing. Each of the preceding techniques is used to remove wrinkles, improve sun-damaged facial skin, and decrease acne scars. The results of each technique vary depending on the patient's skin texture and tone. Patients who are very fair skinned may remain pink for months after any resurfacing technique. Patients with dark complexions are prone to hyperpigmentation (Fig. 25-8). Temporary skin hyperpigmentation, whitehead formation (milia), and allergic skin flare-ups occasionally occur during the healing process.

FACIAL INJECTIONS

The injection of materials into facial laugh lines, smile lines, and glabellar lines has become popular. The number of injectable materials has exploded, and some of the products are not safe or proven. The most common injectable is hyaluronic acid, a gel that causes the body to generate collagen. As individuals mature the amount of facial fat as well as bone structure diminish. Hyaluronic acid is a natural building block in human tissue. Injectable hyaluronic acid injection can augment facial structure and is exceptionally safe. The proper placement of hyaluronic acid can temporarily correct facial wrinkles as well as minor nasal deformities (Fig. 25-9) (see also Chapter 24).

Fat works in restoring facial volume (Fig. 25-10A,B). Approximately 50% of the injected fat remains after the treatment. The addition of platelet enriched plasma (PRP) is a new emerging field in cosmetic surgery. In using PRP, a small amount of the patient's blood is mixed with a collagen matrix. The platelet

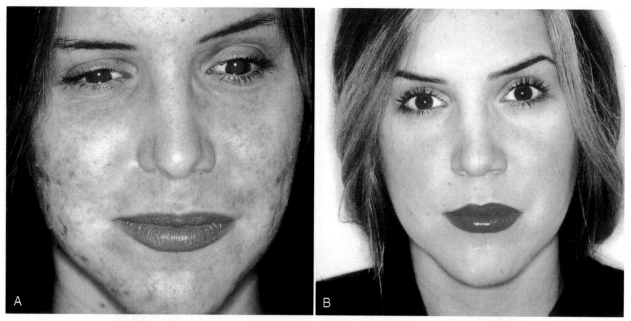

FIGURE 25-8   A Preoperative view of a 25-year-old female patient with severe active acne of the face. **B** Postoperative view of the patient after full face laser surgery.

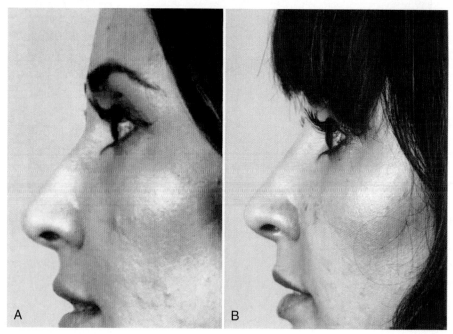

FIGURE 25-9   A, Preoperative and **B,** immediate postoperative views of a patient who had a hyaluronic acid injection to remove appearance of a nasal bump. The bump has been camouflaged and was not removed.

enriched plasma can maximize healing under facelifted skin or the liquid PRP when combined with fat generates stem cells that rejuvenate the face when injected in areas needing augmentation or rejuvenation. The field of stem cell fat grafting is frequently called "liquid facelifts." The long-term efficacy of this new frontier is not yet known, but it appears to be very promising (see Fig. 25-10). The duration of fat grafting with PRP range from 6 months to more than a 5-year correction.

BOTOX

Complete removal of all facial wrinkles is impractical. Temporary reduction of forehead wrinkles and crow's feet has been obtained with Botox, a purified neurotoxin complex that has been in use since 1980 for blepharospasm (involuntary eyelid twitch). Botox binds to small nerve endings and when injected into frown lines or crow's feet, eliminates the muscle activity for 4 to 6 months. Botox can be used two to three times a year (see also Chapter 24).

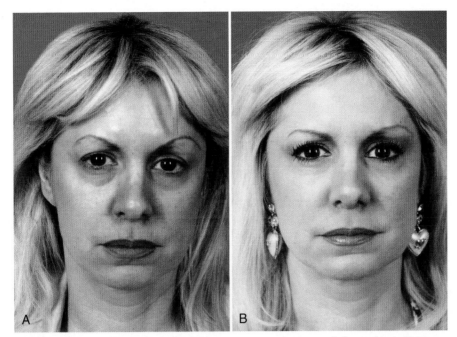

FIGURE 25-10 **A,** Preperative view of a patient prior to stem cell fat grafting. **B,** Two year postoperative view after stem cell fat grafting to enhance the cheeks.

COMPUTER IMAGING

3D computer imaging combined with 2D digital; photography facilitates improved communication between the patient and plastic surgeon. Facial features and body asymmetry can be visualized and intelligently discussed before surgery. Potential operative results can be simulated. Although the predictability of achieving results varies from patient to patient, potential surgical improvement can be presented. The imager can vary the percentage of facial correction produced in the image that can help avoid an implied guarantee and provide an improved patient-doctor relationship

CONCLUSION

Cosmetic facial surgery is becoming more popular. Every year thousands of men and woman undergo cosmetic plastic surgery and are pleased with the results. The reason for choosing cosmetic plastic surgery is unique to each individual. Techniques for reducing noticeable signs of aging are available. Continuing research of existing technology has resulted in predictable surgical as well as nonsurgical results.

Many imperfections of the nose, ears, cheeks, and chin are amenable to improvement with advancing techniques as well as minimal scar surgery. Facial cosmetic surgery may be the first step a person takes to enhance his or her overall improvement. Many patients with an improved facial appearance are encouraged to maintain their new image through lifestyle modifications with exercise, diet, skin, eye, and dental care.

REFERENCES

1. American Society of Plastic Surgeons Bylaws, Arlington Heights, IL, p. 37.
2. American Medical Association Accreditation for Medical Graduate Education, Chicago, p. 243.

Part 5

Esthetic Practice Management

26

Esthetics and Dental Marketing

Edward Zuckerberg

Dental marketing, once embraced by only a small percentage of dental practitioners, is now fully recognized as an essential business tool for a financially successful dental practice. Some of the factors that have transformed the business of practicing dentistry include easier Internet access, changing disease patterns, cost containment policies by business and government, increased unemployment, recession, and the rise of consumerism. These powerful factors, although sometimes cyclic in nature, will continue to affect the profession for some time. As a result, competition among dentists for patients, or for the discretionary income of consumers, has reached historically high levels. In a free market society, marketing is a logical by-product of increasing competition.

HISTORY

Before 1977, when the US Supreme Court ruling in *Bates v. State Bar of Arizona*[1] legalized advertising by attorneys, professional marketing essentially was limited to word-of-mouth patient referrals and fundamental in-office patient relations techniques. Active marketing by dentists was discouraged by organized dentistry, both nationally and at the local level. Soon after the Supreme Court ruling, however, dentistry and other health professions were required by law to allow advertising. The Federal Trade Commission (FTC) applied pressure to state dental boards and other dental organizations to change professional ethics standards and other rules that restricted or prohibited advertising. The FTC's position was that advertising that was not false or misleading would stimulate competition and lower the cost of dental care for consumers. This ushered in a controversial era of conflict between dental professionals and organizations that believed that advertising was unprofessional and those in dentistry and government who argued that it was beneficial and acceptable.

Today, information about individual dentists and their practices is readily available and easily obtainable by both existing and potential patients. Unfortunately, this information may be erroneous and even uncomplimentary. Dentists can either remain passive about this or they can control the image that will be accessed about their practices and themselves.

What Is Marketing?

Marketing encompasses a variety of disciplines and techniques that are intended to motivate a targeted individual or group to take an action that is desired by the marketer. This action may be to purchase a product or service, attend a specific event, vote for a particular candidate, visit a dental office, or elect to have certain dental procedures performed. From 1977 through the early twenty-first century, dental marketing was often a disorganized series of advertisements presented in a variety of media. The most common were print advertisements in Yellow Page directories, newspapers, and local "Pennysavers." Direct-mail campaigns and non-print media such as television and radio were also used. These efforts were generally geared toward attracting new patients and rarely involved more than just a listing or menu of services offered by the practice. The use of coupons or offers, or even the mention of prices for services was initially avoided, but as competition increased among dentists, pricing information appeared. Many dentists elected to avoid advertising or supplemented their efforts to gain new patients by joining insurance company preferred provider organizations (PPOs), whereby their participation and willingness to accept reduced pricing was advertised through the insurance company's print and subsequent online directories.

There are many marketing methods in addition to advertising, however, that can be used to reach a specific audience. Of particular relevance to dentists are two basic marketing approaches: external marketing and internal marketing. An understanding of these two approaches will aid in designing a marketing program that is in harmony with the individual dentist's philosophy.

EXTERNAL AND INTERNAL MARKETING

Two basic goals of dental marketing are to attract new patients to the practice and to keep existing patients active within the practice. Marketing techniques designed to attract new patients can be categorized as external techniques. Those designed to keep existing patients active, pursue necessary and elective care, and motivate them to refer others to the practice are internal techniques.

External Marketing

External marketing techniques encompass any marketing activities designed to attract consumers into the dental office so that they will become active patients. In addition to the methods of advertising previously listed, today's astute dental marketers use a variety of online tools, including search engine optimization (SEO), maintenance of an attractive practice website, and a social media presence to interact with existing and prospective patients. Dentists can also offer to speak to various community groups to educate the public and create visibility for their practice as well as network with other local businesses and dentists to encourage referrals of potential new patients. Of these methods, an increasing number of practitioners are relying on the electronic media, seeing these as a way to reach their target market at a much more reasonable cost than the formerly traditional print, television, and radio media.

Search engine optimization (SEO) is the method whereby a practice gains a greater likelihood of being listed closer to the top results of a search that a patient conducts with Google or other search engines (Fig. 26-1).

For example, if a dentist wishes to increase the number of patients making appointments for cosmetic dental procedures, the practice website, Facebook page, online directory listings, and so on should all include keywords such as cosmetic dentistry, laminates, veneers, ceramic crowns, and bleaching. This will enhance the likelihood that when a patient types: "cosmetic dentist, your town" into the search engine, your practice will appear earlier, and therefore will be more likely to be viewed in the resulting list as opposed to being buried several pages later. Google and other search engines use algorithms that search the Internet to find how often the terms listed in the search appear together with the most regularity to determine your ultimate placement in the search. Of course, there are also paid methods to obtain a more favorable placement in a search result, such as use of Google's AdWords program, which allows you to purchase a high placement in searches that employ these terms. There are also a large number of companies that will perform SEO for a fee, and whether dentists choose to optimize on their own or pay someone else depends on time, budget, and personal expertise. Many practices today employ an individual solely to manage the practice's electronic communications. Similarly, dentists wishing to advertise or promote the implant or pediatric areas of their practice can use the same tools.

Business websites have existed since the turn of this century and although they are an excellent tool for presenting information about a practice and as such are enormously helpful

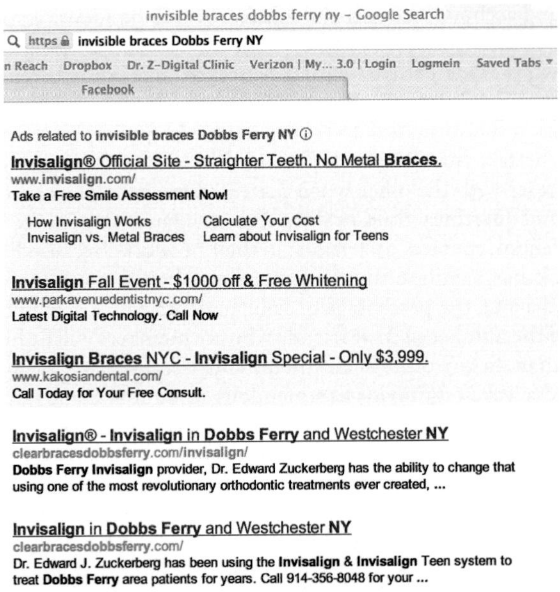

FIGURE 26-1 To promote Invisalign on Google without paying for AdWords, the author uses terms like *invisible braces* and *clear aligners* in the body of his/her Facebook and Web pages to garnish the top two free spots in the search for invisible braces in his/her community. Note that the three higher-shaded links are paid advertising.

in attracting prospective new patients, they are not an effective means of communicating with existing patients (see the section on Internal Marketing).

The final tool for external marketing is the use of social media, such as Facebook. Facebook in particular has huge advantages over other forms of social media, because of its sheer number of members, currently approaching one billion users worldwide. The most desirable referral a dentist can obtain is one that is initiated by a satisfied patient. The referred patient arrives with a preconceived sense of trust and confidence resulting from the "missionary work" of your current patient who has related to them how exemplary you and your staff are, your convenient hours, and so on. A practice can never have enough of this type of referral. Despite marketing gurus extolling the wisdom of asking existing patients to refer their friends, acquaintances, and loved ones, many dentists are either uncomfortable with this or feel that the appropriate situation to do so rarely occurs. In order for a successful word-of-mouth referral to occur in the traditional sense, your "beloved" and satisfied patients must find themselves in a social setting with someone who not only needs your services but voices that need to them. Further, the patient must be willing to make the recommendation and hopefully have your business card or be able to remember your exact website address.

Social media sites such as Facebook have the unique ability to be considered a trusted referral. Facebook is unique because of the sheer size of its user base. The key to Facebook's success for external marketing begins with getting "fans" (patients) for your office Facebook page. This gives it the unique ability to be considered a trusted referral. This can be accomplished by promoting your site everywhere your address and phone number appears (e.g., business cards, envelopes, online or print advertising, or reception area signage). Hopefully, your Facebook and website addresses will be identical (e.g., www.greatdentist.com and www.Facebook.com/greatdentist). Next, provide patients with a reason to "like" your Facebook page, either through offers for fans only, sending worthwhile news and information to their news feeds, or simply by virtue of the fact that Facebook provides the ability to engage and interact with the office when patients have general or specific dental questions. Studies show that each fan averages over 300 Facebook contacts or "friends" in their network. Because Facebook has significantly more members than any other social media site, the percentage of your patients who are members and the number of their friends who are members will be higher than on any other social media site. Because users of social media websites provide a tremendous amount of demographic information, the ability to selectively target an audience is greatly enhanced. An example of this is Facebook's optional fee-based advertising platform, which allows practitioners to target an ad program using demographics including geographic location, age, gender, income, marital status, interests and many others. In addition, social media websites have the ability to follow connections among members, which can greatly amplify the number of people who will hear about a practice through this trusted referral system. An example is Facebook's ad program that has the ability to market directly to the friends of your fans. If you attain 300 fans on your office Facebook page and they each have 300 friends, this results in access to 90,000 potential trusted referrals using this feature. Facebook will "pull" the name of their friend, who is a fan of your page, into the ad and insert the Facebook thumbs up logo with a message that their friend likes your practice (Fig. 26-2).

Thus, a trusted referral is passively harnessed without requiring your "missionary" patient to be in the same place at the same time as the potential new patient who is in need of your services. Dave Kerpen,[2] author of the *New York Times* bestseller *Likeable Social Media*, calls this use of Facebook's ad platform "word of mouth referrals on steroids!"

Internal Marketing

Internal marketing techniques encompass any marketing or communication activities that take place within the practice setting or that are directed at active or inactive patients with the objective of retaining them in the practice or causing them to become more active and to stimulate referrals. A few examples of internal marketing techniques that dentists have traditionally employed include presenting gifts or acknowledgements to referral sources, providing a comfortable, clean and attractive

Jane Doe likes Edward Zuckerberg, D.D.S..

Edward Zuckerberg, D.D.S.,F.A.G.D.
Professional services

Joe Smith and 3 other friends also like this

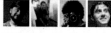

FIGURE 26-2 Friends of Jane Doe and Joe Smith can see from this ad whom they use as their dentist. This enables dentists with Facebook pages to obtain passive word-of-mouth referrals from those who know Jane and Joe.

physical office containing the latest technologies, offering amenities to create pleasant waiting periods for patients such as wi-fi, coffee, hot towels, aromatherapy, and so on. Other examples are supplying educational items such as newsletters and brochures to stimulate patient interest in particular services offered. In addition, one should not overlook details such as showing respect for your patients' time by informing them when the doctor is running late, offering to reschedule them if this would be more convenient, and a post-visit follow up call by the doctor or a staff member to make certain their visit went well. These are all ideas that make your practice more desirable than another office, increase the likelihood of patient retention and referrals, and when effectively employed allow the office to reduce its budget for external marketing as a result of more successful patient retention and increased trusted referrals from your existing patient base.

Another effective internal marketing tool is social media and the ability it provides to engage the existing patient base. Valuable information can be passed on through direct messages and links to Internet articles. The "human" side of the doctor and staff can be portrayed via posts about special achievements or outside activities, new techniques can be publicized, and the patient base can be engaged in meaningful discussions as well as have another outlet or contact point to the office for them to feel more connected to your practice. Hopefully a number of your patients and fans will consistently comment on most of your posts. This should provide an incentive to post useful content to engage them with, which will ultimately be seen by their friends who will learn about your practice. This is the most significant difference between a social media page like Facebook and a practice website. If, for example, you have completed a high-level implant CE course or purchased a CAD/CAM unit, you can, and should, post these items on your practice website. However, the effectiveness of this may be questionable because how many of your patients visit your website regularly and will ever see this content. With Facebook, when you post on your page about these items, they are "pushed" to your fans' newsfeeds so that the information is actively sent to them as opposed to passively viewed on your website. Not only will more of your patients find out about the completed course or new equipment, but also they are likely to engage you about it. This will not only promote your relationship with them, but also potentially spread your message throughout their network.

Managing Negative Publicity

Even the most conscientious practitioner will inevitably encounter a disappointed or disgruntled patient. However, patients will often avoid verbal or telephone confrontations and instead "vent" to friends, family, and colleagues or leave the practice entirely. Social media, on the other hand, provides a more comfortable alternative for them to complain directly with the dentist. This keeps the problem "in house" and provides the opportunity to resolve the dispute and retain the patient.

It is inevitable, therefore, that there will be an occasional negative post on Google, Yahoo, or your office Facebook or Twitter page. Clinicians cannot remove a post from Google or Yahoo no matter how inaccurate it may be; however, they can encourage their satisfied patients to post positive comments on these sites proactively and thus dilute the negative comment(s).

Facebook provides the ability to delete negative posts, but this is often not an effective strategy. The goal should not be to please every patient we encounter, but to take note of these negative comments to learn about possible areas in which the practice or customer service can be improved. Usually these posts are placed by a patient who is unhappy but has not yet left the office and is frustrated by a recent negative experience. Deleting the post sends the message to that patient that his or her thoughts are irrelevant, and will usually result in the patient leaving the practice. Engaging the comment directly, either with a direct response or with a comment that you will telephone them to discuss the matter privately, not only addresses the issue for them, but also establishes to other fans of your page that you care enough to listen to criticism and that the Facebook page is a viable source for interaction. It also demonstrates your responsiveness and approachability. This is of tremendous value to patients who are becoming begrudgingly resigned to "leave a voicemail which will be returned by the doctor or staff member in 24 to 48 hours."

THE FOUR Ps OF MARKETING

The concept of the four Ps was first presented in 1960[3] and is still highly regarded, although from time to time a new "marketing mix" will be proposed to replace this classic formula. The basic principles are still sound and applicable despite the massive changes in the marketing landscape that have occurred since the 1960s, not the least of which is the advent of technology and social media.

The components of the four Ps of marketing your products and services include:

+ Price
+ Place
+ Product
+ Promotion

Price[4]

Determining a fee schedule for services rendered is one of the most difficult tasks facing any dentist. Dentists can adopt a strategy of differentiation, setting a relatively high fee for services justified by superior quality and added extra value. To be successful the higher fee must be perceived by the customers of the practice or potential customers as a worthwhile investment compared with lower fees offered by the dentist's competitors. Using some of these strategies, dentists can create the perception that the value for their services is fair.

Price competition is another approach to determining fees. "Cost is everything" and fees are set relatively low, or set by insurance companies that the dentist affiliates with such as in PPOs. Dentists adopting this strategy will have an easier time generating new patients and keeping busy, but will have to treat more patients and work longer hours to earn the same income as their higher fee charging peers and will generally not be as successful in retaining patients. Of course, these two examples demonstrate the opposite ends of the spectrum; most practices will fall somewhere in between.

When it comes to setting fees, dentists have three options. Cost-plus is the most analytical method and the one generally employed by most practices. The process involves the calculation of fixed costs (those unaffected by the number of patients treated) divided by the number of hours the office is open to determine the fixed hourly cost of doing business. Determination of variable costs is more challenging but will include extra staffing during busy times, inventory utilization that is based on traffic (both administrative and treatment related), and procedure-specific costs such as laboratory fees that do not apply to all services. The total hourly cost of doing business is then divided by the number of practitioners who generate revenue (dentists, hygienists) to determine the hourly fees that must be generated to break even. At this point fees for each procedure are calculated by determining how much hourly profit the owner wants to generate and the time that each procedure takes to complete. This exercise needs to be repeated semi-annually to be certain that fees are consistent with expenses.

The second most common method employed is market pricing or benchmarking. This approach requires the availability of fee information from comparable practices, which can then be customized as desired. This is a simplistic approach that does not take into account differing costs of doing business and profit goals as well as many other factors, which can vary among offices, such as the time required to complete procedures.

The last and arguably most effective approach involves a combination of the two methods. Each practice should know its cost of doing business but if, after carefully determining a fair price using the former method, the resultant fee varies greatly from the prevailing fee, an alteration upward or downward might be indicated for individual procedures. As counterintuitive as it sounds, undercharging can often lead to reduced sales and numerous studies have shown that consumers' perceptions of the quality of service are diminished if the service is underpriced. Overpricing a service may also lead to reduced sales, but creates a dilemma when the fee in question has been calculated to be fair using the cost-plus method. It might be necessary to raise marketing awareness of the special skills the dentist might possess to justify the fee or to lower the cost of producing a particular service to allow the fee to be reduced and maintain the desired profit.

Once pricing is set, special pricing that is either provisional or permanent may be established to influence consumer purchasing on select services. Examples of this might include two-for-one whitening for a soon-to-be-married couple or complimentary whitening when bundled with orthodontic aligner therapy. Although these offers may minimize profits, they often lead to additional purchases by the consumer.

The range of payment options that an office offers will also influence treatments that a patient purchases. The number of patients who can afford a large immediate cash outlay for a cosmetic treatment plan is smaller than the number who can afford a smaller monthly payment expanded over time. The willingness of an office to either extend credit or pay an upfront commission to a patient financing program will increase the treatment acceptance on larger treatment plans. The 5% to 6% commission payable by the office on financing through companies such as CareCredit and CitiHealthcard is recouped by the smaller number of cancellations during the course of treatment because of patients not having the available funds to make a payment at the time of their visit.[5] Factoring in the cost of same-day cancellations is one of the most difficult calculations an office has in accurately setting fees for services.

Place

Dentists often have misconceptions about the thought process that occurs when patients choose the office where they will have their dental care. Patients are not actually paying for the quality of dentistry, but rather the perception of the quality they receive. This perception is formed by many of the non-dental aspects of the patient experience and can ultimately determine what treatment a patient will consent to and purchase.

For example, consider the upscale department store experience. Customers pay a premium, often for the same brands that can be obtained elsewhere, but come for the entire ambience and shopping experience. For dentists wishing to differentiate their practices and validate higher fees, the "Place" factor has many aspects. When choosing a location, there is more to consider than just the surrounding neighborhood. A starting point would be the style of the practice. A dentist can choose a high-volume, high-turnover practice offering good services; a slower-paced more boutique practice offering more complex treatment options; or some version in between the two. This will lead to a view of the patient type a dentist is attempting to attract. The next step is to identify a geographic location where these types of individuals reside or work. If a dentist is targeting high value-added cosmetic treatments, there must be a patient base near the office that can afford these services. As part of the evaluation, a dentist should assess the number and quality of the competition for the services they wish to offer. The final location dilemma is to decide whether to purchase an established practice or create a new one, and the choice between a physical plant that stands alone or one that may be in a private house, professional building, hospital, strip mall, or general office building.

The style of the practice is another underrated factor. A dentist desiring to differentiate, after locating in an upscale location, needs to carry through the image with high-end decorations, reception area amenities, and a highly attractive exterior consistent with or exceeding other local merchants' presentations. Contrast that with the PPO-based, high-volume practice, which can be located in a shopping mall or other high-traffic area and will feature durable mid-level furnishings that can stand up to the extra volume of patients. The majority of practices fall between these two, and many have unique designs or motifs to set them apart from their competitors.

The exterior of the office is the first thing prospective and current patients will see, and the image portrayed should be consistent from outside to inside. Paint and signage should be neat and current and landscaping should be tidy. Once inside, patients want to feel welcomed to the practice and be able to communicate with the staff. The traditional closed wall and Plexiglas window separating the reception staff from the patient acts as a barrier to this process. Opt instead for an open design and make sure the staff has excellent communication skills for these interactions. Given the nature of the profession, treatment rooms need to be spotlessly clean and tidy and this should carry forward throughout the office with fresh paintwork, seating that is comfortable and without ripped cushions, well-arranged magazines, and presentable artwork. Washroom cleanliness and amenities is another area that makes an impression on patients. The appearance of staff members should mirror the image of the office as well. The goal is to create a highly favorable impression of the practice that will influence patients' perceptions of the quality of care that is rendered and ultimately determine the type and quantity of treatment they will purchase. Remember the old saying, "You only get one chance to make a first impression, so make it a good one!"

Product

Product combines the range of treatments that a practice offers and the customer service the patients receive from the dentist and staff. Decisions on what treatments a practice will offer reflect the skill levels and experience of the dentist, the type of practice, and the targeted patient population. A dentist can be completely health motivated in service options or may target factors such as self-esteem and confidence when developing a menu of available treatments. It is vital to understand that simply satisfying customers is not enough to cause patients to refer their friends and family or create a relationship that will not be altered by a change in their economic situation or an inconvenient geographic relocation. To achieve that, dentists must develop a treatment and service package that will exceed the expectations of their patients.

Some practices have succeeded with offerings of services that differentiate their practices and fall into the categories of holistic practices, cosmetic specialty practices, general practices with a focus on preventive care, and general practices with a focus on cosmetic dentistry. For example, the decision to establish a holistic practice is often attributable to a clinician following personal beliefs, but there are also good economic reasons for adopting this approach. With a well-defined practice image, potential customers can easily determine if the practice suits them and inspires them to talk about the practice with their friends and colleagues, making it easier to gain referrals of like-minded consumers. Typically, the atmosphere of the practice promotes relaxation using soft lighting, soothing music and water features, and additional offerings such as homeopathy, acupuncture, reflexology, and nutritional advice.

The cosmetic specialty practice caters to the more affluent and image-conscious consumers and the dentist will need to be viewed as a cosmetic expert and must be certain that the fees charged and appearance of the office match the services offered. In addition to cosmetic dental procedures, this type of practice is likely to offer a range of facial rejuvenation treatments such as Botox and Restylane, and an endless array of amenities including post-treatment relaxation rooms and a place for patients to reapply makeup and fix their hair before leaving.

The practice with a focus on preventive care will emphasize services such as mouth-guards for sports, enhanced oral cancer detection screening, and early caries detection using laser- or fluorescent-based systems appealing to preventive-oriented consumers.

The general practice with a cosmetic focus stresses metal free restorations wherever feasible, emphasizes image enhancement with procedures such as invisible aligner therapy and laminate veneers. Many offer the convenience of one-visit restorations using CAD/CAM technology to differentiate themselves from other practices.

Promotion

Promotion is the tool that assists customers through the buying process and is wholly effective only after the other three Ps are in place. Promotion not only makes consumers aware of the products and services the practice offers, but also makes it easier for them to obtain further information about them, including how they can purchase the product, as well as to educate about services of which they may be unaware (Fig. 26-3).

It also encourages repeat use of some services. Finally, effective promotion encourages customers to recommend the

Edward Zuckerberg, D.D.S.,F.A.G.D. posted an offer.
May 3

FREE! 36 pack of travel size Aquafresh! Checkin on your smartphone at your May dental appt

Expired · 89 claimed

Like · Comment · Share   👍3 💬1 📄1

956 people saw this post

FIGURE 26-3 The author dealt with an oversupply of free toothpaste samples by asking customers to promote his practice by checking in to Facebook with their smart phones.

products or services to other people resulting in referrals. For a practice with a busy schedule, the need for new patients can be reduced with a successful patient retention program and promotion of services to the existing patient base. Brochures to explain treatment options, custom newsletters, and educational videos playing in the reception area and treatment rooms can all be used to educate existing patients about services they may have not realized were offered. An office Facebook page can easily and efficiently promote services offered through updates into existing customers' news feeds. Staff members, often the first to hear of patients' concerns, can be a source of information about services offered as well and can encourage patients to view or "like" the Facebook page. For practices desiring an influx of new patients, advertising is a form of promotion geared at attracting new patients to the practice.

PRODUCT VERSUS SERVICE MARKETING

To properly focus marketing programs on education, motivation, and fulfilling the needs and wants of individuals, it is important to distinguish between product marketing and service marketing.

Product marketing focuses on the actual products being sold. For example, in a television, magazine, or Web advertisement for an automobile, the focus of the visual, auditory, and written message is the particular car being marketed, including its most prominent features. In dentistry, product-focused marketing would emphasize the actual "product" being delivered to the patient, such as a crown, veneer, or composite resin restoration. Many dentists and staff, in their marketing materials and treatment presentations, focus on the actual restoration.

Service marketing focuses on the actual service being provided. The product being sold is secondary to the service and attendant benefits that the product provides. In the dental setting, the "services" and benefits of cosmetic dentistry might include such services as a more attractive smile, a better chance for career advancement, a better social life, and more self-confidence. The actual "product," the veneer or crown, is merely the vehicle for providing that service and achieving a benefit. In a society in which people are extremely conscious of their appearance and use discretionary dollars to have their hair professionally coiffed and colored and use Botox to remove facial wrinkles on a regular basis, dentists who fail to place emphasis on improving their patients' appearance are missing a large economic opportunity.

CLINICAL TIP

Dental marketing should be primarily service-focused marketing, because a service approach more clearly focuses on the patient's individual needs and wants and the ways in which treatment can meet those needs and wants.

In the world of marketing, perception is reality in the mind of the patient. If patients perceive that they have a need, then they definitely have that need, even if the dentist does not have the same perception. The public generally is not as interested in the product, or type of restoration, that is to be provided as they are in the benefits of treatment. These benefits must be tailored to individual needs and wants. The correct focus can mean the difference between gaining patient acceptance of treatment and losing the patient's interest (and thus losing the patient). For example, a product-focused brochure, which simply lists the "products" available, forces the patient to take that information and somehow determine if these products meet his or her needs. In contrast, a service-focused approach does not demand extrapolation by the reader. It explains the benefits of cosmetic services in lay terms. It shows how cosmetic dentistry is the means to an end. It motivates the patient to accept treatment because such treatment is the answer to personal wants and needs.

The following excerpts are brief examples of product- and service-focused marketing statements.

- *Product-focused brochure.* Our office is proud to provide the most advanced cosmetic dental technology. Ask Dr. Jones or our staff about Invisalign, tooth-colored crowns, porcelain veneers, and tooth whitening services that we offer.
- *Service-focused brochure.* Our office can give you a beautiful smile using the latest cosmetic dental technology. Ask Dr. Jones or our staff how we can work together to create an attractive smile that can help your career and your social life.

These are simple examples, but they illustrate the difference in approach between product and service marketing. The first example focuses on specific procedures and restorations, whereas the second example focuses on the patient's needs. Specific individual needs can be determined during patient interviews and in-office discussions and then can be addressed during the treatment presentation. Each staff member, as well as the dentist, should pay close attention to what patients say from the moment they come into the office. A great deal of information about individual needs and desires can be gained from patients' posted comments about their teeth and what they expect from dental visits. Many patients also change offices because of a previously unsatisfactory relationship. In eliciting their past dental history, discovering why a previous relationship failed can help provide clues as to how to best approach the patient and the pitfalls to avoid. In addition, the smile and appearance of the doctor and staff members must reflect the image of the care presented to the patients. If the office desires to provide more Invisalign services, each staff member should have to undergo or have completed Invisalign therapy themselves if they did not have a proper smile in the first place. They then become models for your patients' future smiles, and if any staff member is undergoing current treatment, he or she can share how comfortable and undetectable the aligners are with your patients. Similarly, while trying to promote a whitening system, all staff members should have completed whitening treatment and have bright, white smiles.

DESIGNING A MARKETING PROGRAM

Goals and Objectives

The goals and objectives of the marketing plan are related to the goals and objectives of the practice as a whole, but they consist of the specific goals and objectives of the office's marketing program (i.e., exactly what is to be accomplished with the use of marketing techniques). Are you trying to attract a specific number of new patients each month? Are you trying to target a specific age category of patient, such as the elderly? Are you trying to increase the number of veneers placed per month by a specific amount? It is crucial to identify specific rather than general marketing goals and objectives.

Target Audience

The target audience most likely to satisfy the marketing goals must be identified. For example, if one goal is to increase the number of implants performed each month, then individuals over the age of 55 might constitute a large part of the target audience. If the goal is to increase the number of veneers placed per month, the primary target audience might be women age 18 to 55. A secondary target audience might be men age 21 to 55. This does not mean that people older than 55 do not want veneers, or that men are not interested in veneers; it simply means that it is more likely that women age 18 to 55 will make the decision to invest in veneers for cosmetic reasons. If the surrounding community is composed predominantly of one demographic group, for example a retirement community, the target audience must necessarily reflect that fact (or marketing to other communities may be necessary). Often a target market not normally considered "primary" requires a different marketing focus to motivate them to take action. The purpose of determining a target audience is to provide a tangible, well-defined "target" for the marketing efforts, a target with the highest likelihood of response.

Budget

The techniques to be used and the size of the target market depend on available funds. A typical budget for marketing is 2% to 5% of gross practice revenues. Aggressive dental marketers budget 6% to 8% of revenues or more. A budget sufficient to accomplish the goals and objectives of the marketing plan must be allocated in the formal plan and must be dispensed according to a time schedule as determined by the plan.

Specific Marketing Techniques

Within the confines of the plan's budget, specific marketing techniques should be selected that will best accomplish the marketing goals. Both internal and external marketing techniques can be used, depending on the marketing plan and the philosophy of the practice.

Time Frame for Implementation

Once a plan is in place, be sure to assign an individual who is responsible for verifying that deadlines are met and the plan is executed.

Monitoring Results

Many dentists institute impressive marketing programs but fail to monitor the results of individual elements within the program. Monitoring systems that record results are imperative if the program is to be evaluated and improved. For example, the practice is likely to use a variety of target sources for its advertising program, including Yellow Pages, Facebook ads, direct mail, and others. During the intake of new patient information, the exact source of the referral should be recorded or the means by which the patient discovered your office should be noted into the practice management system (PMS) in in a manner in which revenues can be tracked for a particular referral source. If an office runs an especially successful marketing campaign, new patients might list multiple sources for how they discovered the practice, and a worthwhile feature in a PMS would be the ability to relate multiple referral sources for a particular patient (most allow tracking of only one). In this manner, the cost of the advertisement program can be weighed against the income generated.

> ### CLINICAL TIP
>
> If after a predetermined period of evaluation (perhaps 6 to 12 months) the advertisement does not generate sufficient fees, it should be changed or replaced with another marketing technique.

Continual monitoring of the marketing program is essential if the program is to optimize cost-effectiveness.

> ### CLINICAL TIP
>
> Contingency funds should be 5% to 10% of the total budget allocation.

TREATMENT PRESENTATION

Many marketing techniques can be used to build the cosmetic dental practice. Because each technique has advantages and disadvantages, the final choice depends on many factors. Each practice must decide which techniques are consistent with its philosophy and are appropriate for the goals and objectives of the practice.

One technique common to all practices is the individual patient treatment presentation. Many dentists do not equate the treatment presentation with marketing. Some use a formal treatment presentation, which takes place in an area of the office specially designed for maximum patient comfort and communication. The treatment presentation follows a specific format, and every aspect of the presentation is planned to gain patient acceptance of treatment. Some dentists approach treatment presentation informally, with little preplanning and no prescribed format. However, treatment presentations, in whatever form they take, represent one of the most powerful types of internal marketing available to every dentist.

It is during the treatment presentation that the dentist and staff must educate the patient about his or her individual oral health needs and, most importantly, motivate the patient to accept and pay for needed treatment. If the patient leaves the treatment presentation without a firm commitment to treatment, that patient may be lost.

Patient Motivation Profile

Use of the patient motivation profile can greatly improve the patient's motivation and inclination to accept treatment. Addressing these concerns may motivate a patient to undergo necessary treatment.

From the time a patient first enters or telephones the office, each staff member, as well as the dentist, should carefully monitor the importance to the patient of each of these four areas of concern[6]:
1. Money
2. Love
3. Self-preservation
4. Appearance

CLINICAL TIP

By classifying patients as closely as possible into one or more of the primary areas of concern (E.G., money, love, self-preservation, appearance), it becomes possible to target the treatment presentation to the individual, greatly improving the chances for patient acceptance of treatment.

Treatment Presentation Using the Patient Motivation Profile. For example, an elderly man presents with some missing teeth and one fractured tooth. The dentist, who has not taken the time to analyze the patient's motivating emotions, stresses the economic advantages of the treatment plan, emphasizing that it will save the patient money in the long run by preventing further deterioration of his oral health. The dentist takes this approach because currently the dentist's personal concerns center on money and achieving financial independence. The dentist assumes that the patient is thinking in the same terms, particularly because of his age and the need for financial security in his retirement years. The dentist is surprised when the man shifts uncomfortably in the chair and says he will "think about it" and call later.

If the dentist, receptionist, or other staff members had noticed that during the initial office contact, the man did not mention money or financial concerns but did mention a magazine article he had read about "dental cripples" who had lost all their teeth, a clearer picture of the patient's emotional "trigger" would have been possible. When the man pointed out that his own mother had "pyorrhea" and had lost all her teeth and that he did not want to lose his teeth, too, this should have alerted the dentist to the fact that this person's emotional profile was "self-preservation," not money. Knowing this, the dentist would logically take another approach during the treatment presentation by explaining that treatment would prevent further tilting of the teeth adjacent to the missing spaces and would prevent the fractured tooth from breaking more extensively. The man's chewing would be more efficient, thus aiding in overall systemic health, and his entire mouth would be healthier. With proper home care, as instructed by the hygienist, the patient would significantly improve the likelihood of retaining his teeth for the rest of his life.

When the treatment presentation is keyed to the patient's motivation profile, the patient is far more likely to respond positively to the treatment plan. For the cosmetic dentist, the emotions associated with money, appearance, and romance can be targeted in a powerful way during treatment presentation. A more attractive smile can enhance one's career, thus providing the opportunity to make more money, and it can improve one's social life, thus meeting a patient's need to appear attractive or find romance.

MARKETING TECHNIQUES

Many marketing techniques can be used by dentists in a professional manner. The number of techniques available is limited only by the imagination of the marketer.

Referrals

Referrals have been and remain the most effective marketing tool available. Special effort and a definitive plan should be devoted to stimulating referrals from both patients and outside sources. Good outside referral sources include related health professionals, cosmetologists, realtors, and local business people, who meet the public and often are asked for recommendations about dentists and community services. Strong referral sources should be thanked in a noticeable way. A first- or second-time referral source may simply be sent a personalized thank you note. Those who continue to refer patients can be sent a special gift, such as flowers, concert tickets, or some other tasteful gift. With flowers, it is especially effective to send them directly to the referring individual's place of business. Everyone in the referring person's office will see the flowers and notice who sent them, which expands the marketing effort.

Civic Lectures by Dentists and Staff

An external public relations technique, the civic lecture is highly educational and benefits the entire profession, as well as the individual office. It is a strong marketing tool if the dentist or staff member is enthusiastic and a good speaker. Effective public speaking can be learned through practice.

Practice Newsletter

A newsletter is an internal and external public relations technique. The content should be focused on services and benefits offered by the practice, and is an opportunity to inform patients about many services the practice offers of which they may be unaware. Content should be interesting and informative and contain information about practice basics such as hours, names and roles of staff members, a team photo, contact information, including not only address and phone, but also website and Facebook page URLs. The newsletter should be sent to both existing and potential new patients in a variety of formats; the more valuable it is, the better the chance that it will be successful and will be shared with others.

CLINICAL TIP

Avoid putting sections such as "Did You Know?" in a newsletter. This is mainly filler material for which the patient has little practical use.

It is important to adhere to a publication schedule and not to publish erratically. With any type of publication, consistency is important, because it gives the reader a sense of continuity and dependability. If patients come to expect a dental practice newsletter at a certain time, such as every quarter, it becomes part of their routine. This consistency reinforces the doctor's name in the minds of the patients and hopefully translates into consistency of office visits. From an in-office standpoint, if a fixed publication schedule is not established, the newsletter quickly becomes a task that "we'll get to when we can." This usually means that it will cease publication after a few erratically timed issues. A quarterly publishing schedule usually is sufficient and not too burdensome for the office staff. Finished newsletters should be e-mailed directly to a database maintained by the office that will include predominantly patients but should also include individuals who may be in the position to refer new patients to the practice. Hard copies can be included with statements and other mailings and should be sent to all patients for whom the office does not have an e-mail address. If the procedure is beyond the capabilities of the office, there are services that automate this task, as well as provide recall reminders and appointment confirmations by text and e-mail, send birthday greetings, and solicit patient endorsements and survey completions. The availability of competent staff members and the budget will determine the best approach for each office. *Solution Reach*, *Demand Force*, *Sesame Communications*, and *Einstein Medical* are some of the companies that specialize in providing these services for dental offices.

Direct Mail

An external advertising technique, direct mail can be expensive if not properly targeted.

> ### CLINICAL TIP
>
> Direct mail experts usually agree that a 1% response is strong, although this can vary according to how well the mailing is targeted.

The best results are obtained if target groups are clearly defined and the contents of the direct mail package are focused on the needs of that group. A response mechanism should be included, such as a reply card or a request to call the office for more information.

Yellow Pages Advertisement

Yellow Pages advertisements are an external advertising technique. The results from these advertisements vary across the country. Dentists interested in this technique should try a test advertisement and monitor the results closely. The decision to renew should be based on results. As a rule, larger advertisements work better, but it is important to determine the size of other advertisements that will run on the same page. In a page full of large advertisements, more graphic creativity is required if the advertisement is to stand out. The Yellow Pages representative or a graphic artist should be consulted about various graphic techniques that can improve the response.

Because of the marked decline in the use of print directories, many Yellow Page companies now offer companion services that integrate Internet campaigns, SEOs, and targeted Web pages in addition to the print edition. Many of the older generation of patients are not computer savvy and rely more heavily on print directories, so a campaign that targets that population, such as one for dentures, implants, crowns, or fixed partial denture, should include the use of this medium. However, the value of print directories is continuously declining.

In-Office Educational Materials

An internal marketing technique, in-office educational materials such as educational brochures, photograph albums of cosmetic treatments, and video presentations are highly effective if combined with direct dentist-staff-patient interaction. Whenever possible, the dentist's own treatment results should be used with personal testimonials from the actual patients. These aids represent an excellent opportunity for patient education.

Current technology allows enhanced presentation of these materials using digital photo frames, iPads or patient education service such as Caesy, Guru, or Digital Clinic. These software packages can play pre-programmed loops of dental procedures, on-demand specialty procedures as directed by a staff member, or provide a variety of news and office-specific social media content on a large-screen TV in the reception area.

Radio and Television Advertisements

Although some large dental clinics have successfully used the external advertising technique of radio and television commercials, their effectiveness and feasibility for the average dental practice is questionable. Creation of an advertisement that maintains professionalism and generates new patients requires special talent, such as a professional advertising agency. This can be a very expensive investment, but done properly can generate increased awareness of the practice in the community and could lead to a large volume of new patients.

ELECTRONIC MARKETING

It is clear that the Internet will be, if it is not already, the number one source for media, news, and information. As such, practices that do not embrace the Internet and the digital life will be obsolete in the future. The number of businesses designed to enhance dental marketing can be overwhelming. Knowledgeable practices can perform many of the necessary tasks in-house, but the creation of a department or a specific job title to oversee the practice's electronic medium participation has been embraced by very few practices to date. The tasks that fall under this umbrella include but are not limited to the following:
1. Recall reminders
2. Appointment confirmations
3. Responding to appointment requests made electronically
4. Management of the practice's social media presence
5. Creation and management of the practice website
6. Distribution of the practice newsletter
7. Search engine optimization
8. Patient insurance eligibility verification
9. Insurance claim submissions and tracking
10. Payment management of accounts receivables and payables

These are the top 10 uses of the Internet and cellular technology, but there are many others, and new services to automate and digitize tasks that were previously performed manually are becoming available every day. Individual offices must determine their own comfort level with technology and decide which tasks they will service in-house and which require outside services consultants.

Staff as Marketers. A motivated, enthusiastic staff is one of the most powerful internal and external marketing tools a practice can use. Dentists should make a special effort to train the staff in proper telephone technique and patient interaction techniques. Each staff member should have a business card to distribute at outside functions. Regular staff meetings should be devoted to improving staff-patient relations.

CONCLUSION

One of the greatest satisfactions a dentist can receive occurs at the completion of a cosmetic treatment when a patient views his or her new smile, is thrilled with the treatment outcome, and expresses joy and appreciation. The reality is, however, that a job well done, both technically and cosmetically, results in a patient who is unlikely to require future cosmetic services for many years. Dentists rely on that satisfied patient to spread the word about them and keep them busy and profitable; however, the reality is that most patients, although satisfied, either will not have the opportunity, or if it presents itself, will not make the referral. As a result, dentists need to continually find new sources for their future cosmetic treatments. A successful marketing program is a requirement for all dental practices, no matter the skill level of the dentist. There is an old marketing adage, "Market or Die," which may not be literally true in the treatment of all dental practices, but there is no doubt that the vast majority of practices will not be truly successful without a highly efficient and productive marketing program.

REFERENCES

1. US Supreme Court: *Bates v State Bar of Arizona*, 433 US 350, 1977.
2. Kerpen D: *Likeable social media: how to delight your customers, create an irresistible brand, and be generally amazing on Facebook (and other social networks)*, New York, 2011, McGraw-Hill.
3. McCarthy EJ: *Basic marketing: a managerial approach*, Homewood, IL, 1960, Irwin.
4. Blue Horizons Marketing: http://www.bluehorizonsmarketing.co.uk/articles/private-dentistry/the-4-ps-of-marketing-number-one-price.html. Accessed June 2012.
5. Kleiman S: Preserving wealth: planning steps for your state of life, Inside Dentistry Volume 2, Issue 8, 2006. https://www.dentalaegis.com/id/2006/10/practice-building-and-wealth-management/preserving-wealth-planning-steps-for-your-stage-of-life. Accessed October 2013.
6. Garn R: *The magic power of emotional appeal*, Englewood Cliffs, NJ, 1960, Prentice-Hall.

27

Esthetics and Dental Jurisprudence

John P. Little and Burton R. Pollack

BRIEF HISTORY OF RISK MANAGEMENT

Until the mid-1970s, the term *risk management* was not part of the dental lexicon. Today it is part of everyday conversation in dental circles. The health profession became interested in risk management during a medical malpractice crisis in the early 1970s. Many hospitals instituted in-house programs to reduce liability by providing quality assurance in the provision of health care, identifying risk areas, changing hiring policies, reviewing patient complaints, studying incident reports, and purchasing insurance.

The concept of risk management spread from hospitals to physicians and dentists' offices. Programs for dentists began in the late 1970s and early 1980s, when legal actions against dentists increased dramatically, and settlements and jury awards escalated beyond expectations.

The literature at this time was flooded with risk management articles. Risk management presentations were included at most dental meetings. Insurance companies began risk management educational sessions, either as a benefit for insured dentists or so that they could qualify for premium discounts. Continuing dental education and risk management became linked.

RISK MANAGEMENT IN COSMETIC DENTISTRY

The importance of risk management in dentistry continues to increase given the advances in esthetic and restorative dentistry and the changing patient demographics that are creating a greater patient need for these services. Many of these treatment modalities require a greater level of skill and training and due to their nature potentially create greater legal risks to clinicians. Examples include providing some form of orthodontics (e.g., Invisalign, appliance therapy, or a form of rapid tooth movement), performing more challenging endodontics because of

nickel titanium files and rotary handpieces, using cone beam Computed Technology, injecting Botox and dermal fillers, placing and restoring implants and performing associated surgeries such as sinus lifts, using in-office CAD-CAM to fabricate restorations, using various oral or intravenous sedation techniques, and employing specialists and anesthesiologists.

Therefore it is imperative that each dentist develops individualized risk management policies that address the legal needs and patient management aspects of each individual practice. These policies should be created in conjunction with an attorney knowledgeable about dental practice issues.

Cosmetic dentists should also consider hiring a practice management consultant or firm with cosmetic dental practice experience to help incorporate systems such as staff training, patient education, and treatment presentation. Patient dissatisfaction with the progress of care and the results of care increases the risk of a patient filing a suit or complaint. An unsatisfactory result according to the patient is not always unsatisfactory to the dentist.

> **CLINICAL TIP**
>
> Too often patients fail to realize the limitations of dentistry, a scenario that is particularly true when cosmetic results are important.

> **CLINICAL TIP**
>
> A patient's perceived lack of care or concern by the dentist or staff can also influence a patient's subjective view of the treatment.

Special precautions must be taken because subjective opinions of what is actually involved in the treatment process and about the outcome of care may determine whether a patient sues. The nature and content of the consent given before care begins may determine whether the patient initiates a suit. Patient expectations must be realistic if a dentist wishes to avoid problems when the care is completed. Predictable limitations in outcomes must be incorporated into the consent form and presented at a separate consultation visit. (See the sections on Informed Consent and Consultation Visits.) Documentation is essential. According to a study conducted by Princeton Insurance Company, for claims reported January 2001 through December 2009, "Communication with the patient was a contributing factor most of the time in treatment related claims and was directly attributed to a lack of or inadequate informed discussion about the risks of the procedure in treatment alternatives."[1.]

PROFESSIONAL RESPONSIBILITIES IN RISK MANAGEMENT

In developing a risk management program, cosmetic dentists have some basic responsibilities, which include the following:

1. Purchasing professional liability insurance (See section on Professional Liability/Malpractice Insurance.)
2. Knowing and obeying the laws that regulate dental practice and remaining informed about changes
3. Continuing to become educated and remain knowledgeable about advances in the profession through membership in professional organizations, attending continuing dental education programs, subscribing to professional journals, and possibly joining hospital staffs and the faculty of dental schools. This is especially critical if a cosmetic dentist undertakes procedures usually performed by a specialist (e.g., placing implants) or by a physician (e.g., injecting Botox).
4. Being aware of areas of legal vulnerability in dental practice by reading appropriate literature, exchanging information with colleagues, and attending continuing education courses
5. Fully investigating new materials and techniques and then, only after proper clinical and practice management training, slowly introducing these into practice
6. Limiting care to areas of competence and making necessary and appropriate referrals
7. Carefully evaluating treatment selection by trying to determine whether both the objective dental results and subjective patient expectations can be met
8. Maintaining good interpersonal relationships with, and showing care to, patients and ensuring that the staff does the same by monitoring what they say and how they relate to patients
9. Carefully hiring, training, and supervising competent personnel
10. Having a well thought out patient financial policy to help patients in understanding their financial responsibility prior to beginning treatment
11. Carefully considering patients' responses if they were to be referred to a collection agency or sued for nonpayment of fees. This is one of the major causes of malpractice suits.

CLINICAL TIP

If a dentist is unsure of how to properly implement the previous points then she or he should consider hiring a practice management consultant with experience in advising a cosmetic practice.

12. Obtaining proper consent before initiating treatment and having a separate consultation visit; then, keeping patients informed about their treatment status and any problems arising during treatment (See the section on Informed Consent.)
13. Taking careful health and dental histories and updating them at appropriate intervals (See the section on Health and Dental History.)
14. Keeping proper records for each patient and fastidiously documenting all actions. Keeping patient records forever or as long as possible (See the section on Records.)
15. Never parting with an original record or radiograph unless ordered to do so by a court or an agency having subpoena powers
16. Never altering a patient record after becoming aware that a malpractice suit is being contemplated or initiated by a patient or a patient's attorney
17. Notifying the insurance carrier at the earliest time after becoming aware that a patient intends or has threatened to sue or after becoming aware that an action taken during treatment could result in a malpractice suit (See the section on Procedure for Handling a Malpractice Suit.)

COMMON MALPRACTICE CLAIMS

1. Restoration-related claims such as restorations breaking or falling out, infection under a restoration, or damage to the tooth during preparation
2. Allegations that the teeth were "over-prepared" during veneer or crown/fixed partial denture restorations leading to the need for endodontic therapy.
3. Failure to diagnose, refer, or treat (e.g., periodontal disease or oral cancer), or treatment of a patient beyond the competence of the dentist or that permitted by the applicable dental practice act
4. Osteonecrosis secondary to extractions on a patient with a history of bisphosphonate use
5. Paresthesias caused by injections, extractions, or overextrusion of endodontic obturation materials
6. Failure to inform the patient of an untoward event that occurred during treatment, such as a root tip fracture or an irretrievable broken instrument or file becoming lodged within a root canal
7. Problems associated with the temporomandibular joint allegedly caused during dental treatment
8. Implant failures
9. Orthodontic treatment with unfavorable results, as well as patients having periodontal and caries neglect and root resorption
10. Faulty patient history taking, resulting in allergic responses, drug incompatibilities, injuries, and in rare instances death
11. Extraction of the wrong tooth, broken root tips, or infections after extractions
12. Patient complaints of ill-fitting dentures
13. Failure to obtain informed consent
14. Adverse outcomes caused by the administration of intravenous or oral sedatives
15. Abandonment of a patient by prematurely discontinuing care or not attending to the needs of a patient under treatment

Cosmetic dentists should be aware of the results of the previously mentioned Princeton Insurance Company report, for claims reported January 2001 through December 2011.[2] This report showed that the most common malpractice claims were related to "unsatisfactory restorations." In this report, "unsatisfactory restorations" referred to dental work that "fails to meet the patient's expectations with respect to appearance, fit and comfort."

CLINICAL TIP

A risk management program must include a process whereby the patient is adequately informed and a dentist should not undertake treatment unless confident that both the objective dental results and the patient's subjective expectations can be met.

BRIEF REVIEW OF CONTRACT AND MALPRACTICE LAW

The relationship between a treating dentist and a patient has its foundation in contract law, which governs when the relationship begins and ends; and tort law, which governs malpractice or negligence lawsuits.

CONTRACT LAW

Dentist-Patient Relationship

When the Relationship Begins. The dentist-patient relationship begins when a dentist, in a professional capacity, expresses a professional opinion or recommends to a specific individual a course of action on which the patient may rely. Whether a fee was charged does not affect the relationship.

The relationship or contract of care between a dentist and patient does not have to be in writing to be enforceable. Unfortunately, except in orthodontics, written contracts in dentistry are rare. In dentistry a "written contract" should consist of a treatment plan/financial arrangement form and an informed consent form.

When the Relationship Ends. The dentist-patient relationship ends in the following circumstances:
1. The patient or dentist dies.
2. The patient voluntarily seeks the services of another dentist.
3. The patient files a lawsuit or licensing board complaint against the dentist.
4. The dentist unilaterally terminates the care according to the steps later discussed.

Abandonment. One of the implied duties in the dentist-patient relationship is for the dentist to continue treatment until one of the previously stated conditions occurs. To unilaterally discontinue treatment and avoid liability for abandonment, the following generally accepted rules apply:
1. The dentist should not discontinue treatment if a patient's health may be compromised. This is a professional judgment and there are very few situations in dentistry in which this could occur.
2. The dentist recommends that the patient seeks substitute care. It is best not to recommend another dentist or even to supply patients with a list from which to choose. To do so may create a link with the new dentist should the new dentist be accused of malpractice. The link could be a claim for negligent referral or joint care.

An example of a referral for substitute care would be one in which a patient needs a cosmetic dental "makeover" and the dentist believes that this is beyond the level of his/her skill and expertise, or that the patient's subjective expectations cannot be met. This is legally different from a general dentist referring a patient to a specialist. In that situation the general dentist is still the general dentist of record unless the relationship is terminated in accordance with the steps previously stated.

3. The dentist should inform the patient that he/she will provide emergency care for a reasonable time during the period in which the patient seeks care elsewhere. What constitutes "reasonable" depends on the availability of dentists in the community. A dentist should contact a local health care attorney to determine what is recognized as "reasonable" in the particular community. For example, in New Jersey it is commonly accepted that 30 days is "reasonable."
4. The dentist should inform the patient that he/she will cooperate with a new dentist by making copies of records, radiographs, reports, and other information available. The dentist should never send the original records or radiographs.
5. The dentist should inform the patient that seeking care elsewhere is in the patient's best interest, not the dentist's.

CLINICAL TIP

Do not charge a patient for copying records. This only creates ill will that could be a deciding factor in having a patient file a licensing board complaint or seeking an attorney to begin a malpractice complaint.

Patients should first be informed verbally regarding the previous guidelines and should then receive a notice by certified mail that includes the same information. A dentist may refuse to accept a patient and may discontinue the care of a patient for any reason, without fear of abandonment, except for reasons of race, color, religion, or national origin. As a result of the enactment of the Americans with Disability Act of 1990, which declared a dentist's private office as a "place of public accommodation," a dentist who refuses to treat a patient solely because the patient is HIV positive or is disabled in any other way may be found guilty of discrimination and subjected to severe penalties (i.e., a large fine and possible restriction or loss of the license to practice). Although the Americans with Disability Act makes it clear that federal, state, and local human rights agencies have jurisdiction over what a dentist does in the office (in relation to accepting or refusing patients), it is not clear exactly what constitutes discrimination within the meaning of the law (e.g., wearing two pairs of gloves, restricting office hours, referring patients to special health facilities). However, to be legally safe, it is best to treat all patients exactly the same. Additionally, dentists should consult with a health care attorney regarding state law in this area.

Guarantees

CLINICAL TIP

An important risk management caveat is to never guarantee the outcome of care. To do so is foolish because health care guarantees cannot be truthfully made.

In many instances guarantees lead to unrealistic expectations from the patient. When a patient claims that a dentist breached a contract because a guaranteed result was not achieved, the lawsuit may be subject to contract law. In contract law cases the patient does not have to produce an expert, whereas in malpractice law cases the testimony of an expert must support the patient's claim.

CLINICAL TIP

The considerations regarding guarantees should be strictly observed by dentists who practice cosmetic dentistry. When giving written or verbal information regarding the treatment, it is recommended to include or make an express statement that "No guarantees or warrantees of any nature have been given regarding the treatment to be performed." Similarly, if clinical imaging is used, the dentist should include or make a statement that "Before and after images are for illustrative purposes only and do not guarantee any actual results." Ideally, the chart should include some written documentation that this was communicated to the patient and that the patient understood this. Similarly, the dentist and staff should avoid making any oral statements that could be construed as a guarantee or warranty.

Implied Duties in the Dentist-Patient Relationship

Implied duties are obligations that exist as a result of the dentist-patient relationship. These implied duties do not have to be explicitly stated or written to be legally enforceable.

Dentist's Implied Duties. The dentist automatically gives certain warranties to the patient, including the following:

1. The dentist uses knowledge and skill with reasonable care in the provision of services as measured against customary (acceptable) standards of other dentists of the same school of practice in the community. The definition of *community* by the courts has undergone major changes. Previously it was strictly defined as the *local community* in which the defendant dentist practiced. As communication and travel became more accessible, most courts changed the definition to mean a national standard of care.
2. The dentist is properly licensed and meets all other legal requirements to engage in the practice of dentistry.
3. The dentist employs competent personnel and ensures that they are properly supervised.
4. The dentist maintains a level of knowledge in keeping with current advances in the profession (e.g., participates in continuing dental education programs, subscribes to professional journals, and attends professional meetings).
5. The dentist does not use experimental procedures or drugs without the patient's knowledge and written consent. No clear definition explains what constitutes an experimental procedure or drug. However, from a practical standpoint, no dentist should ever employ any new or experimental procedure or material unless a dentist is working in a dedicated research capacity.
6. The dentist obtains the some type of consent (implied, verbal, informed, written, etc.) from the patient before beginning any examination or treatment; and keeps the patient informed about the progress of the treatment.

7. The dentist does not abandon the patient.
8. The dentist keeps accurate records of the examination and treatment of the patient.
9. The dentist maintains confidentiality and abides by all HIPAA, federal and state privacy laws.

CLINICAL TIP

The American Dental Association publishes a HIPAA handbook that can greatly help a dentist to comply with HIPAA.

10. The dentist requests consultations when appropriate and makes referrals for care when indicated.

Patient's Implied Duties. The patient also gives certain warranties to the dentist, including the following:

1. The patient keeps appointments and notifies the dentist (the office) in a timely manner if appointments cannot be kept.
2. The patient provides honest answers to health and history questions and informs the dentist if changes in health status occur.
3. The patient cooperates with the dentist in care (e.g., follows home hygiene instructions; prescription medication schedule; diet and nutrition instructions; and instructions regarding alcohol, smoking, and drugs).
4. The patient pays fees in a timely manner.

A patient's failure to follow his/her implied duties give a dentist cause for terminating a relationship and additionally may serve as a defense should the patient ever file a complaint or suit.

TORT LAW

Elements of Dental Malpractice

In order to establish and maintain a case for dental malpractice, a patient must prove the following:

1. That the dentist owed a duty to the patient,
2. That the dentist breached a duty to the patient,
3. That the breach of the duty caused an injury to the patient, and
4. The injury was significant enough to be compensable.

Duty and Breach of that Duty. As stated previously, dentists owe patients a number of implied, general duties that are inherent in the practice of dentistry. Most of the implied duties are codified in laws and enforced by the applicable dental licensing board. However, in most instances of alleged malpractice, the malpractice complaint focuses on the actual treatment or diagnosis, or lack thereof. In malpractice cases, the "duty" owed to the patient is to practice within the "standard of care." The generally accepted definition of the standard of care is that the dentist uses knowledge and skill with reasonable care, in the provision of services as measured against customary (acceptable) standards of other dentists of the same school of practice.

The question of what exactly is the standard of care and whether the dentist failed to act with that standard depends on the treatment performed and the facts of the case. Consider the following (oversimplified) hypothetical fact pattern: A patient presents to a cosmetic dentist with a desire to have unaesthetic 8-unit porcelain fused to metal fixed partial denture replaced. The patient does not like the shade of the fixed prosthesis or the fact that he can see "dark lines" at the gum line. The dentist restores the patient with an all-porcelain fixed partial denture. The question of whether the dentist followed the standard of care depends on many factors, all of which are established in the literature and courses. For example, some of these factors include: Did the dentist use appropriate radiographs? Were diagnostic casts and a diagnostic wax-up indicated? Was a face bow transfer and mounting necessary? Were the proper interocclusal records made? Were the teeth underprepared or over-prepared? Did the patient have the proper periodontal condition to support the restoration? Was all porcelain or the type of porcelain even indicated? Did the dentist follow technical standards regarding the number of pontics and length the restoration for the porcelain system used? Did the definitive restoration have the proper occlusion? Did the dentist need to over adjust the porcelain and weaken it? Was the correct cement used for the type of porcelain used? Did the definitive restoration meet acceptable esthetic criteria with regard to size and length of the teeth, contour, emergence profile, midline, lip-line, and phonetic considerations? Were all margins sealed? If the dentist failed to perform any of these steps, then there is an argument that the dentist breached the standard of care.

Causation and Damages. The next issue is whether the patient suffered any damages as a result of the dentist's failure to perform all the steps required by the treatment and universally accepted in providing an all-porcelain fixed partial denture. If the dentist failed to follow many of the beforementioned steps, but the restoration did not fail or the patient did not suffer an injury, then a malpractice case cannot be successful.

Consider the following three scenarios: (1) The patient's restoration has caries to the point of failure after 3 years; (2) The patient's restoration fractures after 3 years; (3) The patient undergoes the loss of an abutment after 3 years and the restoration fails. In all three situations, the patient did suffer an injury; however, the question becomes whether the dentist's act(s) or failure to act was the cause of the loss of the fixed partial denture. Obviously, there are multiple questions that would need to be investigated and the causation could become quite complicated to determine. However, the causation question would be much clearer if the dentist did in fact follow the standard of care and, more importantly, documented this in some manner in the clinical record. This could be a combination of charting, precementation fit check radiographs, postoperative photographs, and retaining copies of laboratory prescriptions and any other communication. (See the section on Records.)

Additionally the patient's actions may have contributed to the fixed partial denture failure. For example:
The patient may have not have followed adequate home care instructions regarding the fixed partial denture.
The patient may have failed to appear for regular hygiene visits.
The patient may have developed a medical condition that decreases salivary flow and led to caries.
The patient may be regularly consuming foods or beverages containing sugar or other cariogenic ingredients.
The patient may have habits such as ice chewing.
Therefore, it is essential to maintain detailed records concerning the patient's behavior.

CLINICAL TIP

Document all patient actions or nonactions that could ever contribute to problems, such as missing appointments, poor hygiene, poor nutrition, and oral habits. This documentation is often overlooked by the staff; however, such documentation can provide evidence of contributory negligence by the patient and can be critical if the actions/nonactions were the cause of the patient's dental problems.

Furthermore, the law recognizes that dentistry and medicine are not exact sciences and that dentists are not liable for "bad results" or a "failure to cure" if the standard of care has been met. A simple example of this is when endodontic therapy fails and a tooth is extracted despite the fact that all canals were located, properly shaped, and obturated to the apex. In this situation there are damages but not necessarily a breach of the standard of care. Consider the opposite scenario: There are numerous instances in which, at least radiographically, poorly performed endodontic therapy presents no clinical problem. Therefore a malpractice case is never filed.

PROFESSIONAL LIABILITY/ MALPRACTICE INSURANCE

It is recommended that a dentist purchase an "occurrence" policy with the highest available limits from a company with the highest rating (i.e., an A++ rating from A.M. Best), if available. An occurrence policy provides malpractice protection if the act that gave rise to the claim occurred when the policy was in force. A claims-made policy will only provide malpractice protection if the claim was filed while the policy is in force. For example, suppose a dentist provides endodontic treatment in 2010, has insurance with ABC insurance company in 2010, but switches to an occurrence policy with XYZ insurance company in 2011 and a lawsuit for negligent endodontic treatment is filed in 2012. If the policy from ABC insurance company was an occurrence policy, ABC insurance company must provide defense and coverage. If the policy was a claim-made policy, then ABC insurance company would not provide defense and coverage unless the dentist purchased a "tail" policy to defend against any claims filed after the claims-made policy was terminated. In addition, XYZ insurance company would only provide coverage if it was a claims-made policy with a prior acts rider. If the dentist did not purchase a tail, the dentist must pay for the full amount of legal defense, and damages, if the case is lost.

CLINICAL TIP

If available, purchase an "occurrence" policy with the highest available limits from a company with an A++ rating from A.M. Best.

CLINICAL TIP

Insurance companies may include "nose" coverage when switching from a claims-made policy to an occurrence policy. "Nose" coverage includes acts that occurred prior to the issue date of the new policy. This removes the need to purchase tail coverage for the old claims-made policy even if the new policy is purchased from a different insurance company.

CONSENT AND INFORMED CONSENT

Consent

Examining or treating a patient without the patient's consent constitutes unauthorized touching (i.e., a trespass against the person) and creates potential liability in a civil suit or criminal action. However, the courts have stated that to sustain an allegation of battery, it must be shown that intent to harm was present in the commission of the act. This essential element can rarely be shown in cases brought against dentists. The trend in most courts today is to treat allegations of faulty consent as professional negligence (malpractice). However, some courts have stated that if the dentist obtains no consent at all, a charge of battery may be appropriate. In this situation the defendant dentist is at a distinct legal disadvantage and may not be covered by malpractice insurance, may be subject to criminal action, and may be assessed punitive damages.

The fact that the act on which the suit is brought may have been necessary and beneficial to the patient does not affect liability. Similarly, liability is not altered if the act was gratuitous.

Only if a true emergency exists at the time the service is provided can the dentist proceed at no risk without the consent of the patient. Most jurisdictions state that an emergency exists when care must be rendered immediately to protect the life or health of the patient. When these conditions are met and time is of the essence, consent need not be obtained directly from the patient; the law implies consent.

Most courts also consider two other factors: (1) whether consent would have been given if the patient was able to grant consent, and (2) whether a reasonable person in the same situation would have granted consent.

Consent may also be implied by the actions of the patient. For example: a patient enters a dentist's office, complains of a toothache, and asks to be examined. The dentist tells the patient that radiographs of the teeth will be taken. The patient allows the radiographs to be taken without objecting. Consent is implied by the action, or inaction, of the patient. The key elements are that (1) the patient was aware of the nature of the problem or the need for the treatment (examination), and (2) the patient made no objection when treatment began.

Informed Consent

Age and Competency Issues in Informed Consent.
Treating a patient without consent is different than treating a patient without informed consent. As stated previously, treating without any consent may constitute battery. Therefore it is better to obtain questionable consent than no consent at all.

For consent to be valid, it must be informed and obtained from a person who is deemed competent to grant it. The person must be an adult of sound mind. It is questionable whether a patient under the influence of alcohol or other drugs has the sufficient mental acuity to grant a valid consent. A patient under stress presents similar problems. Should the patient appear to be under the influence of drugs or alcohol or overly apprehensive or indecisive, treatment should be postponed. Because of varying state laws, a dentist should consult a local health care attorney to determine the law on obtaining legal consent for adults with an *intellectual disability*.[3]

Informed consent for minors presents a number of issues. Only the parents can grant valid consent for care of the minor.

Consent given by siblings, grandparents, or any relatives other than the parents or legal guardians is not valid. However, in most states, the parents may authorize another party to grant consent (e.g., the administrators of a resident school, a neighbor during the parents' absence).

By common law, a minor is anyone who has not reached his or her twenty-first birthday. The age has been reduced by statute to 18. In many jurisdictions special statutes grant *emancipated* minors the right to consent to health care without the consent of the parent. Generally a minor who is financially independent of parental support is emancipated. Many states such as New York have codified common law and may list the conditions under which a minor becomes emancipated. These conditions usually include marriage, pregnancy, or living outside the parent's home. Consent granted by an adult child for a parent or by a sibling for another sibling also is not valid.

When properly executed, consent given over the telephone is acceptable to the courts. However, it must contain all the elements that constitute a valid consent and should be properly documented. When obtaining consent for a minor, the dentist should not treat the minor unless a parent is present and signs a consent form. In an emergency situation or where a minor comes to the office without a parent (e.g., a 17 year old who has a driver's license), the dentist must use his/her judgment as to whether to obtain oral consent from the parent. The dentist should contact the parent(s) or guardian(s) of the minor and tell them that a third party is listening on an extension. The parents should be informed about the situation and the need for treatment, as well all the facts that are required to obtain a valid consent. After the consent is received, appropriate notes should be made in the patient's chart, which should then be signed by the person who obtained the consent and countersigned by the listening third party. The dentist should then have the parent come to the office as soon as possible to acknowledge the consent by signing an appropriate consent form to help provide proof of the preoperative consent.

Studies have shown that patients do not always remember the information they verbally receive. The content of an oral consent and whether or not it was actually obtained can be challenged. Oral consent is recognized by the courts but it is harder to prove than written consent. Therefore a written and signed informed consent is preferable.[4]

CLINICAL TIP

If there is any question as to whether the patient is not mentally competent or not legally old enough to give a legally valid consent; the dentist should postpone treatment until a satisfactory determination can be made. This may require a call to an attorney to determine the applicable laws of that particular state and the necessary documentation needed to establish legal competency or guardianship

A problematic situation can arise when parents are still the financial supporters of young adult "children" (plus 18 years of age) and want to give their own permission for treatment options and costs, and become angry when not given the opportunity to be part of the treatment discussion. This often occurs when the young adult sees the dentist without the parent being present. Privacy laws prevent the dentist from discussing the treatment with the parent. Therefore it is recommended that the young adult either sign a release allowing the dentist to speak with the parent or have the young adult bring the parent with him/her to the consult or treatment visit.

Consent must be freely granted to be valid. Courts have declared consent invalid because to secure needed care, patients were required to consent to conditions not in their best interest. These types of consents are known as *adhesion contracts* and have been declared unenforceable by many courts.

The courts also look unfavorably on consents that contain exculpatory language (i.e., language that relieves the dentist of liability for negligence). An example is a consent that contains the following provision: "I accept this treatment with the understanding that I will hold the doctor harmless for any negligence in the performance of the treatment." The courts have stated in strong terms that exculpatory language in health care consent forms is void as against public policy.

LEGAL ELEMENTS OF INFORMED CONSENT

Basic to the concept of informed consent is that the patient must be given, in understandable language, enough information about the proposed treatment to make an intelligent decision about whether to proceed with the proposed treatment and have an opportunity to ask questions and have them answered.

Both the courts and the legislatures in most jurisdictions have provided specific guidelines regarding the required elements of informed consent. In general for consent to be valid and effective, the following conditions must be met:

1. The consent must be freely given.
2. The proposed treatment and its prognosis must be described.
3. The patient must be informed of the risks and benefits of the proposed treatment.
4. Reasonable alternative treatment(s) to the one suggested (including no treatment); and their risks, benefits, and prognosis must be described.
5. The patient must be given an opportunity to ask questions and have them answered.
6. All communication with the patient must be in language the patient understands.
7. The consent must be obtained from a person legally authorized to grant consent.

One element causing problems for the courts and the dentists concerns the amount of detail the dentist should use when explaining the treatment and options to the patient. Two different standards are applied by the courts. One holds the doctor to the standard of what other doctors in the community tell their patients in the same or similar circumstances (the professional community standard). The other standard requires the dentist to provide the patient with sufficient information for the patient to make an intelligent decision about whether to proceed with the proposed treatment (the reasonable person standard). When using the reasonable person standard, some courts apply an objective standard, which is, "Is the information provided sufficient for a reasonably intelligent person to make an intelligent choice?" Other courts apply a subjective standard, considering only what the patient was told, which is, "Was this person given enough information to make an intelligent decision?" Almost all jurisdictions follow the reasonable person standard. In the reasonable person standard, the risks to be communicated to the

patient are described as *material*. Based on court decisions, it appears that the more invasive the procedure or the greater the risk attached to it, the more detail regarding its risk the doctor is required to disclose for the consent to be informed.

Another issue for cosmetic dentists is whether the type of materials used need to be included in the informed consent. Consider the following hypothetical situation: whether a dentist has to advise a patient of what porcelain system is being used; i.e., CAD/CAM in office or a laboratory fabricated, lithium disilicate or all-zirconium, etc. Based on the reasonable person standard, it would seem that the dentist would not be legally obligated to discuss materials if the material (porcelain system in this instance) is being used within the standard of care for the restoration type and will meet the patient's subjective expectations regarding esthetics. For example, if the patient is having laminate veneers on teeth #'s 7 to 10 for purely esthetic reasons, all-zirconium is likely not indicated and need not be discussed. However, if the patient is a bruxer, then material limitations will need to be discussed based on fracture potential versus esthetics. Adequate informed consent is very case specific and therefore there is no clear-cut answer. However, as a general guide, if the materials being used will create either an objective dental compromise or subjective patient compromise, not only should it be discussed with the patient, but also the dentist should strongly consider not treating the patient.

Court decisions have addressed the issue of who should provide the information to obtain the consent. Options include the treating dentist, an associate, a hygienist, an assistant, or a receptionist. The courts have stated that it is the scope of the information given to the patient that was important, rather than the identity of the person who relayed the information; and the dentist is not required to obtain the consent.

Dentists, however, should keep in mind certain caveats before delegating the responsibility. The staff member should be trained in obtaining informed consent, and the degree of invasiveness and potential risks of the procedure should dictate who should answer questions asked by the patient about the procedure. Dentists who delegate the responsibility to obtain consent to someone else should be available to answer questions asked by the patient.

CLINICAL TIP

Informed consent for cosmetic dentistry can be established in a two-pronged fashion: (1) The dentist should always get an explicit informed consent and treatment plan/payment arrangement form prior to any treatment. Written signed consent is preferred. Additionally, the new patient registration form should have a clause in which the patient consents to the examination, taking of radiographs, diagnostic casts, and photographs. (2) Prior to any cosmetic or elective procedure, the dentist should have a separate consultation with the patient.

CONSULTATION VISITS

A separate consultation visit is essential prior to beginning any cosmetic treatment unless the treatment is very minor, no other realistic treatment options exist and there are no other circumstances such as medical or financial issues that warrant discussion. There are multiple reasons why a consultation visit is important.

During the consultation, the elements of informed consent (as listed previously) should be discussed with the patient. Ideally, the patient would be shown examples of other restorations (preoperative and postoperative photographs), diagnostic casts and a diagnostic wax-up (if indicated by the type of cosmetic treatment being performed), the patient's radiographs (if relevant to the treatment to be performed), and a patient education video. Additionally, the dentist should stress that no guarantees regarding the results of treatment have been made and that if clinical imaging has been used, that the imaging is for illustrative purposes and is not a representation of the definitive result. Details of the consultation visit should be recorded in the patient's chart.

The consultation visit gives the dentist time to reevaluate the patient from a clinical standpoint to help ensure the objective dental results of the treatment plan can be achieved. The consultation visit also gives the dentist an opportunity to see if the dentist can satisfy the patient's cosmetic expectations based on the patient's personality, demeanor and prior history. If there are any doubts about whether the objective dental results can be accomplished or whether the patient's subjective expectations can be satisfied, then the dentist should advise the patient that he/she (the dentist) cannot proceed with treatment.

The consultation visit will also allow the dentist or dedicated staff member to discuss fees with the patient. For a number of reasons, some practice management consultants advise that a dedicated treatment coordinator discuss fees with the patient. If there is any doubt as to whether or not the patient can or will pay for the treatment, then the dentist should not begin any treatment and advise the patient that he/she (the dentist) cannot proceed with treatment. Many licensing board complaints and malpractice complaints are instituted by patients in response to dentists seeking to collect an unpaid balance due.

Once a patient and dentist jointly decide on a treatment plan, a patient will need to consent to treatment as well as the financial arrangements.

CLINICAL TIP

The dentist should use two separate documents, an informed consent form and treatment plan/financial arrangement form if a written consent is used.

The treatment plan/financial arrangement form is critical in rebutting any allegation by a patient that he/she was not informed of the fees.

RECORDS

When a conflict arises between what a patient reports and the notes made by the dentist on the patient's record, the attorney for the patient (after reviewing the record) is likely to dissuade the patient from suing, provided the entries on the record and the entire record appear to be valid.

CLINICAL TIP

Properly maintained patient treatment records are the best defense against a claim of negligence when there has been no negligence, especially records that outline the compliance with the standard of care for a particular course of treatment. Records that are neat, legible, and appear to be accurate representations of treatment can positively influence plaintiff attorneys, juries, and judges.

In many states, there are laws that explain how long the dentist is required to retain the records and what the record must contain. Dentists can contact the appropriate state agency or a local attorney to obtain this information.

Financial information should not be kept on the treatment record. The treatment record should be reserved for treatment and patient reactions to treatment. Financial information should be kept on separate sheets and placed within the chart or computer chart. The presence of financial information on the treatment record may affect the outcome of a case. For example, if a juror believes the fees were excessive, it may influence the juror's decision on matters unrelated to the fees. In addition, any financial information appearing on the treatment record cannot be kept from the jury. The exception to this is if a patient refuses recommended treatment for financial reasons. When a patient refuses or postpones recommended treatment, the dentist should document the reason, including if the reason was financial.

The following rules should be followed regarding patient treatment records:

1. The records should be legible, written in black ink or black ballpoint pen. Pencils should not be used.
2. No erasures should appear on the record.
3. Erroneous entries should not be blocked out so that they cannot be read. Instead, a single line should be drawn through the entry with a note stating, "error in entry, see correction below." The correction should be dated at the time it is made.
4. Entries should be uniformly spaced on the form. The record should contain no unusual or irregular blank spaces.
5. On records in which more than one person is making entries, the entries should be signed or initialed.

In addition to treatment information, the following should be included in every patient record:

1. Documentation that informed consent to care was obtained before treatment was begun and documentation of any remarks made by the patient during the discussion
2. Documentation of all instances in which the patient fails to comply with the previously stated list of implied patient duties such as cancellations, failure to comply with home care instructions, etc.
3. Documentation of the failure of a patient to comply with the dentist's or other dentist's recommendations
4. Documentation of all referrals to, or requests for, consultations with other health professionals.
5. Documentation of all conversations held with other health professionals relating to any consultation about or care of the patient
6. Documentation that the patient was informed of any adverse occurrences or untoward events that took place during the course of treatment. The law recognizes that medicine and dentistry are not exact sciences and that undesirable results

can occur that are not necessarily negligent. Most rational people want to be informed of what is happening during treatment and these otherwise rational people could become upset if information is withheld. This could lead to loss of trust and malpractice or licensing board complaints.

7. Documentation of an initial health history, initial dental history and updated periodic health histories (See the section on Health and Dental History).

Subjective evaluations, such as your opinion about the patient's mental health, should not be entered on the treatment record unless you are qualified and licensed to make such evaluations. The law allows patients copies of their records and such notes may be counterproductive to the dentist. Notes about the patient's mental state or other personal evaluations should be made on a separate sheet.

Do not surrender the original records or radiographs to anyone unless ordered to do so by a court. Do not even surrender the original records to a specialist to whom you have referred a patient. In one court case, failure of the defendant to produce the original radiographs was interpreted as an attempt to conceal information and resulted in a decision against the dentist. In addition, retaining the original records, including radiographs, is required by law in some states.

CLINICAL TIP

Never tamper with a record once legal action is suspected from a patient. This is fraud and may result in severe punishment by the courts. Additionally, this may sway a jury against the dentist even if the dentist did not actually commit any malpractice.

HEALTH AND DENTAL HISTORY

Obtaining a patient's history verbally, with no written documentation of questions asked and answers given, is not a responsible office practice. Only a written history meets a "reasonable standard of care" in taking a patient's history.

Malpractice suits have involved failure to obtain an accurate health history. Some of the problems involved self-administered forms that required patients to check boxes or circle items to indicate "yes" or "no" as answers to various health questions. In one case, conflicting testimony surrounded who actually made the check marks or circled the answers. To prevent these problems, the questionnaire should be designed with open-ended questions to which the patient writes a response. Additionally, as with informed consent, age and competency issues arise as to who can give a legally valid health history. If a minor or legally incompetent person gives an erroneous health history and suffers injury because of dental treatment (e.g., osteonecrosis after extraction because the patient did not disclose bisphosphonate use), the dentist may be found liable.

The errors most commonly associated with medical problems are the following:

1. Failure to discover a potential drug incompatibility
2. Failure to learn of a drug allergy or potential drug allergy
3. Failure to discover a medical condition that may result in serious injury to the patient as a result of dental treatment (e.g., heart valve replacement).

Ideally, the treating dentist should take the history. However, if the responsibility of history taking is delegated to another person, the following rules should be heeded:

1. The person to whom the task is delegated should be specially trained in history taking.
2. The treating dentist should review the history with the patient and document that the dentist reviewed the history with the patient.

In offices with multiple dentists who treat patients, each dentist should review the patient's health history before treatment begins. The same is true for informed consent. It is not sufficient to rely on the ability of others in the office, even another treating dentist or hygienist, to obtain an adequate health history or a valid consent. The rule is that the person who provides the care is responsible for ensuring that (1) the care provided is compatible with the health of the patient and (2) informed consent was obtained.

All history forms should include the following: The patient's name; signature; the signature of the party completing the form if the person is not the patient; the signature of a witness to the patient's signature; and the signature of the dentist who reviewed the form with the patient. The form and all signatures should be completed in black ink or with a black ballpoint pen supplied by the office.

No law or fixed rule delineates how often the medical history should be updated; it is a professional judgment the dentist should make with each patient. For an apparently healthy teenager with uncomplicated dental problems, the dentist may decide to update the health history at every recall visit. For a geriatric patient with a history of diabetes, the dentist may decide to update the health history each month during an extended dental treatment process. Based on professional judgment, it may be sufficient to ask, "Has there been any change in your health since your last visit to the office?" If the dentist thinks that this is sufficient, it must be documented in the patient's record that the question was asked and the answer given by the patient.

CLINICAL TIP

The patient's medical and dental conditions should be monitored at intervals appropriate to the patient's age and medical and dental status.

When a formal update is required, the patient should be given a copy of the most recently completed self-administered history form for review. If the patient states that no changes have developed, this should be noted in the patient's record or on a form specially designed for that purpose. If the patient indicates that changes have occurred, it may be advisable to have the patient complete another history form and for the dentist to repeat the entire history-taking process.

Dental History

A written dental history form should be obtained from the patient at the initial visit. The dental history form should contain open ended questions such as "please list anything about your teeth or your dental appearance that wish you could change," "please list any concerns you have regarding dental treatment," and "please list any dental work that you do not like the appearance of." Additionally, the dental history should inquire as to prior treatment or prior dental problems such as periodontal issues or temporomandibular joint/orofacial pain issues. A thorough dental history can aid significantly in treatment planning, case selection, and ultimately malpractice defense.

Before beginning any cosmetic dentistry, a thorough evaluation of the patient's attitude toward dental care is essential. The dentist should design suitable questions to determine the patient's expectations and perspective. The questions and responses should be accurately documented on the dental history form or in the record. Forms alone are not enough for the dentist to properly and safely formulate a treatment plan. The dentist should also discuss the patient's expectations and demeanor with staff members who interact with the patient. For example, some patients feel more comfortable sharing their concerns with an assistant or hygienist. A discussion with the patient after the completion of the forms is essential; and a separate consultation visit should be scheduled for most cosmetic cases.

STATUTE OF LIMITATIONS

The statute of limitations defines the time within which a lawsuit may be brought. It is designed to prevent the threat of a suit from lasting forever. In addition, the statute takes into account fading memories and the unavailability of witnesses as a result of death or relocation. If the statute has expired, the patient cannot maintain a suit.

Basic issues of the statute of limitations are the following:
1. When does the time begin?
2. Which events or conditions toll (delay) the running of the statute?
3. How long does the statute run?

No nationwide standard has been set for these issues. Therefore dentists who want to know the times related to a statute should consult a local attorney. Following are some generalizations about the statute of limitations as it applies to malpractice suits against dentists.

Commencement

The statute of limitations may begin when the act of negligence takes place, regardless of whether the patient is aware of the negligence at the time it occurs. States that follow this rule are called *occurrence states*. However, some states consider the statute of limitations to start when the patient discovers or should have discovered that an act of negligence caused an injury. States that follow this rule are called *discovery states*. Additional possibilities for the start of the statute of limitations include the following:
1. When the course of treatment in which the negligent act took place ends
2. When the dentist-patient relationship ends
3. When the patient discovers or should have discovered that a foreign object was erroneously left in the body

All states have some combination of the previously listed starting dates.

Tolling

The statute of limitations is tolled during infancy and generally does not begin to run until the individual reaches majority (18 years of age). However, during the malpractice crises of the 1970s and 1980s, states enacted tort reform legislation in an attempt to control the growing number of malpractice suits. Some changes modified the tolling of the statute of limitations for infancy and placed a maximum on tolling years, regardless of when the individual reached adulthood.

Expiration

Even if the statute of limitations has run out, the patient may still file a suit against the dentist. It then becomes the dentist's burden, through an attorney, to answer the initial filing of the claim with an affirmative defense addressing the statute of limitations. Then the court will rule on whether the suit can continue.

The time in which suit may be brought is controlled by state law and varies between 1 and 5 years, with most states using a 2- to 3-year period. The time in which the statute begins and how long it runs create confusion and lack of uniformity. For example, in a state in which the statute does not begin to run until a patient discovers that a fractured root tip was left in the bone during an extraction, the statute may not begin to run until several years after treatment. In effect, the statute of limitations may be for an indefinite period. In another state in which the statute begins at the time of the incident (i.e., the breaking of the root tip), the statute begins to run without the knowledge of the patient and continues for the time set by local law.

FRAUDULENT CONCEALMENT

Courts look unfavorably on dentists who withhold information from a patient about an act of negligence committed during the course of treatment. Many states have enacted legislation on this issue. In those states, the statute of limitations does not begin to run until the patient discovers or should have discovered the fraud, and the statute of limitations for alleged fraud is applied. Therefore even in an occurrence state with a fixed statutory limit, a dentist who withholds a fact from the patient may be charged with fraudulent concealment to extend the period in which the patient may bring suit.

> ### CLINICAL TIP
>
> When unexpected results occur during the course of treatment, inform the patient. Document the event in the record and document that the patient was informed. This fixes the time the statute will begin to run, offers time-related protection to the dentist in discovery states, and prevents tolling of the statute of limitations as a result of fraudulent concealment.

FORMS AND RELEASES

The increase in paperwork in the modern dental office has become oppressive to many dentists. Although electronic records and "paperless" offices are decreasing the amount of actual paper, the dentist still must keep the same records and forms in electronic format. Further complicating dental practice are third-party insurance programs and other forms of third-party payment programs. Although many cosmetic procedures are not technically covered, the dentist may be contractually obligated to charge the patient a contracted fee. This interplay can complicate the practice management aspect of dentistry and needs to be understood to avoid any potential patient misunderstandings that could lead to complaints to insurance boards or licensing boards. Complete and carefully designed record keeping systems are essential in all modern practices as part of the risk management program.

Necessary forms:
1. Medical-Dental History
2. History Updates
3. *Release of information form.* To enable the dentist to obtain health information about the patient from other dentists and health facilities
4. *Permission to take photographs, slides, and videos form.* To allow the taking, use, and publication of photographs, slides, or videos. For both this form and the *release of information form.* The dentist should obtain the American Dental Association's HIPAA guide in order to help Ensure that these forms are HIPAA compliant.
5. Informed consent form.
6. *Follow-up of Telephone Consent.* To document that an informed consent was given to a parent of a minor if the parent was not present.
7. *Release of all claims form.* An essential form that must be signed before a fee is returned to a patient.
8. *Informed refusal form.* To document that the dentist has informed the patient of the consequences of not following the dentist's advice regarding recommended care, referrals, and specialty treatment; particularly useful when periodontal consultation or treatment is recommended and refused by the patient.

Additional needed forms:
1. Treatment Plan and Financial Arrangement. Most dental software has built in, customizable forms that are adequate.
2. Notice of Privacy Practices and Acknowledgement of Receipt of Notice of Privacy Practices. These forms are required by HIPAA law and additionally, state law may influence the requirements and nature of these forms.

PROCEDURE FOR HANDLING A MALPRACTICE SUIT

The shock of a malpractice suit may result in various inappropriate responses. Among them is psychologic denial, possibly causing a dentist to ignore the suit completely. Unfortunately, deadlines must be met. A dentist may want to phone the patient or contact the patient's lawyer. These are both improper because all professional liability insurance contracts contain a clause that requires the dentist to cooperate with the insurance company and to refrain from any activity that may compromise the suit.

The following are some guidelines for what *not* to do when faced with a malpractice suit:
1. The dentist should not respond to questions about the case or the treatment of the patient with anyone not known to be a representative of the dentist's malpractice insurance company or the dentist's attorney.
2. The dentist should not surrender original records to anyone except the dentist's attorney, the dentist's insurance company, or an official government agency with subpoena powers or court order signed by a judge.
3. The dentist should not speak to a dentist who has treated or is currently treating the patient or wrote a report about the case.

4. The dentist should not alter or add any notes to the patient's treatment record.
5. The dentist should not lose any of the patient's records, radiographs, test results, or reports.
6. The dentist should not agree to see or speak to the patient, regardless of the reason. Once the patient elects to file suit, the dentist-patient relationship ends and unfortunately, the adversarial relationship begins. The dentist should notify his or her own attorney for advice if the former patient contacts the dentist.
7. The dentist should not make any entries on the patient's record about the lawsuit or any other matter relating to the suit, such as receipt of the summons, demand for records, or communications with the insurance company or attorney. All notes related to the case should be recorded on a separate sheet and labeled *confidential.*
8. The dentist should not tell anyone about current insurance coverage.
9. The dentist should not speak to anyone about the case except the attorneys representing him/her. All information about the case must remain confidential. The dentist's attorney is in charge and should decide all actions to be taken.

The following are some guidelines for steps to take when faced with a malpractice suit:
1. The dentist should remain calm.
2. The dentist should record the manner in which the suit was served (not on the patient's record, but on a separate sheet headed *confidential*).
3. The dentist should make a copy of all the papers that were included in the service.
4. The dentist should contact all malpractice insurance carriers if the carrier changed during the patient's treatment and notify each carrier of the suit by certified mail, return receipt requested, as soon as possible. The dentist should send the original of all papers included in the service of the suit, including the envelope, if it was sent through the mail (after making copies).
5. The dentist should make a copy of all records and radiographs related to the care of the patient and secure the originals in a safe place.
6. The dentist should write a detailed narrative description of all treatment provided to the patient using the records to help. The sheet should be titled *confidential*. The dentist should include all that can be recalled about conversations held with the patient and statements made about the treatment. The narrative should be dated and signed and a copy sent to the insurance carrier. The original should be locked in a safe place.
7. If the amount of the suit exceeds the limits of the dentist's policy, the dentist should retain a separate attorney to safeguard all his or her financial interests.

CONCLUSION

Services that fall within the dentist's scope of practice have dramatically expanded, largely because of the advancements in restorative materials that have contributed to improved esthetics. Expanded techniques have kept pace with the new materials. The services available to patients, particularly in the field of cosmetic dentistry, have therefore increased.

A concurrent increase in litigation has accompanied the expansion in services. The present legal environment has demonstrated that good professional care is not enough to prevent a lawsuit. A comprehensive risk management program is essential for preventing and protecting against malpractice and licensing board complaints. Patients are entitled to decide which procedures should be done and to have enough information to make an intelligent informed decision about them before the procedures are carried out. Guarantees about outcomes or patient satisfaction should not be made. Case selection is critical. Treatment should not be attempted if there is any doubt that both the objective dental criteria and patient's subjective cosmetic expectations can be met. Documentation is essential in a lawsuit defense. Communication with patients to keep them informed about the care is essential. Because cosmetic dentistry is elective and evaluation of its results is rather subjective, special care must be taken to ensure that all legal preventive measures are followed when cosmetic dentistry is part of the treatment. Finally, good risk management is as important as good professional care. Without both, dentistry becomes a high-risk profession.

REFERENCES

1. Dental Specialty Report: Claims reported January 2001 through December 2009. Dental Specialty Report, Spring 2011. Princeton Insurance Company.
2. Rosa's Law. S.2781. 111th Cong. (2009-2010). Replacing the term "mental retardation" with "intellectual disability" in all Federal Laws.
3. Ferrús-Torres E, Valmaseda-Castellón E, Berini-Aytés L, Gay-Escoda C: Informed consent in oral surgery: the value of written information, *J Oral Maxillofac Surg* 69(1):54-58, 2011.

28

Esthetics and Psychology

Fred B. Abbott and Nellie Abbott

Recent advances in dental materials and procedures have greatly increased the ability to provide esthetic treatment. The wide array of available options increases the need for understanding the patient as a person and places greater emphasis on effective communication. Personality, motivations, desires, expectations, self-esteem, ability to accept change, and willingness to cooperate are important factors for successful treatment.[1,2] An awareness of self theory and a broad application of psychologic and sociologic principles can greatly enhance a dental practice that emphasizes esthetics.

HISTORY OF PSYCHOLOGY AND DENTAL ESTHETICS

As early as 1872 White reminded the dental profession of the need to relate esthetic appearance to the laws of nature, that is, facial contours, age, and temperament.[3] White later attempted to apply this theory to tooth selection; temperamental forms of teeth were produced as "named sets."[4] The term *named sets* refers to the categorization of maxillary anterior teeth.

The search for teeth that would enhance personality and appearance continued. In 1895 a prominent American dentist and artist, J. Leon Williams, expressed concern that the teeth available for dentures did not look lifelike. He carried out extensive research on teeth shape and size. He adopted White's "named sets" idea and classified anterior maxillary teeth as square, ovoid, tapering, or a combination of these types. A newly emerging company (now called Dentsply International, Inc.) used his research to create a mold guide system and techniques that made it possible for the first time for the dentist to select the size and form of teeth that would look best on the patient.[5] It was believed that Williams had discovered nature's law of the face-form–tooth-form harmony.[6]

M.M. House refined and expanded upon the work of Williams to include form and color harmony into denture esthetics.[7] The theories of Williams and House still serve as the frame of reference for tooth selection as taught in many dental schools today. A study by Brown failed to support Williams' and House's face-form–tooth-form theory.[8]

In 1937 House classified patients into four types based on psychologic assessment.[9] According to House:
1. The philosophic patient accepts his [or her] lot in life, copes with frustration, and is well organized with respect to time and habits.
2. The exacting individual is very methodical, accurate, demanding, and extremely precise in life's activities.
3. The indifferent patient is unconcerned, apathetic, and unmotivated.
4. The hysterical patient is emotionally unstable, highly excitable, and extremely apprehensive.

Although House's classification furnishes guidelines for diagnosing patients, the psychologic assessment of a patient goes beyond simple categorization.

"Dentogenic" Movement

In the 1950s the "dentogenic" movement became popular. *Dentogenics* was defined as the convergence of art, practice, and techniques that enabled a denture to add to a person's charm, character, dignity, and beauty in a fully expressive smile.[10] As proponents of dentogenics, J.P. Frush and R.D. Fisher placed great emphasis on projecting a denture wearer's personality, sex, and age. In collaboration with the Swissedent Foundation, they stressed the need to avoid the "denture look." They added to face-form and tooth-form the *SPA factor*: sex, personality, and age.[11]

They hypothesized a personality spectrum ranging from vigorous to medium pleasing to delicate. Based on their experience, Frush and Fisher believed that about 15% of the population was the vigorous type. These individuals tended to be male. About 5% were delicate, and they tended to be female. The remaining 80% were the medium-pleasing type, composed of both sexes.

Tooth selections and characterizations for prostheses were partially guided by the perceived personality type.[11] Frush and Fisher placed great emphasis on the need for sculpting the tooth and for selecting the color and position, to enhance the masculinity or femininity of the patient. They stressed the use of characterization to enhance age and gender.[12] Enhancing age means to make someone appear more youthful; enhancing gender means to make a "rugged" masculine type appear more ruggedly masculine or a "delicate" feminine type appear more delicately feminine, for example.

Recent studies, however, do not support the belief that tooth shape and size have identifiable masculine or feminine characteristics.[8,13] In a study of 300 diagnostic casts (equal numbers of male and female) judgments of gender were made by a layman, dental students, and dental faculty. The results showed an inverse relationship between correct judgment of the sex of the patient and the level of dental knowledge and experience of the judge.[13] However, from an artistic perspective, the consummate delicacy of femininity and the ruggedness of masculinity remain as accepted guidelines reinforcing the dentogenic theory.

THE CONCEPT OF SELF

Evolution of Self Theory

Humankind has long sought to understand the causes of behavior and to create a sense of identity. The term *self-concept* has a twentieth-century origin. Most discussions of self before the twentieth century were embedded in philosophic and religious dogma.

A precursor to self theory goes back to antiquity. Synthesizing ideas from classical Greek medicine and astronomy, a theory of temperaments evolved that prevailed for many centuries. In essence, it stated that an individual's personality type was predetermined by physiology. In the mid 1800s the temperament theory of personality was still in vogue, although it had been modified somewhat. Four classifications of temperaments were believed to exist[14]:

1. *Sanguine.* This type of personality radiated good humor and enthusiasm for life. It was believed to result from a predominance of blood over other body humors (fluids).
2. *Choleric.* This type of personality was irritable and found it difficult to establish a positive relationship. It was believed to result from a predominance of yellow bile over other humors.
3. *Melancholic.* This type of personality was serious, introverted, and cautious and often preferred to do things themselves. This was believed to result from a predominance of black bile over other humors.
4. *Phlegmatic.* This type of personality was characterized by torpor and apathy. It was believed to result from a predominance of phlegm over other humors.

In the clinical situation it is common to find patients whose personalities fall into these categories. The sanguine personality is certainly easier to relate to; the other two may pose a challenge. The choleric type usually is harder to satisfy, and it may be difficult to obtain active involvement on the part of the phlegmatic type. The dentist must develop skill in recognizing personality types early in the data collection stage.

Near the turn of the century, William James postulated that the empiric self includes four components, which he classified in descending order of impact on self-esteem:

1. *Spiritual self.* By "spiritual," James meant thinking and feeling. This is the center around which all other aspects of the empiric self are clustered. He perceived it to be the source of interest, effort, attention, will, and choice. In other words, the spiritual self is a composite of intellectual, religious, and moral aspirations from which a sense of either moral superiority or inferiority or guilt could arise.
2. *Material self.* The material self refers to the clothing and material possessions that an individual views as an important part of himself. Many people define themselves by what they own rather than by what they do.

3. *Social self.* The social self refers to the various aspects of personality that are reflected in the individuals and groups to which one relates. These aspects are designed to serve social ends, such as gaining love and admiration or obtaining influence and power.
4. *Bodily self.* The bodily self was placed last in importance by James; others question this placement. This aspect refers to body image. Achieving an awareness of the self begins with experiencing one's body and feelings, often via the reactions of significant individuals. An individual who has a high degree of self-awareness is often perceived to be "more alive."

These four components interrelate in unique ways to constitute each person's view of his or her empiric self.[15]

The development of self theory was temporarily sidetracked by the ascendancy of behaviorism and its emphasis on the scientific method. During this period, psychology was directed to a rigorous study of only those aspects of behavior that were observable and measurable. However, around 1930 the focus shifted, and the importance of internal events was reintroduced into research and therapy. By the middle of the twentieth century the self concept was firmly established as an important construct in the study of human behavior.[16-18] Since then a massive amount of theorizing and experimenting has occurred in all components of self theory.

Self Theory: Relevant Constructs

Self theory might be defined as that evolving constellation of self-referent constructs that are used to attain a more plausible and complete theoretical account of human conduct. Some of the relevant constructs of self theory are the following:

1. *Self-awareness.* Self-awareness has been defined as knowledge of one's own traits or qualities, insight into and understanding of one's own behavior and motives.
2. *Self-concept.* Many contemporary psychologists ascribe a key role to self-concept as a factor in integrating personality, motivating behavior, and achieving mental health. Volumes have been written on this subject.[19-22] Essentially, self-concept is one's view of oneself, including feelings and perceptions about oneself.
3. *Self-image.* Self-image is the self that one thinks oneself to be. It is not a directly observed self-object but rather a complex concept of personality, character, status, body, and bodily appearance. It may differ greatly from objective fact.[14] A concept closely related to self-image is body image.
4. *Self-esteem or self-evaluation.* Self-evaluation is the process by which individuals examine their performance, capabilities, and attributes according to personal standards and values, which have been internalized from society and significant others. These evaluations promote behavior consistent with self-knowledge. For example, an individual who firmly believes that he has unattractive or ugly teeth may develop speaking patterns or behavioral mannerisms that keep the teeth concealed. He may avoid pursuing certain vocations that, in his opinion, require a certain degree of attractiveness because of face-to-face contact with the public. The image a person has of himself may or may not coincide with reality. A person may be more or less attractive than conceptualized.
5. *Self-actualization.* The most recent development in self theory stresses the importance of a drive labeled "self-actualization." Abraham Maslow proposed that self-actualization results in a striving to develop one's capacities, understanding of self, and acceptance of self in accord with one's "inner nature."[23,24] Maslow looked to a more positive side of nature than many of his contemporaries. He believed that human nature was essentially good and, as personality

unfolded through maturation, the creative powers manifested themselves ever more clearly. If people became neurotic or miserable, he felt that was caused by the environment. Humans became destructive or violent only when their inner nature was twisted or frustrated. Maslow assumed that basic needs, such as physiologic needs, safety, love, belonging, and esteem must be satisfied before self-actualization can be achieved (Fig. 28-1).

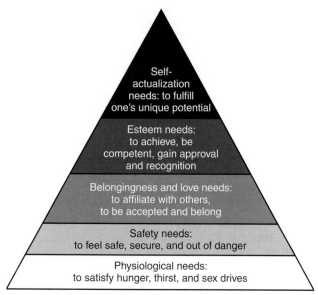

FIGURE 28-1 Abraham Maslow's hierarchy of human needs. (Adapted from Rubin Z, McNeil EB: *Psychology of being human*, ed 4, New York, 1985, Harper & Row.)

Although it is well established that people who have not satisfied their basic physiologic needs are not likely to be interested in much else, the relative order of some of the other needs may vary from person to person. Also, several different needs may motivate behavior at any given time.[25]

PHYSICAL AND PHYSIOLOGIC INFLUENCES

Facial Appearance

A study in 1921 highlighted the importance of facial appearance by proposing that the physical characteristics of individuals exert a profound influence over their associates.[26] However, researchers did not quickly adopt this concept. Some speculate that our society's emphasis on egalitarianism may have contributed to this omission. In other words, the belief that a person's appearance ought not to make a difference in opportunities for development and success may have produced an "ostrich effect."[27]

It was not until the 1960s that studies of facial appearance began appearing in the literature. In the 1970s research on the social psychology of facial appearance became more frequent. Although a vast number of studies have been reported, the quality of most of these studies is questionable.[28] However, a growing body of information is now accumulating on facial appearance. Facial attractiveness has an important impact on an individual's life, a fact increasingly recognized by dentists and physicians.[29]

Few studies of facial appearance have investigated in a scientific manner those dimensions of the face and teeth that are responsible for a pleasant or an unpleasant face. In general, individuals in our society tend to reject the open bite facial

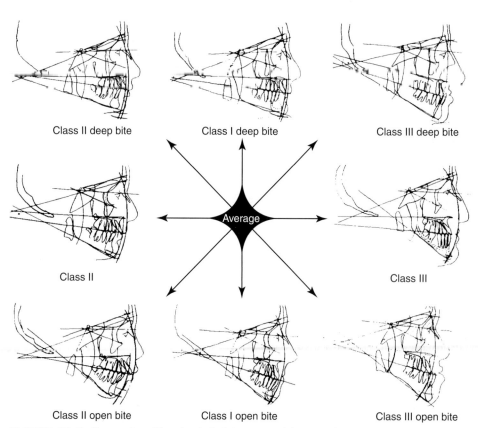

FIGURE 28-2 Composite of four basic facial types and their combinations. (From Sassouni V: A classification of skeletal facial types, *Am J Orthod* 55:120, 1969.)

types (either Class II or Class III) but more readily accept the deep bite facial type (Fig. 28-2).[30,31]

Regardless of the results of studies relating facial attractiveness to success in academics, careers, or interpersonal relationships, the personal testimonies of patients suggest that improved appearance is a goal worth pursuing, as the following situation clearly demonstrates.

The patient is a 49-year-old real estate agent. He originally presented with a dour, morose appearance and was somewhat argumentative. Over the years he had abraded his teeth through bruxism until they were no longer visible when he talked or smiled. Eating was no longer enjoyable because of the significant loss of vertical occluding dimension, which led to facial distortion when he chewed. He was embarrassed by his image. He hoped for a "quick fix" to his problem.

A provisional diagnostic acrylic splint was placed to determine his tolerance for a restored vertical occlusion. The attractive splint dramatically changed his appearance. Composite resin veneers further enhanced the esthetics (Fig. 28-3).

Over the next few weeks the patient's personality gradually changed. He began to smile and appeared more relaxed. When questioned about this perceived change, he stated, "You're absolutely right. You can't believe how good I feel inside. I want to smile at everybody. I can't pass a mirror without stopping to look at my new teeth. I can hardly wait to get my permanent restorations. Already I've started on a self-improvement program, losing a few pounds and toning up. Business has become a pleasure, and I feel more confident in social situations."

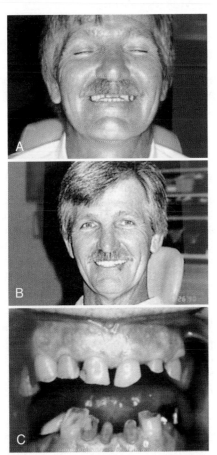

FIGURE 28-3 A, Patient before treatment. **B,** Patient after restorations. **C,** Pretreatment photograph that convinced a patient of the need for treatment.

The Mouth and Oral Cavity

The mouth has long played a prominent role in psychologic theories (e.g., Freud incorporated the "oral" stage of development into psychoanalytic theory). Throughout life the mouth assumes a prominent role in our link with the outside world—nutritionally, sexually, and through verbal communication.[32] When individuals first meet, the mouth is often the first body part noticed. Given the prominence of the mouth, it is surprising that more people do not show sufficient concern for the appearance of their teeth and mouth.

Sex and Age

Many stereotypes regarding sex have changed over the years. Still, the sexes have major differences that must be considered in a dental practice. The dentist needs to be aware of how patients view their own sexuality and the degree to which they wish to emphasize their masculinity or femininity.

The dentist also must consider a person's age, both psychologic and chronologic. Through the use of veneers and bleaching, a more youthful appearance may be created. Although many people wish to appear more youthful, this is not universally true. As one woman so emphatically stated, "I am a little old lady and I want to look like one."

PSYCHOLOGIC INFLUENCES

Personality

An individual's personality is the result of many factors. The degree to which facial, and specifically oral, appearance contributes to personality is difficult to ascertain. We have referred to just a few of the many attempts to broadly classify personality. The individual dentist must choose an approach for determining personality. Because personality is the filter through which relationships take place, an accurate assessment of a patient's personality can be critical to the successful outcome of dental treatment.

Measurement and Evaluation

A number of studies in the dental literature include personality variables in the assessment of patient satisfaction with their current dental condition,[33] as well as with treatments involving complete dentures,[34-37] partial dentures,[38] temporomandibular disorders and chronic pain,[39] orthognathic surgery,[40] prosthetic surgery,[41] and orthodontics and prosthodontics.[42]

Many of these studies deal with captive audiences (e.g., veterans or patients at dental school clinics). Therefore the results are not extensively generalizable. Findings from one study sometimes conflicted with findings from another. No clear picture emerges. Very few studies have been done relating personality characteristics to esthetics, per se.

A variety of tools and techniques have been used to obtain information from patients. They include self-designed questionnaires, focused interviews, projective figure drawing, and standardized tests. Some specific tests that have been recommended include the Cattell 16 PF questionnaire (Form C)[35] and the Cornell Medical Index.[34] Dentists considering using standardized psychologic tests should seek the assistance of a psychologist trained in measurement and evaluation.

A decision is needed regarding how psychologic information will be obtained and recorded.[43] Will it be an informal process based on an interview and observation of the patient, or will it be more formal? Will special forms be used to collect specific information? How will the forms be presented to patients in an effort to gain their cooperation? Who will interpret this information? How will this information be used?

Motivations, Desires, and Expectations

A host of factors may bring patients to a dental office initially, as well as cause them to return. Motivations may include the following:

1. The desire to be better able to eat and enjoy food
2. The desire to improve speech patterns
3. The fear of losing teeth through decay or fracture
4. The desire to be free of pain and discomfort
5. The desire to have fresh breath
6. The desire to enhance appearance or self-image to compete more effectively for attention or advancement

Not all patients are motivated by self-actualization; however, some may be moved in that direction.

In some instances the patients' expectations are unachievable. Patients may have personality problems or interpersonal problems that they believe will be corrected or improved by the desired dental treatment. The dentist must be on guard for this problem and avoid getting into an unresolvable situation. The dentist should not promise more than can be delivered. The dentist should be sensitive to cues that the patients or those accompanying the patients reveal during the initial examination and interview process. The quintessential question that the practitioner must seek to answer is, "What motivated these patients to seek dental treatment?" If the patients are concerned primarily about appearance, what is the underlying motivation? If a particular problem has existed for a long time, what change in their lives caused them to seek help now?

The patients' motivations or concerns form a starting point for developing a proper treatment plan. When patients realize that the dentist is truly listening to their concerns, they will be more likely to also consider the dentist's limitations. For example, if the patient's primary concern is the ability to eat, the most appropriate treatment—to improve mastication—should be addressed first. To achieve that objective, a complete or partial denture may be required. Once that need is addressed, improved esthetics will be incorporated later in connection with the design.

Determining motivation, coupled with a fairly accurate personality assessment, is crucial to successful treatment planning and ultimately to patient satisfaction with the treatment.

CLINICAL TIP

Often it is input from sensitive staff members that provides insight into the patient's needs and desires. Patients often perceive the dentist as an authority figure and have difficulty expressing themselves to someone in that role.

Basic information should be obtained from the patient upon entry into the office. This usually is obtained by means of a form. Auxiliary personnel set the tone in the manner in which they request this information from the patient. Much can be learned from observations of how the person studies the form, from unanswered questions, and from conversations with significant others while filling out the form. Seeking clarification or using information from this form to initiate conversation may elicit valuable information that can illuminate the patient's personality and motivations. This can also help to determine whether the patient is able to articulate expectations in a clear manner.

Developing a Trusting Relationship

CLINICAL TIP

Make a judgment regarding whether the patient can form a trusting relationship. When an individual is suspicious of every suggestion and asks an inordinate number of questions, it may indicate an inability to form a positive relationship.

At times, patients find it difficult to reveal all the relevant aspects of their lives. The dentist may need to gain patients' trust to enable them to open up and be forthright and honest. Roger's client-centered therapy[18] provides three qualities that help to engender trust:[44]

1. Accurate empathy involves the dentist's sensitivity to patients' feelings and an ability to communicate this awareness and acceptance of patients as unique individuals.
2. Nonpossessive warmth refers to the dentist's nonjudgmental acceptance of the patient regardless of behavior. Patients should not be criticized for allowing their oral health to deteriorate.
3. Genuineness implies an openness and spontaneity on the part of the dentist.

Decision-Making Ability

Efforts should be made very early to engage patients in decision making. To the extent possible, patients should be active participants in their treatment.

CLINICAL TIP

When the patient cannot make decisions, it is important to identify a "significant other" in the patient's life and include that person in the process.

Cooperation and Follow-Through

Optimal oral health and a beautiful smile require cooperation from the patient, as well as persistence in maintenance activities. Some people are "starters" but not "finishers." Before initiating treatment, the dentist must adequately inform the patient of the need for follow-up care. Some reconstruction patients, for example, fail to accept responsibility for maintenance and end up losing all benefit of their extensive treatment.

Abnormalities and Problem Patients

Occasionally, "troubled" or "difficult" patients with irrational perceptions of self seek treatment or esthetic alterations that are unrealistic. They may be narcissistic, depressed, paranoid, or have labile or hysterical personalities. Often these individuals are skillful at masking their condition, especially during the interview process.

Only by careful listening over a period of time can the patients' problems be identified. Patients may have unrealistic expectations or may be unable to internalize information provided by the dentist. These patients may be obsessed with perceived or minor flaws or may be unable to develop a trusting relationship.

Once a relationship has been established between a patient and a dentist, termination of that relationship must be handled very carefully to avoid a possible charge of abandonment (see Chapter 27). Treatment undertaken must be completed at least to the point at which the patient is not left in a precarious position. Before terminating a relationship, the dentist must make every effort to correct the problem, improve communication, and gain cooperation. These efforts may not be successful.

If the patient's psychologic problems are severe, the dentist may determine that professional help is needed. Psychologic therapy does not fall within a dentist's scope of practice without training and certification in this field. However, the dentist must appreciate the delicate nature of making a referral to a mental health professional; the referral should be made with care, empathy, and tact.

Not all problems can be anticipated and prevented. The dentist must think about the type of problems faced in an esthetic dental practice and consider an approach to dealing with these problems. It is logical to believe that the following problems are likely to occur:

1. The patient has an unrealistic esthetic expectation that cannot be satisfied.
2. The patient expects that an esthetic improvement will remove or correct deep-seated psychologic problems.
3. The patient is not satisfied with results that are technically and esthetically correct—in other words, the "it's not me" phenomenon.
4. The patient is satisfied with the results, but family and friends are not.
5. The patient does not wish to have esthetics enhanced, and the dentist does.

In dealing with these problems the dentist must be explicit in what the proposed treatment can and cannot do. Active involvement of patients and family members in the treatment phase increases the chance of acceptance (e.g., have them select shades and shapes of teeth). Multiple joint esthetic evaluations may be required. The dentist and the patient may not agree on what is perceived as esthetically appropriate.

CLINICAL TIP

As long as no physiologic or ethical principles are violated, permit the patient to make the definitive esthetic determination.

Patients' views of their esthetic appearance are paramount, because dentists may be unaware of the extent to which patients have psychologically compensated for their esthetic shortcomings.

CULTURAL INFLUENCES

Anthropologists have shown us that standards of beauty vary widely not only from society to society but also locally. Even in societies in which it is fashionable to go naked, the face is extremely important. Malinowski has pointed out that the naked Trobriand Islanders of the Western Pacific devoted tremendous energy to the decoration and elaboration of the face.[33]

The desire to alter the face is universal. In many primitive societies painful elaborations were undertaken not only in pursuit of beauty but also for ritual significance (see Chapter 1). In Australia and New Guinea the native peoples celebrated the achievement of adulthood and maturity by having their two maxillary anterior teeth removed. This custom also prevailed in South Africa, where adults who still had all their teeth were considered ugly. In Borneo, teeth were blackened and holes were drilled

through the facial surfaces of the six maxillary anterior teeth. Plugs of brass with outer ends shaped like stars were inserted. In the East Indies the mesial, distal, and incisal aspects of the teeth were filed off and shaped into points as part of the ceremony of marriage, puberty, or mourning. This custom prevails today among the pygmies of central Africa, specifically the Efe group.[45]

Within the United States today, many cultures exist. The practicing dentist should become aware of the various cultural groups represented in the patient population. In each community, certain ethnic groups have developed traditions of eating and self-care that have implications for dentistry. The dentist can become aware of these groups by subscribing to a local newspaper, becoming involved in community affairs such as health fairs, and communicating with other health professionals who may be a part of the ethnic groups. It may be necessary to use or develop teaching materials geared specifically toward the customs and traditions of these groups.

Mores and Values

Our mores and values have changed a great deal from those in vogue when the country was founded. At that point in history, plainness and austerity were the norm. Individuals who stressed beauty often were ostracized.

Gradually, our society has broadly accepted the idea that health and beauty occur simultaneously. Religious and psychologic barriers have been lowered. The "natural look" is popular. Styles have been modified to expose more of the body. Feeling good about oneself now is acceptable behavior. In fact, the pendulum has almost swung too far in the opposite direction. People who pay little attention to their personal appearance often instill confusion in others.

SOCIOLOGIC INFLUENCES

A number of sociologic trends in our society are believed to contribute to the ability and willingness of individuals to seek out esthetic dentistry.

Affluence

An increasing number of individuals are obtaining more discretionary income. Available funds, coupled with the newer emphasis on self-actualization and the freedom to spend money on self, has led to an increase in the demand for self-improvement, including esthetic dentistry.

CLINICAL TIP

The patient's socioeconomic status can be misleading. Some patients who appear to be able to afford treatment may not value oral health or appearance enough to incur the expense. Other patients with limited resources are able to rearrange their priorities and mobilize resources. Therefore do not initially consider the patient's socioeconomic status, but rather present the ideal treatment as well as acceptable alternatives.

Emphasis on Health, Wellness, and Fitness

After decades, and perhaps even centuries, of basing health care on a sickness model, the changes in recent years have been dramatic. Escalating health care costs, coupled with a national effort to curtail these increasing costs, have resulted in more emphasis on the prevention of illness, physical fitness, and health maintenance.

The dental profession has been at the forefront of this wellness movement. In the 1960s scientific evidence supported the efficacy of fluoridation. Dental disease was perceived to be preventable. Dentists were asked to change their clinical perspective from disease orientation to health orientation, and many did. As newer concepts have been accepted, chair time has been used increasingly for maintenance of health and esthetic dentistry.

Media Influence

Possibly the greatest single factor responsible for increased esthetic awareness among the public is the media. Television, radio, and magazine reports and advertisements daily bombard our society with news of the newest advances in bleaching, bonding, veneering, crowns, implants, orthodontic therapy, and surgery.[46]

Changed Attitudes Toward Medical and Dental Treatment

No longer willing to allow the physician or dentist to solely determine their needs and how to address those needs, many patients expect to be active participants in the analysis and planning phases of their care. They want to know what options are available and the pros and cons of each option.

Attitudes toward the cost of treatment are also slowly changing. Just as the expense of a college education is considered an investment, so is esthetic dentistry viewed as an investment by some individuals who are convinced that their success in life depends on appearance. Quality of life is becoming a value for the elderly.[47]

CLINICAL PRACTICE

Interaction Between Dentist and Patient

To some extent, psychologic bonding occurs between the patient and the dentist. Early in the relationship it is important to determine that a positive relationship can exist. The personalities of the patient and dentist must be compatible. The patient must have confidence in the dentist and believe that the dentist not only understands what the patient desires or needs but also has the creativity, knowledge, skill, and state-of-the-art equipment and materials to meet these needs. One dentist who had gone to great pains to design a modern office in which all extraneous items were kept out of sight was surprised to learn that a patient believed he was not fully equipped. She was accustomed to traditional offices, in which the counters were filled with instruments and materials.

Following the diagnostic work-up, the clinical information is integrated with the psychologic and sociologic information relevant to the patient. A detailed, written treatment plan is formulated. The plan sets forth the optimum treatment, as well as possible acceptable options. In other words, usually more than one way exists to achieve the treatment objectives. Choices must be made. Economics, as well as personality factors, influence which specific plan is selected.

CLINICAL TIP

Carefully structure the presentation of treatment options. If possible, schedule it at the close of the day when time is available for discussing and exploring alternatives. By learning specific treatment options along with the rationale for each, patients are able to recognize their active role in the treatment planning process.

The dentist should be prepared for some negative reactions to the comprehensive treatment plan. In some instances the plan can be overwhelming and even devastating. Patients who have ignored their oral health for years often have such great needs that they may say, "Why don't you just pull out all my teeth and give me some dentures?" They see that as the solution to their problem, not realizing that they are opening the door to a host of other problems. The dentist must be frank with the patient, explaining the many problems that they could face with dentures (e.g., problems with stability, pressure, potential inability to eat certain foods, and the need for relines). In addition, the dentist must point out the ethical and legal problem related to the extraction of teeth with adequate root structure.

Other patients may be more philosophic. They may say, "Well, this didn't happen overnight. Let's get on with the treatment." Sometimes their treatment can be extended over time.

Still others may not wish to be too involved. They may claim to be "confused" by the various options. They say, "Just tell me what I need to have done." In this decision-making role, the dentist must be guided by conscience and the Golden Rule, considering the options and arriving at the most permanent, most physiologic, and most esthetic treatment to address the need. The rationale should be explained to the patient and recorded in the chart. This approach assumes that the dentist is knowledgeable of state-of-the-art dentistry. (See the Clinical Tip in the section on Decision-Making Ability.)

A.G. Cheney suggests that the dentist avoid standardized treatment plans. To obtain greater patient acceptance, he believes that each treatment plan should be customized, based on an assessment of the patient's personality, needs, wants, and desires.[48] He utilizes the psychologic construct known as locus of control to help determine the individualized treatment plan for a given patient.

To the degree possible, the patient's needs, wants, and desires are incorporated into the treatment plan; however, both dental and physiologic limitations may prevent the dentist from fulfilling the patient's esthetic demands. For example, a patient may have a diastema that he wants closed. Treatment options include orthodontic treatment, crowns, composite resin restorations, or porcelain veneers. The treatment of choice is orthodontic treatment. The patient does not want this treatment, yet he insists that he does not want the anterior teeth to be larger than they are now. The dentist is faced with a dilemma. A provisional restoration could be placed to allow the patient to see whether he could accept it. Once the treatment plan has been agreed upon, the treatment phase should proceed as expeditiously as possible to reinforce the patient's motivation and to achieve the desired results. On the other hand, the patient's efforts to expedite the treatment should be resisted if this will compromise the desired results. This can be accomplished by explaining to the patient the specific steps required to achieve a plan of treatment (e.g., if a provisional removable partial denture is indicated, immediately placing a cast removable partial denture can result in poor function and esthetics).

CLINICAL TIP

Avoid shortcuts that will adversely affect quality, in spite of outside pressures.

Interaction Between the Dentist and Dental Laboratory Technician

The relationship between the dentist and the technician is crucial to success. In addition to the knowledge and skill that each possesses, psychologic factors enter this relationship. Mutual respect for each other as individuals should exist, as well as a clear understanding of the role that each plays in patient treatment. Dentists must seek out a technician with whom they can communicate, must set the tone for collaboration, and must provide for a two-way evaluation process that fosters progressive excellence. Both oral and written lines of communication must be kept open. Work authorization forms may need to be redesigned.

CLINICAL TIP

Whenever possible, visit the laboratory. It is helpful to know the laboratory personnel and be personally reassured of the quality of their work.

When the dentist and the technician collaborate on a difficult restoration and the results are pleasing, each gains satisfaction and the relationship is strengthened. Any gestures of staff appreciation should include the technicians, even if they are not on the premises of the dental practice.

Photographs give visual feedback to the technician, especially "before" and "after" views. They show color and texture dimensions that cannot be seen on the stone casts alone.

CLINICAL TIP

Send the technician photographs of completed restorations. This type of evaluation serves as a motivator and may enhance the status of the technician in the eyes of co-workers.

Certain personality characteristics are needed for esthetic dentistry practice. The success of esthetic dentistry depends upon discipline and consistent adherence to procedures. Many newer esthetic materials are very technique sensitive.

PRACTICE MANAGEMENT

The entire dental practice should take into consideration psychologic and sociologic principles. It should function as a well-integrated system.

Physical Environment

An esthetic dental practice should operate in an attractive, neat, clean environment. The patient should be surrounded by pleasing colors and textures that complement each other and suggest that the treatment provided in this setting will be competent and esthetic. Colors, however, should be carefully selected and placed so that they do not interfere with tooth shade selection (muted colors are most desirable). Employing an interior decorator may be a worthwhile investment in creating the proper physical environment. If background music is played, it should be carefully selected to help create the mood for the office. Odors should be carefully monitored and controlled.

Care should be given to the selection and arrangement of furniture. Adequate space should be available in the reception area to provide a display area for teaching materials that highlight the esthetic nature of the practice (e.g., photographs, videotapes).

Psychologic Environment

A greater use of technology in the practice mandates a greater need for the human touch. A sincere caring and concern should emanate from each member of the office staff toward the patient. Patients should be made to feel important. They should be treated with dignity and respect. Staff members should radiate concern for their comfort, privacy, and time. This is manifested in how patients are addressed, where conversations take place, and how the scheduling process is managed.

Scheduling appointments presupposes that the proper amount of time is budgeted and that necessary laboratory work has been completed. The patient should know what to expect and approximately how long it will take. Verifying appointments in advance and alerting patients to possible delays reinforce the value of the time that has been set aside specifically for them. Coordinating treatment between various specialties is another way to reduce stress for the patient and to ensure a more successful outcome.

Personnel as an Extension of the Dentist

Although members of the dentist's staff have unique characteristics, a conscious effort should be made to select individuals who complement the dentist's practice philosophy. Just as the physical environment of the office is important, so is the appearance of each member of the team. Attention to small details such as hair, nails, uniforms, shoes, weight, and smoking will reap rewards. Above all, the staff members should have good oral health. Educating by example yields rewarding results.

Careful planning should go into patient communication. The burden of education must not rest entirely upon the dentist but rather should be shared, when appropriate, with other members of the team. Resources to facilitate understanding must be carefully selected. For example, a variety of teaching materials, ranging from three-dimensional models to photographic displays to brochures, booklets, and videotapes should be available. Informed consent implies patient understanding.

Critical points for communication are at consultation, diagnostic work-up, presentation of the treatment plan, and initiation of treatment. Although technical terminology may be used, it should be translated into the layperson's language.

Communication

Specific terms, such as "white teeth," may need to be clarified before the implementation of treatment. If the dentist has a bias against restorations that lie outside the parameters of the natural color of teeth, this must be made clear. A significant difference may exist between a patient's expectations and the dentist's philosophy or attitude. This point was illustrated when a dentist interacted with a patient who desired "white teeth." The patient was not swayed when the dentist explained that the shade the patient wanted was not natural. She replied, "I bleach my hair blond, put rouge on my cheeks, and mascara on my eyelids; I paint my lips red. These are not natural. So give me white teeth!"[49]

If the request or desire of the patient does not conflict with ethical codes and does not cause physiologic harm to the oral environment, then the dentist has freedom to cooperate. (See also the section on Abnormalities and Problem Patients in this chapter.)

> ### CLINICAL TIP
>
> Upon initiation of treatment, verify the treatment plan with the patient. Clarify any misconceptions that have arisen between the time of the treatment conference and initiation of treatment.

Styles of communication vary widely. Some people communicate directly and honestly; others play games with their communication.[50,51] They may or may not be aware of this game playing. An understanding of transactional analysis therapy may facilitate true communication. This is not to say that the dentist should be a therapist, however. The objective is to get the patient to communicate as an adult and for the dentist not to be trapped into a "child" or "parent" communication style, but rather to also be able to communicate as an adult.

Financial Considerations

Clinical treatment should be separated from the business aspects of the practice. In other health-related disciplines, treatment is not determined by the patient's ability to pay. Avoiding a discussion of fees at the time of treatment planning allows for a more objective discussion of options. Other than helping to decide the fee structure, the dentist should avoid getting involved in this aspect of the practice. This is not to say that the patient's decision will not be largely influenced by cost. However, cost may not be the most crucial consideration. Patients may be willing to invest more time and money than dentists have previously assumed. (See the section on Affluence in this chapter.)

The team member responsible for the financial dealings must be psychologically strong and able to help the patient to view esthetic dentistry as an investment. Money and time will be expended on self-improvement, which has potential payoff in meeting some of the patient's goals and dreams, for example, to help get an advancement or better sell a proposal and win a contract. To accomplish this, the business manager must be aware of the patient's personality and socioeconomic status and relate to each patient in a manner consistent with the philosophy of the practice.[52]

Photography and Computer Technology

Some patients who have become complacent about their deteriorating oral health are shocked when they see a photograph[53-55] (see Chapter 22). For example, the patient described early in the chapter exclaimed, "Is that me?" when he saw a picture of his mouth; this helped to motivate him to pursue treatment. A fairly recent breakthrough in dental photography is the color video intraoral camera, which has the capacity to store images as well as to alter them to present different treatment options[55] (see Chapter 22.)

Ethics, Quality Assurance, and Risk Management

Clinical dental ethics focuses on decisions, both the decision-making process and the outcome, as they are reached in everyday practice.[56-58] Dentists are legally and morally obligated to the following:

1. Benefit the patient's health.
2. Do no harm to the patient.
3. Help the patient weigh the risks or harms of treatment against the anticipated result.

Responsible treatment decisions must weigh the costs of the care against the anticipated benefits.

Although it is important to discern what a patient desires as a treatment outcome, desires may not always be consistent with treatment goals. For example, a patient may desire esthetic restorative dentistry for the maxillary anterior teeth without replacing mandibular posterior teeth. To provide the desired treatment would be unethical because it is doomed to failure. Continuous occlusal trauma of the mandibular anterior teeth will result. When a patient's cosmetic preferences compromise professional standards, the dentist faces a moral dilemma. Even if the patient is willing to take calculated risks, inappropriate treatment should not be undertaken. The dentist is not legally protected from charges of inappropriate treatment, even when the patient signs a release (see Chapter 27).

CONCLUSION

The patient and the dentist each bring to the relationship unique personalities, values, expectations, and motivations, which have been shaped by their respective backgrounds. Dentists have the educational responsibility to learn about psychologic and sociologic concepts and to incorporate them into their practice. If they assume this responsibility, the practice will be enriched. Quality esthetic dentistry rendered to appreciative patients has lasting psychologic rewards for all involved.

ACKNOWLEDGMENT

The authors wish to recognize the editorial assistance of Marc B. Appelbaum, Morristown, NJ.

REFERENCES

1. Abbott FB: Psychological assessment of the prosthodontic patient before treatment, *Dent Clin North Am* 28:361, 1984.
2. Murrell GA: Esthetics and the edentulous patient, *J Am Dent Assoc* (special issue) No. 58E, 1987.
3. White JW: Aesthetic dentistry, *Dent Cosmos* 14:144, 1872.
4. White JW: Temperament in relation to teeth, *Dent Cosmos* 22:113, 1884.
5. Williams JL: A new classification of tooth forms with special reference to a new system of artificial teeth, *Dent Cosmos* 56:627, 1914.
6. Clapp GW: How the science of tooth form selection was made easy, *J Prosthet Dent* 5:596, 1955.
7. House MM: Full denture techniques. Notes of study Club No. 1. Unpublished notes on course given by MM House, 1937.
8. Brown F: *Doctoral dissertation*, Washington, DC, 1975, Howard University.
9. House MM, Loop FL: *Form and color harmony in the dental art*, Whittier, Calif, 1939, Monograph.
10. Frush JP, Fisher RD: Introduction to dentogenic restorations, *J Prosthet Dent* 5:586, 1955.
11. Frush JP, Fisher RD: How dentogenics interprets the personality factor, *J Prosthet Dent* 6:441, 1956.
12. Frush JP, Fisher RD: How dentogenic restorations interpret the sex factor, *J Prosthet Dent* 6:160, 1956.
13. Abbott FB: *Unpublished study*, Philadelphia, 1986, Temple University.
14. English HB, English AC: *A comprehensive dictionary of psychological and psychoanalytical terms*, New York, 1958, David McKay.
15. James W: *Principles of psychology*, New York, 1890, Holt.
16. Lewin K: *Field theory in social sciences*, New York, 1951, Harper & Row.
17. Combs A, Snygg D: *Individual behavior: a perceptual approach*, New York, 1959, Harper & Row.
18. Rogers CR: *Client centered therapy*, Boston, 1951, Houghton Mifflin.
19. Bums RB: *The self concept: theory, measurement, development and behavior*, New York, 1979, Longman.

20. Fitts W: *The self concept and self actualization: studies on the self concept and rehabilitation,* Nashville, 1971, Dede Wallace Center.
21. Wegner D, Vallacher RR: *The self in social psychology,* New York, 1980, Oxford University Press.
22. Wylie R: *The self concept: a critical survey of pertinent research literature,* Lincoln, NE, 1961, University of Nebraska Press.
23. Maslow AH: *Motivation and personality,* New York, 1954, Harper & Row.
24. Maslow AH: *Toward a psychology of being,* Princeton, 1968, Van Nostrand.
25. Rubin Z, McNeil EB: *Psychology: being human,* ed 4, New York, 1985, Harper & Row.
26. Perrin F: Physical attractiveness and repulsiveness, *J Exp Psychol* 4:203, 1921.
27. Hatfield E, Sprecher S: *Mirror, mirror . . . the importance of looks in everyday life,* Albany, NY, 1986, State University of New York Press.
28. Bull R, Rumsey N: *The social psychology of facial appearance,* New York, 1988, Springer Verlag.
29. Bersheid E, Gangestad S: The social psychological implications of facial physical attractiveness, *Clin Plast Surg* 9:289, 1982.
30. Sassouni V: A classification of skeletal facial types, *Am J Orthodont* 55:109, 1969.
31. Sassouni V, Sotereanos GC: *Diagnosis and treatment of dento-facial abnormalities,* Springfield, IL, 1974, Charles C Thomas.
32. Ruel-Kellermann M: What are the psychosocial factors involved in motivating individuals to retain their teeth? *Int Dent J* 34:105, 1984.
33. Liggett J: *The human face,* New York, 1974, Stein & Day.
34. Bolender CL, Swoope CC, Smith DE: The Cornell Medical Index as a prognostic aid for complete denture patients, *J Prosthet Dent* 22:20, 1969.
35. Reeve P, Watson CJ, Stafford FD: The role of personality in the management of complete denture patients, *Br Dent J* 156:356, 1984.
36. Smith M: Measurement of personality traits and their relation to patient satisfaction with complete dentures, *J Prosthet Dent* 35:492, 1976.
37. Silverman S, Silverman SI, Silverman B, Garfinkel L: Self-image and its relation to denture acceptance, *J Prosthet Dent* 35:131, 1976.
38. Watson CL et al: The role of personality in the management of partial dentures, *J Oral Rehabil* 13:83, 1986.
39. Oakley ME et al: Dentists' ability to detect psychological problems in patients with temporomandibular disorders and chronic pain, *J Am Dent Assoc* 118:727, 1989.
40. Kiyak McNeill RW, West RA et al: Predicting psychologic responses to orthognathic surgery, *J Oral Maxillofac Surg* 40:150, 1982.
41. Reeve P, Stafford GD, Hopkins R: The use of Cattell's personality profile in patients who have had preprosthetic surgery, *J Dent* 10:121, 1982.
42. Albino JE, Tedesco LA, Conny DJ: Patient perceptions of dental-facial esthetics: shared concerns in orthodontics and prosthodontics, *J Prosthet Dent* 52:9, 1984.
43. Warman E: Psychological aspects of the patient's history, *N Y J Dent* 46:52, 1976.
44. Mittelman JS: Getting through to your patients: psychological motivation, *Dent Clin North Am* 32:29, 1988.
45. Bailey RC: The Efe: archers of the rain forest, *National Geographic* 176:683, 1989.
46. Sheets CG: Modern dentistry and the esthetically aware patient, *J Am Dent Assoc* (special issue) 103-E, 1987.
47. Giddon DB: Psychologic aspects of prosthodontic treatment for geriatric patients, *J Prosthet Dent* 43:374, 1980.
48. Cheney HG: Effect of patient behavior and personality on treatment planning, *Dent Clin North Am* 21:531, 1977.
49. Ibsen R: *Advances in conservative porcelain bonded restorations,* Cerinate Laboratories seminar, Washington, DC, September 21, 1989.
50. Berne W: *Games people play,* New York, 1964, Grove.
51. Kotwal KR: Beyond classification of behavior types, *J Prosthet Dent* 52:874, 1984.
52. Goldstein RE: Survey of patient attitudes toward current esthetic procedures, *J Prosthet Dent* 52:775, 1984.
53. King M: Photos reinforce change in smile, *Dentist* 67:27, 1989.
54. Leinfelder KF, Isenberg BP, Essig ME: A new method for generating ceramic restorations: a CAD-CAM system, *J Am Dent Assoc* 118:703, 1989.
55. McCane D, Fisch S: Dental technology: knocking at high tech's door, *J Am Dent Assoc* 118:285, 1989.
56. Nash DA: Professional ethics and esthetic dentistry, *J Am Dent Assoc* 117:7E, 1988.
57. Siegler M, Bresnahan JF, Schiedermayer DL, Roberson P: Exploring the future of clinical dental ethics: a summary of the Odontographic Society of Chicago Centennial Symposium, *J Am Coll Dent* 56:13, 1989.
58. Simpson R, Hall D, Crabb L: Decision-making in dental practice, *J Am Coll Dent* 48:238, 1981.

Part 6

Esthetics and Social Issues

29

Esthetic Dentistry and Eating Disorders

Stanley Bodner and Kenneth S. Kurtz

According to the National Association of Anorexia Nervosa and Associated Disorders, it is estimated that in the United States, approximately 24 million persons suffer from some form of an eating disorder.[1] During the course of a lifetime, it is estimated that approximately 0.6% of American adults will present with symptoms of anorexia, 1% will present with bulimic symptoms, and nearly 3% will suffer a binge-eating disorder.[2] Furthermore, during their lifetimes, women are three times more likely than men to contract anorexia or bulimia and are also more likely to develop a binge-eating disorder.[2] The average age of onset for anorexia nervosa is 19 years old, and approximately two-thirds of sufferers do not receive treatment.[3]

Dentists, as well as other oral practitioners, are among the first in line to encounter patients who may be experiencing an eating disorder.[4] Oral manifestations or signs associated with eating disorders (ED) may be evident during a routine dental exam. As a consequence, examination of the mouth and aspects of the face and its contours as well as the general appearance of the patient is an integral initial step in secondary prevention of eating disorders. The latter relates to lessening the prevalence of full-blown eating disorders through early detection, referral, and intervention.[5,6] Prodromal or orodental manifestations correlated with anorexia nervosa (AN) and bulimia nervosa (BN) might be detected approximately six months subsequent to persistent caloric constriction and regurgitation.[7]

CHARACTERISTIC SYMPTOMATOLOGY OF EATING DISORDER SUBTYPES

Anorexia Nervosa

Anorexia nervosa[3] is characterized by extreme thinness (emaciation) and a relentless pursuit of thinness; an adamant unwillingness to maintain a body weight at or above a minimally normal weight for age and height; a deep fear of gaining weight or becoming fat, despite being underweight (with accompanying body image distortion); amenorrhea; a flagrant denial of the seriousness of low body weight; restrictive body eating repertoires; and self-esteem concerns heavily motivated by the individual's misperception of his/her own body weight and shape.

Anorexia includes two subtypes: *restricting* and *binge eating/purging*. In the restrictive type, there is no binge eating or purging (self-induced vomiting or abuse of laxatives, diuretics, or enemas). During the active phase of the binge-eating/purging type, there is no misuse of laxatives, diuretics, or enemas, but there is self-induced vomiting. Binge eating consists of consuming an extreme amount food in a short period, often with little enjoyment and often in a compulsive fashion.

Many practitioners are stymied when attempting to ascertain the distinction between the binge/purging subtype of anorexia nervosa and bulimia nervosas. There is, in fact, symptomatologic overlap. The key distinction between these two similar eating disorders hinges on the patient's body weight. The clinical presentation of any form of AN, by necessity, relates to a significantly underweight individual. Such is not the case with an individual who is diagnosed with BN. Bulimics tend to be either of normal weight or slightly overweight. Thus when an individual presents with either binging or purging tendencies while meeting the diagnostic criteria for AN, the diagnosis of AN (binge-eating/purging type), not BN, is assigned. The diagnosis of AN supersedes the diagnostic assignment of BN because there is a greater fear of mortality for a patient with AN.[8]

Bulimia Nervosa

Bulimia nervosa[3] is characterized by frequent and recurring episodes of binge eating. The nature of the binge eating is such that within a discrete span of time, for example, a 2-hour period, an amount larger than would be eaten by an average individual is consumed. The consumption and the quantity of what is consumed are undertaken without a sense of self-control. Recurring and inappropriate compensatory behaviors, such as purging or excessive exercising, are undertaken in order to counteract significant weight gain. Bulimia nervosa is categorized as either the *purging* or *nonpurging* type.

Purging Type. In this subtype, during a discrete cycle of BN the person steadily misuses laxatives, diuretics, or enemas or launches into episodes of self-induced vomiting.

Nonpurging Type. In this subtype, during a discrete cycle of BN the individual engages in other forms of inappropriate behaviors such as fasting and excessive exercise. However, the individual does not engage in self-induced vomiting; neither does he/she induce any body evacuation procedures.

There is a prevalence with BN of 0.5% for females and 0.1% for males. The average age of onset is 20 years old and is rarely observed in persons under the age of 14.[9] A particularly high at-risk group for the development of BN are competitive athletes, especially in sports in which weight is correlated with performance and in which low body weight is glorified. Specific at-risk groups include (but are not limited to) jockeys, wrestlers, body builders, figure skaters, cross country runners, and gymnasts.[8]

Binge Eating or Eating Disorders Not Otherwise Specified

This category represents eating disorders that do not necessarily meet the criteria encompassed in the previous classifications. Examples of eating disorders not otherwise specified include: (1) AN symptomatology in a female patient who experiences a normal menses or displays normal body weight; (2) BN symptomatology with fewer binge-eating episodes or an individual exhibiting inappropriate compensatory behaviors of a generally shorter duration period; (3) self-induced vomiting in an individual with a normal bodyweight subsequent to the consumption of a small quantity of food; (4) a binge-eating disorder in which there are recurring episodes of binge eating in the absence of the typical inappropriate compensatory mechanisms found in BN, such as purging or laxative usage.

Modifications of the eating disorder classifications are presented in the current (fifth) edition of the American Psychiatric Association's Diagnostic and Statistical Manual of Mental Disorders (DSM-V) published in May, 2013.[10] A significant enhancement in the updated DSM edition relates to the clarification of criteria describing the symptomatology of Binge Eating Disorder. The revision points relate to recurrent episodes of binge eating that are characterized with the following features: recurrent episodes occurring during a discrete time frame, the quantity of food consumed during such periods is significantly more than the average person would eat and the individual exhibits an inability to control his/her consumption. In addition, there must be at least three of the following five features present during a binging episode:

1. Eating with rapidity
2. Eating until one feels uncomfortably full
3. Gratuitous eating
4. Solitary eating because of the anticipated experience of being embarrassed if others observed the quantity of food consumed
5. A feeling of disgust, self-loathing, guilt, or depression in the aftermath of a binge episode.

Furthermore, the individual experiences significant distress during a binge episode and binge episodes, on the average, occur once a week during a typical span of 3 months.

ORAL MANIFESTATIONS OF EATING DISORDERS

Bulimia nervosa can result in nutritional deficiencies and metabolic impairments. Nutritional deficiencies or metabolic impairment can result from a lack of emphasis in performing personal hygiene, underlying psychologic disturbances or the use of certain medications. It is conceivable that changes in the oral cavity can also be rooted in the lack of attention given to personal hygiene or the use of certain medications.

Dental Alterations

Perimylolysis, or decalcification of the teeth from chronic exposure to regurgitated gastric acid, is usually observed on the lingual surfaces of the maxillary anterior teeth as a consequence of purging action.[11] Amalgam restorations on affected teeth may appear "raised" above tooth surface (Figs. 29-1*A,B*).

In eating disorders that involve frequent purging, perimylolysis[12] is often associated with the excessive self-induced vomiting that occurs (Figs. 29-1*C,D*).

Sufferers of ED often consume an excessive amount of caffeinated and/or carbonated drinks, sweetened beverages, sweets, and/or sugared chewing gum (often used to quickly boost energy levels and to decrease reflex hunger pangs through inducing stomach dilation.)[9]

Chronic purging can lead to dental erosion on all tooth-related surfaces (palatal, labial, lingual, and buccal surfaces).[12] The eroded enamel has a texture that is smooth, shiny, and hard and if extensive enough the yellowish color of the dentin becomes more prominent and observable and the teeth might become hypersensitive to temperature changes.

Mucosal Lesions

Mucosal lesions may lead to generalized mucosal atrophy, stomatitis and oral ulcers.[13] Oral lesions are particularly evident on the tongue, buccal mucosa, and the floor of the mouth.[14]

In eating disorders, erythematous mucosal lesions of the soft palate may be the direct result of gastric acid contact during vomiting (epithelial erosion) or the trauma caused by the object used to induce purging such as fingers, fingernails, toothbrushes, etc. (Fig. 29-1*E*).

PERIODONTAL MANIFESTATIONS

Periodontal manifestations are more frequently observed in adults, but can also be detected in teen and pediatric ED sufferers. Compromised oral hygiene can lead to gingival inflammation and future periodontitis.[15] Based on the clinical and anecdotal observations of the author, patients prone to depression and who binge eat and/or purge, often care little about proper oral care.

Salivary and Salivary Gland Manifestations

Sialadenosis, a noninflammatory enlargement of the salivary glands caused by peripheral autonomic neuropathy can be a marker of ED (Fig. 29-2*A*).

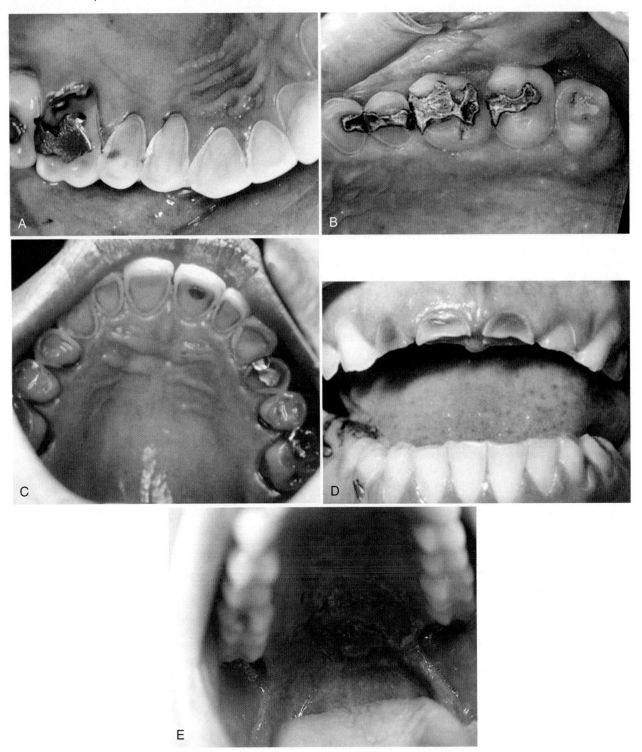

FIGURE 29-1 A, Erosion. Palatal surfaces of the maxillary dentition in which the exposed dentin exhibits a concave surface and a peripheral white line of enamel. The patient had bulimia. **B,** In teeth affected by erosive tooth substance loss, amalgam restorations may stand proud of the remaining tooth surface. **C,** Bulimia. The lingual surfaces of the maxillary teeth show loss of enamel because of constant contact with regurgitated acidic stomach contents. **D,** The destruction of dentition in the mouth of this 26-year-old woman was caused by the eat-and-purge syndrome **E,** Clinical photograph shows a broad, shallow, ulceration of the posterior left hard palate that crosses the midline. The mixed red and white lesion has ragged borders and measures approximately 1.5 × 2 cm. (**A,** From Neville BW, Damm DD, Allen CM, et al: *Oral and maxillofacial pathology*, ed 3, St Louis, 2009, Saunders. **B,** From Walmsley AD, Walsh TF, Lumley P, et al: *Restorative dentistry*, ed 2, London, 2007, Churchill Livingstone. **C,** From Sapp JP, Eversole LR, Wysocki GP: *Contemporary oral and maxillofacial surgery*, ed 2, St Louis, 2004, Mosby. **D,** From Christensen GJ: *A consumer's guide to dentistry*, ed 2, St Louis, 2002, Mosby. **E,** From Solomon LW, Merzianu M, Sullivan M, et al: Necrotizing sialometaplasia associated with bulimia: case report and literature review, *Oral Surg Oral Med Oral Pathol Oral Radiol Endod* 103(2):e39-42, 2007.)

This often results in acinar enlargement and functional impairment. In addition, salivary flow may be reduced.[9] At times dry mouth may be associated with medications used in the treatment of ED (e.g., Prozac (fluoxetine) and Lexapro (escitalopram oxalate) or the earlier generation of tricyclic antidepressants (e.g., amitriptyline).[16-18]

In addition, necrotizing sialometaplasia has been reported to be associated with bulimia.[9]

Dermatologic Manifestation

Self-induced vomiting by finger stimulation of the palatal gag reflex can result in callouses on the knuckles (Russell's sign; Fig. 29-2B).[19] This occurs when the incisal edges of the maxillary anterior teeth repeatedly contact the knuckles during this manipulation.

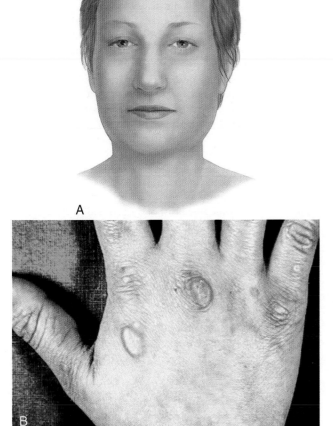

FIGURE 29-2 A, Parotid hypertrophy resulting from chronic vomiting. **B,** Calluses caused by self-induced vomiting (Russell's sign). (**A,** From Stern TA, Rosenbaum JF, Fava M, et al: *Massachusetts General Hospital comprehensive clinical psychiatry,* Philadelphia, 2008, Mosby. **B,** From Russell GFM: Bulimia nervosa: an ominous variant of anorexia nervosa, *Psychol Med* 1979;9:429-448.)

CONSIDERATIONS WHEN APPROACHING A PATIENT PRESENTING WITH SUSPECTED SYMPTOMS OF AN EATING DISORDER

Generally speaking, when a covert disorder or disturbance is suspected on either a sensitive medical or dental issue manifest in a discussion with a patient, a defensive posture or response on the part of the patient is to be expected. If a dental practitioner raises concerns with a patient that an eating disorder may be present, such emotional responses as resentment, denial, or resistance towards suggestions for treatment intervention is to be expected. Notwithstanding such possible negative or avoidant responses on the patient's part, the practitioner has a professional obligation to address potential or probable medical or health concerns. For example, if a patient presents symptoms suggestive of COPD, the dentist should address this concern, including follow-up recommendations for appropriate care. No less concern should be registered when an eating disorder is suspected.

What is most distressing concerning patients who appear to meet criteria consistent with a diagnosable eating disorder is that, based on one comprehensive study, fewer than half actually obtain medical care from a medical provider, and only approximately 28% consulted with a mental health care professional.[20] Furthermore, treatment delay tends to be extraordinarily significant; the median duration of this delay can be approximately 10 years in instances of bulimia and 15 years for anorexic conditions.[7,14] It is to be expected that even when an individual is interested in seeking professional assistance, a procrastination period generally ensues.

There is no prevailing "best practice" approach to follow when broaching concerns with respect to a suspected eating disorder. The individual "facts and circumstances" regarding the patient's persona and life circumstances should be taken into account, as best as possible, and must be carefully contemplated. However, what is of paramount significance is that the practitioner must realize that avoidance of expressing legitimate and objective concerns may possibly lead to unpardonable patient neglect. Hence the following considerations should be weighed when confronting a patient with what appears to be symptomatology suggestive of an eating disorder:

1. If the patient appears to have experienced a significant weight loss since the last office visit, expressing this observation and ferreting out causation is in order, especially when other symptoms are manifest. Medical conditions other than eating disorders must be ruled out.

2. If the patient's face presents a visage of "chipmunk" cheeks or a jowly appearance; or if calluses are observed on hand knuckles; or if there is evidence of dental discoloration or of other suspicious oral signs—a discussion is in order. Some initial dialogue that may be expressed is scripted below:

"In my experience, when I see swelling of the cheeks..."

Or,

"The type of structural changes on the surface of the teeth that I observe in your mouth [or any other oral indication of concern]..."

And/or,

"When I see such knuckle calluses...that usually tells me that the person is doing a lot of vomiting. I'm really concerned. Do you want to share anything or discuss anything with me today?"

Any of the above suggested initial statements, of course, must be expressed in soft and measured tones and in a sympathetic manner. Whether or not an honest response is evoked from the patient, it is entirely appropriate to refer the patient to a primary care physician. Referral to a mental health practitioner who specializes in eating disorders is also warranted if positive indicators are present.

Regardless of how considerate of the patient's feelings a clinician's attempts may be, the patient may respond in anger, in abrupt denial, or with resentment. A defensive or self-protective response should not be considered poor or improper patient care or patient mismanagement. If the patient responds in anger or expresses themes of righteous indignation, an appropriate response might be:

"I did not mean to upset you, and I am genuinely sorry that you're upset . . . . I fully understand, but I felt a professional obligation to raise the questions I asked . . . . it would be wrong of me not to . . . . I really hope you understand . . . ."

3. The practitioner should not expect that there will be immediate resolution despite actually having addressed suspicions of an eating disorder. Resolution and relief from such disorders takes time, because its facets are complex in that many factors may be involved (e.g., medical, dental, psychologic, social, and familial).

4. It is essential that the dental/oral practitioner adopt a nonjudgmental, respectful, and calm demeanor when addressing the patient regardless of clinical impressions or suspicions.

5. In large measure, the essence of patient resistance in complying with recommendations to follow-up with appropriate professional care is that the patient may have to "work through" feelings of shame, fear of weight gain, or perceiving oneself as someone who has an uncontrollable emotional disorder. As a consequence, it is appropriate to offer genuine and supportive messages such as:

"I know this is hard for you . . . . Is there anything I, or my staff, can do to help? I will keep in touch with the doctor you will see . . . ."

6. At the onset it is imperative that the oral clinician does not overwhelm a patient who presents with a suspected eating disorder with a flurry of information, facts, suggestions, or heightened alarm. As alluded to earlier, the patient needs first to absorb what has been expressed by the practitioner and must be willing to accept that there is a need for professional help and follow-up.

7. Whatever the patient's reaction tends to be, a follow-up appointment is recommended to allow for further or necessary discussion.

Frank concerns expressed by the dental practitioner can serve as the initial staging point for the patient's road to recovery and might truly mark the initial phase in rescuing a patient from a genuinely life-threatening situation.

CLINICAL TREATMENT OF A BULIMIC PATIENT*

A 21-year-old female bulimic was referred by a periodontist for treatment of teeth exhibiting perimylolysis. Her medical history was noncontributory except for a history of BN. The patient was informed that some teeth may require endodontic therapy because of the pulpal proximity to the lingual external surfaces of the affected teeth. However, endodontic therapy was not ultimately required.

Upon clinical examination, the patient was asymptomatic with regard to sensitivity, but was concerned with visible incisal edge chipping (Fig. 29-3A). The patient was unaware of the severe palatal erosion (Fig. 29-3B) of the maxillary anterior teeth that was the causative factor for the incisal edge chipping. In this instance three-dimensional tooth movements occurred because the extrusion of the mandibular anterior teeth resulted in occlusal contact with the eroded maxillary anterior dentition. There was also compensatory supraeruption of the maxillary anterior teeth owing to the palatal tooth surface loss. The restorative dentist must carefully evaluate the patient's occlusal vertical dimension and existing excursive mandibular movements prior to making definitive treatment decisions. Upon evaluation the patient had lost anterior guidance and had achieved an occlusal scheme resembling the "bilateral balance" of a complete denture occlusion (Fig. 29-3C).

The gingival architecture was deemed to be atypical and the patient was referred to a periodontist for clinical crown lengthening from the maxillary right first premolar to the maxillary left first premolar. The anticipated gingival architecture was accomplished by a trial surgery of the diagnostic cast, combined with a wax-up of the anticipated restored clinical crown morphology. This activity was duplicated and a vacuform matrix of the desired clinical crowns was provided to the periodontist to serve as a guide for the surgical procedure (Fig. 29-3D)

Following a 2-month healing period, the maxillary anterior teeth were then prepared for all ceramic crowns. Because of the palatal erosion, the only necessary palatal preparation was a rounded shoulder finishing line. The rest of the tooth had conventional reductive tooth preparation for an all-ceramic crown.

One month later the provisional crowns were removed from the asymptomatic teeth and impressions were made. Casts were articulated and sent to the dental laboratory for fabrication of lithium disilicate pressed ceramic full crowns (IPS e.max, Ivoclar Vivadent). A cross-mounted cast of the provisional restorations was provided as a guide for the laboratory technician. The incisal edge position of the maxillary teeth was indexed from the provisional cast, which enabled the technician to exactly duplicate the edge position in the e.max restorations. The definitive restorations were luted into position with conventional resin-ionomer cement. Because the preparations had adequate retention and resistance form, an adhesive bonding approach was not favored for this patient. Adequate tooth morphology and appropriately reestablished anterior disclusion was accomplished, allowing for appropriate esthetics and phonetics (Fig. 29-3E).

---

*The section, Clinical Treatment of a Bulimic Patient, was written by Kenneth S. Kurtz.

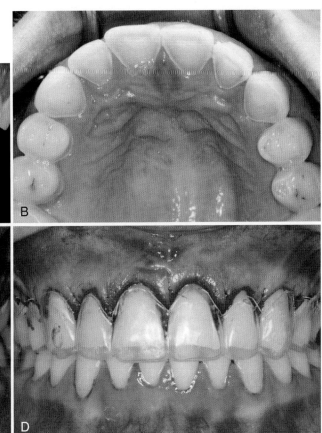

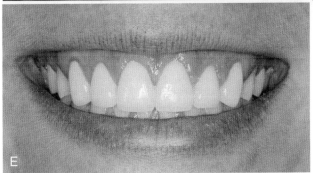

FIGURE 29-3 Treatment of a bulimic patient. **A,** Preoperative frontal view. **B,** Preoperative occlusal view. **C,** Frontal view showing lost anterior guidance. **D,** A surgical guide in place to aid the periodontist during surgery. **E,** The completed restorations.

REFERENCES

1. The Renfrew Center Foundation for Eating Disorders: Eating disorders 101 guide: a summary of issues, statistics and resources, Philadelphia, 2003, Renfrew Center Foundation.
2. Hudson, JI, Hiripi E, Pope HG, et al: The prevalence and correlates of eating disorders in the National Comorbidity Survey Replication, Biological Psychiatry 61:348-358, 2007.
3. American Psychiatric Association: Diagnostic and statistical manual of mental disorders, ed 4, text rev., Arlington, VA, 2000, APA. doi:10.1176/appi.books.9780890423349
4. Milosevic A: Eating disorders and the dentist, Br Dent J 186(3):109-113, 1999.
5. DeBate R, Tedesco L, Kerschbaum W: Knowledge of oral and physical manifestations of anorexia and bulimia nervosa among dentists and dental hygienists, J Dent Educ 69(3):346-354, 2005.
6. DeBate R, Tedesco L: Increasing dentists' capacity for secondary prevention of eating disorders: identification of training, network and professional contingencies, J Dent Educ 70(10):1066-1075, 2006.
7. National Eating Disorders Association: Eating disorders information. At: http://www.nationaleatingdisorders.org. Accessed August 2012.
8. Butcher JN, Mineka S, Hooley JN: Abnormal psychology, ed 13, Boston, MA, 2007, Pearson/Allyn & Bacon, pp 315-317.
9. Frey PD: Bulimia nervosa. January 15, 2007. Available at: http://www.minddisorders.com/Br-Del/Bulimia-nervosa.html. Accessed September 23, 2013.
10. *Diagnostic and Statistical Manual of Mental Disorders* (DSM-5), Feeding and Eating Disorders, © 2013 American Psychiatric Association. http://www.dsm5.org/Documents/Eating%20Disorders%20Fact%20Sheet.pdf. Accessed Sept 10, 2014.
11. Lo Russo L, Campisi G, Di Fede O, et al: Oral manifestations of eating disorders: a critical review, Oral Dis 14(6):479-484, 2008.
12. Holst JJ, Lange F: Perimylolysis: a contribution towards the genesis of tooth wasting from non-mechanical causes, Acta Odontol Scand 1:36-48, 1939.
13. Dahlén G, Ebenfelt A: Necrobacillosis in humans, Expert Rev Anti Infect Ther 9(2):227-236, 2011.
14. Robb ND, Smith BG, Geidrys-Leeper E: The distribution of erosion in the dentitions of patients with eating disorders, Br Dent J 178:171-175, 1995.
15. Personal oral communication with Dr. Harry Dym, Chairman of the Department of Dentistry and Oral and Maxillofacial Surgery, Brooklyn Hospital, Brooklyn, NY, December 31, 2012.
16. *PDR Drug Guide for Mental Health Professionals*, ed 3, Montvale, NJ, 2007, Thomson Healthcare.
17. Capasso A, Petrella C, Milano W: Pharmacological profile of SSRIs and SNRIs in the treatment of eating disorders, Curr Clin Pharmacol 4:78-83, 2009.
18. Jackson CW, Cates M, Lorenz R: Pharmacotherapy of eating disorders, Nutr Clin Pract 25:143-159, 2010.
19. Strumia R: Dermatologic signs in patients with eating disorders, Am J Clin Dermatol 6(3):165-173, 2005.
20. Oakley Browne, MA, Wells JE, McGee MA: Twelve-month and lifetime health service use in Te Rau Hinengaro. The New Zealand Mental Health Survey. *Aust NZ J Psychiatry* 40: 855-864, 2006.

30

Esthetic Dentistry and Domestic Violence

Dawn LaFrance, Jung Yi, and Chelsea Dale

Domestic violence (DV) is a national health concern that affects many patients who enter a dental professional's office. It causes severe consequences to the individual involved and his or her entire family. In many situations the violence escalates in severity over time and can even result in death. Dental professionals are sometimes the only health care providers victims have access to or to whom they feel comfortable speaking. Therefore dentists may have a unique opportunity to intervene. Since head, face, and neck injuries are common in DV, the dental team may be the first to notice signs of the abuse (Fig. 30-1).[1] Often, they are in the important position of screening for DV and taking steps to prevent future occurrences.[2]

DOMESTIC VIOLENCE DEFINED

Domestic violence is defined as violent behavior against a family member, or other violence taking place within a home.[3] Child abuse, spousal/partner abuse, and elder abuse are included in this definition. Although not always obvious, DV is an epidemic that affects individuals in every community[4] and occurs in every population regardless of race, ethnicity, class, sexual orientation, gender identity, religious affiliation, age, or income level.[2] Although child, elder, and partner abuse are all problems that dentists may encounter, partner/spousal abuse is the most common.[3] Intimate partner violence (IPV) is violent behavior occurring within an intimate partner relationship.[1] In the past violence toward women was tolerated by society and even supported. Now, the legal system views violence more seriously. For instance, most states have established laws that designate state health care professionals, including dentists, as mandated reporters of these acts.[5]

Both men and women can be victims of DV; however, approximately 85% of DV victims are women (see Fig. 30-1).[6,7] Data indicate that more than 1 million women and 150,000 men are victims of DV each year in the United States,[8-11] with 20% to 30% of women and 7.5% of men having been abused by a partner.[12,13] One in every four women will experience domestic violence in her lifetime.[14] Women of all ages are at risk for domestic and sexual violence, and those 20 to 24 years of age are at the greatest risk of experiencing nonfatal IPV.[15]

Because of the high rates of IPV toward women, health care providers have established the term *battered woman syndrome* to describe it—a "symptom complex occurring as a result of abusive actions directed against a woman by her male partner."[3] Power and control issues pervade the relationships between battered women and their abusers (Fig. 30-2). Most abusive partners of battered women deliver severe and frequent abuse resulting in a wide variety of physical injuries.[2] Perpetrators are likely jealous and possessive and desire absolute and complete knowledge of everything about their partners. Drug and alcohol use are common among batterers and they commit violence to assert control over their partners. Attempts are usually made by the victim to minimize the violence, but the battered individual is unable to appease the partner.[16]

Victims of abuse suffer more than physical consequences. There can be long-term psychologic effects, including low self-esteem and feelings of inadequacy.[16] Battering episodes are estimated to account for one-third of all female suicide attempts.[1] Health problems appear frequently in IPV victims.[2] These women are 80% more likely to suffer a stroke, 70% more likely to have heart disease, 60% more likely to have asthma, and 70% more likely to abuse alcohol than women who have not experienced IPV.[17]

DENTAL ASSESSMENT OF DOMESTIC VIOLENCE

Despite the widespread nature of DV and the negative consequences resulting from it, most DV situations are never reported to the police.[18] Some IPV victims only seek health care from their dentist and avoid other health care professionals. According to a 1998 national survey, 9.2% of the women who sought health care for physical assault by an intimate partner

550

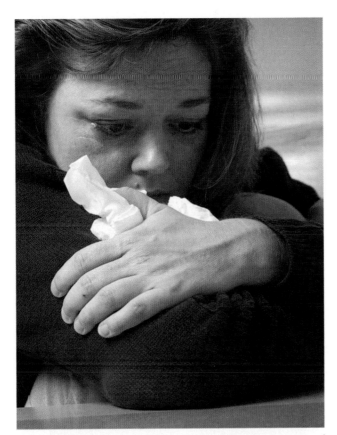

FIGURE 30-1 Physical abuse is the most common cause of injury to women in the United States. Battering occurs in all ethnic, religious, and socioeconomic groups. Although the batterer is unprovoked, the woman is made to feel it is her fault. (From Psychiatric Mental Health Nursing © 2007 Jupiter Images Corporation).

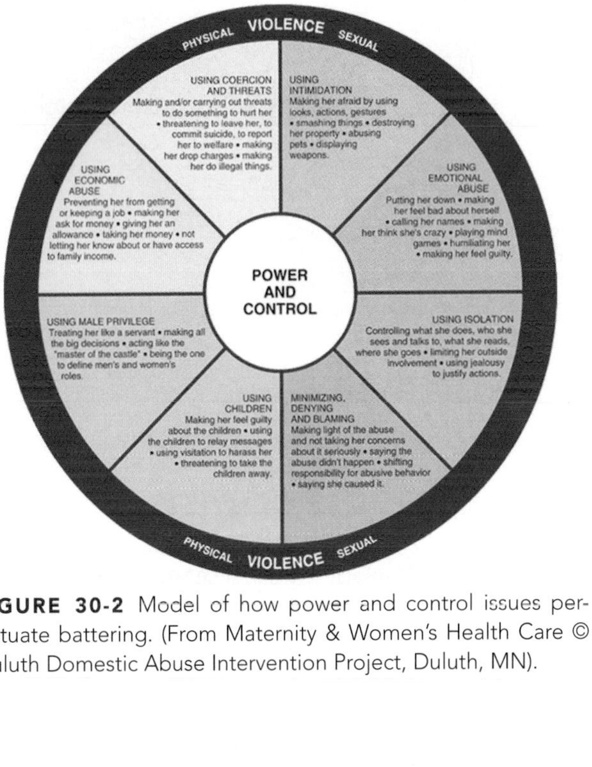

visited a dentist.[19] Unfortunately, data shows that the recognition and reporting rates for IPV are substantially lower than the actual prevalence. Records indicate that dentists report less than 1% of these cases.[5] Low reporting rates have been attributed to health care professionals' lack of knowledge of the problem and its manifestations, ambiguous reports from victims, and practitioners' inattention or distraction.[1] Dentists can improve their ability to prevent ongoing abuse associated with DV by learning to recognize the signs and symptoms.

Approximately two-thirds of all adults in the United States have an annually scheduled dental consultation,[19,20] in which a routine dental examination involving an inspection of the head, neck, and oral cavity may reveal signs of abuse[19,21] (Fig. 30-3; also see Fig. 30-1).

In a study conducted in Brazil, IPV was the third most common cause of traumatic dental injury, after domestic accidents and sporting activities. In this study of 7750 police-recorded physical violence reports, 2% were traumatic dental injuries caused by IPV (22 injuries). The most frequently injured teeth were the maxillary incisors, followed by the mandibular incisors and then the maxillary canines. The reports indicated that 59.1% of the teeth were fractured, 27.2% were luxated, and 13.7% were avulsed.[22] In another study including 85 IPV cases, 14% exhibited neck injuries, 21% had facial injuries, 29% suffered lip injuries, 5% reported tongue trauma, 5% lost teeth, 7% had a fractured jaw, and 3% reported other injuries.[23]

Evidence of violence may be detected in a number of areas, including the oral and perioral structures, through lip trauma, fractured or subluxated teeth, fractures of the mandible or maxilla, or severe bruising of the edentulous ridges (Figs. 30-4 and 30-5).[24]

Indicators of prior trauma may be detected through fractures to the zygomaticomaxillary complex, eye injuries, orbital fractures and facial tissue bruising.[19,25] If a battered woman is presenting to the dental office for treatment of maxillofacial injuries, it is likely that the violence has occurred over a long period of time.[1]

FIGURE 30-2 Model of how power and control issues perpetuate battering. (From Maternity & Women's Health Care © Duluth Domestic Abuse Intervention Project, Duluth, MN).

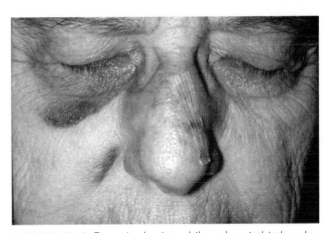

FIGURE 30-3 Forensic dentistry: bilateral periorbital ecchymoses (raccoon mask) and fractured nasal bone in a 77-year-old white female victim of physical elder abuse. (Courtesy Dr. John D. McDowell, 2009. From Neville BW, Damm DD, Allen CM, et al: *Oral and maxillofacial pathology*, ed 3, St Louis, 2009, Saunders.)

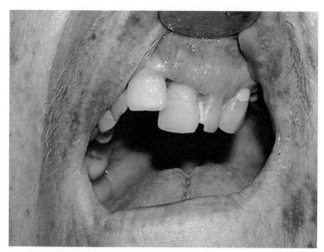

FIGURE 30-4 Dentoalveolar fracture associated with elder abuse at home. (From Panagiotis Kafas P: Do you always believe a provider of home care? Br J Oral Maxillofac Surg 46(4):344, 2008.)

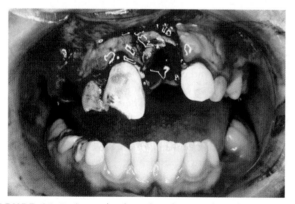

FIGURE 30-5 An avulsed tooth, a fractured tooth, and a torn facial frenum associated with orofacial injuries in physical child abuse. (From Neville BW, Damm DD, Allen CM, et al: *Oral and maxillofacial pathology*, ed 3, St Louis, 2009, Saunders.)

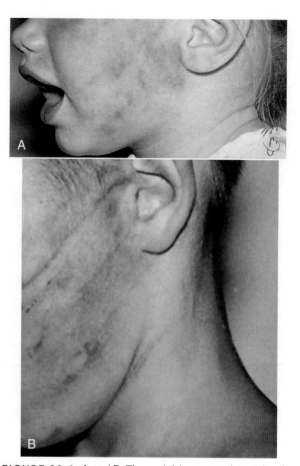

FIGURE 30-6 A and **B,** These children were slapped so forcefully that the outlines of their abuser's fingers are clearly evident. (From Zitelli BJ, McIntire SC, Nowalk AJ: *Zitelli and Davis' atlas of pediatric physical diagnosis*, ed 6, Philadelphia, 2011, Saunders.)

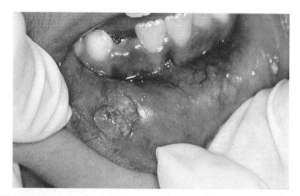

FIGURE 30- 7 Condyloma acuminatum. The presence of condyloma acuminatum in a child is strongly suggestive of sexual abuse. (From Ibsen OAC, Phelan JA: *Oral pathology for the dental hygienist*, ed 6, St Louis, 2014, Saunders.)

In addition to screening adults (often women) for IPV, it is vital that dentists also evaluate for signs of abuse when working with children and elderly patients. Most states have laws outlining the obligations of mandated reporters, stating that a report should be made for any child suspected of being a victim of abuse or neglect.[19,26] More than half of physically abused children have sustained a head and/or neck injury. These areas are often visible to a perceptive dentist.[19,27] Signs of abuse can include oral and perioral injuries, tearing of the frena, isolated laceration of the soft palate, multiple fractured, discolored, nonvital or avulsed anterior teeth (see Fig. 30-6) and odd malocclusions or different levels of occlusions (nonreduced old jaw fractures). Gag marks evident in commissural abrasions/contusions may be present. Circular bruises on both sides of the lower face from grab marks, parallel contusions running diagonally across the face from slap marks (Fig. 30-6) bruises on the ears, or bite marks are also indicators. Finally, oral lesions from sexually transmitted diseases may be detected (Fig. 30-7).[28]

LEGAL ISSUES FOR DENTISTS

Dentists have a legal responsibility to report child abuse. All fifty states, and the District of Columbia, have enacted laws that require the reporting of suspected child abuse.[28]

For example, in New Jersey, any person having reasonable cause to believe that a child has been subjected to abuse or acts of abuse should immediately report this information to the State Central Registry (SCR).[29] Any person who knowingly fails to report suspected abuse or neglect according to the law or to comply with the provisions of the law is considered "a disorderly person" under the law and subject to prosecution. However, the law also provides that any person who, in good faith, makes a report of child abuse or neglect or testifies in a child abuse hearing resulting from such a report is immune from any criminal or civil liability as a result of such action. Calls can be placed to the hotline anonymously. (1-877-ABUSE (652-2873), information available at http://www.nj.gov/dcf/reporting/how/index.html).

Additionally, a recent New Jersey Appellate Division case appears to establish a legal duty for emergency room physicians to report child abuse or risk being held liable for negligence and damages.[30] The full ramifications of this case for emergency room physicians is not clear. However, it appears that at some point in the near future that dentists may be held liable for failure to report child abuse.

Therefore from a legal and ethical standpoint, it is recommended that if a dentist or staff member encounters a situation of suspected abuse, it would be prudent to approach the situation with a two-pronged approach: (1) Have a list of available resources to offer an adult victim; and (2) notify the appropriate agency under the applicable state law.

DISCUSSING DOMESTIC VIOLENCE WITH THE PATIENT

The following information for the remainder of this chapter is provided only as background information and in no way is intended to establish a standard of care for dentists.

When signs of DV or IPV are present, it can be uncomfortable to initiate a discussion with the patient and to determine how to proceed further. As part of office policies and procedures, the protocol to be used when approaching a DV victim should be shared with all staff members to encourage consistent responses. A list of referrals and resources for immediate access and dissemination should be included with these procedures. A comprehensive list of resources is available through The Family Violence Prevention Fund on the Internet at http://www.futureswithoutviolence.org/userfiles/file/Consensus.pdf.[27] These resources may be vital if the patient chooses not to return to the dentist's office.[28]

Psychoeducational posters about DV that are multicultural and multilingual along with handouts about resources for victims of DV could be placed in examination rooms, reception areas and rest rooms. It is beneficial to include both local DV and IPV resources as well as the telephone numbers of the National DV Hotline (800) 799-SAFE, TTY (800) 787-3224. In addition, providing specific resources (e.g., teen, ethnic, or homosexual) that are sensitive and/or specialized to serve specific groups can be helpful to the patient.[2]

Routine inquiries of all patients about DV could be conducted rather than only when indicators of abuse are present. Face-to-face interviews or initial paperwork can include a few specific DV and IPV questions. In order to be prepared to react if there is evidence of abuse in response to these routine inquiries or visible signs of abuse, training about IPV should be considered. Training covers the dynamics of this issue, teaches proper consideration of the balance between victim autonomy and safety, and explores the communication of culturally competent responses. A facet of this training should include hypothetical situations that allow for practice before encountering

an actual abuse situation. However, a general understanding of the procedures is helpful for all team members.

With appropriate informed consent, descriptions of injuries or photographs are encouraged if the dentist is legally required to report the abuse and if the location of the injuries is within the areas routinely examined by dentists.[31] The physical signs observed by the dentist should be recorded in some way, such as taking color, scale photographs of the injuries. The patient should be informed that the photographs will become a part of the treatment record and can only be released with written permission from the patient (at legal age and when deemed to be a competent adult) or pursuant to law.[28]

All patients with indicators of abuse (either by responses to the routine inquiries or by visible signs) should be screened privately or through a more comprehensive intake form with framing questions relating to DV. Whether or not the dentist wants to implement this in his/her office should be based on the dentist's postdoctoral training in the area and based on maintaining the safety of both the patient and staff. When the victim is first evaluated by a person trained in this area such as a licensed psychologist or social worker, questions on a form can be brief, such as those included on the HITS,[31] a short DV assessment tool developed for physician family practices is available at http://www.orchd.com/violence/documents/HITS_eng.pdf. The HITS asks individuals to rate the frequency of abuse www.futureswithoutviolence.org/userfiles/file/Consensus.pdf.[27]

Office procedures can provide for the separation of IPV victims from partners who may be abusing them and are present at the office visit. Risks involved must be assessed and if it cannot be done safely, other options should be considered. For instance, if there is a threat of safety, the victim could be given a packet of health care materials including a pamphlet about DV and important contact telephone numbers. If it is deemed safe to intervene, the suspected abuser should be asked to leave the room during the examination as long as this request does not aggravate a potentially violent situation. After more information is gathered, assistance could be offered and provide the victim with helpful resources.

CLINICAL TIP

It is not recommended that the suspected abuser be questioned by the dentist; rather, the authorities can do this once a report has been filed.[27]

When there is a language barrier, having access to trained interpreters is recommended and may be a legal requirement.[32]

When the suspected victim is an adult, the interviewer should plan to speak with the individual privately. When interacting with victims who exhibit signs of injury, it is important to build rapport in order to build trust.[16] This will likely take more time with new patients. Once it appears that a good relationship has been established, the questions about IPV must be carefully framed in an attempt to prevent defenses from forming.

Instead of asking a question, the interviewer can state, "Many people have injuries like this and often these injuries are caused by a family member or loved one." The interviewer should tell the victim that there are resources that can help him or her.[29]

Listening to the Patient

It is extremely important to listen to the patient. Although providing resources and medical care are necessary, listening can show the victim that someone has a genuine concern and can be the first step in the healing process.[29] It is also important to understand that victims of DV are considering risk, safety, and opportunity factors that may be very confusing and frightening for them. Victims should be given a range of options and the interviewer should respect their frame of reference.[2] It can be difficult to translate one's thoughts into words when confronted with an abuse situation while maintaining the victim's well-being as the priority. Below are some examples of what an interviewer might say during an intervention:

Nonjudgmental Framing Statements

+ We ask all of our patients with injuries if they are experiencing any violence in their relationships. Did these injuries occur when you were with your partner?[28,31]
+ We see violence affecting many families, and it can cause physical and emotional problems for the parents and children. There is help, and we have some referrals and resources available for anyone who needs it.[31]
+ Screening questions to use after a framing statement that are direct and focus on specific behaviors:
  + Are you with somebody who hurts you sometimes or makes you feel afraid?
  + I am concerned that someone may have caused these injuries on your face. Did someone ever try to hit or slap you? Alternatively, has someone ever pushed you or grabbed your neck?
  + Many people come in with injuries like yours, and oftentimes they get them from someone hitting them. Did something like this happen to you?
  + Has your partner threatened you or your children?
  + Has your partner ever threatened to use a gun or weapon on you or your children when he/she was angry?
  + Has your partner ever forced you to have sex?
  + Do you feel like sometimes you're being controlled by your partner?[31]

When a patient states that he/she is experiencing DV, provide messages that are therapeutic and nonjudgmental. A dialogue should be started and then ask for a description of what happened. Listen to the story to begin the healing process and clarify the referrals that must be made. Then validate the patient and offer resources. Say something such as, "I am really glad you told me." Validate the patient's experience by offering assurances, such as "I want you to know that you do not deserve this and that you are not alone. Please let me give you the name/number of a person/place to call."[31]

Formulating a Safety Plan

A safety plan is a set of steps that a victim will take to prevent further violence. Depending on the situation, this will likely include having emergency phone numbers easily accessible and identifying a safe place to stay.

Assisting Victims with Safety Planning

+ When you can assist victims with safety planning, talk to them about the safety plan and attempt to attain their consent to contact the police or emergency personnel.

+ Discuss any discharge instructions with the victim.
+ Make appropriate referrals and follow up with the victim.
+ Carefully document all steps taken.[31]

There are many instances in which victims should be encouraged to talk with a local IPV/DV advocate for a safety plan. These include when the abuser: is abusing children, is making threats to kill the victim or himself/herself, is stalking the victim, is showing serious signs of jealousy, communicates with the victim against his/her will, has hurt the victim before, has made threats against the victim if he/she leaves the relationship, or has access to a gun. The abused victim should be encouraged to contact an advocate if pregnant, has unsuccessfully attempted to leave the relationship, has plans to leave/divorce, or has sought help to stop the abuse. It is also important to be cautious and find an advocate when the violence has been escalating.[31] Advocates are often listed in the front of the telephone book. There are times when an IPV victim who shows evidence of abuse will deny it. In these instances, indirect questions may be used, such as the following:

+ Your health is important, and I am asking you about this because I am concerned about your safety.
+ Are you having some problems with someone at home? Do your fights turn physical?
+ Sometimes people act significantly differently when they have been drinking. Does your partner change sometimes and start to act violently after drinking?[31]
+ Has anyone ever prevented you from visiting a doctor?[28]

If a victim seems offended following an indirect question, you can say, "I did not mean to offend you. I'm sorry, but it's just that I have seen many people with injuries like yours caused by IPV and they won't tell me about what happened unless I ask them questions." or "Domestic violence happens to many people." When there is continued denial and future interactions with the victim are possible, you may want to offer the following statement: "I know sometimes people are afraid or embarrassed to talk about being hit, and I understand that."[31]

It is vital that the case is documented properly. Victims' statements should be documented in their own words. Avoid judgmental or pejorative language and include the date, time, and location of the injury. Objects or weapons used in an assault should be included as well as the names of people who have witnessed the assault. Documentation should include any discussion about resources and referrals made as well as any follow-up appointments or arrangements.

CONCLUSION

It is important that all members of the dental team become aware of the signs and symptoms of domestic violence in order to best help their patients. Dentists should preplan how they will intervene with DV situations so that they are prepared to ask the appropriate questions should the situation arise. Getting specific training is encouraged and dentists should contact local, state, and national dental societies for more information and guidance. Additionally, dentists must make themselves aware of reporting regulations to ensure compliance with the applicable law. Dentists have a unique opportunity to help DV patients receive the help that they may desperately need.

REFERENCES

1. Senn DR, McDowell JD, Alder ME: Dentistry's role in the recognition and reporting of domestic violence, abuse, and neglect, *Dent Clin North Am* 45:343, 2001.
2. Mehra V: Culturally competent responses for identifying and responding to domestic violence in dentist care settings, *J Calif Dent Assoc* 32:387, 2004.
3. McDowell JD, Kassebaum DK, Stromboe SE: Forensic dentistry. Recognizing the signs and symptoms of domestic violence: a guide for dentists, *J Okla Dent Assoc* J 88:21, 1997.
4. National Coalition Against Domestic Violence: *Domestic Violence Facts*, [Web page] Washington, DC, 2007. Available at: http://www.ncadv.org/. Accessed on December 4, 2013.
5. Rappaport HM: Traumatic injuries of the teeth sustained by battered women and children, *J N J Dent Assoc* 67:19, 1996.
6. Rennison CM, Welchans S: Bureau of Justice Statistics Special Report, Intimate Partner Violence, U.S. Department of Justice, Office of Justice Programs, May 2000.
7. Bureau of Justice Statistics: *National Crime Victimization Survey: Criminal Victimization*. Washington, DC, 2008, U.S. Department of Justice. Available at: http://www.bjs.ojp.usdoj.gov/content/pub/pdf/cv08.pdf. Accessed December 4, 2013
8. Berrios DC, Grady D: Domestic violence: risk factors and outcomes, *West J Med* 155:133, 1991.
9. Monahan K, O'Leary KD: Head injury and battered women: an initial inquiry, *Health Soc Worker* 24:269, 1999.
10. Bureau of Justice Statistics: *Violence against women*, Washington, DC, 1994, U.S. Department of Justice.
11. Centers for Disease Control and Prevention: Adverse health conditions and health risk behaviors associated with intimate partner violence, *MMWR* [Web page], February, 2008. Available at: http://www.cdc.gov/mmwr/PDF/wk/mm5705.pdf/. Accessed December 4, 2013.
12. McCauley J et al: The "battering syndrome": prevalence and clinical characteristics of domestic violence in primary care internal medicine practices, *Ann Intern Med* 123:737, 1995.
13. Dearwater SR et al: Prevalence of intimate partner abuse in women treated at community hospital emergency departments, *JAMA* 280:433, 1998.
14. Tjaden P, Thoennes N: Extent, nature and consequences of intimate partner violence: findings from the National Violence Against Women Survey, National Institute of Justice and the Centers for Disease Control and Prevention. 2000. Available at: https://www.ncjrs.gov/pdffiles1/nij/181867.pdf. Accessed December 4, 2013.
15. Catalano S: Intimate Partner violence in the United States, U.S. Department of Justice Bureau of Justice Statistics. 2007. Available at: http://bjs.ojp.usdoj.gov/content/pub/pdf/ipvus.pdf/. Accessed December 4, 2013.
16. Matlin MW: *The psychology of women*, New York, 1987, Holt Reinhart Winston.
17. Centers for Disease Control and Prevention: Adverse health conditions and health risk behaviors associated with intimate partner violence, *MMWR* February, 2008. Available at http://www.cdc.gov/mmwr/PDF/wk/mm5705.pdf/. Accessed December 4, 2013.
18. Frieze IH, Browne A: Violence in marriage. In Ohlin, LE, Tonry, MH, editors: *Family violence*, Chicago, 1989, University of Chicago Press, pp 162-218.
19. Lowe C, Gerbert B, et al: Dentists' attitudes and behaviors regarding domestic violence: The need for response, *J Am Dent Assoc* 132:85, 2001.
20. U.S. Department of Health and Human Services, Centers for Disease Control and Prevention. *Oral health for adults*. Available at: http://www.cdc.gov/OralHealth/Publications/factsheets/adult.htm. Accessed December 4, 2013.
21. Ochs HA, Neuenschwander MC, Dodson TB: Are head, neck, and facial injuries markers for domestic violence? *J Am Dent Assoc* 127:757, 1996.
22. Garbin C, Queiroz A, Rovida T, Garbin A: Occurrence of traumatic dental injury in cases of domestic violence, *Braz Dent J* 23:72, 2012.
23. Nelms AP, Gutmann M, Solomon E, Dewald J, Campbell P: What victims of domestic violence need from the dental professional, *J Dent Educ* 73:490, 2009.
24. McDowell JD: Elder abuse: the presenting signs and symptoms in the dental practice, *Tex Dent J* 107:29, 1990.
25. McDowell JD: Diagnosing and treating victims of domestic violence, *N Y State Dent J* 62:36, 1996.
26. Mouden LD, Bross DC: Legal issues affecting dentistry's role in preventing child abuse and neglect, *J Am Dent Assoc* 126:1173, 1995.
27. The Family Violence Prevention Fund, National Consensus Guidelines. On identifying and responding to domestic violence victimization in health care settings. Available at: http://www.futureswithoutviolence.org/userfiles/file/Consensus.pdf. Accessed December 4, 2013.
28. Connell M, Golding S, Morgan L, Niland J: Expert opinion—Does mandatory reporting trump attorney-client opinion? *American Psychology-Law Society News* 24(3): 10-13,15, 1998.
29. State of New Jersey, Dept. of Children and Families: How and when to report child abuse/neglect. Available at www.nj.gov/dcf/reporting/how. Accessed September 13, 2014.
30. L.A., as Parent and Legal Guardian of S.A., a minor and L.A. individually, Plaintiff-Appellant, v. New Jersey Division of Youth and Family Services, et al. and Jersey Shore University Medical Center and Danuel Yu, M.D. N.J.A.D. A-27236-11T1 (2012).
31. Sherin K et al: HITS: a short domestic violence screening tool for use in a family practice setting, *Fam Med* 30:508, 1998.
32. Surprenant Z, Harris J: *Medical staff training guide for California physicians*, Tucson, AZ, 2006, Medical Directions, Inc.

Appendix A: Custom Staining

*Kenneth W. Aschheim**

FUNDAMENTALS OF CUSTOM STAINING

A fundamental understanding of hue, value, chroma, complementary hue, and the color wheel is essential before attempting custom staining (see Chapter 2—Fundamentals of Esthetics and Smile Analysis and Chapter 4—Color Modifiers and Opaquers).

Dominant Hues

Hue is the name of the color. *Chroma* is the saturation or intensity of color (hue); therefore chroma can be present only when there is hue. *Value* is the relative whiteness or blackness of a color (hue). A light tooth has a high value; a dark tooth has a low value (for detailed definitions, see Chapter 2).

The dominant hue is the principal color of the "body" porcelain. Before custom staining is done, the dominant hue of a restoration must be determined. Shades are then altered from this baseline. The dominant shade is represented only in the middle one third of a tooth. The incisal edge usually is more translucent and the gingival one third more heavily stained.

Known Shades. If a standard shade is selected, a simple reference table can be used (Tables A-1 to A-3).

Unknown Shades. Unknown shades should be evaluated under three different lighting situations or in the lighting situation most appropriate for the individual (see Chapter 2). Certain basic rules apply to the process of determining the dominant shade:
1. Avoid staring at a shade for a long period; the first glance usually is the most accurate.
2. The longer one stares at a shade, the grayer the shade appears to the eye.
3. Focus only on the middle one third of the tooth.

CLINICAL TIP

To aid in determining a shade, mask the incisal and gingival thirds of a tooth with white adhesive tape.

Computerized Digital Shade Technology

Computerized digital shade devices can determine shades accurately regardless of lighting conditions and other elements that typically lead to improper shade measurement (Fig. A-1). Studies have shown that these spectrophotometric devices exhibit a high degree of repeatability of color coordinates for all tooth regions when the same color-measuring device was used.[1,2] (See the section on Computerized Digital Shade Technology in Chapter 2.)

COMPLEMENTARY HUES

The concept of complementary hues allows for certain clinically important modifications. Complementary hues are directly opposite one another on the color wheel (see Chapter 2) (Box A-1).[3]
1. When placed side by side, complementary hues appear to intensify each other. For example, a green stain applied to the incisal edge of a reddish-dominant shade (e.g., Vita-Lumin D-2) intensifies the approximating dominant red hue (Fig. A-2).
2. When blended in equal amounts, complementary hues produce a neutral gray. If a reddish-dominant shade (e.g., Vita-Lumin D-2) is gradually overlapped with its complementary hue (green stain), a neutral gray eventually results. Other complementary pairs (violet-yellow and pink-green[†]) produce similar results.
3. When complementary hues are blended in unequal proportions, the dominant hue will be reduced both in value (look grayer) and chroma (look less intense). When a reddish-dominant shade (e.g., Vita-Lumin D-2) is overlaid with a green stain (but not enough to completely neutralize the red), both the value and chroma of the red shade are reduced.

CHAIRSIDE STAINING
Basic Principles

A few simple steps meticulously adhered to, will produce optimal chairside staining results.
1. The restoration must be meticulously cleaned before and during the staining process.

CLINICAL TIP

Although a 5-minute ultrasonic cleaning with distilled water will sufficiently clean a restoration before staining,[4] the use of a laboratory grade steam cleaner (Reliable i702C Steam Cleaner, Reliable Corporation) will accomplish the same cleaning in only a few seconds.

2. Apply chairside stains before glazing the ceramic.
3. Complete all anatomic and functional adjustment before applying stains.
4. Keep all brushes and instruments clean to avoid contamination.

*A special thanks to Gary Osborne of Ivoclar Vivadent for providing technical and laboratory assistance and Jim Mcguire of Vident for supplying the equipment support with this appendix.

[†]In dental stains, a true red is difficult to achieve and seldom necessary; therefore pink is always substituted.

Table A-1 **Dominant Hue Range of Selected Bioform Porcelain Shades**

B-51 Red-brown range	B-59 Yellow range	B-69 Red-gray range	B-91 Gray range
B-52 Yellow range	B-62 Red-gray range	B-77 Yellow range	B-92 Red-gray range
B-53 Red-brown range	B-63 Red-brown range	B-81 Red-gray range	B-93 Red-gray range
B-54 Red-brown range	B-65 Red-brown range	B-83 Red-brown range	B-94 Gray range
B-55 Yellow range	B-66 Red-gray range	B-84 Red-brown range	B-95 Gray range
B-56 Yellow range	B-67 Yellow range	B-85 Red-brown range	B-96 Gray range

Based on the Bioform Color Ordered Shade Guide, Dentsply International.

Table A-2 **Dominant Hue Range of Selected VITA Classical (Lumin Vacuum) Porcelain Shades**

A-1 Orange range	B-1 Yellow range	C-1 Brown range	D-2 Orange range
A-2 Orange range	B-2 Yellow range	C-2 Brown range	D-3 Yellow range
A-3 Orange range	B-3 Yellow range	C-3 Brown range	D-4 Orange range
A-3.5 Orange range	B-4 Yellow range	C-4 Brown range	
A-4 Orange range			

Based on the VITA classical (Lumin Vacuum) Shade Guide, Vident.

CLINICAL TIP

The use of staining pastes such as IPS e.max CAD Crystall for pre-crystallized IPS e.max Crowns IPS e.max Ceram for pressed and post crystallized e.max Crowns, or IPS Empress Universal Shades, IPS e.max CeramEssence and Shade, or glaze greatly simplifies the staining process (all from Ivoclar Vivadent).

CLINICAL TIP

In order to prevent damage to a crown, it is important to know if the crown had been modified with a cutback and layering technique utilizing a lower-fusing porcelain. If this is the case, then an appropriate lower fusing stain must be used.

5. If a powder/glaze mixture is used, lay out the powders of the stains (the "feeder" supply) on the left side of a clean, dry, glazed porcelain palette.
6. Take care to avoid contaminating the "feeder" supply by accidentally mixing powders or pastes. Mix shades on the right side of the palette to avoid contamination.
7. Mix stains to a thick, toothpaste-like consistency; this can be diluted later to the desired consistency.
8. If a feeder supply dries out, reconstitute it by adding the liquid medium.

CLINICAL TIP

Chairside stains should never be applied intraorally because an absolutely dry field is necessary.

COMPUTERIZED CERAMIC FURNACES

No other component is more important to the success of the chairside color modification procedure than the computerized ceramic furnace, sometimes referred to as a glazing oven (Fig. A-3).

Technical support representatives claim the 20% to 40% calls they receive concerning ceramic problems can be traced to the operation of the furnace.[5] The sole purpose of a ceramic furnace is to heat the ceramic at an optimal rate, in an optimal environment (i.e., complete or partial vacuum) for an optimal period of time. A computerized furnace, when properly programmed, will insure that the manufactures' specifications are followed.

CLINICAL TIP

Although computerize dental furnace have vastly simplified the procedure, it is vital that the proper program is selected and that the furnace is periodically calibrated. Failure to understand the proper operation and maintenance of a dental furnace could lead to restoration failure.

Applying Stains

Armamentarium
- Basic staining setup
- Appropriate staining kit for restoration being stained
- Computerized ceramic furnace (e.g. VITA Vacumat 6000 M Furnace, Vident)

Table A-3 **Trubyte IPN Shade Conversion Chart**

	Shade Match		Shade Correlation		
Portrait IPN	Vita Classic	Vita 3D Master	Bioform IPN	Bioblend IPN	Trublend SLM
P1	A1	1M1	B51		T9
P2	A2	3R1.5	B53	104	T11
P3	A3	3M2	B54	108	T13
P3.5	A3.5	3R2.5	B83	116	T19
P4	A4	4R1.5	B84	118	T20
P11	B1	2M1	B59	100	T2
P12	B2	2M2	B52		T22
P13	B3	3M3	B55		T24
P14	B4	4L2.5	B56	110	T23
P21	C1	2R1.5	B91	102	T10
P22	C2	31.1.5, 4M1	B94		T6
P23	C3	4L1.5, 4M2	B95		T7
P24	C4	5M1, 5M2	B96		T8
P32	D2	3M1	B92		T3
P33	D3		B93		T14
P34	D4		B69	113	T5
P59		1M2	B59	100	T2
P62		2L1.5	B62	102	T10
P65		B65	106	115	
P66		2L2.5, 2R2.5	B66	112	T12
P67		2M3	B67	109	T16
P69		3L2.5	B69	113	15
P77		B77	T17		
P81		4M3, 5M3	B81	114	T18
PW2		0M2, 0M3			
PW4		OM1			
PW7					

(Courtesy Dentsply International, York, PA.)

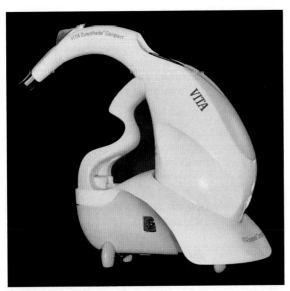

FIGURE A-1 VITA Easyshade Compact is a cordless spectrophotometric device used to determine shades. (Courtesy of Vident, Brea, CA.)

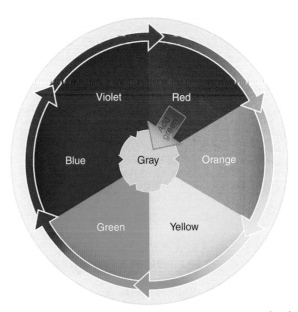

FIGURE A-2 Complementary shades are opposite each other on the color wheel. For example, a green stain is the complementary shade of a reddish hue.

Box A-1		
Dominant Hues vs. Complement Hues		
	Dominant Hue	**Complement Hue**
A Shades	Brown	Blue
B Shades	Yellow	Violet
C Shades	Gray	Gray
D Shades	Red	Green

Adapted from Milnar F: Washington State Dental Association's 2012 Pacific Northwest Dental Conference. A shade selection workshop for the team. June 15, 2012. http://www.wsda.org/storage/pndc-2012-handouts/Shade%20Selection%20Hand%20Out.pdf. Accessed October 2013.

> ### CLINICAL TIP
>
> The use of a computerize oven greatly simplifies the staining process. Although ovens from different manufacturers can be used it is vital that the appropriate firing cycle is programed into the furnace. Always perform a few test firings on non-patient restorations to verify that the furnace is calibrated properly.

+ Red sable brushes
+ Diamond-tipped porcelain restoration pliers or curved hemostat (Tweezers. Ivoclar Vivadent) (Fig. A-4A).
    + Ceramic firing support
    + Shade guide

Editor's Note: Because the temperature and firing times for glazing and staining vary greatly for each type of material, the step-by-step will not give firing temperatures or firing times. Refer to the manufacturer-specific furnace program or protocol before placing any restoration in a porcelain oven.

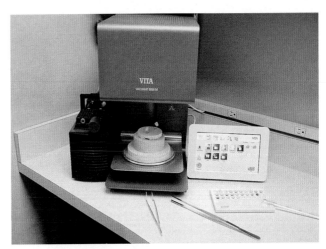

FIGURE A-3 VITA Vacumat 6000 M Furnace.

Clinical Technique
1. Preheat the computerized ceramic furnace to the appropriate temperature.

> ### CLINICAL TIP
>
> The use of a pallet filled with porcelain staining pastes will greatly simplify the staining process (Fig. A-4B)

2. Dilute the surface stains on the working side (right side) of the palette to paint like consistency to allow for easier transfer to the brush. The stain should neither drip nor run.
3. Wet a clean red sable brush with liquid medium, flick off the excess liquid, and draw the brush tip to a point.
4. Wash the crown with distilled water and thoroughly dry it with an oil-free air syringe or hair dryer. Alternatively, use a dental laboratory steamer.

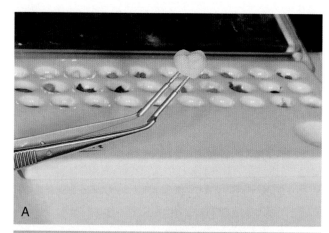

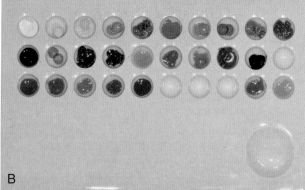

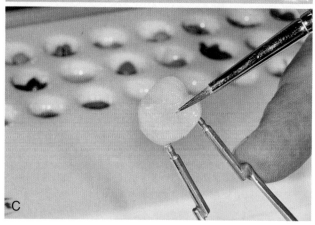

FIGURE A-4 A, Diamond-tipped porcelain restoration pliers hold the restoration in place. B, A palette filled with porcelain staining pastes. C, Stain applied with a light dabbing motion.

CLINICAL TIP

If a restoration has been in the mouth for an extended period, bacteria may adhere to the porcelain surface. If bacteria are not completely removed, they can cause the porcelain to crack when it is heated in the computerized ceramic furnace. Bacteria can be eliminated by soaking the restoration in a porcelain cleaning agent.

5. Hold the restoration securely with locking pliers or a curved hemostat.
6. Apply the stain in a series of light dabbing motions (Fig. A-4C)

CLINICAL TIP

Do not overapply stain. You are looking for the effect of the stain, not the stain itself. Chroma can be controlled by avoiding excess powder in the mixture and by controlling the dispersion of the stain particles with the tip of the brush.

---

7. If the stain extends beyond the intended area, wipe the brush on a tissue until it is semidry and use the tip to absorb excess stain and medium.

CLINICAL TIP

Incorrect stains can be wiped off with a clean tissue, and new stain can be applied.

CLINICAL TIP

Two or three test stainings may be necessary before an acceptable result is obtained.

---

8. After the desired hue, value, and chroma have been obtained, place the restoration in front of the open door of the preheated computerized ceramic furnace.
9. If a programmable furnace is used:
    a. Place the restoration on a ceramic firing support.
    b. Run the appropriate program.
10. If a nonprogrammable furnace is used:
    a. Leave the restoration in place until the liquid medium has evaporated and a powdery film covers the stained surface.
    b. Place the restoration on a ceramic firing support.
    c. Gradually move the restoration into the oven.
    d. When the restoration is in place, close the oven door.
    e. Gradually increase the furnace temperature to the appropriate temperature at the appropriate rate of speed. Adjust the vacuum according to the manufacturer's instructions.

CLINICAL TIP

If high-temperature firing is undesirable (e.g., to avoid thermal stress in a fixed bridge), a lower temperature glaze or stain can be used.

---

    f. Upon completion, slowly remove the restoration from the furnace and allow it to bench cool.
11. Evaluate the case intraorally.
12. Repeat the above steps, if necessary. If necessary, the surface stain can be removed by gently grinding the restoration with a green stone.

ADJUSTING HUE, CHROMA, AND VALUE

Shades should always be adjusted from lighter to darker. The converse can be accomplished only by applying a more opaque stain over the shade to be lightened. This rarely produces an esthetically satisfactory result.

Adjusting Hue

In general, only minor adjustments to hue should be made with custom stains. Adjusting colors with complementary hues also decreases value. If major adjustments to hue are necessary, it is preferable to replace the porcelain with the proper shade.

Armamentarium

• Standard staining setup. See the section on Applying Stains earlier in this appendix.

Clinical Technique

1. Determine the dominant hue of the existing restoration (the "original" hue) (e.g., Vita-Lumin A-1—orange) and the dominant hue to be achieved (the "desired" hue) (e.g., Vita-Lumin D-2—dark orange).

2. Incrementally add sufficient amounts of the complementary hue to the appropriate areas of the restoration until the original hue is neutralized (e.g., the complementary hue of Vita-Lumin A-2 is blue).

3. Apply the *dominant* hue of the desired hue (e.g., the dominant hue of Vita-Lumin D-3 is yellow) until the desired hue is obtained (Fig. A-5A)

CLINICAL TIP

Steps 2 and 3 often can be combined into a single step. Because blue (step 2 above) and yellow (step 3 above) form green when mixed together, this procedure can be done in a single step if a properly proportioned green stain is used.

CLINICAL TIP

If the original hue contains no dominant hue (e.g., Bioform B-91), simply apply the desired stain.

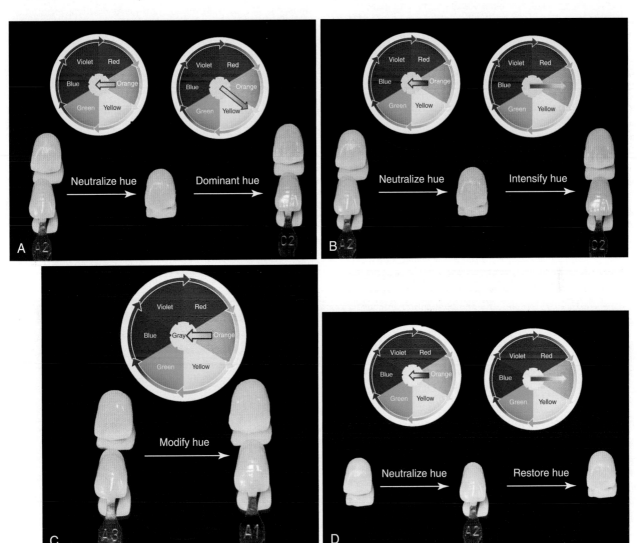

FIGURE A-5 A, First the complementary hue is added to neutralize the unwanted dominant hue. Then the dominant hue of the desired shade is added. Adjusting colors with complementary hues also decreases value. **B,** The dominant hue is added until the desired shade is obtained. **C,** The complementary hue is added until the desired chroma is obtained. Adjusting colors with complementary hues also decreases value. **D,** The complementary hue followed by the dominant hue (if necessary) is added until the desired value is obtained.

4. After the desired result is obtained, fire and glaze the restoration. See the section on Applying Stains earlier in this appendix.

Increasing Chroma

Armamentarium

+ Standard staining setup. See the section on Applying Stains earlier in this appendix.

Clinical Technique

1. Determine the dominant hue of the existing restoration (the "original" hue) (i.e., Vita-Lumin A-2—light orange) and the dominant hue to be achieved (the "desired" hue) (i.e., Vita-Lumin A-4—dark orange yellow).
2. Add the sufficient amount of dominant hue to the appropriate area of the restoration until the desired hue has been obtained (i.e., the dominant hue of Vita-Lumin A-1 is orange (Fig. A-5B).
3. After the desired result has been obtained, fire and glaze the restoration. See the section on Applying Stains earlier in this appendix.

Decreasing Chroma

Armamentarium

+ Standard staining setup. See the section on Applying Stains earlier in this appendix.

Clinical Technique

1. Determine the dominant hue of the existing restoration (the "original" hue) (i.e., Vita-Lumin A-4—orange) and the dominant hue to be achieved (the "desired" hue) (i.e., Vita-Lumin A-3.5—orange).
2. Apply the *complementary* hue to the original hue (i.e., the complementary hue of Vita-Lumin A-4 is blue) until the desired chroma has been obtained (Fig. A-5C).

CLINICAL TIP

Reducing chroma by applying the complementary hue also decreases value.

2. After the desired result has been obtained, fire and glaze the restoration. See the section on Applying Stains earlier in this appendix.

Decreasing Value without Changing Hue

Armamentarium

+ Standard staining setup. See the section on Applying Stains earlier in this appendix.

Clinical Technique

1. Determine the dominant hue of the existing restoration (the "original" hue) (e.g., Bioform B-65—red-brown).
2. Add a sufficient amount of the *complementary* hue to the appropriate area of the restoration until the original hue has been neutralized. This also lowers the value (e.g., the complementary hue of Bioform B-65 is green).
3. Apply the *dominant* hue of the original hue (i.e., the dominant hue of Bioform B-65 is red-brown), if necessary (Fig. A-5D). Because this is applied over the previously neutralized hue, the "added gray" serves to reduce the value without changing the hue.

4. After the desired result has been obtained, fire and glaze the restoration. See the section on Applying Stains earlier in this appendix.

ADJUSTING TRANSLUCENCY

Translucency is the ability of material to allow light transmission. The greater the amount of light transmitted, the greater the "real" translucency. In custom staining, an illusion of translucency can be created called "apparent" translucency.

Increasing Real Translucency

Because real translucency is a quality of the material used, it is impossible to increase real translucency with surface stains.

CLINICAL TIP

It is possible to reduce real translucency with a technique called cutback and layering. In this technique a layer of ceramic is removed and replaced. This technique, although more difficult, can be performed chairside.

Decreasing Real Translucency

Decreasing real translucency is the same as increasing opacity. This usually is accomplished by applying a white stain. This opaque stain can be adjusted to more closely match the desired shade by applying other stains on top of the opaque layer. (See section on Characterization of Teeth later in the appendix).

Increasing Apparent Translucency

Adjustments in translucency are most often required at the incisal edge of the tooth. Changes in apparent translucency are accomplished by altering the amount of blue stain in the incisal area.

CLINICAL TIP

Variants of blue such as blue-violet or blue-green often must be used to adjust translucency because they contain complementary hues that neutralize excess amounts of yellow or pink, which may be visible in the incisal area.

Armamentarium

+ Standard staining setup. See the section on Applying Stains earlier in this appendix.

Clinical Technique

1. Examine the incisal area closely for excess pink, red, or yellow.
2. If pink or red is present, select a blue-green stain.
3. If yellow is present, select a blue-violet stain.
4. Apply the stain to the incisal area (Fig. A-6).

CLINICAL TIP

When placed side by side, complementary colors intensify each other. To further increase the apparent translucency, "rim" the incisal edge with yellow/orange (the complement of violet/blue) or white.

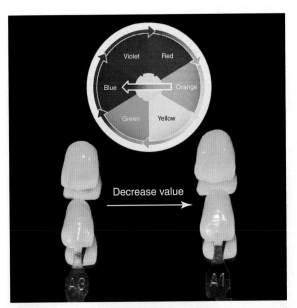

FIGURE A-6 The complementary hue is added until the desired translucency is obtained.

5. After the desired result has been obtained, fire and glaze the restoration. See the section on applying stains earlier in this appendix.

Decreasing Apparent Translucency

A decrease in apparent translucency is accomplished by decreasing the amount of blue by applying its complementary hue, orange. In theory this also decreases value, but because the hues are so dilute, any perceivable change in value is unlikely.

CLINICAL TIP

Translucency alterations are subtle effects. Do not overapply the stain. Begin with very dilute amounts of orange and light applications.

Adjusting the Incisal-Gingival Blend

Often the shade and translucency of a tooth are correct, but the proportion of body shade to incisal translucency is incorrect. The incisal area can be altered by changing the surface area of apparent translucency. If the incisal area must be lengthened, the appropriate amount of dominant body hue should be neutralized with the complementary hue. If the incisal area is too long, a stain should be blended to match the body shade.

CLINICAL TIP

If the dominant hue of the tooth is yellow and the blue incisal area is pronounced, the resultant hue in the incisal area that is being altered may have a greenish tint. If this is unesthetic, it can be neutralized with a small amount of violet stain.

CHARACTERIZATION OF TEETH

Truly esthetic restorations often require the duplication of flaws that exist in adjacent teeth. As patients age, their dentition changes and they may wish to have these imperfections duplicated. Characterization is accomplished with the use of opaque white, brown-gray, and black stains. It sometimes is easier to use a sharp-edged instrument, a trimmed fine point brush, or a single bristle to apply these stains.

CLINICAL TIP

Characterization should be visible but not glaringly obvious. Some applications may be so subtle that one is barely aware of the effect.

Although variations in tooth characterization are limitless, certain types are quite common.

Decalcification

Decalcified areas are common and easy to reproduce.
Armamentarium
+ Standard staining setup. See the section on Applying Stains earlier in this appendix.
Clinical Technique
1. Mix the white stain to a moderately thick consistency.
2. Place the white stain with a brush or pointed instrument (Fig. A-7A).

CLINICAL TIP

Vary the opacity within the opaque area to create a more realistic decalcification effect.

CLINICAL TIP

If additional areas of decalcification are required on the same tooth, differ the shapes and depths of opacity.

3. After the desired result has been obtained, fire and glaze the restoration. See the section on Applying Stains earlier in this appendix.

Enamel Cracks and Checks

Enamel cracks are thin white lines that begin at the incisal edge and extend less than one third the length of the tooth. They generally occur in younger patients. Over time these cracks discolor, and they then are termed *enamel checks*. They range in shade from orange to brown, sometimes with a grayish cast. Cracks and checks often cast a slight shadow along their length.
Armamentarium
+ Standard staining setup. See the section on Applying Stains earlier in this appendix.
Clinical Technique
1. To create a crack, mix a white stain to a moderately thick consistency. For a check, use orange, brown, or gray stain.
2. Press a wetted brush against the porcelain palette to form a flat, "chisel" edge.
3. After picking up the stain, run the chisel edge of the brush from a point one third of the way up the tooth toward the incisal edge. This should be done in a single, fast, light stroke.

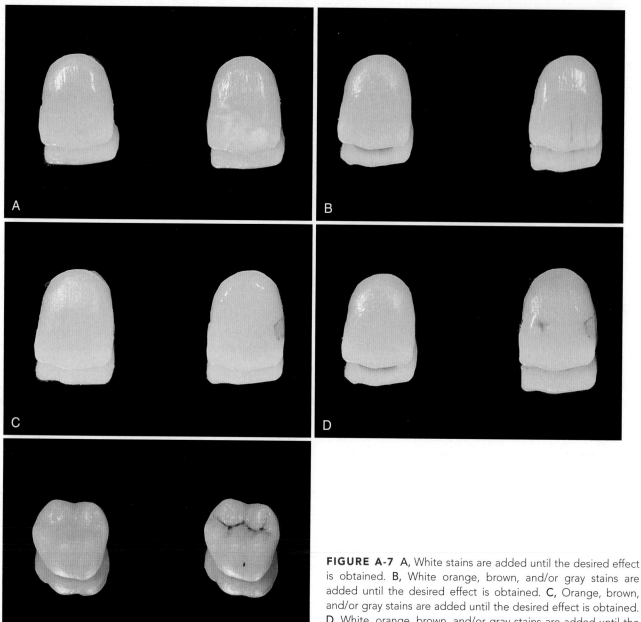

FIGURE A-7 **A,** White stains are added until the desired effect is obtained. **B,** White orange, brown, and/or gray stains are added until the desired effect is obtained. **C,** Orange, brown, and/or gray stains are added until the desired effect is obtained. **D,** White, orange, brown, and/or gray stains are added until the desired effect is obtained. **E,** White, orange, brown, and/or gray stains are added until the desired effect is obtained.

CLINICAL TIP

A sharp edge, a single bristle, or a pointed instrument may be used instead of a brush.

---

4. If the line is too thick or uneven, clean and "point" the brush, wipe it semidry, and run the point along the side of the line to remove excess stain.
5. After a line with the proper thickness has been created, clean the brush, reform the chisel edge, and create a shadow effect by running a faint black line along one side of the white "crack" (Fig. A-7B).
6. After the desired result has been obtained, fire and glaze the restoration. See the section on Applying Stains earlier in this appendix.

Stained Composite Resin or Silicate Restorations

Old anterior restorations tend to be opaque and usually are discolored. In addition, they often exhibit marginal staining.
Armamentarium
♦ Standard staining setup. See the section on Applying Stains earlier in this appendix.
Clinical Technique
1. Determine the dominant hue of the restoration.
2. Mix a white stain to a moderately thick consistency to reduce the tendency of the material to run.
3. With a brush or instrument, create the simulated restoration with the white stain as a base and add gray, black, or other appropriate hues until the dominant hue of the restoration has been approximated.

4. Use orange or brown stain to precisely outline the restoration.

CLINICAL TIP

In younger patients with light translucent teeth, a hairline of black or gray stain may be used as an outline.

5. If discoloration is desired, use a brush to form an uneven halo of orange-brown-gray. The discoloration should not abut the outline, but should fade out in a narrow, uneven, feathery pattern (Fig. A-7C).

CLINICAL TIP

Reflected undermining of teeth may be simulated by applying gray or brown stain, either individually or blended together in a semihalo effect on the incisal portion of the simulated restoration.

6. After the desired result has been obtained, fire and glaze the restoration. (See the section on Applying Stains earlier in this appendix.)

Random Discolorations

One type of characterization consists of slight intensifications of chroma in random areas of the tooth surface. This sometimes is accompanied by a slight change of hue. By varying the amount of medium used to dilute the stains, different degrees of discoloration can be produced (Fig. A-7D).

Pits and Fissures

Characterization of pits and fissures is usually restricted to older patients. It is accomplished by applying thin orange or brown lines to the fissures, grooves, and pits. It is also possible to replicate worn enamel edges of mandibular anterior teeth by using an orange-brown or brown stain to mimic exposed dentin (Fig. A-7E).

REFERENCES

1. Llena C, Lozano E, Amengual J, Forner L: Reliability of two color selection devices in matching and measuring tooth color, *J Contemp Dent Pract* 12(1):19-23, 2011.
2. Khashayar G, Dozic A, Kleverlaan CJ, Feilzer AJ: Data comparison between two dental spectrophotometers, *Oper Dent* 37(1):12-20, 2012.
3. Milnar F: Washington State Dental Association's 2012. Pacific Northwest Dental Conference. A shade selection workshop for the team. June 15, 2012. http://www.wsda.org/storage/pndc-2012-handouts/Shade%20Selection%20Hand%20Out.pdf. Accessed October 2013.
4. Gary Osborne, Ivoclar Vivadent, personal communication.
5. Patrick B: Porcelain and pressing furnaces: understanding the dynamics of modern furnaces and ceramic materials can positively affect the esthetic outcome of restorations. *Inside Dental Technology*, 2(3): 2011.

Appendix B: Ninety Second Rubber Dam Placement

It is highly unlikely that a dentist would be faulted for routinely using a rubber dam. Few procedures in dentistry are more universally accepted. Ironically, the infrequency of rubber dam use demonstrates that few dental procedures are more universally rejected as well.[1]

This paradox is further complicated by the reasons given for the rejection of rubber dam placement as a routine part of the daily practice of dentistry. Those who shun the technique cite patient disapproval, inconvenience, lack of necessity, and additional time requirements as the rationale for rejection.[2] Advocates hold diametrically opposing views, indicating patient preference, work simplification and convenience, necessity, and an overall time savings.[1,3,4] The dental student's early experiences with rubber dam application often are negative because of a typical and expected lack of manual dexterity. The virtually total avoidance of rubber dam use, except during endodontic therapy, routinely begins immediately upon graduation.

A simplified technique, along with the average practitioner's naturally acquired manual adeptness, allows placement of the rubber dam in 90 seconds or less to be a quickly attainable reality. With a minimum of practice, placement time can be reduced even further. The average application time (isolating an average of 4.6 teeth) of five private practitioners who routinely used rubber dam was 50.7 seconds.[5]

RUBBER DAM CLAMP SELECTION

Selection of a rubber dam clamp can be confusing because of the vast array of available clamp sizes and styles. The basic assortment presented in Table B-1, however, can accommodate virtually every clinical situation.

Table B-1 Rubber Dam Clamps

Winged Type	Wingless Type	Indication
14A	W14A	Most adult molars
14	W14	Small adult molars, adult premolars, and primary molars
8A	W8A	More aggressive clamp for adult molars
1	W1	Mandibular anterior teeth
211	212	Maxillary and mandibular anterior teeth (Class V restorations)

Armamentarium (Fig. B-1)

- 6 × 6-inch rubber dam, medium gauge (e.g., Hygenic Flexi Dam Rubber Dam Non Latex 6 × 6 Med, Coltene/Whaledent. Inc.)
- 6 × 6-inch plastic U-shaped rubber dam frame (e.g., Hygenic Rubber Dam Frame 6" (Plastic), Coltene/Whaledent)
- Rubber dam hole punch (e.g., Hygenic Extended Reach Dental Dam Punch, Coltene/Whaledent)
- Rubber dam hole placement template or rubber stamp (optional) (e.g., Hygenic Dental Dam Template, Coltene/Whaledent or Hygenic Dental Dam Stamp, Coltene/Whaledent)
- Stamp pad (optional)
- Dental floss (e.g., Reach Total Care Dental Floss, Johnson & Johnson)
- Rubber dam clamp assortment (see Table B-1)
- Rubber dam clamp forceps (Hygenic Clamp Forceps, Coltene/Whaledent)
- Dental Scissor (Joseph Straight Scissor, Hu-Friedy Mfg. Co.).

Clinical Technique. The approximate time required to perform each step is indicated at the end of the description.

1. Punch a double hole in the rubber dam at the point corresponding to the tooth to be clamped (Fig. B-2A). For a single occlusal restoration, clamp only the tooth to be restored and skip to step 3. For a single multiple-surface tooth restoration

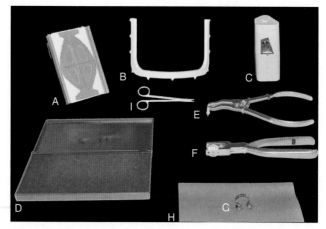

FIGURE B-1 Complete Rubber Dam Armamentarium A, Rubber dam rubber stamp (optional). **B,** 6 × 6-inch plastic U-shaped rubber dam frame. **C,** Dental floss. **D,** Stamp pad (optional). **E,** Rubber dam clamp forceps. **F,** Rubber dam hole punch. **G,** Rubber dam clamp. **H,** Rubber dam. **I,** Dental scissor.

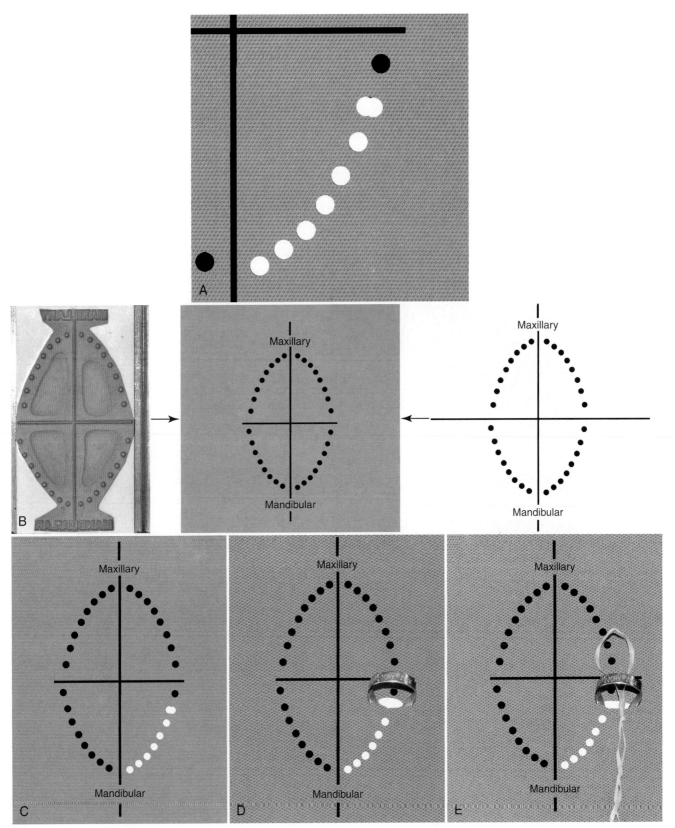

FIGURE B-2 A, A double hole corresponding to the tooth to be clamped facilitates placement of the rubber dam. **B,** Either a rubber dam stamp (*left*) or rubber dam template (*right*) aids in determining the proper positioning of the holes in the rubber dam (*center*). **C,** Normally, floss and rubber dam material can easily be passed through the interproximal contact areas of the incisor teeth. Therefore extending isolation to include one central incisor facilitates placement of the rubber dam. **D,** The rubber dam clamp is positioned in the rubber dam with the open end of the clamp facing mesially. **E,** A loop of dental floss is placed under the bow of the rubber dam clamp.

Continued

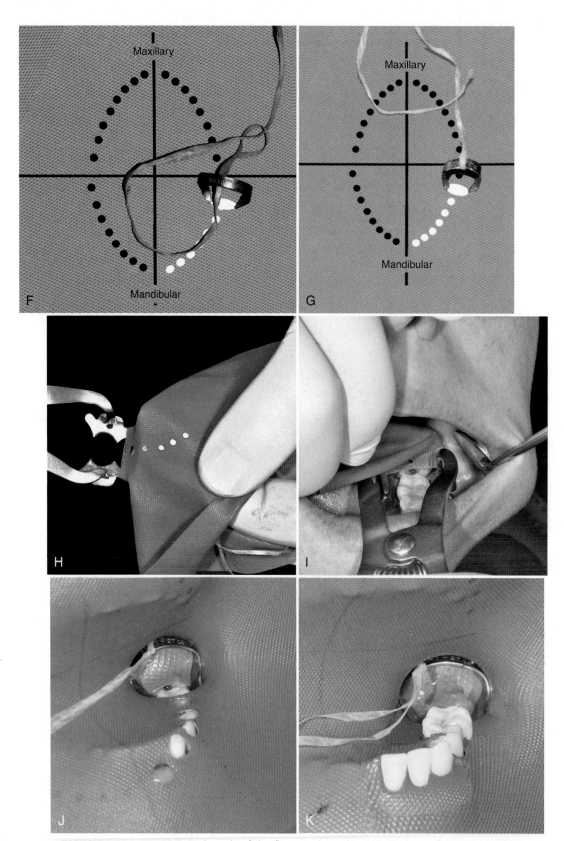

FIGURE B-2, cont'd F, Both ends of the floss are brought over the bow of the rubber dam clamp and through the loop of floss. **G,** The floss is securely tightened in the center of the bow. **H,** The rubber dam clamp forceps are attached to the rubber dam clamp. **I,** After the rubber dam clamp has been attached to the rubber dam clamp forceps, the forceps are held with the dominant hand (e.g., the right hand for right-handed dentists) and the rubber dam material is gathered with the other hand. The "teeth" of the rubber dam clamp should be readily visible. **J,** The rubber dam clamp is placed on the appropriate tooth. **K,** Typically at least one of the anterior interproximal contact areas will readily allow the passage of rubber dam material without the necessity of using dental floss. Often all three anterior teeth can be isolated with one quick maneuver.

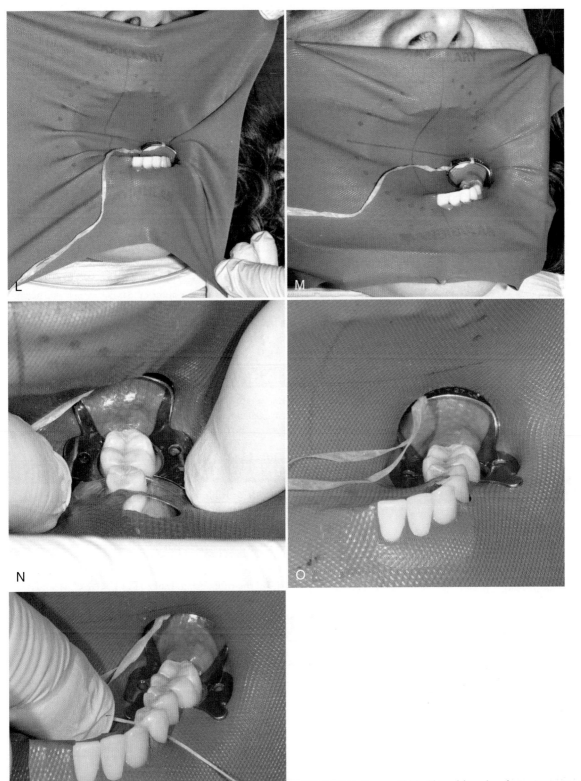

FIGURE B-2, cont'd L, The rubber dam frame is positioned. **M,** The rubber dam material is folded under the top of the frame, **N,** The rubber dam is slipped over the wings of the rubber dam clamp. **O,** Most interproximal contact areas have been negotiated without the use of dental floss. In this case, the contact area between the first and second premolars could not be negotiated. **P,** Dental floss is used to position the rubber dam material between the first and second premolars.

or when restoring more than one tooth, clamp at least one tooth distal to the tooth to be restored, if possible. (3 seconds)

Punching a double-sized hole facilitates the placement of the rubber dam around the clamp (Fig. B-2*B*).

2. Punch single holes corresponding to the positions of the remaining teeth to be isolated (see Fig. B-2*A*). A rubber dam stamp or rubber dam template (Fig. B-2*C*) is helpful for properly positioning the holes. (7 seconds)

CLINICAL TIP

When isolating several teeth, always extend isolation to include one central incisor. This significantly increases the efficiency of rubber dam placement because the interproximal contact areas of the incisor teeth usually are not resistant to the passage of the rubber dam material (see Fig. B-2*C*).

3. Position the double hole in the rubber dam over the bow of the clamp. Push the bow through the hole (Fig. B-2*D*). The open end of the clamp should face mesially. (5 seconds)
4. Tie dental floss to the bow of the rubber dam clamp. (5 seconds)

CLINICAL TIP

The following ligation is easily placed and is more easily removed than a square knot:
A. Place a loop of floss under the bow of the rubber dam clamp (Fig. B-2*E*).
B. Bring both free ends of the floss over the bow of the rubber dam clamp and through the loop of floss (Fig. B-2*F*).
C. Tighten the floss securely in the center of the bow (Fig. B-2*G*).

CLINICAL TIP

Do not ligate the clamp through the holes that often are found on the wings of the clamp. Ligation in this area complicates placement of the rubber dam.

5. Attach the rubber dam clamp to the rubber dam clamp forceps. Hold the forceps with the dominant hand (e.g., the right hand for right-handed dentists) and gather the rubber dam material with the other hand so that the "teeth" of the rubber dam clamp are readily visible (Figs. B-2*H,I*). (5 seconds)
6. Place the clamp on the appropriate tooth (Fig. B-2*J*). (5 seconds)

CLINICAL TIP

Mandibular teeth: If lingual anesthesia has been achieved along with mandibular block anesthesia, position the "teeth" of the rubber dam clamp onto the lingual surface of the tooth. Then gently slide the clamp onto the buccal surface. This sequence provides increased control of clamp placement in the area of the unanesthetized buccal gingiva. *Maxillary teeth:* If buccal anesthesia has been achieved, position the "teeth" of the rubber dam clamp onto the buccal surface of the tooth. Then gently slide the clamp onto the palatal surface. This sequence provides increased control of clamp placement in the area of the unanesthetized palatal gingiva.

7. For single tooth isolation, skip to step 8. For all other situations, position the most anterior three holes of the rubber dam over the corresponding anterior teeth. Attempt to slip the rubber dam through the interproximal contact areas of all three teeth in a single quick maneuver (Fig. B-2*K*). Usually at least one of the anterior contact areas will permit easy passage of the dam material and often all three teeth can be isolated with one quick maneuver. Do not use dental floss at this time. (5 seconds)

CLINICAL TIP

The key to rapid placement of a rubber dam is the flexibility and tear resistance of modern rubber dam material. It can be stretched to the thinness of dental floss and used as such.

CLINICAL TIP

If a template or rubber dam stamp was not used, the holes may be properly spaced relative to one another, but the "arch" of holes may be improperly positioned within the square of rubber dam. Use of a 5 × 5-inch frame and a 6 × 6 inch rubber dam sheet may compensate for this error.

8. Position the rubber dam frame (Fig. B-2*L*). (5 seconds)

CLINICAL TIP

This placement sequence allows for the positioning of the rubber dam frame as soon as possible. Once the frame is in place, rubber dam placement becomes significantly easier and more efficient because unobstructed visibility is assured and both hands are free.

9. Fold any excess rubber dam material that contacts the nose under the top of the rubber dam frame (Fig. B-2*M*). (5 seconds)
10. Slip the rubber dam over the wings of the rubber dam clamp (Fig. B-2*N*). (2 seconds)
11. Isolation for a single occlusal restoration is now complete. For all other restorations, attempt to position the remaining rubber dam material through all of the remaining contact areas in a single quick maneuver. Do not use dental floss at this time. (3 seconds)

12. Forcefully attempt to pass the material through any individual resistant contact areas without using dental floss. Stretch the material until it is as thin as dental floss and use a sawing motion to work it through the interproximal contact area as if it were dental floss (Fig. B-2O). (10 seconds)

CLINICAL TIP

Avoiding the use of dental floss at this time is an important timesaving strategy.

13. Use dental floss to position any remaining rubber dam material that could not be negotiated through the corresponding contact areas (Fig. B-2P). (15 seconds)

14. Use scissors to cut any rubber dam material that could not be negotiated through the corresponding contact area. (15 seconds)

Total time: 90 seconds

RUBBER DAM INVERSION

It sometimes is necessary to invert the rubber dam into the gingival sulcus to achieve better isolation and visibility (Fig. B-3A). This is easily accomplished in the following manner:

1. Stretch the rubber dam buccally so that it does not contact the cervical areas of the teeth (Fig. B-3B).
2. Dry the teeth with compressed air.
3. Slowly release the tension on the rubber dam until it contacts the teeth. The dam usually will "self-invert" (Fig. B-3C).

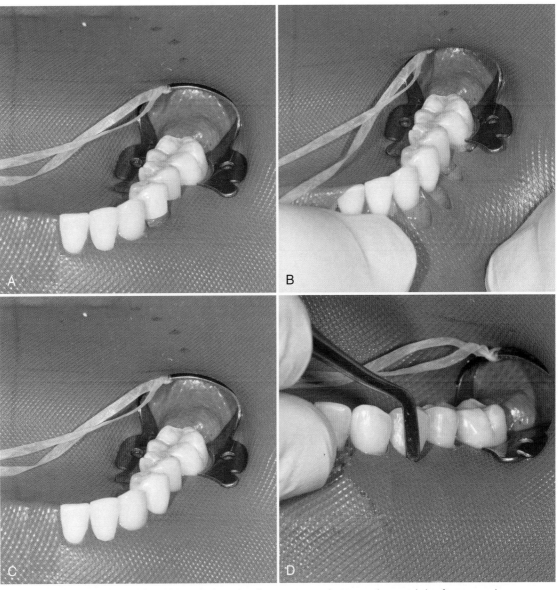

FIGURE B-3 A, The rubber dam material is not properly inverted around the first premolar. **B,** The rubber dam material is stretched away from the cervical area. A stream of air is directed at the cervical region of the first premolar until the area is dry. **C,** When the rubber dam material is slowly released, it "self-inverts" into the gingival sulcus. **D,** A instrument is used to invert the rubber dam material if the above sequence is not successful.

4. Any areas that do not self-invert can be properly positioned with a flat-ended plastic instrument (Fig. B-3*D*).

PATIENT REACTIONS TO RUBBER DAM USE

In a preliminary study, patients were asked to indicate their reactions to the use of a rubber dam during operative procedures compared with similar procedures performed without a rubber dam.[5] More than 87% preferred or were neutral about the use of a rubber dam. Rubber dam use therefore may be a practice builder, especially when it is presented favorably.

The following introductory statements can further reinforce a positive patient response to rubber dam use:

1. The rubber dam prevents tooth structure, decay, debris, and restorative material from being swallowed.
2. The rubber dam prevents moisture contamination, which can adversely affect the properties and longevity of the medicaments and restorative materials.
3. By virtue of its elasticity, the rubber dam reduces the muscle fatigue associated with maintaining an open mouth posture.
4. The rubber dam allows the patient to breathe through both the mouth and the nose. The rubber dam is watertight only around the individual teeth.

5. The rubber dam merely "muffles" the patient's speech, as when a napkin is held to the mouth; verbal communication is still possible.

CLINICAL TIP

The napkin analogy is particularly useful because it relates the rubber dam to a common, nonthreatening, helpful object.

6. The rubber dam clamp should be referred to as a "ring." The sensation caused by clamp placement should be described as "tight and secure."

REFERENCES

1. Going R, Sawinski V: Parameters related to use of rubber dam, *J Am Dent Assoc* 77:598, 1968.
2. Going R, Sawinski V: Frequency of use of the rubber dam: a survey, J Am Dent Assoc 75:158, 1967.
3. Stebner CM: Economy of sound fundamentals in operative dentistry, J Am Dent Assoc 49:294, 1954.
4. Ireland L: The rubber dam: its advantages and application, Texas Dent J 80:6, 1962.

Index